SuperNaturawl Newtrition
The Raw Truth to Longer Living

Your one-stop guide to achieving radiant health & longevity

Karen A. Di Gloria

DISCLAIMER

The information contained herein has been compiled from various sources and is based on the research, training and experiencing of the author. It is provided for informational purposes only. No statement should be taken as medical advice or as a substitute for medical counseling. The body's power and ability to heal depends upon the totality of diet, nutrition, lifestyle and environmental factors. No claim for the cure of any disease is intended or implied. The author and affiliates will not be held accountable for the use or misuse of any suggestions or procedures described therein. Due to the uniqueness of every person and situation, always consult a qualified healthcare professional before starting any new program or protocol.

Special thanks to…

    Kayleigh Walters, Proofreading Edits

    Matthew Yee, Formatting Edits

    Kristina Hanson, Cover Artwork

    Billy Mays III & Heidi Olsen, Photography

    Adam P. Kantrovitz, Granting Me Solitude ☺

Copyright © 2018 Karen A. Di Gloria

All rights reserved

CreateSpace

ISBN-13: 978-1491045428

ISBN-10: 1491045426

A NOTE FROM THE AUTHOR

Dear Reader,

People always ask why it is important to eat organic and as close to nature as possible. The answer: genuinely grown organic foods are richer in vitamins, minerals, phytonutrients and antioxidants. They are not saturated with hundreds of pesticides, herbicides and fungicides which can create undue bodily stress, a plummet in immune system function and an open-door policy to invisible invaders like harmful microbes. That being said, focusing on organics alone may not be enough – especially for the very young, elderly and sick – as the quality of our soil is currently in a critical state of mineral deficiency. Yes, we should definitely be eating organic, but we should also be eating a larger percentage of our foods in their live, raw and natural states. Foods that are both organic and raw have not been unnecessarily destroyed by high heat, over-processing, genetically modified organisms, added chemicals, dyes, antibiotics, preservatives, etc. As a result, essential nutrients have a fair chance at entering the body fully intact.

How well vital nutrients get absorbed and assimilated by the body depends on their environment. Our immune system is our foundation; it governs and protects against disease. So now I ask you: "why, as a society are we settling for less than the best? Why are we putting a price tag on our personal health and well-being?"

What happens when house settling occurs? Cracks can form in the foundation and, if significant, can create instability. What about our body, our metaphorical house that protects our soul and all our vital internal organs? With all the abuse we are putting our external environment through – the chemicals we are spilling into the air, onto our land, and into the waters – we are unwittingly the creators of the cracks developing in our own foundation. Our weakening structure is affecting our future health and longevity and the future generations of those to come. You wouldn't build a second, third or fourth story on a foundation that is structurally unsound, would you? So why then are we allowing this chaos to continue? Do we want to bring more devastation, deficiency and disease into our lives? Do we want this nature of chaos for our children and our children's children?

This book is your guide to restoring foundational health and well-being. I will take you through my personal journey into the raw lifestyle and share a plethora of my research, resources and tips:

- ★ **Quality above all!** Learn why the quality of a food can be more vital than the food itself. Meaning, the place of origin (where it grows), growing and harvesting conditions (grown organically or wild-crafted) and post-harvesting practices (methods utilized for food-processing and preservation).
- ★ **"You are what you eat!"** Gain a better understanding of the biochemistry of food and how it directly affects the biochemistry of the human brain and body – health-lifting versus health-leeching.
- ★ **Live youthfully!** Discover the best of the best in superfoods, superfruits and superherbs; including the absolute "must have" ingredients you will need in your kitchen for preventing and reversing all that contributes to aging. It's never too early, and it's never too late.

- ★ **Have fun with whole foods!** Learn how easy it can be to create living and raw food alternatives to conventional classics. I share well over 250 tried and tested recipes and quick tips to kick-start your journey to rejuvenation. All are as tantalizingly delicious as they are transformative to your health.
- ★ **Take control of your life!** Obtain the knowledge required to truly respect your body and take responsibility for your health. Stop poisoning your mind and body, and don't allow yourself, or someone you love, to fall into the trap of synthetic substances and pharmaceutical drugs.

To your renewed health and longevity,

Karen A. Di Gloria

"The doctor of the future will give no medicines, but will interest his patients in the care of the human frame, in diet, and in the causes and prevention of disease."
– Thomas Edison

This book is dedicated to my dad,
who always inspired me to be the
best I could possibly be and to
never fear rejection when living
with passion and purpose.

ACKNOWLEDGEMENTS

I have spent the past ten years gaining a new perspective on what I learned in school and what I did not learn in school. Thanks to the many leaders in the field of cutting edge nutritional science, a whole new world is open to me.

When it comes to understanding the energy and nutrient content of food (or lack thereof) and how the human body utilizes it (or doesn't), I strongly feel we have been brainwashed. My objective is to bring about a shift in consumer perception that will lead to more health-conscious choices, sustained energy and youthful vitality.

I give tremendous credit to the following individuals, as without their shared knowledge, I may have continued to be part of the problem rather than the solution: Dr. Gabriel Cousens, David Wolfe, Dr. Brian Clement, Dr. Robert Marshall, Dr. Joseph Mercola, Mike Adams, Truth Calkins, Daniel Vitalis, Dr. Bruce Fife, Dr. G. Patrick Flanagan, Paul Stamets, Ron Teeguarden, George Lamoureux, Jeffrey Smith, Dr. Udo Erasmus and Dr. Wayne Coates. I also want to take this opportunity to thank any and all individuals not mentioned who have greatly impacted, and will continue to impact, my educational journey.

Continued Education & Special Thanks

My acknowledgements would not be at all complete if I did not single out and give an extra special thank you to David Wolfe and The Best Day Ever site. Becoming a member of this amazing and dynamic site was by far one of the best things I have done. It has allowed me to gain access to the most cutting-edge health technologies and information in the world without ever having to leave the comforts of my home. There are literally hundreds of audio interviews and video health programs available for listening to and viewing at your convenience. If you are serious about learning health and longevity, then I highly advise becoming a member. It is better than any school (online or in-person). Become a member and you will become empowered just knowing you are among a community of like-minded individuals. They come from all over the globe, and are incredibly enthusiastic about healing and health, and totally dedicated to learning and living the longevity lifestyle. For more information, please visit www.thebestdayever.com.

Table of Contents

A Note from the Author i
Acknowledgements iv
Introduction 1
    Basic Raw Knowledge 101 1
    Why Go Raw: A Few Personal Thoughts 3
    A Bit About Myself & My Personal Journey into the Raw Food Lifestyle 4
    My Life Mission and a Few Words of Advice 7
Chapter 1 The Raw Truth: A Few Secrets Revealed & Myths Debunked! 8
    How Do "Raw Foodists" Get Their Protein? 8
    Why Are Enzymes So Important? 9
    The Dirty Dairy Secret: Does It "Really" Do the Body Good? 12
        Calcium Rich Foods that Giveth, Not Taketh Away! 13
        Breaking the Myth on Bone-Mineral Density 14
    Healthy Gums & Teeth: The Answer Is Not in Your "Regular" Toothpaste! 15
    How to Reap the Vital Benefits of Vitamin D3 15
        Beneath the Expression "Beauty Is Only Skin Deep" 18
        Could This Little Known Endocrine Disrupter Be the Root of Your Thyroid Issues? 19
    Soy Isoflavones & Anti-Nutrients: Another Major Contributor to Thyroid Dysfunction 19
Chapter 2 How to Stock & Prep for Your Raw Food Kitchen Makeover 22
    Let's Go Grocery Shopping, Shall We? 22
        Fresh Produce 22
        Dried Fruits 24
        Nuts & Seeds 25
    Must Have Condiments 29
        Sea Salt, the New Table Salt 29
        Sea Veggies 30
        Miso 31

- Olives 32
- Coconut Amino, a Natural Soy-Free Sauce 33
- Nutritional Yeast 33
- Sweet Flavor for Your Creations, Being Sweet Savvy with Nature's Best 34
  - Green Leaf Stevia 34
  - Xylitol 35
  - Agave 35
  - Coconut Nectar & Crystals 39
  - Sun-Dried Cane Juice Crystals 40
  - Raw Honey 40
  - Lucuma 41
  - Mesquite 42
- Sour Flavors 43
  - Fruits with a Kick 44
  - Start Eating for Internal Balance! 44
  - Don't Forget to Drink Your Water! 46
  - Apple Cider Vinegar 47
  - Coconut Vinegar 48
  - Sauerkraut & Kimchi 49
  - Miso 49

Chapter 3 Fats Can Be Your Friends, when You Choose to Get to Know Them 50
- Breaking Fats Down – Literally! 50
  - Understanding Types of Fat: Saturated & Unsaturated 53
  - Beware of the Hidden Toxic Fats Lurking in Your Everyday Foods! 58
  - Aim to Thrive, Not Just Survive 60
  - Back to the Hidden Toxic Fats 63
  - Fats to Avoid 66
  - Mass-Marketed Food, or Mass-Marketed Manipulation? 67
  - Food Processing Industry; a Double Edged Sword 68

Essential Facts About Essential Fatty Acids 70
    What About Fish & Fish Oil? 72
    Factors that Affect Conversion 74
    Improving Omega-3 Potential with Coconut Oil 76
    What About Flax? 77
    Tipping the Scales Back Towards Health 80
    Fats to Eat & Select as Staple Foods 80
Getting to Know Your True "FAT" Friends 81
    Nuts & Seeds 81
    Avocado 87
    Coconut Oil 88
    Olive Oil 96
    Hemp Seed Oil 101
    Wrap-Up 104

Chapter 4 Detoxification is a Lifestyle, Not the Latest Craze 106
Keep Your House Clean; Take the Trash Out! 106
    Beware of the Impostors! 107
    Learning to Listen to Our Body's Intuitive & Intelligent Guidance 109
Chelation & Heavy Metal Detoxification: Wellness Tips and Tools to Live By 111

Chapter 5 The Best of the Best 118
Hemp Seeds 118
Chia Seeds 122
Cacao 127
Anandamide 135
Phenethylamine 139
Tryptophan 140
MAO Inhibitors 141
Theobromine 142
Demystifying Chocolate Myths 144

Aloe Vera 150

MSM 152

Microalgae: Nature's Natural Multivitamins 158

    Chlorella 158

    Marine Phytoplankton 163

    Spirulina 167

Sprouts: Tiny Mighties! 171

    Ten Great Reasons to Start Sprouting Today! 173

    Shedding Some Light on the "Mother of ALL Grains" 175

World-Wide Superfruits: Best Bangin' Berries! 181

    Goji Berries 181

    Golden Berries 184

    Camu Camu 186

    Baobab Fruit 188

South American Superherbs 189

    Maca 189

    Cat's Claw 192

    Pau D'Arco 194

    Chanca Piedra 196

    Yerba Mate 197

Ayurvedic Superherbs 201

    Shilajit 201

    Mucuna Pruriens 204

    Ashwagandha 207

    Turmeric 209

    The Amazing World of Ayurveda 213

Chinese Superherbs 214

    Gynostemma 214

    Schizandra Berries 217

  Ginseng..220
  Medicinal Mushrooms..223
  The Charm of Traditional Chinese Herbalism........................227

Chapter 6 Tools of the Trade..229
 The Raw Necessities..229
  When to Use Which Blender..230
  When to Use a Food Processor over a Blender........................232
  Kitchen Measurements & Equivalent Conversion Charts........232
  Tips of the Trade: What You Need to Know............................234

Chapter 7 Rawlicious Recipes..239
 Blending Herbs & Spices..239
 The Rawkin' Spice Blends..241
  Italian Blend..241
  Mediterranean Blend..241
  Poultry Blend..241
  Pumpkin Pie Blend..242
  Apple Pie Blend..242
  Curry Blend..242
  Spicy Infusion Blend..242
  Garam Masala Blend..242
  Taco Blend..243
  Chili Blend..243
  Asian Blend..243
  Moroccan Blend..243
  Creole Blend..244
  Cajun Blend..244
 All-Day Breakfast Foods..245
  Quick Smoothie Tips..246
 Rawk Star Smoothies..250

Fruit Smoothies 251
    Pow-Wow Cacao Smoothie 251
    Orange Screamsicle Smoothie 252
    Choco-Cherry Smoothie 252
    Choco-Mint Smoothie 253
    Chunky Monkey Smoothie 253
    Banana Split Smoothie 254
    Almond Joy Smoothie 255
    Strawberries & Crème Smoothie 255
    Blastin' Berry Smoothie 256
    Inflammation Soother Smoothie 256

Green Smoothies 257
    Apple-Avocado Green Smoothie 257
    Pear-Avocado Green Smoothie 258
    Orange-Banana Green Smoothie 259
    Pear-Mango Green Smoothie 259
    Apple-Berry Green Smoothie 260
    Banana-Mango Green Smoothie 260

Karen's Superfood Spoonable Smoothies 261
    "Brain on Bliss" Cacao Spoonable 261
    Super Sunwarrior Spoonable 262
    Muscle Mania Spoonable 263
    Power Pumpin' Spoonable 264

Raw Prana Parfaits 266
    Quick Parfait Tips 266
    Nut-Berry Parfait 267
    Raw Berry Jam 268
    Raw Apricot Jam 268
    Raw Fig Jam 269

- "Just Peachy" Parfait 269
- Kiwi-Pineapple Parfait 270
- Pumpkin Spiced Cranberry Parfait 271

Cereal of Champions 272
- Quick Cereal Tips 272
- Raw Nuts N' Berries Cereal 273
- Go-To Nut Mylk 275
- Go-To Seed Mylk 276
- Coconut Mylk (short cut) 276
- Strawberry Mylk 276
- Hazelnut Chocolate Mylk 277
- Apple Cinnamon Cereal 277
- Banana-Blueberry Cereal 278

Crunch Chewy Grawnola 279
- Quick Grawnola Tips 280
- Go-To Grawnola (dehydrator needed) 280

Jubilant Juices 283
- Quick Juicing Tips 284

"It's Alive!" Juices 285
- Go-To Juice 285
- Go-To Juice + Add-ons 286

Healing from the Inside Out! 287
- Ulcer Eliminator 287
- Colon Cleanser Juice #1 287
- Colon Cleanser Juice #2 287
- Ultimate Green Hulk Detoxifier 288
- Kidney Cleanser Juice #1 288
- Kidney Cleanser Juice #2 288
- Kidney Cleanser Juice #3 289

- Kidney Cleanser Juice #4 289
- Kidney Cleanser Juice #5 290
- Bladder & UTI Buster 290
- Liver Cleanser Juice #1 290
- Liver Cleanser Juice #2 290
- Liver Cleanser Juice #3 291
- Liver Cleanser Juice #4 291
- Citrus Gallbladder Squeeze Juice #1 291
- Citrus Gallbladder Squeeze Juice #2 291
- Lymphatic Lifter Juice #1 291
- Lymphatic Lifter Juice #2 291
- Blood Buster Juice #1 291
- Blood Buster Juice #2 292
- Lung Rejuvenator Juice #1 292
- Lung Rejuvenator Juice #2 292
- Skin Beautifier Juice #1 292
- Skin Beautifier Juice #2 292
- Skin Beautifier Juice #3 293

Souper Scrumptious Soups 293
- Quick Soup Tips 293

Savory Soup Ideas 295
- Creamy Cucumber Soup 295
- Thai Cucumber Soup 295
- Carrot Curry Soup 296
- Carrot Ginger Soup 296
- Cream of Bell Pepper 297
- Spicy Bell Pepper 297
- Creamy Tomato Basil 298
- Creamy Corn Soup 298

- Bali-Flower Soup 299
- Creamy Cauliflower Soup 300
- Cream of Choice Soup 300
- Fiesta Chili 301
- Macho Gazpacho 302
- Beet Borscht in the Raw 303
- Red Beet Borscht 303
- Sweet Potato Soup 304
- Zucchini Noodle Soup 304
- Sea-Veggie Miso Soup 305

Sweet Fruit Infusion Soup Ideas 307
- Pineapple Chiller 307
- Tahitian Sunrise Soup 308
- Papaya Blush Soup 308
- Spiked Blueberries & Crème Soup 309

Splendid Salads, Slaws & Rawghetti 309
- Quick Recipe Tips 310

Sumptuous Salads 311
- Step 1: Go-To Garden Salad 311
- Step 2: Go-To Salad Dressing 312
- Prawma Sprinkle (my raw version of parmesan sprinkle cheese) 312
- Tuscan Spinach Salad 314
- Miso Caesar Salad 315
- Greek Isles Salad 316
- Curried Cruciferous Salad 317
- Asian Cabbage Salad 318
- Sweet & Zesty Cabbage Salad 319
- Mexican Spring Corn Salad 320
- Fennel & Grapefruit Salad 321

- Sprouted Quinoa Salad 322
- Massaged Kale & Avocado Salad 322
- Massaged Kale & Tropical Fruit Salad 323
- Spiraled Beet Salad 324

Splendiferous Slaws 325
- Cabbage Slaw 325
- Asian Root Veggie Slaw 326
- Broccoli Slaw 327

Rawlicious Rawghetti 329
- Zucchini & Summer Squash Rawghetti 329
- Kelp Noodle Rawghetti 330
- Arame Seaweed Rawghetti 330
- Rawghetti Sauce & Dressing Options 331

Mouthwatering Stove Stoppers 332
- Quick Recipe Tips 332

Protein Packed Pâtés 336
- Brazilian Sunrise Pâté 336
- "Hold the Chicken" Salad Pâté 336
- "Hold the Egg" Salad Pâté 337
- "Hold the Tuna" Salad Pâté 338
- Re-Fined Bean Pâtés 339
- Raw Rancho Taco Pâtés 340
- Italian Stallion Pâtés 341
- Greek Gyraw Pâtés 341
- Marvelous Mediterranean Falafel Pâtés 342
- Rawkin' Burgers (dehydrator needed) 343

Nut Crèmes & Cheezes 345
- Sour Nut Crème 345
- Mozzarawlla Cheeze 346

- "Betta than Feta" Cheeze 346
- Macho Nacho Cheeze 346
- Crème Cheeze 347

Delectable Dips, Side Dishes & Condiments 347
- Guacamole 347
- Fresh & Spicy Tomato Salsa 348
- Veggie-Style Rice 348
- Mashed Turner Tots 349
- Pecan Mushroom Gravy 349
- Cranberry-Goji Holiday Relish 350
- Island Pineapple Chutney 350
- Genie Zucchini Hummus 351
- Hemp Tabouli Salad 352
- Maconaise 352
- Pucker-Up Mustard 353
- Snazzy Ketchup 354
- Zany BBQ Sauce 354
- Sicilian Tapenade 355
- Curry Spread 355
- Cilantro Pesto: for Heavy Metal Cleansing 356

Sexy Sauces & Dressings 357
- Hemp Pesto Sauce 357
- Popeye's Pesto Sauce 357
- Alfrawdo Sauce 358
- Marawnara Sauce 358
- Enchilada Sauce 359
- Asian Dipping Sauce 360
- Asian Dressing 360
- Miso Caesar Dressing 361

Hemp Caesar Dressing	362
Ranch Dressing	362
Thai-Hini Dressing	363
"A Thousand Islands" Dressing	363
Cucumber Tahini Dressing	364
Very Berry Vinaigrette Dressing	365
Citrus Gold Vinaigrette Dressing	365
Decadent Desserts & Sweet Treats	**366**
Quick Dessert & Sweet Treat Tips	367
Raw Cakes, Frostings, Icings & Pies	**370**
Basic Cheeze Cake	370
Chocolate Topping	372
La-Caramel Topping	372
Strawberry Topping	373
Raspberry Topping	373
Blueberry Topping	373
Cherry Topping	374
Karen's Chocolate Crème Cake	374
Chocolate Hazelnut Dream Cake	377
Tiramisu Crème Cake	378
Vanilla Cake Envy	380
Chocolate Cake Envy	381
Carrot Cake Envy	382
Vanilla Crème Frosting	383
Crème Cheeze Frosting	384
Spiced Walnut Crème Frosting	384
Vanilla Icing	384
Chocolate Icing	385
Go-To Raw Icings	385

Pecan Pie	386
Lemon Chia Pie	388
Sweet Potato Pie	390
Amazing Apple Pie	391
Brawnies, Rawkies, Bars & Bites	**392**
Quick Recipe Tips	393
Fudge Brawnies (raw brownies)	394
Oreo Rawkie Bars (my raw version of Oreo-like cookie bars)	396
Key Lime Bars	397
Amazonian Energy Bars	398
Hemp Fudge Power Bites	399
Chocolate Chip Rawkie Dough Balls (real, raw cookie dough)	399
Maca-Roons	400
Mulberry Maca-Roons	401
Christmas Goji-Roons	401
Jungle Peanut Balls	402
Goji Christmas Balls	402
Chocolate Hazelnut Snowballs	403
Halvah	404
Rawklava (my raw version of the Greek favorite: baklava)	405
Afternoon Delight Scones (nut free)	406
Super Seed Power Balls	407
Chocolate Fudge Truffles	408
Go-To Rawkies (raw cookies)	409
Pure Indulgent Puddings & More!	**410**
Bliss Kiss Pudding	410
Vanilla Lime Pudding	411
Maca Mineral Pudding	412
Matcha Pudding	412

- Chia "Tapioca" Pudding ... 413
- O-Mega Yougurt (my raw & dairy free version of yogurt) ... 414
- Fruit N' Nut Crumbles ... 415
- Spirulina Pear-Mango Pudding ... 416
- Souped-Up Applesauce ... 416

Luscious Raw Ice Creams ... 417
- Quick Recipe Tips ... 417
- Dreamy Vanilla Bean #1 ... 418
- Dreamy Vanilla Bean #2 ... 419
- Jacked Up Jackfruit ... 419
- Succulent Strawberry ... 420
- Black Forest Cherry ... 420
- Chocolate Exotica ... 421
- Luscious La-Caramel ... 421
- Chocolate La-Caramel ... 422
- Majestic Mocha ... 422
- Maca Madness ... 423
- Chocolate Malt ... 423

Raw Chocolate Pleasures ... 424
- Quick Recipe Tips ... 425

Fabulous Fudges ... 426
- Chocolate Ecstasy Fudge ... 426
- Chocolate Malt Fudge ... 426
- Chocolate Peanut Butter Fudge ... 427
- Mocha Fudge ... 427
- Vanilla White Chocolate Fudge ... 427
- La-Caramel White Chocolate Fudge ... 428
- Goji-Orange White Chocolate Fudge ... 428
- Matcha Green Tea White Chocolate Fudge ... 428

Maple Walnut White Chocolate Fudge 428
  La-Caramel Pecan White Chocolate Fudge 429
 Homemade Chocolates & Barks 430
  Raw Chocolates (using cacao powder & coconut oil) 430
  Raw Chocolates (using cacao powder & cacao butter) 431
  Raw Chocolates (using cacao paste & coconut oil) 431
Chapter 8 Dehydrated Pizza Crusts, Craks & Chips 435
  Quick Recipe Tips 435
 Go-To Pizza Crust 438
 Savory Craks & Chipz 440
  "Seeds of Change" Craks 440
  Cabbage N' Carrot Craks 440
  Cheezy Craks 441
  Mediterranean Pita Chipz 442
  Chili-Lime Tortilla Chipz 442
  Rosemary Craks 443
  Bell Pepper Quinoa Chipz 443
  Cheezy Kale Chipz #1 445
  Cheezy Kale Chipz #2 446
  Italian-Style Kale Chipz 447
  Thai-Style Kale Chipz 447
 Sweet Craks & Chipz 449
  Chocolate Chia Craks 449
  Spiced Green Apple Chipz 449
  Sweet N' Berry Craks 450
  Chocolate Kale Chipz 451
  Sesame Honey Kale Chipz 452
 Savory Snackin' Sides (Dehydrator Needed) 453
  Rawkin' Friez 453

    Italian Batter of Choice 455

    Other Savory Veggie Batter Favorites! 459

  Sweet Snackin' Sides (Dehydrator Needed) 460

    Coconut-Fruit Crepes (nut free) 460

    Candied Nuts & Seeds 462

Chapter 9 Longevity Elixir Drinks & Teas 464

  Quick Recipe Tips 464

  Mind Altering Mochaccino 466

  Vanilla Caramel Chaga Latte 467

  Spicy Mayan Infusion 467

  Hormone Balancing Macaccino 468

  Matcha Tea Latte 469

  Chocolate Hemp Nog 470

  Chocolate Orange Hibiscus 471

  Endocrine Elixir 472

  Anti-inflammatory Elixir 472

  Longevity Iced Tea 473

  Morning Chlorella Detox Elixir 475

  Digestive Elixir 475

  Candida Kicker Elixir 476

Brewing Loose-leaf Tea Is Easy 477

  Basic Black Tea Brewing Instruction (including pu-erh) 479

  Basic Oolong Tea Brewing Instruction 479

  Basic Green Tea Brewing Instruction 480

  Basic White Tea Brewing Instruction 480

  Basic Tisane Brewing Instruction (rooibos & other herbal infusions) 480

  Basic Yerba Mate Brewing Instructions 481

  Hot Brewing Method for Iced Tea 481

  Cold Brewing Method for Iced Tea, Simply Delicious! 481

How to Kick Caffeine from Your Cup Right at Home 482
    Simple Decaffeination Method 482
    Answers to Commonly Asked Tea Questions 483

A Final Word 484
    Will You Take the Red Pill or the Blue Pill? 484
        Our Body, Our Temple 484
    Above All, Do No Harm 486

Take the 21-Day Challenge! 488
    Week One 488
        Days 1-5 488
        Days 1-5 or Days 6 & 7 489
    Week Two 489
        Days 8-14, 8-21 or 8-24 489
    Week Three 490
        Days 15-21, 22-28 or 25-31 490
    Week Four & Beyond 490

Appendix A 491
    The Commingling of Business & Politics 491

Appendix B 492
    For the People, or for Profit? 492

Appendix C 493
    What Is Estrogen Dominance? 493
        Progesterone Deficiency: A Problem for Both Sexes 493
        What Are Xenoestrogens? 495
        What Are Phytoestrogens? 495
        Getting to the Root of the Problem 496
        In Closing 497

Appendix D 499
    Food Combining for Optimal Digestion 499

    Quick Tips 500
  Fruits 501
    Quick Tips 501
Appendix E 503
  Acid-Alkaline Foods for Optimal Health 503
    Quick Tips 505
Appendix F 506
  Ayurveda Made Easy 506
    The Three Doshas: Vata, Pitta, & Kapha 506
    Determining Your Dosha(s) 508
    Balancing the Doshas Through Taste 516
    The Six Tastes: Sweet, Sour, Salty, Bitter, Pungent & Astringent 517
Appendix G 519
  Yin-Yang Balance 519
    How to Balance Yin (cold) 521
    How to Balance Dampness 521
    How to Balance Yang (heat) 521
    How to Balance Dryness 521
    Quick Tips 527
About the Author 528
Rebel with a Cause! 529

INTRODUCTION

BASIC RAW KNOWLEDGE 101

What Is a Raw and Living Food Diet, and What Does a "Raw Foodist" Eat?

A raw food diet, or more appropriately termed, raw food lifestyle, is primarily comprised of uncooked, unprocessed, sustainable and often organically (whenever possible) grown plant-based foods. These include raw fruits and vegetables, nuts, seeds, sprouts, fresh and low-temperature dried herbs and sea vegetables. Raw foodists also drink fresh fruit and vegetable juices and some include a moderate amount of lightly processed items such as cold-pressed oils, raw nut/seed butters, un-pasteurized fermented foods, etc. Most raw foodists do not consume animal products of any kind, nor foods containing chemically processed, refined, pasteurized or irradiated ingredients. While some raw foodists include raw (unpasteurized) dairy products, raw meat, raw eggs and sushi into their diets, the majority of those who self-identify as raw foodists are mostly vegan or vegetarian. The exact definition of raw may vary slightly when it comes to cut-off temperature and enzyme/nutrient preservation, but a basic guideline to follow is that the food should never be heated or dehydrated above 115°F.

What Are Some of the Benefits of Such a Lifestyle?

The benefits of going raw are numerous! For some, going raw is the most natural way to achieve and sustain weight loss goals. Eating raw and living food will enable you to enjoy delicious, guilt-free meals and sweet treats while shedding excess weight effortlessly, efficiently and healthily. For others, going raw is simply the best way to eat healthily and naturally improve digestion and the absorption and assimilation of nutrients. Many raw foodists happily proclaim a remarkable change in their overall appearance. Their complexion clears and their skin becomes firmer, more radiant and youthful. They tend to glow from the inside out! What's more, many experience a significant increase in energy, endurance and stamina, and excitedly attest to feeling years younger. No matter who you are or what your age, you can start to experience all these benefits by incorporating more raw and living foods into your life. It's never too late to renew yourself!

In addition to helping you feel your best inside and out, studies have shown that when you eat foods that are raw and living (meaning, rich in vital nutrients and enzymes), your body is much better equipped with the necessary tools it needs to build and strengthen the immune system. When your immune system is finally functioning properly, it can help to alleviate many illnesses already present in the body and prevent a host of potential health conditions from ever arising. Some of the minor to severe illnesses, conditions and symptoms that have been healed or alleviated include: obesity, diabetic hyperglycemia and hypoglycemia, Crohn's disease, ulcerative colitis, diverticulitis, diverticulosis, acid indigestion, heartburn, acid reflux, gas, bloating, constipation, diarrhea, Candida overgrowth, chronic fatigue, fibromyalgia, arthritis, migraine headaches, back, neck and joint pain, minor to serious allergies, asthma, mood swings, depression, anxiety, high blood pressure (hypertension), high cholesterol, minor to severe acne, skin diseases, cancers and many more!

What Nutritional Principles Do Raw Foodists Generally Follow?

Raw foods (especially organic) are packed full of natural dietary fiber, phytochemicals (aka phytonutrients), antioxidants, viable vitamins and minerals and live enzyme. Enzymes are proteins that act as catalysts in order to regulate the digestive process in the body.

- ★ When you heat, warm or dehydrate food above the maximum of 115°F, the enzymes which aid in the digestive process begin to degrade. When food is cooked (baked, broiled, nuked, fried, etc.), the enzymes are completely destroyed.
- ★ Once vitamins, minerals and enzymes are destroyed, the human body takes on the task of having to digest these <u>dead</u> foods without the aid of the enzymes nature provides naturally. This causes the body to work much harder, drawing from other important bodily processes and depleting the body of energy – which can make you feel drained and tired.
- ★ In the long-term, consuming foods depleted of essential nutrients, and without enzymes, can contribute to the following: excess food consumption due to malnourishment that may lead to diabetes and obesity, inflammation in genetically predisposed and weakened areas of the body, toxicity within the body (toxemia), and the accumulation of more and more nuisances, deficiencies and acute illnesses with the potential to become serious and chronic.
- ★ Raw and living foods that are wild and organically grown have a much higher nutrient value than conventionally grown foods, and a much, much, much higher nutrient value when compared to foods (organic or conventional) that have been cooked, refined, pasteurized, irradiated or manipulated in any way, shape or form.
- ★ When you are hungry and eat organic, raw and living foods that naturally have a higher nutrient content, the "I'm satisfied!" button rather than the "I'm full!" button is turned on sooner. Hence, people will tend not to overeat like they do when they consume cooked, processed and refined foods. This is due to the body being properly nourished and, as a result, properly satisfied.
- ★ Raw and living foods contain good bacteria and helpful microorganisms that stimulate the immune system and enhance digestion by populating the digestive tract with beneficial flora.

WHY GO RAW: A FEW PERSONAL THOUGHTS

This book is a guide to a realistic approach to achieving your optimum weight, health and wellness goals while never having to feel deprived of the sweet tastes and savory, rich flavors that can bring joy, satisfaction and pure ecstasy! We can be inspired and motivated to explore healthful raw and living food alternatives to traditional and conventional ingredients by delving into the many natural foods, superfoods and superherbs nature gives us.

You Need Never Feel Like You're Cheated Again!

Going raw – or at least making a conscious choice to incorporate more natural, raw and living foods into your life – does not have to be boring. I assure you, there is a lot more to raw foodism than just rabbit food.

Do I believe we at least can be thinking about and aiming for the very best possible fuel to fill our precious self-healing machines? Of course! We are given only one body, and I feel we need to treat it with respect if we want to spend our years living a quality life, rather than dying a slow death through processed foods and pharmaceuticals. Nevertheless, we must be realistic in the process. We should also be patient with ourselves and always remember that any change in a positive direction is still progress, no matter how big or small, no matter how slow or fast. Some individuals can become inspired and make extreme changes overnight – never to look back again – while others may need to take baby steps. It's all good!

"To get through the hardest journey we need take only one step at a time, but we must keep on stepping." – Chinese Proverb

Chances are (if you are like most) you have struggled or are struggling right now, not just with foods and the question "what exactly do I eat to lose weight and gain energy while successfully controlling temptation and cravings," but possibly with other issues that involve social eating with family and friends. These issues may include: how to handle social situations and the holidays; what to bring to an event or simple gathering; how to make healthy eating fun for children; what to do during times of travel; how to deal with cravings for old favorites or comfort foods in times of stress; how to make changes in habitual and routine eating because it is second nature; where to look for answers to nutritional questions and concerns; how to sort through conflicting information; what to expect during periods of cleansing and detoxification when eliminating processed sugars, allergy provoking foods, hydrogenated oils and the many other hidden, toxic ingredients typically found in the standard America diet (SAD).

To capture the true meaning of what going raw can do, I must end this segment by sharing the following affirmation: going raw is not just about making some healthy dietary changes, clearing up a few food sensitivities or allergies, or even healing and preventing disease in the body – which are all huge and life changing in and of themselves. Going raw is truly about transforming your entire being. Your skin glows and your eyes sparkle, your joints feel juicer and more flexible, and your energy, endurance and stamina increase. You reach your optimum weight naturally, your reflexes are faster, you look and feel more youthful, your immune response is swifter and stronger, your mind is sharper, your thoughts are clearer, you feel more productive and you smile a lot more. You discover the true meaning of gratitude and love and what it really feels like. I could go on and on! Many people reveal that when they start truly respecting themselves by putting the right raw nutrients into their bodies a switch is flipped, and suddenly their whole world starts to take on new meaning. They become more in-tune and aware of what their true purpose is on this planet. Synchronicities are noticed, accepted and taken more seriously, opportunities are accepted and conquered with a fearless attitude, and better choices are made with positive outcomes that follow. Going raw the right way is truly about balancing one's physical, emotional, mental and spiritual well-being; because when the whole person is in a state of balance, health, healing and continued growth can happen more naturally and with ease.

A Bit About Myself & My Personal Journey into the Raw Food Lifestyle

I was born and raised just north of Boston, Massachusetts. I attended college at the University of Massachusetts with a major in nursing and a minor in psychology. I vividly recall being drawn to learning about health and the human body at a very young age. I also remember how much I truly enjoyed taking the initiative to help others. For instance, I can remember at age four handing my grandfather his cane, taking his other hand, and telling him it was time for his walk. That being said, my desire and mission to someday work in the healthcare field didn't fully develop until I watched my grandmother painfully suffer and die from her battle with stomach cancer a few years later. So, you can only imagine when I graduated with a Bachelor of Science Degree in Nursing, and then went a step further to become certified in Oncology/Hematology, I truly thought all my dreams had come true; that I was going to live my life helping others achieve a cancer-free life. When I landed a position in one of the best teaching hospitals in Boston (working on the Bone Marrow Transplant Unit as well as the Oncology/Hematology Units), I thought I had reached my ultimate career goal. In retrospect, all I can honestly say is that I received quite a wakeup call instead.

Sadly, I witnessed most patients return; and more times than not their condition was worse than the first time. As I started to question and research every single drug, their actions and interactions and then all their side effects, I grew more and more disenchanted and disheartened by conventional medicine and the pharmaceutical industry as a whole. I realized that by administering chemotherapy (a toxic poison) into the human body, the stage was being set for a complete immune system crash. I experienced firsthand how chemotherapy and pharmaceuticals can actually be more harmful, damaging and devastating to every biological system (sometimes beyond repair) than you can bear to imagine. I endured many sleepless nights just thinking to myself, "there has to be a better way." I knew I was never going to find the answers I was desperately seeking if I kept swimming in the same pool of insanity; therefore, I decided to leave nursing and the whole field of conventional medicine entirely.

Not long after, I became certified as a Personal Fitness Trainer. I found it to be a fitting short-term career change strategy that came naturally to me, since I've always been very disciplined and passionate about working out every day – either with cardio, weight training or yoga. I love that it gave me the extra time to seek and find my true calling. It was the perfect transitional road along my journey (after my awakening to the truth) that ultimately guided me to the straight path. My quest for a preventative and natural approach to true health, inner contentment and longevity was finally in sight.

Throughout my journey, with all life's twists and turns along the way, I never stopped searching for the true answers to a disease-free life – or at least what it takes to have the capability to naturally heal, reverse and dramatically lessen the degree of disease in the body. I would ask, "if the human body has the ability to heal itself when given the right tools, then what are the most important building blocks and major players that make it all possible for the body to do so?"

I felt compelled to learn and seek out as much as I could about natural and whole food nutrition, Eastern and Ayurvedic herbal treatments and holistic and alternative approaches to medicine. It became an addiction to say the least. I was utterly fascinated!

Lo and behold, it led me to the healing power of raw and living foods, superfoods, superfruits and superherbs. It seemed that all my research kept pointing to one major issue as to why one's health starts to decline, and eventually fails, if they do not take action – Inflammation! Evidently, the primary cause of disease in the body can be traced back to stressors (outside forces) and stress (how one relates and copes with the stressors). How well one deals with stressors and stress (physically, emotionally, etc.) will determine how much calcification, inflammation and toxicity develops in the body as a result. With the tremendous amount of stress many find themselves under today, which is then compounded by an increased number of outside stressors, our endocrine, immune and other body systems are regrettably taking a major hit and becoming weakened. If these systems continue to be stressed to the max, they will eventually go haywire (and may even shut-down) and leave the human body susceptible to a host of diseases and disorders.

What Causes Inflammation, You Ask?

EVERY POSSIBLE FORM OF STRESS! A sampling (key word here) of the stressors that greatly impact our health and overall well-being include:

- ★ Cooked foods, processed and refined foods, pasteurized foods, irradiated foods, conventional meat, poultry, fish and seafood, eggs and dairy, and some other allergy provoking foods not already mentioned – such as wheat, gluten, processed soy and corn, some beans, peanuts (due to aflatoxins) and most grains (due to mycotoxins).
- ★ Lack of sleep or poor sleep quality, negative or toxic relationships and unmet needs, and other negative emotions and thoughts such as anger, fear, guilt and sadness.
- ★ Synthetic pharmaceutical drugs, over-the-counter medication and vaccinations being over-prescribed and advised in current society.
- ★ Synthetic materials we wear as clothing and all the personal care and beauty products with which we lather ourselves.

> ★ Dyes, heavy metals (mercury, lead, cadmium, aluminum, etc.), pesticides (including herbicides, fungicides and larvicide), molds, petrochemicals, plastics and plasticizers, and so on and so on.

All of these environmental toxins are contributing to the non-stop pollution of the air we breathe, the land we walk on, and the arenas from which we eat. Consider our soil, farms, gardens, plant life, animals and other wildlife. In addition, we must consider seriously the water we drink, bathe in and swim in, including our oceans, rivers, lakes and streams, not to mention our sea life.

> *Did you know that practically every disease, such as cancer, heart disease, rheumatoid arthritis and diabetes (to name just a few), is caused by inflammation in a part of our bodies?*

Greatly impacted and inspired to make changes by what I was learning through all my research, I decided to be my own test subject by slowly transitioning into a lifestyle of eating only raw and living foods, superfoods, superfruits and superherbs (which took me approximately two years to achieve). I must admit, this transition did not come without self-discipline, hard work, willpower and periods of trial and error before getting it just right for my specific needs. However, now I can speak from personal experience and proudly state that I have never felt more exuberant, mentally sharp and physically fit and flexible than I do today! And if that's not enough, I have more energy and zest for life than I ever thought possible!

Through this process, the biggest lesson I learned was how to truly listen to my body's cries for help. When your body becomes clean from consuming organic, raw and living foods – and finally clears itself of all the gunk, junk and sludge – it is then able to absorb and assimilate nutrients much more efficiently. Having such a sharp and clean running machine, your body can also immediately signal you when you have eaten a food (or more likely a food ingredient or additive) that may be potentially harmful and toxic to your particular system. Although you may not think so in the moment, this is truly a blessing in disguise. Accept it as your body's red light signaling you to stop.

Another important piece to the puzzle is to understand and recognize that your body is not craving an actual food product – such as a donut, candy bar, hotdog, french fries or hamburger – but rather the minerals, vitamins, amino acids, essential fatty acids, neurotransmitters and other nutrients your body may be deficient in and in desperate need of receiving. This constant search for the proper nutrients tends to lead many to overeat. Why? Because the human body will never get what it needs to thrive on from cooked, overly processed, chemical-laden, nutrient-devoid and mineral depleted substances. The human body may be able to <u>survive</u> for a period of time before disease rears its ugly head, but it certainly will not <u>thrive</u>. Why simply survive when you can thrive?

As a testimony to what I have witnessed – first with myself and then with everyone I have been fortunate enough to work with – I am convinced that eating organically grown, raw and living plant-based foods as much as possible, along with the right superfoods, superfruits and superherbs is where it's at. Eating this way makes reaching ultimate levels of wellness, optimal weight control and the very best state of physical, emotional, mental and spiritual health possible. So, what are you waiting for? Get excited – take charge – take control!

What Is the One Major Factor in Daily Living that Is a Constant?

FOOD! We can literally spend all day thinking about what to eat, when to eat, how much to eat. Then, once we have eaten, we find ourselves questioning how we feel (physically and emotionally) about what we just ate and when we should eat again.

What Is the Single Most Controllable Lifestyle Change We Can Make that Would Have the Greatest Impact on Our Health as a Whole?

To make a conscious decision and heart-felt attempt to eat a diet rich in whole, organic, raw, nutrient dense, enzyme rich and life-giving foods. As the old saying goes, "we are what we eat." Commitment to a raw food lifestyle is also as green as it gets when it comes to improving the health of our environment. It is truly the most sustainable way to live overall!

MY LIFE MISSION AND A FEW WORDS OF ADVICE

To this day I am very excited and committed to continue learning and sharing information. Every day, I look forward to challenging myself to reach new levels and breakthroughs, and to helping my clients do the same. I've combined my years of experience as a Registered Nurse, Certified Personal Fitness Trainer and Raw Food Lifestyle and Whole Life Coach, into long-term goals (or shall I say lifelong goals) involving living out each and every one of my passions: empowering others to take control of their health and happiness and sharing knowledge and exchanging experiences with the world. I'm doing what I love, eating what I love and enjoying it raw!

I always tell people, "for every cooked food there is a raw alternative." At the end of the day it's not about giving up what you love, but about making a better choice that can energize you and give you the "biggest bang for your buck." Everyone's body is unique and everyone's nutritional needs differ – even when it comes to the most immediate and closest of family members. There is no one diet, one food or one herb out there (even in the raw food realm) that will fit all and work for everyone. But there are better and <u>best</u> food choices, as well as combinations of foods and herbs, that can work wonders for each of our unique machines. It takes being your own private detective and acting on what your body needs at different stages in your life. Start by adding more raw and living foods into your day-to-day life (a little at a time and in any way you wish); and by all means, have a blast experimenting with some raw alternatives to traditional and cooked food favorites. The rest will start to fall into place when the time is ripe!

CHAPTER 1
THE RAW TRUTH:
A FEW SECRETS REVEALED &
MYTHS DEBUNKED!

"Let food be thy medicine and medicine be thy food."
– Hippocrates 460-377 B.C.

The information contained herein has been compiled from various sources and is for informational purposes only. No statement should be taken as medical advice. The body's power and ability to heal depends upon the totality of diet, nutrition, lifestyle and environmental factors. No claim for the cure of any disease is intended or implied. Always consult a healthcare professional before starting any new program or protocol.

How Do "Raw Foodists" Get Their Protein?

This is probably the most frequently asked question regarding a plant-based diet. First, we must understand that amino acids are the building blocks of proteins, and out of the 22 amino acids found in the body, eight must be derived from food. All eight are abundantly available in raw and living plant-based food, which are the true body builders – especially organic greens and homegrown sprouts! Their nutrients are bio-available, meaning that the nutrients are readily absorbed and become available to the target bodily system(s) soon after ingesting. Examples of animals that build enormous musculature on green leafy vegetation include: gorillas, giraffes, hippos, elephants and horses. People think they need flesh protein to build flesh protein. If that were true then cows would need to eat flesh to get protein. Learn to cut out the middle man (or animal in this case) and go straight for the bio-available nature of plant-based protein sources.

Great sources of plant-based protein, all of which happen to be my personal favorites that I rotate every other day and consume on a daily basis, are: hemp seeds and hemp protein powder, chia seeds, spirulina powder, chlorella powder, bee pollen, Sunwarrior protein products, Surthrival colostrum and pine pollen powder, jungle peanuts, avocados, and, of course, large amounts of green leafy veggies and homegrown sprouts. Some other superfoods I love adding to my morning smoothie are maca, mesquite, goji berries and golden berries – as they are surprisingly rich in amino acids as well. I also enjoy making creamy dressings with a variety of sprouted nuts or seeds a couple times per week, which I often pour atop kelp noodles, spiraled veggies or rich, colorful salads.

The simple fact with humans is that we taught ourselves to eat everything. Human beings are not natural flesh (aka meat) eaters. Don't take my word for it; there are a ton of scientific facts and research out there to back this truth. We eat meat because as a society we have been conditioned and trained to like it and think we need it.

> *"Although we think we are one, and we act as if we are one, human beings are not natural carnivores. When we kill animals to eat them, they end up killing us because their flesh, which contains cholesterol and saturated fat, was never intended for human beings, who are natural herbivores."*
> – William C. Roberts, M.D., editor, American Journal of Cardiology

WHY ARE ENZYMES SO IMPORTANT?

I will save the <u>much</u> longer answer to this very important question for the great resources out there exclusively dedicated to this subject matter. Keeping it understandable and as brief as I can, I will start by stating – "life cannot exist without enzymes." Period!

- ★ Enzymes are found in all living cells: animal cells, human cells, plant cells – you name it!
- ★ Enzymes are large and complex energized <u>protein</u> molecules needed for every chemical reaction that takes place in the body.
- ★ Enzymes are catalysts; they are connected to every working organ in our body and run our life's processes.
- ★ Enzymes presence and strength can be determined by improved blood and immune system function.
- ★ Enzymes are needed by vitamins and minerals to accomplish their delivery within the body.
- ★ Enzymes are required by all food for digestion, which is why it is so important to not destroy them by cooking and processing food at high heat and with chemicals.
- ★ Enzymes can prevent partially digested proteins from putrefying, carbohydrates from fermenting and fats from turning rancid within our system.
- ★ And last but not least, enzymes from a raw and living plant-based food source become active as soon as they enter the body. For this reason, why not eat more raw and living foods!

> *A very important benefit of eating a diet primarily of raw and living foods is that these foods contain their own enzymes so the body does not have to put extra fuel and energy into making them. This helps the body hold on to its reserve in place from birth and take advantage of a well-deserved break.*

Our bodies naturally produce both digestive and metabolic enzymes as they are needed. Surplus enzymes can be stored by some organs for later use and used as fuel for the brain. **Metabolic Enzymes** speed up the chemical reaction within the cells for the ongoing detoxification and production of energy, which the body needs on a regular basis in order to remain in a healthy and balanced state. Metabolic enzymes enable us to see, hear, feel, move and think. Every organ, every tissue and all 100 trillion cells in our body depend upon metabolic enzymes for their very survival.

Digestive Enzymes can be introduced to the body without necessarily having to be body created, but only through the raw and living foods we eat. Therefore, depending on the percentage of raw and living foods we eat, this will in turn determine if there are enough enzymes to support the body's natural ability to build, cleanse, energize and heal without overly taxing our vital organs. For instance, relying on a piece of wilted lettuce on a hamburger is clearly not enough, not even close! Why? A substantial number of enzymes would still need to be drawn from the limited reserve given at birth.

Any time our body has to produce its own metabolic or digestive enzymes – due to overeating and primarily relying on a diet of cooked and processed foods and synthetic/chemical substances we label as food – it puts a tremendous strain on the liver, pancreas, gallbladder and other organs. This is why what we choose to eat (enzyme and nutrient-devoid foods versus enzyme and nutrient-rich foods) and how we choose to eat it (raw and living versus cooked/processed and dead) is the key to our health and longevity. It would be a good idea to start taking preventative steps now rather than waiting for signs and symptoms of a problem to creep up. It's always much easier to prevent a problem than it is to reverse one.

The cooking or processing of food destroys all of its enzymes, and if the enzymes are no longer active, vital nutrients have no way of breaking down and getting into the blood stream to do their necessary jobs.

Since most of the foods we eat are either cooked, processed or chemically altered in some way – and the raw foods we do eat contain only enough enzymes to help in the breakdown of that particular food – our bodies are constantly being called upon to produce an excessive and unnecessary number of digestive enzymes. Sure, we can take supplemental enzymes, which can be a great support, but they are not the ideal long-term solution for our overall health and well-being – especially if our food choices continue to be less than ideal. A band-aid on any problem is never the solution.

The three main digestive enzymes include: lipase for breaking down fats, protease for protein and amylase for carbohydrates and starches. The body cannot make cellulase, an enzyme necessary for proper digestion of cellulose/fiber, so it must be introduced through raw and living plant-based foods. Unfortunately, our bodies were not designed to make the massive number of enzymes needed in order to eat the standard American diet (which we were never designed to eat in the first place). After about 30 years or so of constantly overworking the liver, pancreas, gallbladder and other organs – by eating mostly cooked, processed, chemical-laden foods and substances – these organs begin to fail and become "tapped out." This is when negative health signs and symptoms start to become noticeable and trouble can set it.

Could What We Call "Aging" Simply Be a Case of Enzyme Deficiency?

Digestion will always take precedence over nearly everything else – no matter what; and this eventually results in a lowering of our body's disease-fighting capability and a general weakening of the body's ability to mend itself. Once again, I stress that a large part of this is due to so much of our enzyme potential having to go into the making of the digestive enzymes necessary to break down our choice of foods. Therefore, as we age we begin to run short, and our ability to keep up with the demand and requirements for digestive enzymes begin to suffer. This deficiency will eventually lead us down a path of malabsorption, malnourishment, digestive issues and complaints. Picture this happening: undigested food collects in the colon, poorly digested protein putrefies, fats turn rancid and carbohydrates ferment. These undigested food particles leak back into the bloodstream from the colon and create further toxicity. As we use up and abuse our enzyme potential, we begin to slow down and lose energy. Furthermore, our body loses the ability to fight disease and remedy its own naturally-occurring malfunctions. This all leads to inflammation, disease and eventually death. We associate this scenario with the "aging process," yet it may be more accurate to associate it with the highly self-induced depletion of metabolic and digestive enzymes and enzyme activity happening inside us.

Please Note: If you are interested in understanding more on enzymes and the role they play in our health and longevity, I suggest *Enzyme Nutrition* and *Enzymes for Health & Longevity* by Dr. Edward Howell.

The Big Picture

It is hard to comprehend how enzyme depletion, mineral deficiency and malnourishment can be at the very root of so many conditions, when at the same time we have more restaurants, fast food chains, supermarkets and grocery stores popping up more than ever before. Add to this equation the sad and disturbing fact that obesity in America has become a major health problem and public health threat. It truly makes you wonder (or at least it should): what is really going on here?

As a nation, we need to question. Not just the superficial facts – meaning the food we see with our eyes and the ingredients we read (yet can hardly pronounce) listed on the packaging – but every synthetic item, every chemical, every hidden ingredient and every secret substance that went into the whole production (from start to finish) of a food, right up until the time we put it in our mouth. We also need to be a bit more concerned about how all this affects our short and long-term health. Where and how do we start, you ask? By becoming more responsible, respecting ourselves more, empowering ourselves with knowledge, asking lots of questions and demanding real, solid answers with real, strong evidence to back it up. We can do this by investigating who is behind the study and testing of our food.

I find this to be particularly important today, when man is making so many of the ingredients we call food – not to mention the many nutritional supplements and pharmaceutical drugs so many consume on an everyday basis. Sadly, there is a staggering amount of artificial food and drink items being made in laboratories through the use of chemical manipulation and genetically modified organisms (GMOs). Just think about it: we ingest more synthetics and pharmaceutical drugs than ever before. Pharmaceutical drugs only mask symptoms rather than getting to the core of the primary issue at hand. How we can get so excited to see lab results that have been unnaturally manipulated by drugs is baffling to me; especially when we haven't done a thing to figure out the root problem. On top of this, we are eating more and more meat and dairy from filthy factory farms due to mass production, which has been created through greed and negative intentions. The injecting of antibiotics and hormone pumping is also a major concern. Not to mention the increased amount of feces, worms, parasites and diseases allowed into our food chain from sick and poorly treated animals.

Although I'm grateful for much of the intelligent and ingenious technology we have today, let us get back to the basics on this one. FOOD DOES MATTER! So, get started by eating more wild fruits, vegetables and herbs from mother earth, organic foods from quality mineral-rich soil, and eating the majority of them whole and raw as nature intended.

THE DIRTY DAIRY SECRET: DOES IT "REALLY" DO THE BODY GOOD?

For someone who loved cheese in every style (and on everything), I tried my hardest to justify why I should keep a certain amount in my diet (even raw cheese); but as I dug and dug, the statistics, research and results made it harder and harder for me to consume anything that involved dairy. I don't want to write an entire book on this issue, but I would like to plant the seed for further investigation on your part. Get the facts and become aware of the scary connection between dairy and osteoporosis, dairy and weight gain and diary's association with numerous diseases and common allergies. If you haven't heard about or yet read *The China Study* by Dr. T. Colin Campbell, I highly suggest it.

> *"The association between the intake of animal protein and fracture rates appears to be as strong as the association between cigarette smoking and lung cancer." – Dr. T. Colin Campbell*

Dairy products are loaded with synthetic hormones, antibiotics, bacteria, pus, chalk and tap water, then pasteurized, homogenized, x-rayed (aka irradiated), and placed in chemical leaching, hormone-disrupting plastic containers. Ponder that for a moment!

Dairy is such a mucous-forming, acid-forming food, that it actually causes osteoporosis. In an effort to neutralize and buffer our internal acidity and keep our blood healthily balanced, alkalizing minerals – such as calcium and magnesium – are literally robbed from our bones, tissues and bodily fluids.

In *Breaking the Food Seduction* by Dr. Neal Barnard, the scientific basis for the "addiction" and "cravings" that most people feel toward dairy foods (especially cheese, being the most concentrated) is well-documented.

Did you know that the mother's milk of a species is naturally laced with opiates to trigger the habit of suckling/nursing? The release of opiates in our bodies is not enough to be labeled as a drug, but it is significant enough to hook us, creating a strong "addiction." Hence, our strong "cravings" for cheese, ice cream and many other foods derived from milk and dairy products.

> *"It is hard to turn on the television without hearing commercials suggesting that milk promotes strong bones. The commercials do not point out that only 30 percent of milk's calcium is absorbed by the body or that osteoporosis is common among milk drinkers. Nor do they help you correct the real causes of bone loss."* – Dr. Neal Barnard

More fine quotes to ponder by great doctors who truly take "first, do no harm" seriously.

> *"Milk, it now seems clear, is not the solution to poor bone density. To the contrary, it's part of the problem."* – Dr. Charles Attwood

> *"The primary cause of osteoporosis is the high-protein diet most Americans consume today. As one leading researcher in this area said, 'eating a high-protein diet is like pouring acid rain on your bones.'"*
> – Dr. John McDougall

Calcium Rich Foods that Giveth, Not Taketh Away!

Mature green leafy vegetables are calcium rich. The many choices include: spinach, collards, kale, Swiss chard, dandelion greens, mustard green, turnip greens, arugula, parsley, watercress, broccoli and many sprouts. Also, you may be surprised to learn that sesame seeds, numerous sea vegetables, raw olives, figs, several dried fruits, oranges, berries, baobab, raw mesquite powder, garlic and many raw nuts and seeds all contain a significant amount of calcium that is easily digested, assimilated and absorbed.

Please Note: If you are prone to kidney stones or gallstones, you may want to limit or even avoid certain foods that contain oxalic acid (aka oxalates) – beets and beet greens, dandelion greens, spinach, Swiss chard, cranberries and strawberries, for example. According to much research, this may only be a concern when cooked, but not when eaten raw or juiced. Please read the box below.

> In *Fresh Vegetable and Fruit Juices* by Dr. Norman Walker, oxalic acid is only a concern if it is cooked or processed. According to Dr. Norman Walker, the oxalic acid found in raw and living foods is in its <u>organic</u> state, having no negative effect on the body. Actually, Dr. Norman Walker claims that <u>organic</u> oxalic acid is an important element necessary for peristalsis stimulation and bowel toning. However, when these same foods are cooked or processed, the oxalic acid they contain becomes <u>inorganic</u>. Oxalic acid in its <u>inorganic</u> state is dead and can combine with calcium (even the calcium in the other foods eaten during the same meal), destroying its nutritional value and making it possible to form painful calcium oxalate stones in the kidneys or other organs in the body.

Another helpful tip: vitamin D3, vitamin K2 from non-GMO natto (fermented soy) sources only, magnesium, coconut oil and foods naturally rich in chlorophyll and minerals (like living green superfood powders) can all be a tremendous help in enhancing calcium absorption.

Breaking the Myth on Bone-Mineral Density

Bone density is not increased by eating calcium rich foods and calcium supplementation as the dairy industry would love us to keep believing. Calcium is the "end" (mature) product of a biological transmutation, and <u>cannot</u> be transformed into something else (i.e., absorbed and assimilated to increase bone and bone density). Calcium's true purpose is relaxing smooth muscle tissue and alkalizing and relaxing the digestive tract (stomach and intestines).

Silica, on the other hand, is the "young" product of a biological transmutation and <u>can</u> be transformed by the body to become calcium in bones. It is also known for improving the thickness and strength of skin, hair and nails; stimulating cell metabolism and cell formation; and boosting the immune system. Silica is also an anti-inflammatory and plays a key role in the structure and function of connective tissue. Therefore, for strong and healthy bones, teeth, skin, hair and nails, start increasing your silica intake. You can do this by eating silica rich foods and herbs such as horsetail, nettles, hemp leaf, radishes, romaine lettuce and burdock root. Also, be sure to eat the skins of organic cucumbers, peppers and tomatoes – all of which are also high in silica.

> **Quick Tip:** Always wash your fruits and vegetables with 3% food grade hydrogen peroxide (H2O2) or a good quality, all-natural veggie wash. I also suggest scrubbing all the skins of your fruits and vegetables that are hard and tough enough to take a good scrub. I like using a coconut fiber vegetable brush, which is great for apples, bell peppers, carrots, cucumbers, tomatoes and more.

Due to horsetail being one of the richest sources of silica, it has the amazing ability to enrich our blood, knit calcium in the bones and form collagen – an important protein found in connective tissue, skin, bone, cartilage and ligaments. Therefore, horsetail can be used to help mend broken bones, sprained tendons and as a supplement to treat and prevent osteoporosis.

Horsetail – specifically *Equisetum arvense* – is an herb with a tremendous amount of medicinal value; therefore, as with any herb taken as medicine, be sure to do your due diligence and consult an herbal specialist or naturopath trained in the field of botanical medicine. You always want to be sure to avoid any possible side effects and/or interactions with other herbs and medications you may be taking. For instance, long-term use of horsetail can lead to a deficiency of vitamin B1 (thiamine); therefore, it would be wise to supplement with a <u>natural</u> B vitamin supplement like Max B-ND by Premier Research Labs.

Healthy Gums & Teeth: The Answer Is Not in Your "Regular" Toothpaste!

Neem bark and neem oil support healthy gums and teeth, which includes tightening of the gum tissue. For centuries, millions of people in India and Africa have been using neem bark as disposable toothbrushes. The practice is said to clean the teeth of plaque and phlegm particles, rendering the mouth clean and pleasant.

I use Herbodent Herbal Toothpaste. It is made of rare herbs, fruits, extracts and the oils of natural ingredients such as neem, clove, babool, majuphal, coriander, ginger, lemon, spearmint, etc. The natural ingredients in Herbodent are based on ancient, well-documented Ayurvedic medical formulations and years of indigenous research. You can find it at www.healthandyoga.com. I also make a habit of rubbing a few drops of neem oil into my gums after brushing my teeth each night, right before bedtime. My favorite brand is by Premier Research Labs, as I can count on them for purity and quality.

Other Great Natural Tips for Dental Hygiene

Re-mineralize your teeth by chewing on organically grown wheatgrass or parsley (like you would a piece of gum), as both are super rich in chlorophyll and minerals. Yes, I said chewing rather than juicing. If you have a cavity, I suggest chewing directly on the site. This will help activate the nerve and prevent damage as it alkalizes and kills bacteria. In my experience, I have found parsley to be just as powerful, if not more powerful, than wheatgrass.

Use coconut oil or fresh coconut water (not pasteurized) for its great antimicrobial, antibacterial, antifungal and antiviral properties in place of mouthwash. Rub it on your teeth and gums and leave it there, or just swish it around! At least you don't have to be afraid of swallowing this style of mouthwash. I use coconut oil for almost everything! I eat it, use it on my body and face as moisturizer, and even rub it into the ends of my hair. I always keep a small amount in a glass container right in my bathroom.

Use 3% food grade hydrogen peroxide (H2O2) and aluminum free baking soda (Bob's Red Mill brand) either separately or together to naturally whiten your teeth at home.

Please Note: Do not use hydrogen peroxide for teeth/gums if you have amalgam (mercury) fillings. It can cause metals to oxidize and lead to increased mercury exposure and absorption.

Always remember to protect your precious tooth enamel/dentin by rinsing your mouth after eating high sugar or high citric acid fruits (dried fruits, lemons, limes, etc.).

How to Reap the Vital Benefits of Vitamin D3

Have you ever wondered why we are seeing an alarming increase in vitamin D deficiency and related diseases? Haven't we been told to stay out of the sun and wear sun protection at all times for several years now? What about the fact that one of cholesterol's many functions in the body is to act as a precursor to vitamin D, and, by inhibiting the synthesis of cholesterol, we also inhibit the synthesis of vitamin D? What role do you think the increase in "low cholesterol" diets prescribed by physicians, the media advertising "cholesterol free" products, and the pharmaceutical industry's push for consuming cholesterol lowering drugs potentially plays in this?

A lack of vitamin D, specifically vitamin D3, has been associated with osteoporosis and an increase in bone fractures, certain cancers, diabetes, heart disease, obesity and autoimmune disorders such as multiple sclerosis (MS), arthritis, depression, fatigue, infertility and PMS – to name just a few.

Contrary to popular belief, the best time to be in the sun for vitamin D3 production is roughly between 10 A.M.-2 P.M.

Exposure to natural sunlight is an important source of vitamin D3. Our bodies do not make vitamin D; therefore, we must get it from the sun, food or supplements, with the sun being the optimal source. If you must rely on a supplement, I suggest a natural liquid source of D3 over capsules. Due to D3 being a fat-soluble vitamin, I suggest taking it with meals. My favorite is a live source of natural D3 in a serum by Premier Research Labs.

Please Note: If you rely on supplementation for your D3 needs, please be sure to have your 25-hydroxy vitamin D levels tested and monitored on a regular basis. Optimum levels have been noted to be between 50-75ng/ml.

Sunscreens with a sun protection factor of eight or greater will block UVB rays. However, UVB is responsible for producing the vitamin D3 we so desperately need. How ironic!

Did you know that vitamin D3 is formed from exposure to UVB rays, whereas UVA radiation actually destroys vitamin D? UVA increases oxidative stress in the body and ages our skin. Also, you may not have known that UVA radiation has a longer wave length than UVB and can penetrate materials much more easily – such as the earth's atmosphere and window glass.

Once again, it is all about balance – and Mother Nature knows best!

This is why it is so important to get outside and in touch with Mother Nature. When you spend time <u>outside</u> your body has the intuitive nature to balance and protect itself from overdosing on vitamin D and harmful UVA rays. On the other hand, when you spend most of your time <u>inside</u> and expose yourself to sunlight filtered through window glass (either at home, work or in your car) you get all the UVA rays but virtually none of the beneficial UVB rays.

Please Note: This is not an invitation to sunburn your skin and cause inflammation through too much exposure. Moderation and balance is the key! And this does not just go for sun exposure, but everything in life.

How Much Sun Is Enough for the Production of Vitamin D3?

Optimal exposure time will be different depending on your skin type, weather conditions and other environmental factors. The objective is to get enough exposure without burning. For a light-skinned person, up to 20 minutes of exposure is a good guideline to follow. Olive-skinned and dark-skinned people will need to be outside longer, possibly significantly longer, in order to obtain optimal levels. This could be up to two hours, especially for people with very dark brown skin.

Antioxidants & Sunburn

Did you know that the number of antioxidants you have in your skin plays a major role in your development of sunburn?

Yes, that's right! The more antioxidants you have in your system the better protection you have against sunburn. Eat a healthy diet rich in fresh, raw vegetables, fruits and berries (such as blackberries, raspberries and blueberries), medicinal quality goji berries, medicinal mushrooms (especially melanin rich chaga mushroom), antioxidant rich raw chocolate, and drink plenty of green and white loose-leaf teas loaded with polyphenols. Do this and you will be on your way to helping your cells regulate light absorption, which can protect from over-exposure and lower your risk of burning quickly.

Dr. Joseph Mercola released an awesome article titled "Shocking Update – Sunshine Can Actually Decrease Your Vitamin D Levels," posted May 12, 2009, on www.mercola.com. In this article he explains the connection between exposure to sunshine, vitamin D3 and showering. I found the information very interesting with tremendous "food for thought." The following is a segment from the article.

> **WHAT DOES SHOWERING HAVE TO DO WITH YOUR VITAMIN D LEVELS?**
>
> First, it's important to understand that vitamin D3 is an oil soluble steroid hormone. It's formed when your skin is exposed to ultraviolet B (UVB) radiation from the sun (or a safe tanning bed). When UVB strikes the surface of your skin, your skin converts a cholesterol derivative in your skin into vitamin D3.
>
> However, the vitamin D3 that is formed on the surface of your skin does not immediately penetrate into your bloodstream. It actually needs to be absorbed from the surface of your skin into your bloodstream.
>
> The critical question then is: how long does it take the vitamin D3 to penetrate your skin and reach your bloodstream?
>
> If you're thinking about an hour or two, like I did until recently, you're wrong. Because new evidence shows it takes up to 48 hours before you absorb the majority of the vitamin D that was generated by exposing your skin to the sun!
>
> Therefore, if you shower with soap, you will simply wash away much of the vitamin D3 your skin generated and decrease the benefits of your sun exposure. So, to optimize your vitamin D level, you need to delay washing your body with soap for about two full days after sun exposure.
>
> Not many people are going to avoid bathing for two full days. However, you really only need to use soap underneath your arms and your groin area, so this is not a major hygiene issue. You'll just want to avoid soaping up the larger areas of your body that were exposed to the sun." – Dr. Joseph Mercola

Beneath the Expression "Beauty Is Only Skin Deep"

Your skin is the largest organ of your body and can be viewed as a kind of litmus paper to your general state of health. For instance, when your skin comes into contact with something you're allergic to, it may react by breaking out with hives or a rash. When you're not feeling well, your skin may either turn pale and become cold and clammy, or become hot, flushed and sweaty.

> *Did you know that it has been reported that 95% of all products marketed for skin, hair and personal care and beauty contain chemicals linked to cancer or skin disorders?*

What's important to remember about the skin is that it is a living part of your body, with several well developed and interconnected circulating systems such as the blood, sweat, sebum, nerve and lymph systems. Any one of these vital systems can be damaged by the absorption of chemicals or enhanced by a good skin care protocol. It is vital to get into the habit of reading labels. If a product lists an ingredient you would not ideally or typically put in your mouth, eat or drink, then think twice before slathering it all over your body or bathing in it. This also goes for bathing and swimming in chemical and chlorine filled hot tubs and pools, not to mention the chemicals and chlorine coming out of our faucets and shower heads that we wash and shower in every day.

Could This Little-Known Endocrine Disrupter Be the Root of Your Thyroid Issues?

Bromides are chemicals; they are toxic and they are all around us! Bromide is so dangerous because it competes for the same receptors that are used in the thyroid gland to capture iodine and as we know, iodine is crucial for thyroid function. When bromide dominates, our iodine diminishes.

Iodine affects every tissue in your body – not just your thyroid. Every day we are exposed to and absorb toxic bromides in more forms than one: Methyl Bromide is a pesticide used predominantly in the California areas, especially on strawberries; Brominated Vegetable Oil (BVO) is added to citrus drinks (for example, Mountain Dew and Gatorade) to help suspend the flavoring in the liquid; Potassium Bromate is a dough conditioner found in commercial bread and bakery products, as well as some flours. Almost every time you eat bread in a restaurant, or eat hamburger or hotdog buns, you are consuming toxic bromide. Potassium Bromate is also found in many dental products such as toothpaste and mouthwash. Bromides can be found in fire-retardant fabrics all over the home and in cars; in textile dyes and hair dyes; in plastics, like those used to make computers; and in medications such as certain brand name inhalers, nasal sprays and anesthesia.

SOY ISOFLAVONES & ANTI-NUTRIENTS: ANOTHER MAJOR CONTRIBUTOR TO THYROID DYSFUNCTION

Anti-nutrients are natural or synthetic compounds that interfere with the assimilation and absorption of one or more nutrients. Soybeans contain a number of natural anti-nutrients. These include: soyatoxin, protease inhibitors, phytic acid and oxalic acid (all of which can interfere with the enzymes needed to digest protein), along with high levels of soy isoflavones (which can create goitrogenic and estrogenic activity).

All unfermented soy products, such as tofu, bean curd, soy drinks and milks, soy ice cream, soy infant formula, soy protein powders and soy meat alternatives (e.g., soy sausages and soy veggie burgers made from hydrolyzed soy powder), should be avoided at all costs! If the soy isoflavones and other anti-nutrients they contain is not a good enough reason, then what about the fact that over 90% of the soy grown in the U.S. is genetically modified (GM)?

So, What Is Wrong with Eating Unfermented Soy You Ask? Let Us Count the Ways!

The following information was obtained primarily from two articles: "This 'Miracle Health Food' Has Been Linked to Brain Damage and Breast Cancer," by Dr. Joseph Mercola, posted September 18, 2010, on www.mercola.com, and "The Truth about Unfermented Soy and Its Harmful Effects," by Teya Skae, posted February 12, 2008, on www.naturalnews.com.

- Soy contains one of the highest amounts of phytic acid, which in large amounts can block the absorption of essential minerals in the intestines. These minerals include calcium, cooper, magnesium, iodine, iron and zinc.
- Soy is high in oxalic acid, which may increase your risk of developing calcium oxalate kidney stones if you are predisposed to this condition.
- Soy contains goitrogens that can block the synthesis of thyroid hormones and interfere with iodine metabolism.
- Soy contains a hormone-like compound called genistein (aka plant estrogen or phytoestrogen), which has been found to impair immune system function. Mice that were injected with genistein showed a drop in immune cells. In addition, the thymus gland (where immune cells mature) actually shrank.
- Soy can cause a severe and potentially fatal allergic reaction due to an overreaction of the immune system.
- Soy contains phytoestrogens, which can mimic and sometimes block the effects of our own estrogens. Drinking two glasses of soy milk daily for only one month has been shown to have enough of this compound to alter a woman's menstrual cycle.
- Soy is one of the most detrimental foods you could feed any baby, infant or child. It has been estimated that babies and infants, exclusively fed soy formula, receive the equivalent of five birth control pills of estrogen every day. The estrogens in soy may then irreversibly harm their underdeveloped reproductive system.
- Soy formula has over 1,000% more aluminum than conventional milk-based formulas. Aluminum doesn't just affect soy formula, but all processed soy products, as soybeans go through an acid washing process in aluminum tanks. Aluminum is an extremely poisonous substance that can accumulate in the body's tissues and can be highly toxic to the central nervous system, digestive system and kidneys.
- Soy increases the body's requirement for vitamin B12 and vitamin D3.
- And more!

So, are there any safe and healthy soy products that one can consume? Yes, but only if they are organic (GM free) and properly fermented. These include miso, natto and tempeh. Once soybeans have been properly fermented, all the anti-nutrients (phytic acid, oxalic acid, goitrogens, estrogens, etc.) are reduced, making their beneficial properties readily available.

Simple Tips on How to Heal & Support Your Thyroid Naturally

- Let's start with sea vegetables! All sea vegetables, such as dulse, nori and wakame, will provide you with necessary iodine, but kelp takes first place in my opinion. Sea vegetable flakes or powders are a great and simple way to obtain your iodine needs naturally. They are also super high in minerals and can add that salty flavor to soups and salads – so start sprinkling!
- Increase your intake of essential fatty acids EPA and DHA with algae oils (e.g., marine phytoplankton). Algae oils are a great alternative to fish oils, which may be contaminated despite manufacturers' claims.

- ★ Selenium works in conjunction with iodine and other essential nutrients as part of a natural protocol for boosting your thyroid function. Did you know that selenium is one of the minerals that most of us are deficient in? If you consume just 3-5 Brazil nuts per day you will get your daily dose of selenium.
- ★ Adding organic, raw, extra virgin coconut oil to your diet will be another great inclusion to this natural protocol. Coconut oil stimulates the production of hormones, gets your growth factor going and enhances immunity and absorption of nutrients. For instance, consuming coconut oil (in a smoothie, raw soup or salad) along with hemp seeds, chia seeds, chlorella, marine phytoplankton, spirulina and algae oils, can maximize your omega-3 potential. What's more, the unique medium chain fatty acid molecules that make up coconut oil can actually protect against myocardial infarctions (aka heart attacks) and strokes and does not have a negative effect on cholesterol.
- ★ One final suggestion I will leave you with is to start experimenting with raw maca powder in your smoothies, desserts and raw chocolate treats. Among the many amazing properties maca possesses, it is a natural hormonal rejuvenator and balancer, providing great health benefits for both men and women. Maca is definitely worthy of some online research time if you are unfamiliar with it. I also get into maca and its benefits under "South American Superherbs" (page 190).

CHAPTER 2
HOW TO STOCK & PREP FOR
YOUR RAW FOOD KITCHEN MAKEOVER

LET'S GO GROCERY SHOPPING, SHALL WE?

I know I mentioned it earlier, but I cannot stress enough just how important it is to shop and buy organic whenever possible. Most health food stores carry organic foods and even many of the larger supermarket chains are beginning to carry more and more organic options as well. On average, organic food is 25% more nutritious in terms of vitamins and minerals than conventional. Organic foods – especially raw and non-processed options – contain higher levels of beta carotene, vitamins C, D and E, health-promoting polyphenols, cancer-fighting antioxidants, flavonoids that help ward off heart disease, essential fatty acids, and essential minerals (such as calcium, magnesium, chromium and iron). These essential minerals are severely depleted in conventional foods grown in pesticide and nitrate fertilizer-abused soil. UK and US government statistics indicate that levels of trace minerals in conventional fruits and vegetables fell by up to 76% between 1940 and 1991.

> *Did you know that it has been reported that more than 400 chemical pesticides are routinely used in conventional farming, and that the residues remain on these conventional foods even after washing?*

But Eating Organic Is Expensive, or Isn't It?

When I hear this, I can only say one thing – "you can either pay now for vibrant health and a good quality of life, or you can pay it out to the medical and pharmaceutical industries later." Organic food's retail price is approximately only 20% higher than that of conventional, chemical laden foods; when you add to this the astronomical hidden costs (damage to your health, climate, environment and government subsidies), eating organic can actually be cheaper.

- ★ Organic food doesn't contain artificial sweeteners (like high fructose corn syrup), contaminants (like mercury), food additives and flavor enhancers (like MSG), or preservatives (like sodium nitrate), that can all cause health problems.
- ★ Eating organic has the potential to lower the incidence of allergies, autism, cancer, coronary heart disease, dementia, hyperactivity, learning disorders, migraines and osteoporosis.

Fresh Produce

Knowing how long your precious organic fresh fruits and vegetables last and where to store them for maximum shelf life leads to wiser purchases. Produce loses its vibrancy over time, so get into the habit of checking it frequently to ensure freshness. By doing this, you will learn to make better decisions about how much to buy of a particular food. You will also be able to use more (if not all) of it before it goes bad.

Leafy Greens: Refrigerate unwashed to avoid premature wilting. I advise washing all your produce just prior to eating it. The excess water can make them wilt or become mushy earlier than necessary. Store your leafy greens in a plastic bag or air-tight container with a slightly damp paper towel to keep them crisp. Avoid storing in the same drawer as apples, pears, etc., which release ethylene gases that act as a natural ripening agent.

> **Quick Tip:** For my smoothie and salad greens, I like to use a Zyliss salad spinner to wash, rinse and drain all my leafy greens (such as lettuces, kale and leafy green herbs). This way, any leftovers can easily be kept right in the strainer inside the salad spinner and in the fridge. Instant crisper until your next usage!

Herbs: When using fresh herbs, store them in the refrigerator in a plastic bag or air-tight container with a slightly damp paper towel on the top and bottom.

Fresh Berries: Store in fridge unwashed in their original container.

Summer Fruits (such as peaches, plums and nectarines): For maximum freshness, store on the counter in a paper bag punched with holes and away from sunlight. Once ripe, you can transfer to the fridge.

Fall/Winter Fruits (such as apples and pears): Store in a bowl on the counter. Once ripe, you may transfer them to the fridge.

Tropical Fruits (such as mangoes, papayas, pineapples and kiwis): Store on the counter until ripe and then transfer to fridge. Mangos will ripen best in a paper bag in a cool place. Transfer to fridge once ripe.

Bananas & Citrus (such as grapefruits, oranges, lemons and limes): Store in bowls on the counter outside the fridge. When bananas get too ripe, you can always peel them and place them in a bag or air-tight container in the freezer; then use them for smoothies or for making raw ice creams.

Avocados: Store in a bowl on the counter. Once ripe, you may transfer them to the fridge.

Tomatoes: Spread them out on the counter out of direct sunlight for even ripening. Once ripe, you can store stem side down in the refrigerator.

Cucumbers: Store in the fridge in a plastic bag or in your crisper. You can also wrap each one with a dry paper towel to keep from getting too soft when they are touching one another (which happens due to the high moisture content of cucumbers).

Celery & Carrots: Store each in the fridge in their own plastic bags. Adding a slightly moist paper towel to the bag will keep them from drying out and losing their stiff crispness. For celery, I find it holds its crispness longer when I wrap a moistened paper towel around the bottom of each bunch.

Asparagus: Cut a small portion of the bottoms off, and then store the stalks in the fridge. You may either place them upright in an inch of water in a cup, or simply store in a plastic bag with a damp paper towel around the bottoms.

Beets: Remove green tops approximately one inch above the crown, and then store in fridge in a plastic bag to prevent moisture loss. Store beet greens in a <u>separate</u> plastic bag.

Bell Peppers, Radishes & Cabbages: Store loose in fridge.

Broccoli & Cauliflower: Store in fridge and in a sealed plastic bag.

Peas: Store in the fridge and in a <u>perforated</u> plastic bag.

Zucchinis & Summer Squashes: Store in the fridge and in a <u>perforated</u> plastic bag. You can also wrap each one with a dry paper towel to keep from getting too soft when they are touching one another (which happens due to the high moisture content).

Summer Melons & Winter Squashes: Store at room temperature on the counter.

Onions & Garlic: Store in the pantry away from light, heat and moisture.

Dried Fruits

When storing dried fruits, I suggest always keeping them in an air-tight jar or container (preferably glass) in your pantry away from light, heat and moisture.

Dried and dehydrated fruits definitely have a place and serve a purpose in a raw food lifestyle. They are great when you need a sweet snack or want to add some natural sweetness to a food or drink. Their sticky texture can help bind ingredients together (especially in dessert making), and they can be great as part of a trail mix blended with nuts and seeds.

Some of my favorite dried fruits to work with are goji berries, golden berries, Hunza golden raisins and mulberries (always); cherries, currants, Turkish apricots and Turkish figs (on occasion) and dates (rarely).

Personally, I have learned to stay clear of certain dried fruits. Some are a little too sweet and set off my addictive nature for eating sweet and sugary foods. For instance, I will not eat dates or use them in any recipes for myself. In addition, many found in the grocery store are not "truly raw" (they can be either pasteurized – to inhibit mold growth; heat-treated – to produce lower moisture content; or steam-treated – to increase moisture and plumpness). Although I love them so, I use these facts to justify my reasoning behind staying away from them. When I want to treat myself (maybe once a year, if that) I go the extra mile by ordering all my dates from either The Date People (www.datepeople.net) or Flying Disc Ranch (www.flyingdiscranch.com). The quality and taste of every date variety is unsurpassed!

Before I purchase any dried fruits, I always look for the following things to make sure their beneficial vitamins (like vitamin C) or minerals have not been destroyed by a high heating, blanching or drying process:

- ★ They must always be 100% certified organic.

- ★ They must always be sun-dried or low-temperature dehydrated to raw food standards.
- ★ They must never be pre-treated with sulfites.

Please Note: Not only does sulfur dioxide destroy thiamine (B1), but many people have allergic reactions to sulfites and should be careful when eating treated dried fruit. <u>Always</u> check under "other ingredients."

- ★ They must always be free of any added sugars.

Buyers Beware: Sometimes sugar is added during the pre-treatment process. This makes dried fruit, which is already higher in concentrated sugars per serving than fresh fruit, even higher in sugar.

- ★ They must be free of any preservatives or color savors/enhancers.

> **Quick Tip:** When working with dried fruits that tend to get a slight coating of natural sugars over them, I like to give them a quick squirt of 3% food grade hydrogen peroxide, rinse them quickly in a strainer, and then soak them for a short period to rehydrate them a bit. This helps cut down on some of the sugar and washes off any surface debris.

Nuts & Seeds

In a nutshell (pun intended), you can generally store most nuts and seeds as follows:

- ★ Store in the pantry away from light, heat and moisture for up to three months.
- ★ Store in the fridge for up to six months.
- ★ Store in the freezer for a year or more.

Personally, I will never purchase nuts and seeds from the bins at grocery stores. Your chances of buying nuts or seeds which have already had their oils go rancid are much higher. With some varieties, you can tell right away by either smelling or tasting them (they will taste either really rank, sour or smell off); with other varieties, it is a bit more challenging.

- ★ First, I don't know how long they have been sitting in those bins. Also, have the nuts and seeds been properly rotated? Have the bins been cleaned out? If the bins are not cleaned routinely, eventually the oily residue is going to spoil and potentially contaminate the fresh batch going in.
- ★ Second, just think of how often those bins open and close day after day; how many people have been touching the scooper (or just digging their hands in). Those poor little nuts and seeds are not just being exposed to air constantly, but to potentially harmful bacteria (depending on where people's hands have been).
- ★ And third, they are almost always in clear plastic bins under direct, bright florescent lighting.
- ★ All of these potential factors have a direct effect on the integrity of the fatty acids within each nut or seed, which then has a direct effect on our health.

I suggest purchasing nuts and seeds in pre-packaging whenever possible. Once you get them home, it would then be best to transfer them into air-tight glass jars before storing in the pantry, fridge or freezer.

I prefer to see certain nuts and seeds with the highest amount of delicate fatty acids stored in the fridge at all times (never in the pantry). These include the following: hemp seeds, walnuts, pecans, pine nuts, sunflower seeds and most store-bought macadamia nuts. I've actually been told to store pecans in the freezer. Therefore, if you're planning to buy more than a pound, yet don't see yourself using them up within six weeks, it may be a good idea to leave a small portion in the fridge and store the rest in the freezer. Personally, I purchase only the highest quality, 100% organic nuts and seeds – most of which have been low-temperature hulled, dried or dehydrated in order to keep their nutritional integrity. For instance, I only purchase "truly raw" cashews from Bali, Indonesia and Vietnam. Unlike the organic cashews in stores, which are labeled "raw" but are actually steamed or fried to remove the shell, organic cashews from Bali, Indonesia and Vietnam are hand-cracked (shelled by hand), and never roasted.

The macadamia nuts I buy are quite unique as well. I purchase them directly from a farm in Hawaii, where the nuts are cracked while green and then low-temperature dehydrated at 105°F in order to preserve the integrity of the nut and the health benefits of its oils. I've been informed by the farmer that their low-temp dehydrated macadamia nuts are best stored out of the fridge. This is because moisture from the fridge can reintroduce moisture to the macadamias, causing them to lose some of their crunch. Therefore, if I know I'm going to be using them within three months, I store them in an air-tight glass mason jar in a cool, dry, dark environment rather than in the fridge.

To Soak or Not to Soak, that Is the Question

One of the questions that I get asked a lot is whether you should soak nuts and seeds. The answer is a definite yes, but for some it is much more necessary than for others. Many nuts and seeds contain enzyme inhibitors, such as phytic acid (aka phytates), which can put a strain on your digestive system if you consume too much. By soaking, you are reducing the amount of enzyme inhibitors (such as phytic acid, oxalic acid and tannins), making them more digestible. This process may take a little extra work, but the benefits can be well worth the wait. Soaking is known to enhance the absorption of calcium, magnesium, iron, copper and zinc, along with more protein and less of the fat found in nuts.

The Science Behind the Soak

Nature has set up a defense mechanism so that nuts and seeds are able to survive insects, microbes, animals and other predators until an environment that is suitable for growing presents itself. One of nature's defense mechanisms includes enzyme inhibitors, which can be naturally removed when there is enough moisture. In nature when it rains, the nut or seed gets wet and can then germinate to produce a new plant. By soaking nuts and seeds in our home, we are actually mimicking what happens in nature. The raw nut or seed recognizes that it is in a suitable, moisture-rich environment, causing it to "wake-up" out of its dormant state. This causes the inhibitors to "shut off" so the enzymes can become activated.

One good rule of thumb I like to follow: is if a nut or seed has a brown coating or skin (tannins) and a slightly bitter taste, it will benefit from soaking. Good examples are almonds, pecans, walnuts, pumpkin seeds and sesame seeds. Soaking also makes them easier to process in your blender or food processor, which is important for specific recipes.

> **Quick Tip:** If not planning to soak nuts or seeds, I suggest giving them a quick squirt of 3% food grade hydrogen peroxide and then giving them a quick rinse. At the very least, give them a quick rinse off in a strainer. This will help remove any surface debris before you consume or make something with them.

General Soaking Schedule for Nuts & Seeds

Nuts that should ideally always be soaked are almonds, pecans and walnuts.

Seeds that should ideally always be soaked are pumpkin, sesame and sunflower.

Some nuts and seeds are not known to have enzyme inhibitors (or at least not enough to pose any real problems); therefore, they don't necessarily need to be soaked (unless you are looking to soften them for a creamier texture in certain recipes such as nut/seed cheeses, dressings and ice cream). As a general rule, the following do not need to be soaked: Brazil nuts, hazelnuts, macadamia nuts, pine nuts, pistachios, chia seeds and hemp seeds.

> **Quick Tip:** If you know you are going to be consuming nuts and seeds that have not been soaked, you can always pop a quality digestive enzyme and extra protease (to maximize protein break down) right before you eat. Personally, I like the quality of Premier Research Labs and always take at least one each of Premier Digest and Premier Protease anytime I'm about to consume a heavy nut/seed dish or dessert. This will relieve some digestive stress (along with some mental stress) and allow you to enjoy your food. Remember, eating this way should be less stressful, and not everyone can always prepare for each and every meal or snack. Just do your best.

If you choose to soak your nuts and seeds, please follow the general soaking schedule below. As a reminder, soaking stimulates the process of germination, which is thought to increase the nutrient content and availability. It helps neutralize the phytic acid present in some nuts and seeds and in the bran of many grains, thereby helping to increase the absorption of minerals. Furthermore, other enzyme inhibitors are neutralized, making the process of digestion gentler.

Almonds	8-12 hrs	**Flax Seeds**	8 hrs
Pumpkin Seeds	8 hrs	**Jungle Peanuts**	6-8 hrs
Sesame Seeds	8 hrs	**Pecans**	4-6 hrs

Walnuts	4 hrs	**Cashews**	1-2 hrs
Sunflower Seeds	2 hrs		

Soaking Instructions:

1. Soak nuts or seeds in a glass jar or bowl covered with a dish towel, cheesecloth or sprouting type screen.

> **Quick Tip:** A sprouting screen is great, because it fits perfectly inside the screw covers that accompany most wide mouth canning jars (with the exception of the really small ones). Mason makes a set of three plastic covers with different sized holes (small, medium and large) which also fit their wide mouth jars.

2. Cover nuts or seeds in a bath of room-temperature, filtered water and stir in up to one teaspoon of sea salt.
3. Soak overnight (or for the recommended amount of time for shorter soaks).
4. Rinse and drain thoroughly when maximum soak time is reached.

> **Quick Tip:** For bigger nuts, such as almonds, walnuts and pecans, I like to use a salad spinner to remove the excess water

5. Transfer them to an air-tight glass container and store them in the fridge. They should keep for up to 5-7 days.

Please Note: When soaking nuts and seeds, they can easily absorb chemicals from the water or container that they've been soaking in, which may be even more of a concern than the phytic acid and protease inhibitors that you're going out of your way to avoid. Therefore, I highly recommend always using a glass container (not plastic) and purified, filtered water. I also recommend slightly acidic water that is room-temperature to slightly warm. According to much research, phytase enzymes tend to function optimally at a slightly acidic pH and at warmer temperatures. In order to make certain that I'm not losing minerals to the soak water, I choose a highly mineralized Himalayan rock salt or sea salt, which is believed to help activate enzymes that de-activate enzyme inhibitors. To make sure the pH is acidic enough, especially if you use alkaline water, you may add (or substitute with) a small splash of lemon juice, raw apple cider vinegar or coconut vinegar. Otherwise, the Himalayan rock salt or sea salt should be all you need to keep the pH low enough, and to help keep the water from wanting to leach minerals from the nuts or seeds.

The Next Three Steps Are Optional

1. If you have a dehydrator, you can dehydrate your nuts and seeds at 105°F for 24 hrs. You will find that smaller seeds are usually done in less time and that almonds sometimes need a few more hours; therefore, feel free to sample a few along the way while rotating and turning the trays a couple of times.

2. When they are completely dry, turn dehydrator off and let them cool off a bit (30-60 minutes or so).
3. Transfer them to air-tight glass containers and store in a cool, dark place.

> **Quick Tip:** I suggest purchasing glass canning jars in several different sizes. They are great, versatile and inexpensive. I highly recommend using "wide mouth" mason jars for storage. They are much easier to fill, scoop, scrap stuff out of and clean.

MUST HAVE CONDIMENTS

The following includes kitchen ingredient "must haves" for adding that SALTY FLAVOR to dishes.

Sea Salt, the New Table Salt

If you have not done so already, please throw away your old table salt. Table salt is highly refined, and what is left after this refining process is almost pure sodium chloride. Due to the high heating process, all the beneficial minerals are stripped away – just leaving very high levels of sodium. Excess sodium intake can cause water retention, high blood pressure, an irregular heartbeat, and can be the underlying cause of some life-threatening health issues such as myocardial infarctions and strokes.

The benefits of switching to a quality sea salt are not just in the taste but in the role it plays in the quality of your nutrition.

- ★ The first benefit of sea salt is that it actually contains less sodium overall. In quality sea salt, the minimal processing leaves a lot of natural trace minerals intact. This in turn reduces the actual sodium content.
- ★ Sea salt contains the necessary minerals of magnesium, calcium and potassium, to name a few.

Choosing a High-Quality Sea Salt

Not all culinary sea salt or rock salt is created equal, so I'm glad to help make this choice simple. My top two choices of all the salts on the market are Premier Pink Salt by Premier Research Labs (which is a combination of two premium, untreated, unheated, solar-dried sea salts: Mediterranean sea salt and pink Alaea Hawaiian sea salt) and raw Himalayan stone-ground crystal salt. I use either one of these two salts in all my recipes, and to add natural electrolytes to my drinking water (especially home distilled water from which everything has been removed). I feel these two quality salts are the purest of all available salts on the market.

> High-quality sea salt or Himalayan rock salt contains a whopping total of 84 major and trace minerals which are good for our health. It helps to regulate the electrolyte balance of cells, prevent muscle spasms and much more!

Please Note: One concern we should have, regardless of which type of salt we prefer to use, is keeping our overall sodium consumption to a minimum. Although there are nutritional benefits to choosing a good sea salt over a table salt, sodium is still sodium.

Sea Veggies

Sea vegetables are nutrient-rich treasure chests filled with vitamins and major and trace minerals –unlike the majority of current land grown vegetables. These superstars of the sea are high in vitamins A, B-complex, C, D, E and K; they're abundantly rich in minerals such as calcium, magnesium, iron, potassium, iodine, manganese and chromium; and they provide great dietary fiber, enzymes and high-quality protein.

Sadly, due to a number of modern soil techniques, our crop land is depleted of many necessary minerals for performing and maintaining our bodily processes. Minerals are vital to the ongoing health of our blood, muscle tissue and nerve cells. They build strong bones and teeth and are needed for turning the food we eat into usable energy. Sea vegetables are extremely abundant in substances our soil now lacks. They are also extremely easy to add to dishes with the use of whole leaf, flake, powdered or encapsulated extract forms.

Aside from being so full of vitamins and minerals, sea vegetables are very alkalizing to the body, and can help bring balance to an overly acidic system. Dis-ease (aka disease) – from the common cold to cancer – thrives in an acid environment. Therefore, we should consume as many alkaline foods as possible.

Sea vegetables are well documented and widely known across the globe as being highly effective in the treatment of heavy metal and radiation poisoning. Did you know that an important function of sea vegetables, in helping our bodies fight radiation poisoning, actually takes place in the thyroid gland? If our thyroid is saturated with organic forms of iodine, it cannot absorb radioactive contaminants. Sea vegetables are an excellent food source of naturally-occurring iodine, with kelp being the most significant source.

How to Store & Eat Sea Veggies

There are many different varieties of sea vegetables, each with their own different flavors, preparation styles and nutritional benefits. Below are some of the most popular of the bunch. You can choose to use whole leaf varieties (either whole or chopped in soups or on salads) or sprinkle flake or powder varieties as a nutritious salt alternative. However you choose to include them in your diet, I recommend purchasing organic and sun-dried sea vegetables to ensure their living nutrient nature. Most of these can be found in your local health food store (Maine Coast Sea Vegetables and Emerald Cove are two widely accessible brands). You will want to store them in an air-tight container in a cool, dark place away from heat, light and moisture.

Nori: You've probably eaten this one before. Although it was most likely the toasted, sheet variety – as they are popular in the traditional making of sushi rolls. Again, I suggest purchasing the organic and sun-dried variety of nori sheets (dark purple-black color). Toasted nori sheets (dark green) often have soy sauce, sugar and salt added.

Dulse: This one is delicious even right out of the bag. It is a great option for a seaweed newbie. Dulse has a soft, chewy texture and a reddish-brown color. On just about any food, dulse makes a great snack in its whole leaf form and a great salt replacement in its flake form.

Kelp: Light brown to dark green in color, kelp is available in flakes or powder form, as well as whole leaf. Kelp is a bit stronger in taste, the highest in iodine of all the sea vegetables (specifically brown kelp), and probably the most beneficial to our overall health. One exciting way to add kelp without the fishy taste is to check out an awesome product by Sea Tangle Kelp Noodle Company. It makes the best spaghetti alternative! This product is virtually tasteless and will take on the full flavors of whatever sauce or dressing you choose to marinate it in. Some questions people ask are: "why is it clear in color?" and "how does it have such a mild taste?" The answer I received when I asked this myself was: because it is actually taken from the inner part of a particular variety of kelp. A perfect analogy I can give is when you fillet an aloe leaf: the tough outer skin is green, but the inner part you scrap out is clear. Using the inner rather than the outer portion of this seaweed is also the reason for its mild flavor.

Kombu: Very dark in color and generally sold in strips or sheets. Often used as a flavoring or base for soups.

Wakame: Emerald green in color and very similar to kombu. Most commonly used to make seaweed salads and as a flavoring or base for tasty miso soup.

Arame: This is a deeply colored and lacy, wiry sea vegetable. As with dulse, arame is sweeter and milder in taste than many other sea vegetables, making it another great choice for a seaweed newbie. It is delicious in miso soup or marinated and tossed in a salad.

> **Quick Tip:** Flakes and powders can be sprinkled on food or eaten raw as is, whereas some of the thicker or tougher whole leaf varieties – such as kelp, kombu and wakame – may need to be soaked for 10-15 minutes to rehydrate and soften them. Check the bag for instructions. If you wish, you can always use the soak water as a base for dressing or a soup, allowing for some of the minerals and natural salty flavor that washed out during the soaking process to be incorporated.

Miso

Miso is a soft fermented paste whose salty taste, buttery texture and unique nutritional profile make it a versatile condiment for many recipes. Traditional miso is made from cultured (fermented) soybeans, but there are many other varieties on the market that feature adzuki beans, chickpeas, barley and others. My personal favorite is an organic chickpea miso made by Organic Miso Master. It is a versatile light miso made with sumptuous chickpeas instead of soybeans. I find it imparts a wonderful sweet/salty flavor and makes a great base and flavor enhancer for many raw soups, dressings, sauces, dips and marinades.

Beware, some miso pastes are pasteurized while others are not. When purchasing a miso, I highly suggest avoiding the pasteurized version and spending your money on organic, unpasteurized miso. By consuming the unpasteurized, truly live, enzyme-rich version, you will reap much more of the health benefits of the culturing process that miso undergoes.

Some scientifically researched benefits of this live food which you may not have been aware of are:

- ★ Miso helps to stimulate the secretion of digestive juices in the stomach.
- ★ Miso is rich in enzymes that assist in the digestion and assimilation of other foods.
- ★ Miso is loaded with beneficial microorganisms that can restore and strengthen the "good" intestinal bacteria (flora) in your gut.
- ★ Miso strengthens the immune system.
- ★ Miso contains many essential amino acids (a live source of plant-based protein).
- ★ Miso is a great plant-based, live source of B vitamins.
- ★ Miso helps to lower LDL ("bad" cholesterol).

Olives

Naturally ripened, raw, sun-dried olives, grown organically, are unlike any other olives you have ever tasted. If you are like me and have only experienced chemically treated and canned olives growing up, you must splurge, as you are in for a real treat! With all their natural oil goodness, meaty texture and salty flavor, raw olives bring a savory depth that compliments many raw food creations. I'm absolutely in love with raw, sun-dried and organic Peruvian "botija" olives (sometimes called "botilla"). If I allowed myself, I could easily go through an entire jar in less than a week. All the natural oils within the olives are untouched, making them rich, plump, juicy and the most superb addition to salads and raw dressings. They are ideal for making a raw olive tapenade. Although I'm infatuated with all raw, sun-dried olive varieties, I must admit, I'm a tad bit partial to the premium olives grown on the coastal desert plains of southern Peru. Part of the reason may be that they are ecologically cultivated, hand-picked and packed with extraordinarily conscientious care.

> Ripe olives and oils made from ripe olives are excellent sources of beautifying oleic acid, as stated in one of my favorite books, *Eating for Beauty* by David Wolfe.

Did You Know…?

Olives have the greatest mucus-dissolving capacity of any food and are also considered a fruit! Furthermore, for their little size, they pack a big mineral punch. For instance, when olives are allowed to ripen naturally and are eaten raw, they provide a natural form of organic calcium that our body can actually recognize and utilize. But, wait! There's more! Ripe, raw, sun-dried olives contain a great amount of natural fiber; high natural amounts of the antioxidant vitamin E (a fat-soluble antioxidant that neutralizes damaging free radicals);

polyphenols and flavonoids (which have anti-inflammatory properties); and large amounts of health-giving monounsaturated fats (found to reduce the risk of atherosclerosis and increase HDL, the "good" cholesterol).

Coconut Amino, a Natural Soy-Free Sauce

A big thank you to Coconut Secret, a company which produces a delicious, soy-free sauce called Coconut Aminos. It contains a whopping 17 amino acids, has a low glycemic index, contains naturally-occurring minerals, broad-spectrum B vitamins, vitamin C and has a nearly neutral pH. I am truly amazed at its resemblance to soy sauce. It is dark in color, and rich and salty in flavor. And I've saved the best part for last – it's made from only raw coconut tree sap and sun-dried sea salt, which has been naturally aged, of course.

It is wonderful when you want to ramp up a salad dressing, a marinade or a simple dipping sauce for your raw nori rolls!

Please Note: Many raw food recipes call for a product called Nama Shoyu, but please beware – Nama Shoyu contains gluten due to the addition of westernized wheat. Individuals with wheat allergies, gluten intolerance or diagnosed with celiac disease (which cumulatively, is a big percentage of the population) cannot consume it. In addition, the products Nama Shoyu and Bragg Liquid Aminos contain naturally-occurring MSG in the form of glutamic acid; so, if you are sensitive to MSG, you will want to avoid these types of soybean products.

Nutritional Yeast

With its savory and slightly salty flavor profile, nutritional yeast is a good substitute for Parmesan cheese. One of the flavors I truly miss is anything cheesy. Nutritional yeast has been the answer to my longings. Nutritional yeast may not be a raw food, but its profile makes it one of the oldest, most valuable, well-known superfoods used by vegetarians, vegans and raw foodies alike. I sprinkle it on salads, zucchini and kelp noodles and into soups. You name it!

Nutritional yeast is an amazing source of multiple nutrients packed into one food!

- ★ Rich in Bio-available Protein (high in amino acids lysine and tryptophan)
- ★ Rich in BCAAs (branched chain amino acids)
- ★ Rich in B Vitamins (a reliable, non-animal source of broad-spectrum Bs)
- ★ Rich in Glutathione (helps boost liver and immune system function)
- ★ Prebiotic (helps support healthy colon flora)
- ★ Rich in Beta 1, 3-Glucans (acts as a free radical scavenger and macrophage stimulator)
- ★ Rich in Trace Minerals (such as selenium, chromium, manganese, copper, vanadium, molybdenum and lithium)
- ★ Very Low in Sodium

What About Candida?

I get asked this all the time and for good reason; there are a lot of misconceptions and misunderstandings regarding the issue of consuming yeast products. Quality sourced nutritional yeast is "primary" grown food yeast containing only a pure yeast strain called *Saccharomyces cerevisia*. It is not pathogenic yeast and does not cause Candida or other yeast infections.

Please Note: Brewer's yeast is not "primary" grown yeast, but instead, a by-product of the beer-brewing industry which does not contain the robust properties of primary grown yeast. In addition, it may contain impure yeast strains encountered during the brewing process. Brewer's yeast may be considered a raw food, but I would avoid this product due to its questionable, inferior quality.

Due to the high level of nutritional ethics and integrity behind Premier Research Labs, I only use Premier Nutritional Flakes. It is truly the finest source of nutritional yeast – specially grown on mineral rich molasses (not petrochemical sludge or refined sugar). The processing method used by Premier Research Labs makes for a superior end product, preventing any intestinal concerns, such as gas and bloating, and – as mention above – will not aggravate Candida related conditions.

SWEET FLAVOR FOR YOUR CREATIONS, BEING SWEET SAVVY WITH NATURE'S BEST

Organic, perfectly ripened fruit is one of Mother Nature's sweetest gifts to us. Fruits are generally high in fiber, water, vitamin C and phytochemicals, and – of course – sugars in their most natural form. Some vegetables and vegetable type fruits also give us sweetness when that balance of flavors is needed. These include: beets, bell peppers (red, orange and yellow), carrots, peas (English, snow and sugar snap) and tomatoes. Let's also remember some of the spices that impart subtle sweetness, such as cinnamon, nutmeg and vanilla bean.

Green Leaf Stevia

Stevia is a South American perennial shrub (*Stevia rebandiana*), a member of the chrysanthemum family (a white-flowered herb) indigenous to Paraguay.

The leaves of stevia contain glycosides which taste very sweet to the tongue, and do not contain sugar, calories or carbohydrates. Therefore, despite its sweetness, stevia does not have a GI (meaning, it's zero on the glycemic index), nor does it affect the body's insulin levels. Stevia has also been shown to assist the pancreas and improve digestion. Excellent for those with diabetes, Candida, seeking weight control, or for those simply wanting to avoid cavities, the stevia herb can be an ideal natural sweetener. Stevia leaves are one of the sweetest substances known in nature, with a sweetness rating of up to 300 times the sweetening power of sugar. A pinch or dash may be all you need.

> **Quick Tip:** When you want to cut down on the GI or sugar content of a sweetener you prefer, you can always use half the called for amount, and then add a small amount at a time of stevia until you've reach the sweetness level you desire. There are many times I will use half the called for amount of raw agave nectar, raw honey or sun-dried cane juice crystals, and then add a small amount of green leaf stevia to cut down on the sugar content, but not the sweet taste.

Please Note: There are many different clear liquids and white crystalline dried powdered extracts of stevia on the market; but I highly suggest purchasing the green leaf stevia (whole leaf or powered leaf) instead. This will ensure you receive not just sweetness, but all the extraordinary health benefits that only the whole green leaf of stevia can provide.

Xylitol

If you are unable to acquire a taste for stevia but want to find a quality low GI sugar, then I suggest giving xylitol a try. Xylitol has the low glycemic index of seven, compared to refined sugar which has a rating of approximately 60.

> **Quick Tip:** Xylitol is a recommended sugar substitute for those on a Candida free diet or for those with a serious health condition, such as cancer or diabetes. Unlike other sugar substitutes, xylitol has no aftertaste at all. You can use it just like sugar and in equal quantities.

Please Note: Xylitol is a natural substance derived from the xylan of birch and other hardwood trees, berries, almond hulls and corn cobs. I recommend purchasing Smart Sweet Xylitol. This brand is a quality product produced in the United States of America from organic hardwood trees – not corn! Therefore, it is guaranteed to be free of any genetically modified organisms (GMOs). Smart Sweet Xylitol is produced in a state-of-the-art facility under strict good manufacturing practice (GMP) guidelines, resulting in the best and purest product available anywhere on the market.

If you experience a laxative effect from xylitol, Smart Sweet produces another 100% pure alternative sweetener called erythritol. Erythritol is also safe for diabetics, but has a high digestive tolerance. Like xylitol, erythritol will not cause tooth decay or encourage the growth of yeast in the body.

Agave

It is a common misconception that the agave plant is a cactus. The truth is: agave is a succulent, closely related to the lily and amaryllis families.

A number of health-conscious people consider agave nectar to be one of the overall best natural sweeteners on the market today, but buyers beware – not all agave nectar is created equal.

Please Note: The focus of the following information is not on the completely fraudulent products out there which have either been cooked, highly processed or had high-fructose corn syrup (HFCS) added to them. Rather, the focus of my information is on the highest quality agave nectar – carefully and skillfully collected from the sweet juice of the Blue Agave Tequilana Weber variety only. Due to my own diligent review of laboratory data and personal research, I not only believe in exposing the facts and placing blame where blame is due, but in praising and supporting the companies who work hard at proving their quality and integrity time and time again by consistently providing consumers with only the best.

Naturally-Occurring Fructose vs High Fructose Corn Syrup (HFCS)

★ Fructose is a natural sugar found in many foods, especially fruit. It was formerly known as levulose.
★ Eating fresh, raw plant-based foods, like whole fruits, or even small amounts of carefully low-temperature processed foods (i.e., raw honey, raw agave and whole ground mesquite pod powder with their naturally-occurring fructose as well as viable fiber, enzymes and nutrients left intact), is not the same as eating the highly manipulated (man-made) fructose in commercially prepared, refined and processed foods.
★ High fructose corn syrup (HFCS) is produced by processing corn starch in such a way that its sugars are changed from glucose to fructose.
★ HFCS is a very popular man-made sugar found in a vast number of commercially prepared and processed products and under a variety of aliases (such as chicory, corn sugar, inulin isoglucose, glucose-fructose syrup and fruit fructose).
★ Man-made fructose comes without the enzymes, fiber and other natural attributes seen in nature.
★ Alone, naturally-occurring fructose causes a much lower rise in blood sugar levels than does sucrose or glucose.
★ Naturally-occurring fructose is broken down more slowly by an enzyme in the bowel, and does not require insulin. On the other hand, dietary sources of glucose are digested, absorbed and transported to the liver, then released into the general blood stream. Many tissues take glucose from the blood to use for energy, and this process requires insulin.
★ Man-made fructose acts more like a fat in the body, and is stored in the same manner.

> **WHAT IS THE GLYCEMIC INDEX?**
>
> The glycemic index (GI) or glucose index of a food is simply how quickly the body absorbs the sugars found in food. Individuals with diabetes and heart disease should focus on low GI foods (55 or less). Moderate GI foods earn a 56-69 rating, while high GI foods will be a 70 or above.
>
> While many different types of foods contain sugars, in some cases the sugars are very slow to be absorbed (most low GI foods). In fact, your body may not even absorb the sugars before they pass through your system (particularly whole foods and high fiber foods). However, in other cases, the sugars are absorbed by your body with amazing speed, and are stored away in the fat cells for later use (high GI foods, refined sugars and processed foods).

It has been reported that the glycemic index of quality processed agave is approximately 11, making this type of agave a low GI food. If you choose agave as your low glycemic sweetener, I highly suggest you purchase and support only 100% certified organic clear agave nectar of the type Ultimate Superfoods distributes. The chemical composition of their "Real" Raw Agave Nectar is far superior in quality when compared to the competition – especially in light of the lack of legal norms and quality control standards in the agave industry as a whole.

Ultimate Superfoods agave nectar production involves removing the leaves from the agave plant, crushing and milling the plant core called the "pina," capturing the precious fluid and then putting it through a proprietary natural process to deactivate specific enzymes in order to keep it from fermenting. The result is "Real" Raw Agave Nectar – the purest on the market.

> *This is the only agave I will use in recipes, the only agave I support, and yes, the only agave I will ever consume myself!*

A quality, processed agave can be a wonderfully pure and natural low glycemic sweetener. It can easily be added to teas, smoothies, desserts and more; but please look for all the qualities I list below before you buy. Only support companies that truly take pride in the health of the consumer, their families and our environment.

- 100% Organic Blue Agave Tequilana Weber variety only (this particular plant has the highest concentrations of minerals as well as a high content of inulin).
- High concentrations of viable minerals.
- High content of natural inulin (a prebiotic fiber that promotes healthy intestinal flora and the absorption of minerals, particularly calcium).
- Never cooked (retaining its natural consistency based on high velocity centrifugal straining of juices – thus keeping the product in a true raw food category).
- Clear in color. Not the golden/amber or dark varieties (which makes me suspect that they have been cooked, changing the molecular structure of their sugars – basically caramelizing them – making them no better than refined and processed sugar in how your body responds to them).
- Thinner than honey in consistency.
- Enzymes or acids never added.
- Temperature always maintained at a low rate (assuring much of the beneficial enzymes, inulin fiber and other natural attributes are still present).
- Certified 100% Organic (free of any chemicals and other toxic substances).

> **Quick Tip:** Please keep in mind, a little agave goes a long way. You can use about 25% less of this raw agave nectar than you would other sweeteners.

What Are Inulins?

I'll break it down: inulins are a group of naturally-occurring polysaccharides produced by many types of plants, which belong to a class of fibers known as fructans. Fructans are polymers of fructose molecules. Although they are not the same, inulins are closely related to fructo-oligosaccharides (FOS), and the terms are sometimes used interchangeably.

Inulins have been a healthful part of our diet for thousands of years and occur naturally in over 36,000 plants, some of which include agave, artichokes, asparagus, chicory, dandelion, green beans, garlic, onions and yacon.

Inulins have some truly unique health properties. In terms of nutrition, inulins are considered a form of soluble fiber and are sometimes categorized as a prebiotic. Because inulin is not digested in the upper gastrointestinal tract, it is allowed to reach the large intestine intact where it is fermented by your intestinal flora.

Acting as a soluble fiber, inulin provides the type of bulk that studies have shown can increase the absorption of several major minerals in the small intestine (calcium, magnesium and in some cases phosphorus), as well as trace minerals (mainly copper, iron and zinc).

Due to the body's inability to digest inulin, it has virtually no impact on blood sugar and will not trigger insulin secretion or raise triglycerides. This makes eating foods with naturally-occurring inulin potentially helpful in managing blood sugar-related illnesses such as diabetes.

Please Note: Only consume foods that contain natural inulin or FOS. Do your body good by not resorting to refined, overly processed or super concentrated forms of any food, herb or man-made substance. This single resolution may just be what makes the difference between damaging your health or building and maintaining it.

PREBIOTIC VS PROBIOTIC

Carbohydrates, such as inulin, are considered prebiotics. A prebiotic is a non-digestible carbohydrate that stimulates the growth of probiotics, otherwise known as the beneficial intestinal bacteria naturally residing in the colon. Probiotic bacteria, specifically bifidobacteria and lactobacilli, promote a healthy colon by inhibiting the growth of harmful pathogens. In turn, the potential for toxins, infections and carcinogens is reduced; the synthesis of B vitamins (including the elusive B12) is increased; and the overall health of the immune system is greatly supported.

Coconut Nectar & Crystals

Another two great products from the Coconut Secret line are Raw Coconut Nectar and Raw Coconut Sap Crystals. They are stated to be 100% pure, low glycemic, enzymatically alive and raw (meaning, low-temperature evaporated at approximately 105°F to remove excess moisture).

Please Note: There are many other coconut palm sugars in granulated form on the market that cannot be considered a truly raw product due to the boiling process used to go from liquid sap to granule state.

When the coconut tree is tapped, it produces a nutrient-rich sap which is exuded from the coconut blossoms of the tree. This sap is very low glycemic (GI of only 35), considered diabetic friendly, and is an abundant source of minerals, 17 amino acids, vitamin C and broad-spectrum B vitamins when carefully processed.

It is also stated that coconut nectar and crystals break down much less rapidly than traditional cane sugar (refined white or brown sugar); therefore, they do not enter the blood stream as fast.

What about the taste? Surprisingly, coconut crystals do not taste like coconut. They taste more like light brown sugar or Sugar In The Raw (which is not truly raw by any means, considering they use a slow boiling process). Coconut crystals can be used in a 1:1 ratio to replace regular cane sugar in any recipe. Coconut nectar, on the other hand, can be used in a 1:1 ratio to replace liquid sweeteners such as honey or agave.

Sun-Dried Cane Juice Crystals

Sun-dried cane juice crystals are considered a healthy alternative to refined sugar. While both types of sweeteners may be made from sugar cane, sun-dried cane juice doesn't undergo the same degree of processing that both refined white sugar and brown sugar go through – not by a long shot! Unlike all the varieties of refined sugar on the market – which are guaranteed to be devoid of nutrients – sun-dried cane juice is nutrient-rich and contains the following minerals: phosphorus, calcium, iron, magnesium and potassium.

I highly advise purchasing only sun-dried cane juice crystals made from 100% certified organic sugar cane. I also suggest that you research your source and only consume cane sugar products that come from the most pristine areas on the planet. For instance, when I want to indulge, I only go for a very particular sugar cane product sourced from Ecuador and put out by New Horizons Health. It is naturally grown in highly mineralized volcanic soil. In addition, I absolutely love that this product is fresh pressed, sun dried and then put through a natural cooling process to crystallize.

Please Note: People who have tried and tested this particular 100% organic, sun-dried cane juice product (in moderation of course) have reported no negative side effects or dangerous medical reactions – even when taken on an empty stomach. So as long as you are not suffering from a blood sugar disorder (like diabetes), or a critical health condition (such as cancer or Candida), then you don't have to deny your desire for something satisfyingly sweet. As long as you use it sparingly, sun-dried cane juice is a natural source of sweetness which can be part of a healthy and balanced diet.

> **Quick Tip:** This product is amazing for making your very own raw chocolate creations. Personally, I prefer sun-dried cane juice crystals over all other sweeteners when it comes to making chocolates and many other sweet treats. It will give your chocolate that perfect snap and desired sheen, as well as a velvety textured mouth feel. Pure ecstasy – Oh Yum!

Raw Honey

Honey is composed of simple sugars (glucose and fructose) that are used quickly by the body. It is considered an excellent substitute for sugar and was actually man's first and most reliable source of sweetener. It has been hypothesized that different floral varieties can impact the GI of honey due to differences in the simple sugar concentrations (particularly the fructose to glucose ratio). According to some internet gathered information on the GI of honey from different floral varieties and origins, it appears honey can range anywhere from 35-87 on the GI. However, the many health benefits of honey – completely unrelated to its carbohydrate/sugar content such as amino acid profile, broad-spectrum B vitamins and array of minerals – make it more of a moderate GI food in the way your body processes it.

A bee's precious nectar, known as honey, is created by the combination of nectar from flowers, enzymes in the bee's saliva and propolis (a tree resin used to seal and protect bee hives from outside contaminants). Hippocrates, the father of medicine himself, always emphasized the nutritional and medicinal values of honey. On the nutritional side of the coin, honey contains the minerals calcium, magnesium, potassium, sodium chloride, sulfur, iron and a small quantity of copper, iodine and zinc. Then we have the amazing medicinal side of the coin: honey's unique antioxidant and microbial properties.

David Wolfe, author of *Superfoods: The Food and Medicine of the Future*, suggests the use of raw, natural bee products of all types for longevity. We need to protect the health and vitality of our precious bees – as bees are vital to the health of our crops. This can be easily done by supporting only organic beekeepers who treat their bees and hives with the utmost respect and care.

Here are just some of the miraculous healing powers of raw honey:

- ★ Provides enzymes and an array of vitamins and minerals.
- ★ Increases calcium absorption.
- ★ Can increase hemoglobin count and treat or prevent anemia caused by certain nutritional factors.
- ★ When combined with raw apple cider vinegar, can help ease the discomfort of arthritic joints.
- ★ Fights colds and respiratory infections of all kinds.
- ★ When used externally, speeds the healing process of skin burns and wounds.
- ★ Can help boost the healing of gastrointestinal ulcers.
- ★ Helps constipation by working as a natural and gentle laxative.
- ★ Supplies instant energy without the insulin surge caused by refined/processed cane sugar.

Please Note: When I speak of honey, I'm not talking about the honey in your plastic honey bear container purchased from your average supermarket. I'm talking about the pure, unadulterated, unpasteurized, pesticide free honey which has not been dangerously heated in order to be removed from the hive. Only raw honey can provide all the healing properties and medicinal power for which it is prized.

In addition, when it comes to moderate to high GI foods of any kind, I highly advise everyone to consume in moderation. Please exercise caution if you are diabetic, dealing with a Candida issues or have been diagnosed with cancer.

Lucuma

Lucuma is a sub-tropical, South American fruit native to Peru, Chile and Ecuador that has been gaining popularity as a healthy, whole fruit sweetener. In fact, it was once referred to as the Gold of the Incas. The lucuma tree is an evergreen that has been cultivated since ancient times.

Although I have never tasted fresh lucuma fruit, I understand it has a similar appearance to a mango, with beautiful golden, orange/yellow colored flesh on the inside. As for the taste, some claim it tastes like caramel custard while others say it tastes a bit like pumpkin. Unlike most fruits, its texture is described as being quite dry and starchy, with a paste-like consistency that melts in your mouth.

> *Did you know if you were to visit Peru, you would most likely find that lucuma flavored ice cream is more popular than vanilla or chocolate?*

In the United States, lucuma can be found and enjoyed in a raw, low-temperature dehydrated form (which I am so grateful we get to experience). The lucuma whole fruit powder can be used as a natural and nutritious low-glycemic sweetener. It has been noted to be about 25 on the GI, making it great for diabetics or anyone who desires a full-bodied, yet subtle sweet taste without the worry of empty calories. Lucuma is absolutely delicious when added to nut mylks, smoothies, chocolates and other raw desserts (e.g., lucuma ice cream or tapioca pudding made with chia seeds). I like to describe the taste as a tropical caramel to somewhat of a maple-like flavor.

Lucuma is an excellent source of carbohydrates, dietary fiber, vitamins and minerals. In addition, it provides remarkable concentrations of beta-carotene (making it a powerful immune system booster), niacin (making it a cholesterol and triglyceride balancer), as well as iron and B vitamins (B1, B2, B3, etc.).

Mesquite

Raw, organic mesquite powder is a nutritious, aromatic condiment ground from the bean pods of the mesquite tree. Traditionally, mesquite pod meal was known to be made into porridge. Due to its sweet molasses-like flavor with a hint of caramel, I love blending it into raw chocolate creations, cookies, crackers, energy bars, granola – you name it! It's also a great addition when making savory soups, sauces and dressings. I also love combining mesquite with maca in my supercharged morning smoothie (see page 189 for more on maca).

Mesquite powder is rich in dietary fiber, amino acids (with lysine being the noteworthy highlight) and minerals such as calcium, magnesium, potassium, iron and zinc. Because the entire mesquite pod is ground, including the protein-rich seed, mesquite powder has been noted to have a considerable amount of protein (11 to 17%).

> **Quick Tip:** With mesquite's high lysine content and nuts being high in the amino acid arginine, adding mesquite powder to your nut dishes and desserts can creates a really nice balance between these two amino acids. Ahh – synergy success!

> *Did you know adding mesquite can support a diabetic diet or help maintain healthy pancreatic insulin secretions in non-diabetics?*

It has been documented that mesquite was a staple food that Native Americans in the Southwest and Mexico relied on for thousands of years. During that time in those particular communities, there was not one reported case of diabetes. It is believed that the elimination of mesquite from their diets is one of the main reasons for the skyrocketing diabetes and obesity rates which now trouble these particular communities.

Mesquite powder has a reported glycemic index of 25 (which is considered low) and a high percentage of dietary fiber (approximately 25%). The substantial amount of dietary fiber found in mesquite pods allows the body to absorb and assimilate the sugars from mesquite powder more slowly.

What's more, mesquite's sugar is in the form of naturally-occurring fructose which is broken down more slowly by an enzyme in the bowel, and does not require insulin. This makes it even easier for the body to maintain constant blood sugar levels for sustained periods of time.

Sour Flavors

The general North American diet tends to have way too many foods with sweet and salty tastes, not enough sour, and definitely not enough bitter, pungent and astringent tastes. In Ayurveda (a system of medicine that originated in India over 5,000 years ago), to restore health and wellness through nutritional balance, it is recommended to include all six tastes at every meal. Below we will get into the "power behind the sour" – so pucker up!

Anatomically speaking, tart and sour flavors are simply acids that are sensed by receptors on the sides of the tongue. In both Ayurvedic Herbal Medicine and Traditional Chinese Medicine (TCM), sour is categorized as one of the six tastes. In Chinese Medicine, the others are sweet, salty, bitter, bland and pungent (aka heating), with pungent actually being _tasted_ in the nose. For instance, chili pepper heat is not a true taste but a sensation caused by capsaicin, a natural compound that is concentrated in the pith of chili peppers. The only difference between the Ayurvedic and Chinese systems is that in Ayurvedic Medicine there is a much stronger interest in the category of astringent foods and herbs (aka cooling, drying and toning), rather than bland-tasting foods and herbs.

Please Note: In much of the literature regarding Chinese Medicine only five basic tastes are identified (sweet, salty, sour, bitter and pungent). The neutral or bland taste is in between these tastes.

In both Ayurvedic and Chinese Medicine, if one is eager to improve and enhance one's quality of life, health, vigor and longevity, then coordinating and balancing all six (or five) tastes must be accomplished daily. (Please refer to **Appendix F** and **Appendix G** for a more detailed look into these ancient philosophies of medicine.)

Fruits with a Kick

Many common fruits, such as lemons, limes, grapefruits, oranges and other citrus, can be utilized in recipes when that tart burst or acidic/sour flavor is desired. Some vegetable fruits, like tomatoes, sun-dried tomatoes and sun-dried olives, have the ability to do the same. Although not considered a common food, a tart and tangy favorite of mine is the glorious golden berry. Golden berries can add that puckery punch with a major burst of nutrients, to boot! Categorized as an adaptogenic food, and enriched with many vitamins and minerals in their natural form, golden berries are easily considered a powerful superfruit (see page 184 for more on golden berries).

> **Quick Tips:** Get the biggest health bang for your buck by choosing foods that give you only the very best from all possible nutritional worlds! For instance, instead of thinking you must cook your tomatoes in order to obtain the highest amount of lycopene – why not eat them in their sun-dried form? Sun-dried tomatoes can give you lycopene – a cancer-preventing antioxidant – without destroying many other vital nutrients through the addition of high heat. There is no need to cook out so many of the essential vitamins, minerals and other nutrients (especially water-soluble ones like vitamin C) just for the sake of one. Thanks to the sun-drying process, and even the process of low-temperature dehydrating, we can preserve the integrity of certain nutrients that are better obtained raw, while gaining access to others that are more accessible when cooked.
>
> Rather than resorting to pasteurized fruit juices, such as store-bought orange juice, get into the habit of juicing them fresh. The heat from pasteurizing can destroy almost every vital nutrient. Better still – why not eat oranges whole for all the wholesome goodness they provide? Taking in just the juice – without the natural fiber and some of the pith – creates a very unnecessary blood sugar spike. This is due to the high amount of concentrated sugar hitting the bloodstream all at once. Besides, oranges give us more than just an abundance of natural vitamin C. Did you know their pith contains a flavanone called herperidin, which is thought to lower both cholesterol and blood pressure? Try peeling, deseeding and then blending oranges whole in the blender for a new take on pulpy orange juice and drink creations.

Did you know that most citrus fruits, such as lemons and limes, have an acidic pH outside of the body, but when consumed, leave an alkaline residue in the body after being metabolized?

Start Eating for Internal Balance!

Before continuing on my list of favorite condiments for that acid/sour flavor, I feel the need to digress for just a moment. I love that more and more people are becoming aware that they need to alkalize their diet and eat less acid forming foods, but I am concerned about the number of individuals that appear to be very conflicted on how to do this properly. It appears that there is much confusion when it comes to comprehending the difference between acid foods, as we know them in nature, and acid forming foods, once processed by the digestive system. I find it unfortunate that so many are reluctant to include the healing acid fruits and vegetables due to either misinformation or a misunderstanding on how the body translates foods and substances as a whole.

To explain it simply, we must look at body chemistry and focus more on the <u>after</u> effects a particular food has on the body rather than whether the food in question starts off acid or alkaline <u>before</u> we consume it.

- ★ All food is so-called "burned" in the body – leaving a residue of ash as the result of the burning (aka digestion).
- ★ The food ash will be neutral, acid or alkaline, depending largely on the mineral composition of the food.
- ★ For optimum health and maximum resistance to disease, it is vitally important that we consume the proper balance between alkaline and acid forming foods on a daily basis. A good guideline to follow is three parts alkaline forming to one-part acid forming. For instance, citrus fruits and tomatoes are acidic, but they have a net alkaline yield once their constituents get to the kidneys. This is due to fresh fruits and vegetables being rich in potassium salts – a natural buffer. By avoiding these foods, we are depriving ourselves of natural potassium, a mineral that protects against hypertension and stroke.

Finding balance in the areas of diet and lifestyle is critical to our body's overall health and wellness, and the best way to achieve balance is through our food choices. When blood pH drops below the ideal range of approximately 7.35-7.45, health issues can arise. Essentially, the body will do anything it can to raise the pH level, putting unnecessary stress on internal organs and their associated functions. For instance, if the body is too acidic – whether it is from mental anguish or fast food consumption – it will leach alkalizing minerals (such as magnesium and calcium) from your bones and teeth in order to maintain overall homeostasis and a normal blood pH of approximately 7.4.

An internal acidic environment will eventually lead to problems such as inflammation, narrowing of the arteries, calcification and corrosion of bodily tissues. A chronic, long-term acidic pH can further lead to cancer, heart disease, diabetes, etc. Most individuals who suffer pH-related health problems do so because of a pH that is chronically too low due to the standard American diet (cooked animal fats and protein, pasteurized dairy, all non-sprouted grains, refined and processed foods, etc.). Other stressors, such as environmental toxins, emotional stress and lack of restorative sleep, are also to blame, but the biggest culprit is the food we fuel our bodies with on a daily basis.

It is considered ideal to make a minimum of 75-80% of the foods we eat alkaline forming and only 20-25% acid forming (remember the 3:1 ratio). Of the alkaline forming foods, approximately 70% are most effective when eaten raw and alive. It is the viable vitamins, minerals, enzymes, amino acids and other health-promoting cofactors which make up a very important part of the equation. When we alter these live, natural nutrients found in our foods by adding chemicals – or by over processing, refining, heating, boiling, cooking, grilling, burning, pasteurizing, irradiating, microwaving, etc. – we inadvertently "strip the locks" or "break off pieces to the puzzle." This makes it very difficult for our body to "key in" or "piece together" what is necessary to "open the door" or "complete the picture" for total health, wellness and longevity!

In summary, because most organic fruits and vegetables are either alkaline in nature or alkalizing and health promoting within the body, an easy way to accomplish our 3:1 ratio is to make fresh, ripe, organic fruits and vegetables the main part of each meal. This is easily accomplished with different salad creations. (Please refer to **Appendix E** for more details on acid and alkaline foods.)

In his book, *The pH Miracle,* Dr. Robert Young discusses the importance of regulating your body's acid/alkaline chemistry and how it can result in weight loss, increased stamina and strength and a stronger immune system. If you are looking for a deeper understanding, this would be one source I recommend.

Don't Forget to Drink Your Water!

The human body is composed of 75 percent water and 25 percent solid mass. To provide nourishment, eliminate waste and conduct all the trillions of activities in the body, we need to drink more natural sources of water. As they say, "the solution to pollution is dilution;" therefore, a healthy balanced diet also includes drinking lots of pure clean water (local spring water stored in glass being the ultimate best). To find the ideal amount for your weight, multiply your weight by 0.66, and then convert to ounces. For example: 150 pounds x 0.66 = 99. Therefore, 99 ounces of pure water should be drunk daily.

Please Note: I find water another topic of much confusion and controversy. I see so many people buying expensive alkaline water and water systems, which in my opinion will, of course, work for a short period (when you look at where most people are starting from). However, they can wreak havoc, causing some major destruction to the function of certain bodily systems. For instance, drinking alkaline water that is not properly balanced can weaken stomach acid and reduce the absorption of dietary minerals. Therefore, alkaline water should never be consumed with mineral supplements or foods requiring strong acidic breakdown. Alkaline water literally dilutes stomach acids, interfering with the proper digestion and proper absorption and assimilation of nutrients. From my understanding, as long as our drinking water is properly balanced and has the right organic minerals as part of its structure, it is okay for it to be slightly acidic (a pH of approximately 7.0 down to 5.6). In my opinion, it is more important that our drinking water be rich in hydrogen, which not only means better hydration to the cells of our body, but when the active hydrogen in hydrogen rich water binds with active oxygen in the body, we decrease our risk of diseases caused by free radical damage and oxidative stress.

> **Quick Tip:** Just remember what I mentioned above about acidifying and alkalizing foods, which can be a much better, more ideal strategy for truly alkalizing the body with real long-term health-promoting benefits. Just start by eating more whole fruits and vegetables; drinking fresh vegetable drinks (from juicing or blending); eliminating refined sugars and processed foods from the diet; and avoiding coffee and sodas. Sodas are highly acidic and corrosive to the body because they contain phosphoric acid. In my opinion, eliminating soda should be the very first thing you do. Once you accomplish this, follow it up with the rest.

Apple Cider Vinegar

Raw, unfiltered apple cider vinegar (ACV) is a popular condiment in the living and raw food realm. It gives salads a kick, makes a great substitute for lemon juice, gives gusto to home-made dressings, sauces and spreads, and can be used to make a zesty marinade to soften tough vegetables such as cabbage, broccoli and cauliflower.

> **Quick Tip:** Accompany apple cider vinegar (or any other acid for that matter such as lemon, lime, other citrus, etc.) with fats such as avocados, nuts, seeds or olives. When an acid is added to an avocado salad, or a mock nut/seed pâté, it can really help the body break down the fats and digest them better. Before using apple cider vinegar, be sure to shake the bottle gently to thoroughly distribute all of the nutrients. Apple cider vinegar does not need to be refrigerated. Just store in a cool, dark place.

By far, my favorite apple cider vinegar is by Bragg. It is certified organic, unfiltered, unheated, unpasteurized and aged in wood. I love that it contains the amazing Mother of Vinegar which occurs naturally as "strand-like enzymes of connected protein molecules."

Raw apple cider vinegar has been highly regarded for many years as a true miracle health elixir for warding off dangerous and infectious diseases and keeps one's general health fit and strong. It can also be used as a simple antiseptic/disinfectant. The reported cures from using apple cider vinegar go as far back as 3000 BC, the great Hippocrates (aka the father of medicine), Babylonia and 15th century England.

Please Note: Many of the home remedies for common ailments listed below call for a tonic of apple cider vinegar made by mixing two or three teaspoons of ACV in an eight-ounce glass of water and drinking this before or during each meal. Check out *Apple Cider Vinegar: Miracle Health System* by Patricia Bragg and Paul C. Bragg to learn more.

Reported <u>internal</u> benefits of apple cider vinegar:

- ★ Is enzymatically alive
- ★ Is a rich source of the mineral potassium
- ★ Helps with allergies, colds, sinus infections, sore throats and the flu
- ★ Relieves heartburn (acid reflux)
- ★ Promotes digestion

- ★ Helps break down fat, leading to better weight control
- ★ Helps control high cholesterol (especially the "bad" cholesterol known as LDL)
- ★ Helps control high blood pressure
- ★ Supports a healthy immune system
- ★ Helps remove sludgy toxins from the body
- ★ Helps control blood sugar levels
- ★ Helps reduce hot flashes and night sweats
- ★ And much, much, more!

Reported <u>external</u> benefits of apple cider vinegar:

- ★ Helps maintain healthy skin when used as a skin toner
- ★ Soothes irritated skin from a variety of conditions
- ★ Relieves muscle soreness from exercise
- ★ And more!

Coconut Vinegar

Raw, coconut vinegar is similar to other naturally fermented vinegars (such as balsamic and apple cider vinegar). It can also be used in a variety of recipes or as a standalone condiment on salads and veggies in exactly the same way as apple cider vinegar (see above). It contains the natural Mother of Vinegar, which is full of living enzymes, probiotics and other health-promoting cofactors. According to some stated claims, it is believed that coconut vinegar nutritionally exceeds other vinegars in its vitamin, mineral and amino acid content. In addition, it is an excellent source of fructo-oligosaccharides (FOS), a prebiotic that promotes digestive health.

The coconut vinegar brought to us by Coconut Secret is my favorite product in the Coconut Secret line (a close second is the coconut aminos). The product is described as follows: 100% organic, gluten free and low glycemic. Moreover, it is a great source of 17 amino acids, minerals, vitamin C, broad-spectrum B vitamins and has a nearly neutral pH.

Coconut Secret's site says that, "the 'sap' collected from coconut blossoms before they form into mature coconuts is universally revered in tropical cultures as the 'lifeblood' of the coconut tree." It also states that their certified organic coconut vinegar (like all their products) is made from small batches to ensure that the raw vinegar made from this natural sap is a "truly" unheated, enzymatically alive product. I also like that the coconut vinegar is naturally aged and fermented for up to one whole year! Many other coconut vinegars are water-based and undergo an assisted fermentation with fermentation starters.

Please Note: When consumed regularly, organic, "truly raw," un-pasteurized and non-distilled vinegars (like the two described above) can actually balance the body's pH – taking it from acidic to neutral in a short period of time. Normally, it would be hard to believe that such an acidic substance could normalize, or even lower, our pH. However, according to the experience of many proponents and the beliefs of holistic practitioners, our digestive system naturally converts this kind of quality vinegar to an alkaline-based substance.

Sauerkraut & Kimchi

From kimchi in Asia to sauerkraut in Germany, civilizations around the world have prepared and relied on organic, raw cultured vegetables as a staple in their diets. Ever since opening our café and raw food marketplace, I've noticed an increased interest in health-conscious people discovering organic, raw cultured vegetables as the perfect health-promoting alternative to cultured milk products such as yogurt. Organic, raw cultured vegetables provide an ideal dairy-free source of lactobacilli, including acidophilus and lactobacillus plantarum (aka the "good" flora that promotes a healthy digestive tract and can alleviate many gastric disorders when consumed regularly). When the intestines are maintained with the proper number of good microorganisms, conditions, such as chronic constipation, irritable bowel syndrome and frequent acid indigestion, can be greatly relieved.

Please Note: If cultured vegetables are not your thing, I highly suggest only the best probiotic blend you can find. The only one I take and promote is by Premier Research Labs, as it undergoes a very unique fermentation process for three whole years with the inclusion of 95 different synergistic herbs for optimum immune and intestinal health. Personally, I like getting both in on a regular basis. "The more, the merrier!"

Raw, organic sauerkraut and kimchi make the perfect tart and tangy condiment to any dish. The taste is slightly sour and salty with a slight crunch depending on the combination of vegetables. My favorite brand is by Beagle Bay Organics, with Rejuvenative Foods being a close second. Why? Because their process of lacto-fermentation (aka culturing) is the most natural, with only sea salt added to the organic cabbage and vegetables. Traditionally, cultured foods are eaten in small quantities of about 1-2 tablespoons at a time. I also love adding a little to my collard or nori wrap and tossing some in my salad.

Considering the total lack of fiber in the standard American diet, I always suggest sauerkraut or kimchi for the raw food newbie who may be having a difficult time digesting all the new roughage in their diet. Cultured food can be extremely helpful, as it is a pre-digested food because of the natural fermentation process it undergoes. This allows for easier and more complete digestion when eaten, thereby allowing for more vital nutrients (i.e., vitamins, enzymes and minerals) to be absorbed and taken to all the cells in the body.

Miso

Depending on the variety of miso you choose and the length of its fermentation process, miso can either impart more of a light, sweet and salty taste or more of a savory, sour and salty taste (see page 31 for more on miso).

CHAPTER 3
FATS CAN BE YOUR FRIENDS,
WHEN YOU CHOOSE TO GET TO KNOW THEM

> According to the results of a consumer study carried out in 16 countries and investigating 6,426 subjects in total, 59% of respondents thought fat should be avoided, 65% thought a low-fat diet was a healthy diet and 38% claimed to avoid foods containing fat. The results of the survey showed that consumers were aware of different types of fats but did not know which ones were healthier. It also showed that omegas had the greatest level of recognition but at the same time many did not even realize that they were fats. Therefore, it was concluded that approximately half of consumers do not know whether fats are good or bad, meaning, they do not know what to eat.
>
> **Reference:** Diekman C, Malcolm K. "Consumer Perception and Insights on Fats and Fatty Acids: Knowledge on the Quality of Diet Fat." *Ann Nutr Metab*. 54.1 (2009): 25-32a

BREAKING FATS DOWN – LITERALLY!

At times throughout this section, you may notice that I tend to use the terms fat(s), fatty acid(s) and oil(s) interchangeably – but in a strict sense, fat is usually defined as a solid at room temperature (approximately 70°F); oil is usually defined as a liquid at room temperature; and fatty acids are the individual fat molecules of which all fats (and oils) are composed. Okay. Now in order to demystify the lingo of fats, I'll start by breaking them down as follows:

All **fats** are a combination of various **fatty acids**. All **fatty acids** fall under one of three categories – **saturated, monounsaturated** or **polyunsaturated.** All-natural fats are a blend of all three. What makes us categorize and call a food just one type – like when we refer to an avocado as being a monounsaturated fat – is a direct result of the higher percentage it contains of one fat group over another. For instance, coconut oil is considered a saturated fat, because it is mostly made up of saturated fatty acids; olive oil is considered a monounsaturated fat, because it is primarily made up of a particular fatty acid coming from this group; and safflower seed oil is considered a polyunsaturated fat, because it is predominantly made up of polyunsaturated fatty acids.

Fatty acids are individual **fat molecules**, each with their own assigned names (a common name, and a technical name) depending on their individual chemical structure and configuration. For example, lauric acid is the common name of a saturated fat found in coconut oil; oleic acid is the common name of a monounsaturated fat found in olive oil; and linoleic acid is the common name of a polyunsaturated fat found in safflower oil.

Depending on the size of the individual molecules, certain fatty acids are further categorized and known as the following:

- ★ **Short-chain fatty acids (SCFAs)** or **short-chain triglycerides (SCTs)** when they have less than six carbon atoms.
- ★ **Medium-chain fatty acids (MCFAs)** or **medium chain triglycerides (MCTs)** when they have 6-12 carbon atoms.
- ★ **Long-chain fatty acids (LCFAs)** or **long-chain triglycerides (LCTs)** when they have more than 12 carbon atoms.

However, essential fatty acids (described below) from a nutritional perspective are considered short-chain if they have 18 carbon atoms and long-chain if they have 20 or more carbon atoms.

Essential fatty acids (**EFAs**) are fatty acids that humans must ingest because the body cannot make them. Like vitamins and minerals, EFAs are vital nutritional components that our bodies need for many functions and require for optimal health. The term "essential fatty acid" refers to fatty acids needed for biological processes – not those which only act as fuel. EFAs can be found in every cell of the human body. They work to regulate the fluidity and flexibility of our cell membranes, which allows for nutrients to flow into and out of the cell; they provide growth of brain cells during infancy and help to maintain cognitive function in an aging brain; and they produce hormone-like compounds called eicosanoids which work in the body to promote immune system responses and regulate inflammatory responses.

The only two **EFAs** known for humans are:

- ★ **Alpha-linolenic acid (ALA or LNA)** – a short-chain omega-3 fatty acid known to have anti-inflammatory properties.
- ★ **Linoleic acid (LA)** – a short-chain omega-6 fatty acid known to have pro-inflammatory properties.

All **omega-3 fatty acids** and **omega-6 fatty acids** are also **polyunsaturated fatty acids (PUFAs)**. As we will soon discover, the chemical properties of polyunsaturated fats (unlike saturated fats) make them fragile and highly unstable – meaning, they spoil easily when exposed to heat, light and oxygen and can turn rancid fast. This means that foods rich in our prized EFAs (omega-3 polyunsaturated fatty acids and omega-6 polyunsaturated fatty acids) can do their best work for us only when consumed in their raw, natural state. They should never be overheated during processing and should technically never be cooked.

Nutritionally important **omega-3 fatty acids** include the following:

- ★ **Alpha-linolenic acid (ALA)** – found in plant-based foods such as green leafy vegetables, nuts, seeds and seed oils.
- ★ **Eicosapentaenoic acid (EPA)** and **Docosahexaenoic acid (DHA)** – found in phytoplankton, algae, algae oil, cold water fish and fish oil.

ALA is a **short-chain omega-3 fatty acid**, while **EPA** and **DHA** are **long-chain omega-3 fatty acids**. Our bodies are quite capable of producing EPA and DHA from ALA according to the research done by the Linus Pauling Institute at Oregon State University, and by Dr. Udo Erasmus and Dr. Wayne Coates. However, in our contemporary Western society, there are some very important influencing factors (most of which involve changeable lifestyle habits) affecting the conversion rate of omega-3 essential fatty acid ALA to EPA and then further to DHA.

One of the major factors affecting conversion is our imbalance of these two EFAs in the typical Western diet. Although some inflammation from omega-6 essential fatty acid LA is essential, because it helps the body repair itself (as in acute injuries such as a muscle strains), too much inflammation can lead to chronic and degenerative diseases. Just take a look at all the highly processed and refined vegetable and cooking oils (such as soybean and corn) found in the marketplace, and it's pretty clear that as a nation we are consuming too little omega-3 essential fatty acid ALA and way too much omega-6 essential fatty acid LA. Soy and corn are abundantly found in packaged snacks, baked products and commercial salad dressings, to name but a few.

Sad to say, but the standard American diet does not contain even close to the right balance of omega-6 to omega-3. Ideally our omega-6 to omega-3 ratio should be between 2:1 and 4:1. While it may appear that we have been cutting back on total fat consumption, our diets are still overloaded with omega-6 fatty acids and deficient in omega-3 fatty acids. We can thank the current state of our food industry for this one. This is why we need to understand what we are eating. Polyunsaturated vegetable and seed oils, such as safflower, sunflower, soybean, cottonseed and corn, contain at least 50 percent omega-6 (safflower containing as high as 75%) and zero to very little amounts of omega-3. Depending on the research study you're looking at, this places the current omega-6 to omega-3 ratio anywhere between 10:1 and 40:1 in the average American diet. This is appallingly high! Talk about tipping the scales towards our own slow death and creating unnecessary chronic and degenerative diseases simply by our food choices! Also, modern factory farming practices significantly decrease the omega-3 content of meat, eggs, dairy and vegetables, contributing even further to our dismal omega-6 to omega-3 ratio. For example, animals that are fed grain, corn, soy, hormones and other additives to fatten them up typically have a ratio of 15:1 (if not higher). When people then consume the meat of these animals, it increases their ratio as well. All of this is another great argument for why I feel everyone should be eating more organic, raw, unprocessed and unrefined plant-based foods as much as possible – and I mean AS MUCH AS POSSIBLE!

Both omega-6 and omega-3 polyunsaturated fatty acids are an essential part of a healthy diet, but it is critically important that they remain balanced. When omega-6 is not properly balanced by omega-3, it can fiercely fuel the inflammatory fires. Omega-6 fatty acids interfere with the health benefits of omega-3 fatty acids, in part because they compete for the same rate-limiting enzymes in our body. Therefore, if we are consuming way too much omega-6, then omega-3 doesn't stand a chance. A less than proper balance of these fatty acids may contribute to the development of diseases, such as myocardial infarctions, thrombotic strokes, arrhythmias, arthritis, osteoporosis, inflammation, mood disorders, obesity and cancers – to name a few. A proper balance can help to prevent disease and actually improve the quality of our health.

> *Did you know that many manufacturers of so-called edible cooking oils intentionally remove omega-3 for the sake of shelf life?*

In summary: Research is beginning to show that the <u>amount</u> of fat consumed may not be as harmful as the <u>type</u> of fat consumed. Different fatty acids have different effects on the body; the health benefits that certain foods, fats and oils offer depends a great deal on their fatty acid composition.

This is where it can get a bit complicated, because how does one know what to eat, how much to eat, and how best to eat it? In the following sections I will do my best to explain in detail why all processed and refined foods should be avoided; why most fats and oils should never be cooked or even slightly heated; and why I feel certain fat containing foods and oils are superior when it comes to achieving a healthier balance for both brain and body. I will also explain why I feel so strongly about consuming not only fats, but all nutrients in their natural, whole and raw state as much as possible.

Please Note: When it comes to how much one should consume, this can vary tremendously, as it all depends on the person and his/her individual needs. Constant as well as changeable factors should always be taken into consideration. These include: sex, age, size, activity level and state of health.

Understanding Types of Fat: Saturated & Unsaturated

In order to better understand the nutritional science of fats on a more chemical and physiological level – with the important role each type can play in boosting and maintaining the health and function of our bodily systems – I decided to mindfully piece together and share a conglomeration of information. Some of the information may get a bit technical, but I feel it is necessary in the grand scheme of things. Throughout this entire book, but especially under the topic of fats, my ultimate goal is to power up some "light bulb moments" – with the hopes of other food-body connections and correlations being made and an even bigger nutritional picture being seen.

My Skinny on Fats

Now, as we continue on, please notice the great deal of focus I place on the specific differences between saturated and unsaturated fats and how they (especially when manhandled by the food industry) directly affect the overall wellness, health and function of our many bodily systems.

Everything I share comes from my years of researching studies and articles, along with years of taking notes when listening to some of my favorite experts in the field, interviewers and authors speak. When it comes to how I developed a deeper appreciation for the topic at hand, I give tremendous credit to Dr. Bruce Fife, David Wolfe, Dr. Udo Erasmus, Dr. Wayne

Coates, Dr. Mary G. Enig and Dr. Mary Newport. I value and hold close to my heart a little something from each and every one. References are given where applicable.

Also, due to my big aha! moment happening at a much deeper level once I read and thoroughly dissected a few articles written by Dr. Ray Peat, I will zealously interject with pieces that I simply recollect or have taken and modified from some of his great written work. You will find me referencing Dr. Ray Peat and his work once we get into coconut oil (page 88). Dr. Ray Peat is an endocrinologist and leading researcher in the area of hormones. He has a Ph.D. in Biology from the University of Oregon, with a specialty in the field of physiology.

Now, without further ado…

You may have already surmised that all oils are also fats; but not all fats (i.e., oils) are created equal. For instance, saturated fats differ from unsaturated fats in terms of their molecular shape/structure, physical form (i.e., degree of solidity at room temperature), and chemical properties (i.e., reactivity to heat, light and oxygen). I know you're probably saying to yourself: "what in the world do I need to know this for?" Please bear with me! It does turn out to be very important if true quality of life and longevity is your goal. All these fat facts and what-not may seem like complicated mumbo jumbo now, but should start making sense soon.

It's now time for me to explain the biochemical differences between a saturated fat and an unsaturated fat. Here we go! I will try and do my best to not put you to sleep.

What Is a "Saturated" Fat?

Saturated fat (e.g., coconut oil, palm kernel oil and butter) means that the fatty acid chain of carbon atoms has <u>all</u> its hydrogen atoms (hence, the term "saturated").

Saturated fat also means that all the individual carbon atoms of the fatty acid chain are bonded together by <u>single bonds</u>.

- ★ In other words, fatty acids are considered "saturated" when the spaces surrounding each individual carbon atom are completely filled with hydrogen atoms. Now, because each carbon atom is completely surrounded by hydrogen atoms, saturated fatty acids are compact in structure, making them extremely stable, even under high temperatures.
- ★ All the links of the hydrocarbon chain are fully "saturated" with hydrogen, making it complete.
- ★ This makes coconut oil very stable, and quite resistant to free radicals, oxidation and rancidity.

What Is an "Unsaturated" Fat?

Unsaturated fat means that the fatty acid chain of carbon atoms is <u>missing</u> some of its hydrogen atoms (hence, the term "unsaturated").

Unsaturated fat also means that the individual carbon atoms of the fatty acid chain are bonded together by either <u>one or more double bonds</u>.

The lack of the extra hydrogen atoms on the molecule's surface typically reduces the strength of the compound's intermolecular forces.

If the fatty acid has <u>one double bond</u> in its chain of carbon atoms, it is called a **monounsaturated fat** ("mono" means one).

In other words, when a fatty acid is missing a couple of hydrogen atoms, it has one double bond between two individual carbon atoms. Now, because there is only one double bond, and the two individual carbon atoms must share this one double bond, we call them monounsaturated fatty acids ("mono," because there is only one double bond).

The one double bond of a monounsaturated fatty acid causes the entire chain of carbon atoms to bend at the double bond – which means that many of these fatty acid chains mixed together do not form a tightly packed structure. Now because of this, monounsaturated fatty acids are usually liquid at room temperature (e.g., olive oil, canola oil and peanut oil). Having only one kink in each chain of fatty acids translates to monounsaturated fatty acids being relatively stable (as long as they are stored away from light and oxygen and not exposed to high heat). But, of course, they cannot be as stable as saturated fatty acids, which are as tightly packed as possible.

If the fatty acid contains <u>more than one double bond</u> in its chain of carbon atoms, it is considered a **polyunsaturated fat** ("poly" means two or more).

Having <u>multiple</u>, incomplete <u>double bonds</u> leaves polyunsaturated fats with the least amount of hydrogen atoms. This means that they are even more "unsaturated" than monounsaturated fats, meaning, more unstable as well.

In other words, the greater the degree of "unsaturation" in a fatty acid (meaning, the more double bonds present), the more incomplete and unstable it is and the more vulnerable it is to lipid peroxidation (rancidity).

Also, if each double bond represents a kink in the fatty acid chain (where it is allowed to bend), and polyunsaturated fatty acids have two or more kinks, what does this make them? That's right, very loosely packed, which is how they can remain liquid even in the refrigerator.

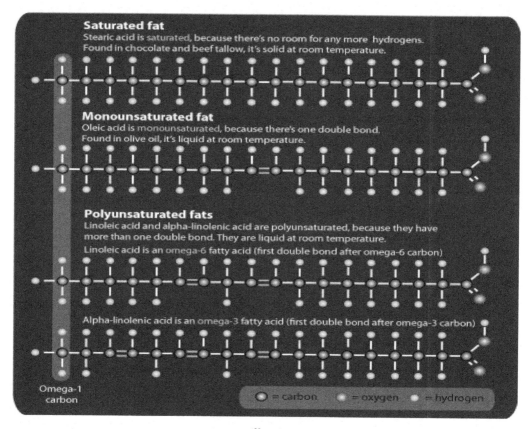

www.gorillaprotein.com

In Summary: Unsaturated fats, especially polyunsaturated fats are missing hydrogen atoms. This means the structure of their molecules are opened up in a way that makes them susceptible to attack by free radical oxidation and rancidity.

> *Free radical induced oxidation is believed to be a causative factor in the formation of atherosclerotic plaque lesions in blood vessel walls.*

What Are Free Radicals?

Free radicals are a part of life and a normal by-product of regular metabolism. Just the simple everyday act of burning energy creates waste. Walking, talking, thinking, breathing, digesting food and circulating blood will all produce waste – and that waste is known as free radicals. However, our bodies are only made to withstand so much exposure to free radicals. So, what do you think happens when we partake in unhealthy lifestyle habits and eating behaviors? That's right – our body's innate ability to fight off free radicals begins to decline and an imbalance between free radicals and antioxidants results, called oxidative stress. Talk about aging at warp speed!

Free radicals are compounds that, when in the body, can travel around in your blood and cause damage to just about everything they touch. Regularly consuming low-quality, mass-marketed monounsaturated oils (e.g., canola and peanut oil) and polyunsaturated oils (e.g., highly processed and refined corn and soybean oil) – all of which dominate our entire food supply – can eventually weaken our immune system's function in ways that are similar to the damage caused by radiation, hormone imbalance, cancer or viral infections.

Free radicals can create a laundry list of problems for the human body. These include: lack of energy, wrinkles and premature aging, poor blood circulation and bruising, arteriosclerosis, atherosclerosis, cardiovascular disease, liver disease, cancer, diabetes, macular degeneration, mental deterioration, Alzheimer's disease, arthritis, multiple sclerosis (MS) and Parkinson's disease.

What Is Rancidity?

Rancidity is the chemical decomposition or oxidation of fats, fatty acids and edible oils.

The three biggest enemies of edible oils are heat, light and oxygen. And in case you didn't know, the rancidity clock starts ticking at the time of production. Along with heat, the use of chemicals in production can cause oil to deteriorate dramatically – or at the very least speed up the rate of spoilage.

Oxidative rancidity is also associated with degradation by oxygen in the air. This primarily occurs with unsaturated fats.

What Is Lipid Peroxidation?

The term **lipid peroxidation** is mostly used when referring to <u>fats in the body</u> that oxidize and become rancid.

Lipid peroxidation refers to the oxidative degradation of lipids (fats). It is the process in which free radicals steal electrons from the lipids in cell membranes, resulting in cell damage.

Lipid peroxidation most often affects polyunsaturated fats.

In other words, when unsaturated fatty acids (specifically polyunsaturated) start oxidizing in the presence of free radicals, they undergo lipid peroxidation, become rancid and form lipid peroxides. An accumulation of lipid peroxides in the cell is associated with diseases and cellular stress. In high concentrations, lipid peroxides can trigger cell death. Elevated concentrations of lipid peroxides are often found in individuals diagnosed with common diseases such as atherosclerosis, diabetes and cancer, and neurodegenerative diseases including Parkinson's and Alzheimer's.

> *Oxidized (rancid) oils can produce damaging chemicals and substances that may not make you immediately sick but can cause a great deal of harm over time.*

Now, I don't know about you, but I sure don't want to fuel my body with foods or oils containing high amounts of oxidizing and already oxidized (rancid) fats. Nor do I want free radicals running rampant in my body setting the stage for a bunch of diseases I'm doing my very best to avoid. Well guess what? If you are eating processes and refined foods, and consuming processed and refined unsaturated oils (aka commercial vegetable or cooking oils), then you are most likely ingesting rancid fats – which can only increase oxidative stress in the body and free radical damage to cells. Impossible, you're thinking – right? You would know by smelling a food or oil if it went bad already – right? Wrong! Only if it were so old that even the preservatives died off. We may like to think that by processing foods and adding chemicals, preservatives and additives in order to extend shelf life, manufacturers are looking out for our best interest – but this is not the case if delicate nutrients have been killed off by the processing and refining itself. The food is already dead – there is no actual life to extend. Take the case of unsaturated oils, for example. Heat and chemical processing destroys delicate fatty acid molecules on contact, leaving us with oxidizing (near dead) to completely dead) oil. Manufacturers then process these oils even further to get rid of the rank-smelling odor before disguising the poor, lifeless oil in a prettied-up bottle. Then we bring the oil home and really finish it off (if it isn't already) by cooking with it.

> When I think of how mass-marketed oils are treated, it compares in a way to a corpse being sent to an embalmer in order to have the decomposing body chemically preserved. Manufacturers of commercial food products are like embalmers in my eyes – they preserve dead, lifeless food, like an embalmer would a corpse, for a lifelike appearance. I know, the analogy may seem a bit gruesome, but it gets the point across – does it not?

Processed and refined foods are made for shelf life – NOT HUMAN LIFE. Eating a bunch of once living, but now dead "stuff" – or something made in a laboratory out of a bunch of chemicals our bodies can't relate to – doesn't make much sense when you really think about it. I don't care how convenient, appetizing and lifelike our modern food production industry wants to make their products look, taste or smell. You wouldn't eat the fake plastic fruit in the fruit bowl – would you? Well, in my opinion, the majority of our modern-day foods and supplements are almost no better than plastic.

Beware of the Hidden Toxic Fats Lurking in Your Everyday Foods!

Rancid oils are toxic and can create a great deal of harm to important bodily systems, including circulatory, hormonal, immune, neurological, etc.

Now that I have your full attention after that lovely analogy above, I want to ask you a question. "Have you ever stopped and wondered – maybe while sitting in your favorite restaurant or café, or walking through your local grocery store – just how much of our food (or ingredients used in and on our food) may already be contaminated with rancid fats?" Well, if we consider the mass amount of food that is processed with high levels of heat (like pasteurization) and ultraviolet light (like radiation) before they even reach the restaurants, grocery stores, etc. – then I'm going to hazard a guess and answer that question: "an amount much greater than we may want to know but should certainly care to know." To think, that before we even take that first bite or get all our groceries home from the market, many of our bulk, packaged and premade foods, bottled sauces, dips and dressings may already be "damaged goods." This is a tough nut to swallow, is it not? I strongly feel that because we do not physically see all the harsh commercial processing methods being applied to our foods, we are totally unaware of their potentially harmful effects to the delicate oils within; therefore, we tend not to envision how they can be impacting our long-term health. It is not the fat itself that is creating obesity, causing disease and killing us, it is the raping and unnecessary man-handling of wholesome foods happening behind the scenes.

> Nearly all commercial foods on the market today contain unstable unsaturated fat – many in the form of highly processed and refined polyunsaturated or partially hydrogenated fats or oils. They are deceivingly being advertised as "healthy," "natural," "vegetarian," "vegan," "cholesterol free," "sugar free," and even "fat free" alternatives.
>
> Some of these foods include: breads, candies, cereals, chips, crackers, coffee creamers, dairy milk and ice cream (and many of their vegan alternatives), dips, dressings, mayonnaise (and many of its vegan alternatives), pastries and most all crunchy snacks.

It's no wonder we hear so much talk about the need for increased antioxidant rich foods in our diets. Nevertheless, few of us are aware that most antioxidants are also destroyed by high heat, light and oxygen.

Buyer Beware: Manufacturers who claim their product is high in antioxidants may only be telling you half the truth. If they have processed, refined or cooked it beyond its resistance to heat, then their claim may no longer be valid, as the nutrients are no longer viable. Between the poor choices of food that conveniently surrounds us, and the deliberately misconstrued facts, we are inadvertently the creators of our own internal oxidation. As a result, we are becoming increasingly unstable (like our foods) at a much faster rate than normal. This is a nice way of saying that we are "rusting" or "corroding" ourselves from the inside out. What a pleasant thought!

What Are Antioxidants?

Antioxidants are molecules capable of inhibiting the oxidation of other molecules.

Did you know that if free radicals are not neutralized by an antioxidant, they can create even more volatile free radicals or cause damage to the cell membrane, vessel wall, proteins, fats or even the DNA nucleus of a cell? Are you aware of the fact that our standard American diet is so dominated by foods that are overly processed, fake and synthetic that it lacks or is completely devoid of natural antioxidants?

- ★ Where are all the rich, fresh, colorful fruits and vegetable in the standard American diet? We are certainly not meeting our antioxidant needs from a wilted piece of lettuce on a lifeless sandwich, fake fruit on the bottom of yogurt, or bowl of artificial fruity pebbles cereal.
- ★ Are we buying our fruits and vegetables organic or have they been sprayed to death with penetrating, cancer causing chemicals?

- ★ Are we eating fruits and vegetables whole and raw as much as possible, or are we cooking the life right out of them?

Even many vegans and vegetarians are not eating enough fresh, whole fruits and vegetables. Where are the vibrant leafy greens and deeply colored berries? All I see is a lot of soy, bread, cooked grains, pasta and rice. Let's not forget about the aflatoxin rich peanut butter, pasteurized almond milk from a box, and beans from an epoxy-lined can. Most vegans and vegetarians are also not getting enough variety in their diet. Furthermore, they're certainly not eating enough foods in their whole, raw and natural state in order to gain enough antioxidant benefits to counteract the effects of what they are eating. I happen to know many vegans and vegetarians who are still eating far too much fast, processed and refined food. Their diets are way off balance, with a colossally high intake of pro-inflammatory omega-6 polyunsaturated fatty acids; a bunch of cooked colorless starches; and totally not enough quality, plant-based proteins, saturated fats or essential omega-3 fats. Then they wonder why their bodies have all of a sudden gone off kilter. After a period of feeling good, they now feel apathetic, weak, sick and tired. Many suffer from being anemic, are deficient in essential nutrients, battle Candida issues and more. The intention may be good, but in order to thrive we must first understand that there is a <u>right</u> and a <u>wrong</u> way to doing everything – even when going vegetarian, vegan or raw.

Aim to Thrive, Not Just Survive

I choose not to eat meat, dairy or eggs, but I make sure to eat a variety of plant-based foods and superfoods that are in their raw state and rich in color (meaning, antioxidants). Therefore, I can feel assured that I'm consuming foods rich in prana (vital life force energy) and natural nutrition. I also pay attention to make certain my staple foods are well balanced in fatty acids and amino acids from the very start (such as hemp and chia seed), and make a conscious effort to synergistically combine these staples with other foods capable of intensifying their unique benefits.

With the exception of drinking warm brewed (below 160°F) loose-leaf teas, tisanes and superfood herbal elixirs, all my foods are eaten in their raw, living, sprouted and fermented state 100% of the time. I also choose to eat only 100% organic, beyond organic or wild-crafted.

> So much of the food in our society today is too rich in "less than the best" ingredients to ever properly be able to support the long-term health and function of our minds and bodies – even some of the ones labeled "organic" and marketed as "health" foods and snacks. I find this extremely deceiving.
>
> Do you think small organic businesses and green companies being snatched up by large corporations could have anything to do with this? Large corporations don't have health in mind; they have shelf life, dollars and cents in mind. We need to keep the small organic businesses and farmers thriving, but first we need to know who they are and where their integrity lies.

Because I strongly feel it is very important to understand our body's physiochemical constitution and the relationship it has with all food constituents, I will continue on my tangent in order to drive home what I feel to be very important points to chew on. Therefore, I ask that you please continue to read on before we get back to the facts on fats. Think "big picture."

Microbiology has taught me that heat is capable of altering, denaturing and destroying <u>every</u> living, organic molecule! We may think this is great for microbes (e.g., viruses, bacteria and other pathogens), but we do not want this purposely being done to the living nutrients in our food that we rely so heavily on to live ourselves.

It doesn't matter whether it's a "health" food or a "junk" food; whenever macro-nutrients (carbohydrates, proteins and fats) and micro-nutrients (vitamins, minerals, phytochemicals and water) are altered, damaged, removed from their natural state or isolated from their vital cofactors and coenzymes, our body knows the difference and will eventually strike back with a vengeance. It is usually just a matter of time before we physically start to notice the outward signs and symptoms.

Whole foods and whole food supplements are in their physiochemical form – which the body recognizes.

On the other hand, manhandled foods and synthetic (isolated) supplements, which have been stripped of vital enzymes, vitamins, minerals and other cofactors, are in forms that are not recognized by the body. As a result, they are treated as toxic foreign substances.

Just because a food or supplement possesses properties that are known to be good for us, doesn't mean our bodies will translate it to mean the same. When it comes to the biochemical relationship between health and nutrition, there are many factors and variables to consider. We must always keep in mind that what we've been told about a particular food or individual nutrient – and its supposed function in the body – may change and perform quite differently once actually in the body.

In other words, even if the packaging of a food is labeled "natural" or even "organic," it doesn't mean that it is free from having been processed beyond its limit or manipulated in some way, shape or form. This means, beyond its natural capabilities to remain nutritionally sound and maintain nutritional stability. When you're going for truly natural and organic, then whole, raw and living foods should always be at the top of your shopping list. The rest is questionable, so fact-find first!

Questions to Ponder Before You Purchase

When it comes to anything you plan to put in your mouth (or on your body for that matter), if you can automatically answer "yes" to any of the following questions below, then I highly advise you do not buy it. Why? Simply stated, you are slowly tipping the scales towards disease. If your answer is "I don't know," then be diligent and look into it. Your body will thank you!

- ★ Has it been manipulated by high heat or radiation at any stage during the manufacturing process? At the start? In the middle? At the end?
- ★ Has it been refined or does it contain refined ingredients?
- ★ Has it been chemically modified, contain chemically modified ingredients or just plain old contain ingredients you cannot pronounce or define?
- ★ Has it been hydrogenated? Partially hydrogenated? Contain trans-fatty acids?
- ★ Are there undesirable synthetics, chemicals and preservatives added?
- ★ Has it been genetically modified (GM/GMOs)?

If true health is your goal, then you need to know that any and all of the above can easily destroy delicate molecules. They can turn a perfectly natural and beneficial food into an unnatural and toxic substance that your body will soon reject.

> **THE BIG PICTURE**
>
> There are huge amounts of misconceptions, myths and half-truths out there – and not just regarding the big "fats" debate. This is why I have wandered away from focusing solely on fats this entire section. I cannot tell you how many times I have heard health and medical professionals – even registered dietitians and nutritionists – tell someone to eat or not eat a particular food, all because of the category it falls under or the general label it has been given by mass media. But when asked to explain why and how a particular food affects the chemistry and physiology of our bodily systems (positively or negatively, in the short or long-term, etc.), the so-called professionals cannot give you the answer. We really do need to start demanding answers to these very important questions. We should be asking: "what is it doing in my body?" and "how will it affect me long-term?" Asking these questions also applies to the many synthetic and isolated forms of nutritional supplements, pharmaceutical drugs and over-the-counter medicines. And please don't forget to question the fillers, binders and preservatives, which are usually listed under "other ingredients."
>
> The same goes for all the products surrounded by a bunch of fad-like media hype and marketing ploys. Start asking the following questions: "Is it really doing for my body what it claims to?" "How viable is the end product once it is processed and packaged?" "Is there enough of the star ingredient for it to be therapeutic?" "Are the main star ingredients diluted down and then just dressed up in pretty packaging?" "Could the long list of impressive looking ingredients be canceling each other out?" Remember, more is not always better. A symbiotic and synergistic relationship is a true science and can be magical with the <u>right</u> premeditated and <u>good</u> intentions; not just at the start, but through to the very end.
>
> As a society, we need to stop focusing on the little that we do know (or think we know) and start digging deeper into the true science behind it all. This is where you can gain a real understanding on how the unique physiochemical make-up of a food or substance can either work for or against the physiology of the human body and, more importantly, the unique and individual nature of <u>your</u> chemical and physiological make-up. There is no such thing as one-size-fits-all!

Back to the Hidden Toxic Fats

Are you eating oxidatively stressed fats and oils that could be contributing to the premature aging of your body's cells? It just so happens that almost every vegetable oil (commonly re-ferred to as cooking oil) is also super high in pro-inflammatory omega-6 polyunsaturated fatty acids. Add to this the following facts, and we have ourselves one fat, ugly picture!

- ★ Chemically speaking, polyunsaturated fats are the most structurally unstable of all fats.
- ★ Unstable fatty acid molecules are delicate and easily destroyed in the presence of heat, light and oxygen, making them highly vulnerable to rancidity.

- ★ Delicate oils that are sensitive to heat, light and oxygen should be handled with care and with health in mind by carefully protecting them during processing, filtering, packaging and storing.
- ★ Delicate oils should never be overheated, exposed to direct light or left open to the air.

So now let me ask you the following question: "why then are these delicate oils almost all high-temperature processed and refined, marketed and used as 'cooking' oils, and found as ingredients in just about every packaged and prepared food that either has been or will be baked, fried, grilled or roasted?" Furthermore, "why are they most often found in clear glass bottles at the grocery store, under the brightest of florescent lights?" What about the long periods of time they sit in commercial restaurant fryers being reused over and over again?

Is the picture becoming clear? Can you see the devil in the details?

If you can believe it, the picture I'm portraying gets a bit uglier. How? Because companies don't have our health in mind, they have shelf life in mind, remember? Not only have many mass-marketed, pro-inflammatory omega-6 polyunsaturated oils been overheated during processing and refining – but we have many that have been subjected to other destructive commercial processing methods with the use of harsh, damaging chemicals. According to Dr. Udo Erasmus, author of *Fats That Heal Fats That Kill,* some of the damaging chemicals used in the process of creating vegetable oils include the following:

- ★ Sodium hydroxide (used to degum)
- ★ Phosphoric acid (used to refine)
- ★ Bleaching clays (used to bleach)

Dr. Udo Erasmus also states that these chemicals create such "malodorous rancidity" that in order to blow off the rank-smelling odor (from damaging these fragile structured fatty acids) one more process is needed:

- ★ Steam or molecular distillation (used to de-odorize)

Remember my manufacturer/embalmer analogy earlier? Now you can better understand where the distrust towards so many food manufacturers in the commercial food industry comes from – especially when just about all mass-produced vegetable oils are rancid before they even reach the shelves. Edible oils (if we dare to call them that) are just one category of food. What about the mass amount of processed and refined foods that contain not just essential fatty acids, but every other essential nutrient?

Remember the big picture here: "dead food equates to dead people." When society is denied access to health enhancing, nutrient-rich, living and raw foods, its health will begin to decline. What does this ultimately create? That's right – a financial bonanza for the medical and pharmaceutical industries that thrive on suffering and disease.

Heat and chemicals de-nature, de-escalate and destroy!

Getting back (once again) to the hidden toxic fats lurking in our everyday foods – next time you are tempted to buy your packaged, prepared, and bottled favorites (even the ones touted as healthy and natural), be sure to question the processing method of not just the food as a whole but every ingredient that went into making it.

The following is an example of a step-by-step approach used by many in the edible oil industry that I feel every consumer should be aware of before they pour.

- ★ Many mass-marketed oils are extracted using harsh chemical solvents that destroy natural flavors and nutrients.
- ★ Many mass-marketed oils are refined in order to disguise impurities in the oils themselves. In addition to the chemical solvents used during the extraction process, more harsh chemicals (like phosphoric acid solvents) are used to refine the oil. This process exposes oils to extremely high temperatures (500°F) in order to remove unwanted odors and colors.
- ★ Many mass-marketed oils go through a post-refining process, where chemical preservatives are often added to prolong their shelf life.
- ★ Many mass-marketed oils are hydrogenated, which creates an unnatural solid from natural liquid oil. **The result:** Trans-fats are formed and are virtually impossible for our body to break down, leading to a host of health problems.
- ★ **Last and probably the most important to remember is the following:** Many packaged, premade and bottled foods contain these destructively overheated and chemically produced oils. Therefore, buyers beware whenever you see safflower, sunflower, sesame, soybean, cottonseed, corn, canola or peanut oil on any food label. The same goes for their partially hydrogenated counterparts.

Please Note: Pasteurization and irradiation methods are two other processing methods many of us are aware of but don't tend to think about as we stroll down the aisles of the grocery store. Not to mention the many other nutritionally damaging food processing and preservation methods that we do not discern, causing us to overlook them as potential prime movers towards countless health consequences? Take, for example, the excessive heat involved in the commercial shelling, drying, pregrinding and milling of our many mass market nuts, seeds, beans and grains.

What Is the Take Home Message?

Oxidative stressed fats and oils can create a major problem for our overall health and long-term well-being. The more oxidatively unstable and stressed our food is, the more oxidatively unstable and stressed we become. We truly are what we eat, absorb and assimilate.

- ★ When unsaturated fats peroxidize, they initiate a free radical free-for-all.
- ★ When free radicals start making their way through our body, they begin damaging everything from cell membranes, to DNA/RNA strands, to blood vessels, etc.
- ★ Consistent exposure to free radicals has been strongly linked to the development of tumors, cancer, cardiovascular disease, premature aging, autoimmune diseases, Parkinson's, Alzheimer's and cataracts.

I don't personally know anyone that would willingly ask for internal bodily devastation, do you? Therefore, we should all want to become more aware of our foods, what our foods are made up of, and how they are being handled. Start by becoming a more educated consumer. Demand high-quality, less processed and chemical free foods. Then reap the rewards by gaining control of your health and well-being.

Fats to Avoid

So, knowing what we know thus far, how do we minimize internal bodily devastation from happening?

Avoid commercially produced, unsaturated vegetable oils such safflower, sunflower, soybean, corn, cottonseed, sesame, peanut and canola. This also includes the massive market of food products and items that contain them. Now that we have a better understanding of how the chemical structure of fats can play a major role in our health, it makes sense to avoid the use of unstable oils that have been subjected to heat processing and refining – along with the packaged and prepared foods that contain them. This is especially true if any part of the oil extracting process involved an industrial plant, multiple stainless-steel vats, a deodorizer, a de-gummer or the harsh, petroleum-derived solvent known as hexane. Yuk!

Avoid oils (and the foods that contain them) that have not been pressed, filtered, filled, packaged and stored under protection from the destructive influences of heat, light and oxygen. This even includes products labeled as "all natural" or "organic." Organic foods are foods that are produced using methods that do not involve modern synthetic pesticides, chemical fertilizers, genetically modified organisms (GMOs), industrial solvents or chemical food additives. This is all great, don't get me wrong, but it still does not mean that all organic products can actually be considered healthy for us. Why? The food (or other ingredients within) may have been severely damaged by overheating during processing or cooking.

Avoid foods deep fried in unsaturated vegetable oils:

- ★ French fries, chips, chicken wings, chicken nuggets, corn dogs, tofu, egg rolls, donuts, mozzarella sticks, seafood, etc.

Avoid powdered foods or foods made with powdered ingredients:
- ★ Powdered milk, cheese and eggs; pancake, muffin, cookie and cake mixes; boxed macaroni and cheese; soft serve ice cream; skim and low-fat milks; coffee creamer; etc.

Avoid cured meats:
- ★ Hot dogs, pepperoni and most luncheon meats.

Avoid meats (such as beef and pork) which have been fed soybeans, corn and other grains.

Avoid all processed soy and corn products.

Avoid all margarine, shortening and other hydrogenated and partially hydrogenate fats.

Mass-Marketed Food, or Mass-Marketed Manipulation?

In the previous section, I spent a lot of time explaining the down side of unsaturated fatty acids with a particular emphasis on polyunsaturated fatty acids (PUFAs); but this is not to say that all unsaturated fats and polyunsaturated fats are bad and should be avoided. Remember, omega-3 essential fatty acid alpha-linolenic acid (ALA) and omega-6 essential fatty acid linoleic acid (LA) are the two essential fatty acids for humans, which just so happen to be polyunsaturated fats. In an ideal world, the only real concern we would need to keep in mind is the fact that all polyunsaturated fats are the most fragile – therefore, the most sensitive to heat, light and oxygen exposure. Common sense would tell us to handle foods higher in these fats with extra care and eat them in their raw, raw and soaked, or raw, soaked and sprouted form as much as possible. That's basically it. But thanks to the food industry complicating everything by selling us on the convenience factor (hmm... how ironic), we have a lot more to concern ourselves with if we truly want to be well. We basically need to unlearn everything we've been taught and reject what we've been conditioned to blindly accept as safe. What are the problems we should be most concerned with? Ahh... I'm so glad you asked!

1. It is the cheap, highly unstable, bottom of the barrel fats the food industry conveniently chooses to use (e.g., soybean, corn, peanut and canola).
2. The grotesque amount of omega-6 fats overloading the typical American diet (e.g., safflower, sunflower, soybean, corn and cottonseed oil), which inevitably leads to a dangerous imbalance between anti-inflammatory omega-3 and pro-inflammatory omega-6.
3. The fact that manufacturers tend to heat process and refine these highly unstable oils, market them as "cooking" oils, and then have them sit in clear glass bottles on supermarket shelves under the brightness of florescent lights.
4. The verifiable truth that fast food chains, and yes, even fancy and remote restaurants, thoughtlessly fry their foods in these delicate oils over and over, day after day. Talk about beating a dead horse.

Put the above four facts together and we can conclude that the majority of the foods we eat are impregnated with highly unstable, low-quality fats – all of which damage quickly and easily. Even more frightening is that all of these fats can damage us quickly and easily, as they create oxidation, inflammation and free radical devastation within the body.

Hmm... there seem to be too many eerie coincidences going on here (or perhaps hidden agendas), don't you think? How is it that the warnings signs are undeniably out there, yet this insanity continues to go on? I clearly see a "death by food" correlation that I find hard to deny; but instead of cleaning up our diets and taking on a healthful lifestyle, what do the majority of us choose to do? Believe our doctor when he/she says it has nothing to do with our food choices, and then give into taking medications that can only mask the madness. It may be just my opinion, but it sounds like a slow death execution strategy if I've ever heard one.

Ponder this... How many of us truthfully know what we are eating and just what it takes to turn a perfectly natural and beneficial food into an unnatural and toxic substance? Let's take nuts and seeds for example. We know they are abundant in excellent, mostly heart-healthy unsaturated fats, vitamins and minerals, as well as a good amount of plant-based protein and dietary fiber, but what happens once we strip away everything but the concentrated liquid fat? We lose a lot of the wholesome goodness which makes them a true health food. Now let's take it a step further. What happens when manufacturers use heat and harsh chemical methods in order to extract, refine and isolate the oil? We end up with damaged, oxidized, rancid fatty acids, which are now no longer good to us at all! We gain no nutritional value and risk a whole lot of toxicological consequences. The same goes for whole nuts and seeds that have been roasted. They may be delicious, but you're eating rancid fats.

Food Processing Industry; a Double-Edged Sword

Yes, there is no denying that processed foods taste better. But this is no accident. All the sugar, salt, artificial flavorings and neurotoxic chemicals added to our foods make us crave them and keeps us coming back for more. Then we have the smells and aromas of cooked foods, which trigger our brain and can have a powerful and controlling effect on our behavior. Don't think for a minute that this is a mistake. Then, of course, we have the deceiving notion that a longer shelf life is desirable, when in reality the food is already dead and smothered in dangerous chemical preservatives. Saving the best for last, we have totally bought into ease of use and convenience. Therefore, we never really have to think long and hard about what we should eat.

Aha! That's it! When things are made easy for us, we don't think. When we don't think, we become neglectful, lackadaisical, irresponsible and dependent. We lose sight of what's right and wrong. Big business has us right where they want us – deliberately dumbed-down, hopeless, helpless and addicted. Like a puppet on a string, government and the food industry are controlling our every move by feeding us biologically addictive substances and over-cooked, over-processed, nutrient deficient food. Then when our bodies become overburdened with toxins and inflammation, government and big pharmaceutical companies have us by the purse strings, willing to pay any amount of money because we feel we have no other choice.

They have us caught up in a vicious cycle. I think it's about time we take back our purse strings and put an end to this cycle.

How many people stop to think about the molecular structure of food? Are you aware that when the molecular structure of food gets distorted – through the addition of heat or chemicals – it can have a negative effect on your health, create disease and speed-up the aging process? Do you think about whether the oil is unsaturated before pouring it into a scorching hot pan? Before eating a skillet omelet or pancakes for breakfast in the morning? Before baking a cake or eating your favorite packaged cookies after dinner? Before gobbling down food deep-fried, pan-fried or stir-fried at your favorite restaurant or snacking on a bunch of rancid – I mean roasted – nuts? I know I sure didn't before putting in long hours of self-study. I certainly didn't learn any of this while going to school to become a health professional. Kind of shameful, isn't it?

Now ponder this...Why do you think it is that we don't look more at our food as being either a medicine or a poison? Why do we constantly hold everyone else responsible for our own personal health rather than ourselves? Could it be that we are too addicted to a bunch of nonsense? Could it be that society has us so distracted and hooked on technology, media and drama that we have forgotten what really matters? We may never live in a perfect world, but it's never too late to change our "heads buried in the sand" attitude.

> *Nature intended for us to consume foods in their whole form – and for good reason. Each and every whole food comes packaged with its own set of raw ingredients (vitamins, minerals, antioxidants, enzymes, etc.) which our bodies recognize and welcome, absorbing and assimilating as a life-giving energy. In other words – as a whole – raw ingredients work synergistically to give our body what it requires for optimal health.*

If you haven't noticed, I do not trust the food industry, not even in the slightest! Government and the food industry will have people thinking that they have made food safer by heat processing it, refining it, adding a bunch of chemicals to kill microorganisms – yadda, yadda, yadda! But is dead food safe? Are foods stripped of vital nutrients safe? Are mass-marketed vegetable and seed oils, stripped of anti-inflammatory omega-3 for the sake of a longer shelf life, safe? Are toxic chemicals added to our food and water, which kill or unnaturally preserve them, considered safe? Are synthetic hormones in our food safe? Are synthetic antibiotics in our food safe? Are chemical substances and flavorings thrown together in a laboratory and passed off as food safe? Are genetically modified animals and crops safe?

Who is to blame for the overload of environmental pollutants, deadly chemicals and other toxins in the first place? What about the bunch of mad scientists who made frankenfood? Government and the food industry may be the instigators, but we're the ones taking the bait. We eat it up like a bunch of blind lab mice.

Who are they really trying to protect? The only thing on the minds of the government and food industries is bigger yield! Real nutrition – found in whole and organic foods and herbs – <u>cannot</u> be patented. This means big business <u>cannot</u> benefit by making <u>big</u> money. Nor does it feed whatever secret agendas they may have.

> *When we strip the food we eat of its innate intelligence, we inadvertently strip ourselves of intelligence.*

I find nothing safe or sustainable about the standard American diet. You know what the truly sad part about this is? It does not have to be this way. Greed is not the answer. There are simpler, safer and more sustainable choices and solutions all around us. We just need to want to embrace the truth by wiping the cobwebs from our eyes.

> *If you are sick and tired of the rollercoaster ride, then get off! There will be no point to running a ride if nobody is on board.*

My father once asked me, "if our food is so bad, then why are we living longer than our ancestors?" My answer to him was – "dying slower does not mean living longer."

Essential Facts About Essential Fatty Acids

The Big, the Bad & the Ugly Has Been Bared, Now Let's Declare the Good!

Did you know that after water, fat is the most abundant substance in our body? Perhaps the most important role of fat in the human body is in the manufacturing of prostaglandins. Prostaglandins are hormone-like compounds that regulate every function in the human body at the molecular level. Due to our tissues' inability to store prostaglandins, each cell needs a daily amount of essential fat.

Other life-supporting functions of fat include: assisting the body in utilizing broad-spectrum B vitamins for digestion, nerve health, mental health and energy; carrying and storing fat-soluble vitamins such as A, D, E and K; converting carotenoids (fat-soluble plant pigments) to vitamin A; increasing calcium levels in the bloodstream so it can be transported to bodily tissues and provide a strong skeletal system, functioning cardiovascular system and cramp-free muscles; insulating and cushioning vital organs, nerves and muscles against shock, heat and cold; helping the body conserve protein in order to rebuild vital tissues; supporting healthy blood clotting; and activating bile flow in order to digest fat.

> *Myelin, the protective sheath that covers communicating neurons, is composed of 30% protein and 70% fat.*

A healthy brain needs healthy fats. In order to build healthy brain cells, we need our essential fatty acids, and we need them in the proper balance. The first essential fatty acid we need is alpha-linolenic acid (ALA). ALA is the foundation of the "omega-3" family. The second essential fatty acid we need is linoleic acid (LA). LA is the foundation of the "omega-6" family.

Omega-3 fatty acids are extremely important for our health and probably the more important of the two. One major reason for this is because they tend to suppress inflammation, which is the leading cause of the many chronic and degenerative diseases that plague us. They do this by countering the pro-inflammatory effects of omega-6.

Nutritionally important omega-3 fatty acids:

- ★ Alpha-linolenic acid (ALA)
- ★ Eicosapentaenoic acid (EPA)
- ★ Docosahexaenoic acid (DHA)

My top choices for healthy, raw plant-based foods rich in omega-3 fatty acids are: microalgae oil, marine phytoplankton, chlorella, spirulina, chia seeds, sea vegetables and dark green vegetables (such as purslane, broccoli, spinach, kale, cabbage, parsley and a variety of other dark leafy greens, including baby spring greens).

Nutritionally important omega-6 fatty acids:

- ★ Linoleic acid (LA)
- ★ Gamma linolenic acid (GLA)
- ★ Arachidonic acid (AA)

My top picks for healthy, raw plant-based foods rich in omega-6 fatty acids are: almonds, Brazil nuts, cashews, hazelnuts, jungle peanuts, pistachios, pumpkin seeds, sesame seeds, sunflower seeds and cacao beans.

My top choices for raw plant-based foods with a healthy balance of omega-6 to omega-3 are: hemp seeds, black walnuts, English walnuts, macadamia nuts, pecans, avocados and a wide variety of living sprouts.

Please Note: Because omega-6 is found abundantly in our world of modern and processed foods, I feel it is particularly important to pay extra attention to the foods with higher omega-3 content, as well as the foods with a healthy balance of omega-6 to omega-3 already built in. Most meat and dairy eaters, vegetarians and vegans alike, are getting more than their fair share of omega-6 without even thinking about it. So please make note of all the foods in your diet that are high in omega-6 and eat them more moderately or even sparingly. This includes all grains (whole and refined grain products) and legumes (such as beans, peas, lentils and peanuts).

To ensure optimal omega-3 absorption and conversion from ALA to EPA and DHA, please read "Factors that Affect Conversion" (page 74), as these are extremely important and require making a conscious effort if we truly desire making a serious shift towards a healthy and quality lifestyle. We also need to be conscious of how we purchase foods containing these delicate fatty acids and take special care in how we choose to prepare them, prepare with them and consume them.

- ★ Pesticides, herbicides and fungicides are often concentrated in fats and oils, so it is best to buy organic whenever possible.
- ★ Heat, light and oxygen are a triple threat, as they speed up free radical induced oxidation and rancidity. Therefore, I suggest buying and consuming only "truly raw" nuts and seeds, cold-processed nut and seed butters and cold-pressed oils. It is the only way to go in my opinion.

According to Dr. Udo Erasmus, omega-3 ALA is five times more sensitive than omega-6 LA when it comes to the destructive influences created by heat, light and oxygen. He also states that omega-3 DHA is five times more sensitive than omega-3 ALA. In other words, when exposed to heat, light and oxygen, omega-3 DHA is destroyed faster than omega-3 ALA, which is destroyed faster than omega-6 LA.

> Unfortunately, with the onset of the industrial revolution and, consequently, the mass refinement of foods and supplements, delicate omega-3 polyunsaturated fatty acids that are essential for all anti-inflammatory functions in the body are either destroyed by heat and chemicals, transformed to toxic compounds during processing (or while cooking) or purposely removed to increase shelf life.

What About Fish & Fish Oil?

Good question! Omega-3 polyunsaturated fatty acids found in fish tend to run the same risk of rancidity as plant-based sources. In fact, according to Dr. Udo Erasmus, EPA and DHA (found in fish and fish oils) are five times _more_ sensitive to destruction from heat, light and oxygen than ALA (found in plants, nuts and seeds). This means the rancidity risk is actually _higher_ with the omega-3 found in fish than with plant-based sources of omega-3.

Cold water fish, like wild caught Alaskan salmon, might be a better source of omega-3's (EPA and DHA) than warm water fish (such as tuna and grouper), but there is one major drawback that all fish in general share: they are all lacking in naturally-occurring antioxidants. Fish must rely on their immune system to prevent damage. In addition, the cold-water temperatures they swim in help slow down the oxidative process. Therefore, in order to prevent fish oils from turning rancid they must be kept very cold during the process of extraction and then carefully encapsulated in such a way to prevent them from the damaging effects of oxygen exposure. This means, that even under the best of processing conditions, by relying on fish and fish oil supplements for omega-3 fatty acids, we now increase our need for more antioxidants to make sure the oils from fish don't oxidize and become rancid inside our body. Without adequate antioxidant protection, oxidation can lead to the formation of unhealthy free radicals, triggering a cascade of adverse health effects.

What About Concerns of Fish Oil Contamination?

YES! Environmental toxins = contaminated waters = contaminated fish. No matter what the fish oil market wants to say, "I ain't buyin' it!" Sad but true, it is a commonly known fact that many companies producing fish oil supplements do not adhere to any rules or regulations and are just selling cheaply sourced fish oil in order to make money. Money is their goal, so please do not think they actually care about the quality of the product. When they encapsulate the oil, most of the time the toxins are still present.

What About Fish Oil that Is Labeled "Pure" or "Molecularly Distilled?"

Remember when I mentioned my hope for "light bulb moments?" Well, here is when one is needed. Not only is molecularly distilling not a guarantee that all toxins will be cleared away, but high heat and chemicals, such as hexane, may be used. This is why I tortured everyone with my technical mumbo jumbo. If EPA and DHA found in fish are also polyunsaturated fats and need to be highly protected from the damaging effects of heat, what effects will the process of molecularly distilling have on the fragile omega-3 polyunsaturated fats found in fish? To think, if the steps prior to molecular distillation haven't already damaged the majority of fatty acids, then you can bet on the heat or chemicals used in this step getting the job done.

I must ask, what is the point of adding a little bit of synthetic vitamin E (or any other synthetic antioxidants they want to boast about throwing in the capsule) if the damage to the fish oil has already been done? It might not seem like a big deal, but there are many individuals taking loads of fish oil per day due to a health challenge that more times than not was brought on by free radicals and oxidative stress in the first place. Do we really want to add more free radical fuel to the fire if we don't have to?

So, what's my overall feeling on fish and fish oil? Well, with a growing body of evidence suggesting that many of our fish oils are either already rancid, contaminated with heavy metals, PCB's or other toxins or partially damaged due to destructive processing methods and steps that must be taken to kill of contaminants – I think it's safe to say that fish oil may not be the safest way to get your daily dose of omega-3 fatty acids. Oh, and let's not forget why many edible oil manufacturers use the molecular distillation step: to "clean-up" the rank-smelling odor of rancid oil. In one of my surfing the net marathons, I distinctly remember reading that in the deodorization step alone, the temperature of fish oils can reach a temperature as high as 428-455°F. If this is true, then ouch! That's hot!

As if we didn't have enough to consider, there is also the fact that in March 2011, the FDA and USDA approved genetically modified salmon. Why in the world do we need a salmon species that can grow more than twice as fast as natural salmon? I find this creepy and deeply disturbing. Imagine if all we had left to eat was the plastic apple in the fruit bowl instead of the real apple as God intended for the human body. Well, with the list of genetically modified (GM) foods continuing to grow, I fear this could be in the future. As of now an estimated 75% of foods in U.S. grocery stores contain GM ingredients. This is devastating! If you don't want this horrific nightmare to continue, I suggest reading and watching *Seeds of Deception* and *Genetic Roulette* by Jeffrey Smith to become fully educated on this issue that affects each and every one of us. Start making a conscious effort to stop buying foods that have been artificially tampered with and mutated. Start demanding the labeling of GM foods; right now, no labeling is required and most people have no idea what they're putting in their mouth – or the mouths of their children. In his books and videos, Jeffrey Smith addresses GM related health problems in both animals and people. You will learn that GM foods can contribute to food allergies, cause cancer, potentially cause damage to your immune system, create super viruses and possibly create outbreaks of Morgellons Disease. What is Morgellons Disease? It is the name that has been given to an unexplained and debilitating condition that has emerged as a public health concern.

According to the article, "Morgellons Disease May Be Linked to Genetically Modified Food" by Barbara L. Minton, posted April 13, 2008 on www.naturalnews.com, individuals suffering with this condition report a range of simultaneous manifestations. These include: crawling, biting and stinging sensations, granules, threads or black speck-like materials on or beneath the skin and skin lesions (such as rashes or sores). Some sufferers also report systemic symptoms such as fatigue, mental confusion, short-term memory loss, joint pain and changes in vision.

For the most comprehensive online education on GMOs, I suggest checking out The Institute for Responsible Technology at www.responsibletechnology.org. With online videos, podcasts, blogs and reports, Jeffrey Smith has made it easy for everyone to obtain accurate and up to date information on GMOs.

Fish Oil Alternatives: What You Need to Know

The body needs a substantial supply of two very important long-chain omega-3 fatty acids: eicosapentaenoic acid (EPA) and docosahexaenoic acid (DHA). Both are required in copious amounts by the eyes and brain for optimal neurological functioning. Since we can no longer rely on fish and fish oil supplements to be the safest form of obtaining healthy omega-3s (EPA and DHA), I find more and more people are supplementing their diet with plant-based sources of omega-3 (ALA). But are we consuming enough and in the proper form to even hit the mark? Most likely, the answer is no. Read on to understand why.

Alpha-linolenic acid (ALA) is a short-chain fat and the precursor (aka building block) to long-chain fats eicosapentaenoic acid (EPA) and docosahexaenoic acid (DHA).

In other words:

- ★ ALA must first be converted to EPA
- ★ This is then transformed into docosapentaenoic acid (DPA)
- ★ Then finally DHA

Plant-based sources rich in omega-3 ALA (such as green, leafy vegetables, nuts and seeds) can be a great alternative to fish and fish oils, except for the fact that ALA is converted to EPA and DHA at varying rates in different people. In general, young women tend to be more efficient than men at metabolizing ALA in order to make EPA and DHA. According to the Linus Pauling Institute at Oregon State University, the better conversion efficiency of young women, compared to men at any age, appears to be related to the effects of estrogen. Because of this, conversion can be even more challenging in older individuals of both sexes.

As we will learn below, much of this conversion business can be boosted by paying more attention to the types of fatty acids we are taking in. We need to watch how we are taking them in (raw/cold-processed vs cooked/heat-processed), and make sure they remain balanced, nutritionally sound and as stable as possible – even through the digestive process.

Factors that Affect Conversion

According to an article written by Dr. Wayne Coates, titled "ALA Conversion to EPA, DPA and DHA – or another way to put it – Factors Influencing Long Chain Fatty Acid Synthesis," it is made pretty clear that there are four factors that essentially affect the conversion of short-chain omega-3 ALA to long-chain omega-3 EPA and DHA.

One influencing factor, which seems to be relatively consistent among individuals, is related to the omega-6 polyunsaturated fatty acid called linoleic acid (LA). If you recall, this is an essential fatty acid and must be ingested. The dilemma lies in the fact that the same enzymes that convert short-chain omega-3 ALA to long-chain metabolites EPA, DPA and DHA, also converts short-chain omega-6 LA into its long-chain metabolite known as arachidonic acid (AA). So, what happens in a diet rich in short-chain omega-6 (as is the case if you eat the standard American diet)? The conversion of short-chain omega-3 ALA into its long-chain metabolites decreases. Why? The two compete for the exact same enzymes that convert them for our usage. Quite the catch-22!

My Solution: Be sure your intake of omega-3 rich foods and oils overrides your intake of omega-6 rich foods and oils. Also, it may not hurt to intentionally consume these two groups of foods separately to make sure they're not competing for the same enzymes at every meal.

The second influencing factor is genetic variations related to the enzymes themselves (delta-5 desaturase and delta-6 desaturase). According to the research done by Dr. Wayne Coates, these variations have been found to influence long-chain fatty acid levels in the blood.

My Solution: It may not be a scientific solution, but I would do everything I could to boost my conversion rate by first increasing my daily intake of omega-3 rich foods and oils. Then I would boost their potential by taking them with coconut oil (see below) and other super-foods that are antioxidant rich. Speaking of antioxidant rich, now would be a good time for me to mention a product I really like, one that may actually constitute being a scientific solution. It's called MegaHydrate by Phi Sciences. Invented by Dr. Patrick Flanagan – who was named "Scientist of the Year" in 1997 – MegaHydrate provides powerful intracellular hydration and is stated to be the most powerful known antioxidant food. According to the literature, the antioxidant power of MegaHydrate can significantly improve intracellular absorption of vitamins, minerals, amino acids, and the delicate omega-3 fatty acids our bodies so desperately need. This is a genius way to effectively keep omega-3 fatty acids from oxidizing during the process of digestion, as well as the more fragile nutrients from breaking down before reaching their purposeful destinations.

A third influencing factor which affects the conversion of fats can be directly related to dietary and lifestyle factors. This is in addition to the typical American dietary imbalance of omega-6 to omega-3 already discussed. It has been shown that high intakes of saturated animal fats, trans-fats, alcohol and caffeine can have a detrimental effect on the role of one of the converting enzymes, called delta-6 desaturase. The result is impaired synthesis of long-chain fatty acids in the body.

My Solution: Simple. Don't consume these foods. Start by limiting them and then slowly phasing them out.

The final influencing factor is the effect other components of the diet have on conversion. Deficiencies of certain vitamins and minerals can have significant effects on long-chain fatty acid synthesis. According to Dr. Wayne Coates, zinc, magnesium, selenium, broad-spectrum B vitamins and vitamin C are all necessary cofactors for certain enzymes (such as elongase and desaturase). Together, these enzymes play an important role on the synthesis of EPA and DHA from ALA.

My Solution: Consume more whole, raw, plant-based foods, superfoods and superherbs that are rich in an array of vitamins, minerals and cofactors, and this will not be as concerning. Also, I would only choose whole food-based supplements. This will help make certain that you are getting all the necessary cofactors needed.

The Short & Sweet of it All

In examining the written work of Dr. Wayne Coates and Dr. Udo Erasmus, along with the extensive research done by the Linus Pauling Institute, there is a sufficient amount of evidence to back up claims that supplementing the diet with sufficient amounts of omega-3 ALA will lead to increased amounts of EPA and DHA in the blood plasma. However, as Dr. Wayne Coates states in his article, the one major factor that must be taken into account (by everyone) is the amount of omega-6 LA in the diet, especially since the imbalance of these two essential fatty acids do indeed seem to affect conversion, as well as the fact that they both compete for the same enzymes.

Successful conversion is vital for the health and function of our neurological system (e.g., mood, memory and ability to concentrate) and our internal electrical energy system (e.g., ability to communicate, coordinate muscles and sense the world around us through sight, sound, smell, touch and taste). So, on that note, I highly suggest making a conscious effort to increase your intake of high-quality, low to no processed algae and plant-based omega-3.

Improving Omega-3 Potential with Coconut Oil

According to Dr. Gabriel Cousens and David Wolfe, scientific research has found that coconut oil can help the body utilize essential fatty acids more efficiently. In addition, coconut oil and omega-3 fatty acids seem to be twice as effective when taken together (see page 88 for more on coconut oil).

So, what do I suggest? It's simple. Start adding the best of the best omega-3 sources to your daily regimen and consume them with some coconut oil. For me, because I choose not to consume damaged, contaminated, antioxidant deficient fish and fish oil, the best of the best includes marine phytoplankton, chlorella and spirulina on a daily basis. These three are great plant-based algae sources of omega-3 EPA and DHA. I also rotate through the many varieties of sea vegetables (dulse, kelp, nori, etc.). For the best of the best when it comes to plant-based omega-3 ALA, I choose chia seeds, hemp seeds, a variety of sprouts and deep green leafy vegetables as my staples.

> In his book, *Spiritual Nutrition: Six Foundations for Spiritual Life and the Awakening of Kundalini,* Dr. Gabriel Cousens states that the conversion from short-chain omega-3 fatty acids (ALA) to long-chain omega-3 fatty acids (EPA and DHA) is easily boosted (1.3% up to 6%) by consuming just one tablespoon of coconut oil per day!

> **Quick Tip:** Adding chia seeds, hemp seeds, spirulina and coconut oil to your smoothies for either breakfast or lunch will help supercharge your omega-3 potential! Also, it's easy to add sea vegetables and sprouts to salads and wraps drizzled with a combo of coconut and chia or hemp seed oil. These are just a few synergistic ideas. The possibilities are endless!

What About Flax?

People ask me all the time why I don't recommend flax as a whole food supplement and source for omega-3 ALA, and the truth is I am not a big flax fan. With so many better choices that provide so much more, I'm going to have to say "flax is not all it's cracked up to be" – at least in my book. A small amount of sprouted or freshly ground flax seeds may have its place on occasion and for some, but I do not recommend flax seed oil at all! Besides being an unbalanced source of essential fatty acids, even Dr. Udo Erasmus admits that the problem with flax seed oil is freshness.

First let's recall that omega-3 alpha-linolenic acid (ALA) is five times more unstable than omega-6 linoleic acid (LA). Therefore, when exposed to heat, light or oxygen, ALA will be destroyed even faster, becoming rancid even quicker.

So, unless you get flax seed oil right from the processor and freeze it until you start using it, it will have already deteriorated by the time you buy it. How many people are getting it straight from the processor? How many methods of shipping use freezers? In my experience, you're lucky if you get a thawed-out ice pack by the time the package arrives at your door. How thoughtful!

Flax seed oil is so unstable, in fact, that when the oil is being pressed from the seeds, it must be pressed in the complete and total absence of light and oxygen. It must be handled in this way straight through to the packaging stage and then quickly refrigerated or frozen. The shelf life of the best available flax seed oil is approximately only two months with refrigeration. How long do you want to guess it sits in warehouse storage before it even reaches the retail shelves of the grocery store? Let's not guess and say we did.

Hemp seeds, on the other hand, are the most nutritious seed in the world! It is one of nature's most perfect foods (hence, the term superfood). In comparing the extracted oil, hemp seed oil comes out on top! Hemp seeds contain more essential fatty acids than flax seeds, is in the ideal balance for supporting optimal health and well-being, and what's more, hemp seed oil actually tastes good! It is nutty in flavor and free from the undertones and aftertaste of flax seed oil (see page 101 for more on hemp seed oil).

Then there are chia seeds, which in my opinion are the second most nutritious seed in the world next to hemp seeds! They are higher in omega-3 ALA than flax seed and super high in antioxidants! Do to their richness in antioxidants, chia seeds do not have the rancidity problems that flax seeds have. In fact, chia seeds have a shelf life of approximately five years when stored away from heat, light, oxygen and moisture. To boot, you do not need to grind them in order to benefit from their omega-3 fatty acids (as you do flax seeds). Whole, ground or made into a gel, all the benefits of chia seeds are readily absorbed and completely digestible. Although I do not specifically reference chia seed oil as I do hemp seed oil, I highly recommend it as a premium omega-3 source and supplement. I hands-down choose chia seed oil over flax seed oil. It may be a bit on the pricey side but well worth it for special recipes and for when that synergistic balancing of fats is desired. My two favorite sources are from Andreas Oil and Foods Alive (see page 122 for more on chia seeds).

Although not as potent as soy, flax also contains something called phytoestrogens, which are a type of phytochemical that have estrogen-like effects on the body. The two major types of phytoestrogens are isoflavones (found in soy) and lignans (found in flax seeds). Phytoestrogens are weak estrogens that mimic estradiol (the main estrogen found in the human body) and bind to our estrogen receptors. Due to estrogen dominance becoming a huge problem all over the world, I do not recommend flax seeds on a regular basis as a way of supplementing your diet with omega-3. We are already consuming and absorbing far too many estrogens from both obvious and hidden sources which are elevating our estrogen levels by way too much. And please do not think this is just a female problem either. Men naturally make estrogen as well, making estrogen dominance a problem no matter your gender or age. (Please refer to **Appendix C** for more on estrogen dominance.)

What Have We Learned?

The long and short of it is: essential fatty acids, as well as their metabolites, have a wide range of functions in the body. They are vital for the structure of flexible cell membranes. Having flexible cell membranes allows nutrients to easily flow into cells and toxins to easily flow out. In short, essential fatty acids are extremely important to life due to the many crucial roles they play in the proper functioning of our many bodily systems. These systems include our cardiovascular system, digestive system, endocrine system, immune system, nervous system, reproductive system and more.

Studies estimate that more than 95% of the American population is deficient in the essential fatty acid omega-3 ALA and its metabolites EPA and DHA, making omega-3s the essential fatty acids and essential nutrients we need to focus on the most.

The excessive amount of omega-6 LA embedded in almost all our food appears to be the causative factor behind the many chronic and degenerative diseases that plague us today. A lifestyle that is abundant in omega-6 and lacking in omega-3 (e.g., our standard American diet) can create the following health issues: Alzheimer's, arthritis, asthma, autoimmune disorders, blood clots, cancer, cardiovascular disease, digestive problems, impaired growth, learning disorders, liver damage, macular degeneration, sterility, violent behavior and weight gain. According to many researchers, this is most likely caused by the overproduction of pro-inflammatory hormones due to an out of balance ratio in favor of omega-6.

Then add to the above the fact that most all our food is being stripped of its vital nutrients (due to modern-day processing and refining methods that use high heat and chemicals), then further damaged when we add additional heat while cooking, and now we really have a recipe for disaster.

I passionately believe this issue of imbalance is critically important for us to understand. Many of us are truly trying to make better choices by choosing more natural and organic alternatives, but our current industries are being controlled by big companies that run on greed. At the end of the day, we are getting only half truths (if that) and certainly not the quality we deserve. I know that for me, if I really want the best of the best going into my body, I need to seek out small companies that have our health in mind rather than large yields and a long shelf life. I want to know that I'm buying from companies that place value on integrity, have a true sense of nutritional knowledge, a passion for whole food and an appreciation for keeping it real, keeping it raw and keeping it enzymatically alive!

It is quite clear that the consumption of omega-3 must increase. How can this be accomplished? Well, since we know that all polyunsaturated fats tend to quickly go rancid when exposed to heat, light and oxygen, these fats truly have no application in mainstream foods. Therefore, I feel we should be turning our attention to more suitable plant-based foods, superfoods and functional food options in their raw form. Again, this includes foods such as quality processed algae oil, marine phytoplankton, chlorella, spirulina, sea vegetables, chia seeds and hemp seeds. And don't forget that we can optimize our omega-3 potential by adding coconut oil to the mix. For more added assurance, I choose to take a quality DHA supplement derived from algae oil by Premier Research Labs. I also suggest taking omega-3 with food sources and supplements high in antioxidants. Think of products such as Dragon Herbs PureTrans Resveratrol and MegaHydrate by Phi Sciences (page 75).

New motto: quality over quantity

Please Note: When it comes to purchasing certain superfood and super green powders (more specifically chlorella and spirulina), I think it is wise to purchase them separately and not all pre-mixed with a ton of other ingredients. When you buy blends, you don't know the processing and quality control of each ingredient. I know pre-mixed blends may be convenient, but I would much rather work with everything separately; unless, of course, I have thoroughly investigated the source and trust their intentions. Otherwise, how does one truly know what they're getting? You could just be throwing your money down the toilet. I also like the idea of being a purist, as you can better tune into your individual needs each day and cycle through different products. This will allow your body to not get too used to any one thing or blend of things in particular. Our bodies are constantly changing, and our need for more or less of certain things will also change. Just as we cycle through exercises and change up our workout routines to prevent stagnation, we could benefit tremendously by doing the same with our foods.

Tipping the Scales Back Towards Health

To make life a bit easier, and without a doubt healthier, I decided to come up with a quick and easy checklist system. Please use this tool and make a habit of asking yourself the following questions before you drop just any food item into your grocery cart.

Do They Set the BAR?

- **Balance:** Is the ratio of omega-6 to omega-3 in the proper balance of 3:1 for vital human bodily processes and overall human health?
- **Antioxidants:** Is it rich in naturally-occurring antioxidants (such as natural vitamin E, C and beta-carotene) that act to naturally preserve and protect?
- **Rawness:** Is it organic, pure and raw? Has it been cold-processed or cold-pressed to keep the fragile fatty acid molecules and the fat-digesting enzymes (lipase) healthfully intact (not to mention all the other vital nutrients and cofactors)?

Fats to Eat & Select as Staple Foods

Eat whole, raw food and healthy raw fats (such as coconut, avocados, olives, nuts and seeds) as much as possible rather than highly processed and refined concentrated oils. Purchase organic nuts and seeds as fresh as possible and always eat them in their raw form with all their natural antioxidants (like vitamin E) intact. Avoid nuts and seeds that are roasted. Practice purchasing all your nuts and seeds from reliable sources that truly understand the value of raw and living nutrients. I also suggest storing all raw nuts and seeds in glass and away from heat, light and moisture, and refrigerating (or freezing) when necessary.

Please Note: If you really like nut and seed butters, only purchase ones that are labeled raw and organic, be sure to check the expiration dates, and always keep them stored in the refrigerator. My personal favorites are by Blue Mountain Organics. All their nut and seed butters are made in small batches using only low-temperature processes. Add one tablespoon to eight ounces of purified, filtered water to make a fast and simple homemade mylk. Use for making quick salad dressings, dips and spreads; but whatever you do – do not cook with them!

When purchasing oils, it would be in your best interest to forego the highly processed and mass-marketed unsaturated vegetable and seed oils (such as safflower, sunflower, soybean, corn, cottonseed, sesame, peanut and canola). As a first choice, I suggest raw, virgin coconut oil instead. As close seconds, only the best quality extra virgin olive oil (due to it being mostly monounsaturated fat and high in antioxidants), a high-quality, cold-pressed hemp seed oil (for a naturally balanced omega-6 to omega-3 oil that is also rich in antioxidants) or a high-quality, cold-pressed chia seed oil (for the highest percentage of anti-inflammatory omega-3). But remember, in order to have the health benefits and claims we constantly hear about, these oils should always be made from 100% pure, unadulterated coconuts, organically grown and fully ripened olives, organically grown hemp seeds or organically grown chia seeds.

In addition, whether you foster raw foodism or not, all should be processed according to raw food standards. Be sure to purchase your olive oil, hemp seed oil and chia seed oil in the darkest bottles you can find. Once opened use them up in a reasonable amount of time. Also, remember to never cook with olive, hemp seed, chia seed or any other plant-based oil containing a higher ratio of either monounsaturated or polyunsaturated fats. If you are going to be heating or cooking, use only a high-quality coconut oil.

Getting to Know Your True "Fat" Friends

Nuts & Seeds

Did you know studies have revealed that eating nuts and seeds five or more times a week can reduce your risk of a myocardial infarction (heart attack) by a whopping 60%? Beneficial effects were found for men, women, the overweight, the underweight, the old, the young, those who exercised and those who didn't. Although many people are hesitant to eat nuts and seeds because they are high in fat, eating small amounts at a time can provide a sense of fullness and satisfaction. Also, contrary to popular belief, research shows that people who eat more nuts and seeds are generally thinner. They also have lower levels of LDL (bad) cholesterol and better bone health. According to studies, eating these tasty, portable, nutrient powerhouses have been linked to a lower risk of cancer, heart disease and inflammation.

Raw, organic nuts and seeds are rich in fiber and phytochemicals and are a great plant-based source of protein and essential fatty acids (omega-3 and omega-6). They provide a good amount of magnesium, potassium, boron and zinc, which are essential for bone health. They are great sources of the antioxidant mineral manganese, vitamin E, folic acid, copper and the essential amino acid arginine, which is a precursor of human growth hormone. The body also uses arginine to produce nitric oxide, which helps keeps blood vessels flexible. Some nuts contain tryptophan, a stimulator of serotonin in the brain that can relieve depression and increase relaxation.

> **Quick Tip:** To avoid going "a little nutty" by eating too many nuts and seeds, I suggest portioning out whichever kind(s) you decide to have that day, and then put them back into your storage space (away and out of your sight) before that uncontrollable urge to keep snacking gets carried away. Nuts and seeds are very nutrient dense foods with a great amount of concentrated heart-healthy fats and protein. No empty calories here – a little truly goes a long way. I suggest if you are making nut/seed pâtés, to limit yourself to a 3-4-ounce scoop. If using nuts and seeds as a topping on a salad or for blending in a trail mix, limit yourself to no more than a good handful at a time. For instance, if I decide to make nuts and seeds my protein source for a meal or snack, I find a ¼ C of nuts and a ⅓-½ C of seeds works for me, with no more than ¼ C eaten at any given time (especially nuts). The amount your body can breakdown efficiently and utilize for energy will vary depending on your age, size, metabolism, activity level, food combining skills, etc. It is highly individualized. Therefore, get to know your body and what works for you.

> When applicable, I highly suggest soaking nuts and seeds to awaken them from their dormant state. Remember, soaking nuts and seeds in room temperature water (with a little Himalayan rock salt or sea salt) will work to neutralize the enzyme inhibitors that are naturally present to prevent them from sprouting prematurely in nature. It will also help encourage the production of beneficial enzymes. In turn, these enzymes will improve digestibility, as well as increase the absorption and assimilation of essential fatty acids, amino acids, vitamins, minerals, etc.

Health Benefits in a Nutshell

- ★ **Nuts & Seeds** are the richest source of natural vitamin E – a powerful antioxidant which can help slow the aging process, increase longevity and prevent many age-related diseases.
- ★ **Nut & Seeds** are rich in B vitamins, which give you energy and promote your metabolism.
- ★ **Nuts & Seeds** are a rich source of the mineral phosphorous, which supports energy production and the formation of nucleic acids such as DNA.
- ★ **Nuts & Seeds** have a low glycemic index which is beneficial for people with diabetes.
- ★ **Walnuts, Hemp Seeds, Chia Seeds & ground Flax Seeds** are especially rich in plant-based omega-3 (ALA), which lowers inflammation throughout the body. For this reason, they are particularly good options for people with arthritis and can even help prevent asthma, Crohn's disease and other inflammatory conditions.
- ★ **Almonds** are rich in nutrients that can help prevent osteoporosis and regulate blood pressure. Approximately ¼ C of almonds contains more protein than the typical egg.

Please Note: If you want the nutritional value and health benefits that almonds can provide, be sure to only purchase and consume truly raw almonds that have not been pasteurized and falsely labeled as raw.

★ **Walnuts** in particular, when compared to other nuts (not seeds), are especially rich in plant-based omega-3 alpha-linolenic acid (ALA), which has been shown to lower LDL cholesterol. Walnuts also contain bio-available melatonin, which helps regulate sleep. Also, like most nuts and seeds, studies have shown that walnuts are effective in preventing gallstones – especially in women.

★ **Pecans** are ranked #1 in antioxidants (for nuts). This makes them a great food for fighting Alzheimer's, Parkinson's, cancer and heart disease. Pecans are rich in fiber and contain more than 19 vitamins and minerals. They are especially rich in one form of vitamin E called gamma-tocopherols, which has been studied and found to be helpful in preventing unwanted oxidation of blood lipids (fats). Pecans also have an impressive number of plant-sterols (known for lowering cholesterol and reducing the risk of heart disease).

Please Note: The native, non-hybridized varieties of pecans are the best, as they are a truly wild food with only the best nutritional integrity.

★ **Sunflower Seeds** are one of the best natural sources of dietary vitamin E (helping to prevent free radical damage and inflammation in the body). They are also an excellent source of omega-6 linoleic acid (LA). Sunflower seeds have been noted to contain tryptophan, an amino acid that helps in the production of serotonin, which is an important neurotransmitter for promoting relaxation and relieving tension.

★ **Pistachios**, like most nuts and seeds, are rich in minerals and healthy fats. Although they cannot be a considered a cure for any joint related pain condition, studies have shown that the nutrients in pistachios may help alleviate joint pain. Pistachios are also a good source of two important carotenoids – lutein and zeaxanthin. These two compounds are known to help ward off common eye conditions (like macular degeneration). Carotenoids are also prized for being strong antioxidants that can help counteract cell injury and damage.

Please Note: Avoid commercial pistachios that have been dyed red (or sometimes green). Instead, enjoy snacking on pistachios which are raw, unhulled and unsalted for the best nutritional benefits.

★ **Pumpkin Seeds** are known for their mild anti-parasitic effect – especially against roundworm and tapeworm. Their high zinc content may be beneficial for the treatment of impotence and prostate enlargement in men. Zinc can also offer protection against osteoporosis in both men and women. According to studies, pumpkin seeds can prevent calcium oxalate kidney stone formation. A ½ C of pumpkin seeds has been noted to contain over 90% of our daily value of magnesium (a mineral in which most Americans are deficient).

- **Sesame Seeds (unhulled, black or tan)** provide the richest and most bio-available source of dietary calcium. For the ultimate in absorption, I suggest sprouting, low-temperature drying and pregrinding. Approximately one ounce of sesame seeds contains as much calcium as a cup of milk. Research has also accumulated on a unique, protective lignan abundantly found in sesame seeds called sesamin. In human studies, sesamin has been shown to have cholesterol lowering, anti-hypertensive, antioxidant and anti-cancer properties – especially for hormonal related cancers. Sesame seeds are also high in copper (strengthens blood vessels, joints and bones) and magnesium (supports vascular and respiratory health), among many other minerals.

    Please Note: Some studies have reported that raw, <u>unhulled</u>, black sesame seeds have three times more polyphenol antioxidants than <u>hulled</u>, white sesame seeds. Because of this, raw, <u>unhulled</u>, black sesame seeds are my first choice; raw, <u>unhulled</u>, tan sesame seeds are my second choice; and last (or not at all) would be the <u>hulled</u>, white sesame seeds. Sesame skins may be a bit bitter in taste, but they act as a natural protective shield to all the essential, health-giving oils within. Also, the sesame skins are what make sesame seeds such a rich source of beneficial nutrients (especially calcium). As a little side note, some have claimed that eating black sesame can actually keep the gray out of your hair. Good to know!

Raw Nuts & Seeds with Honorable Mention

- **Brazil Nuts** are a truly wild food from the Amazonian rainforest. Brazil Nuts are a great plant-based source of complete protein. They are rich in sulfur-bearing amino acids and provide the richest dietary source of selenium. Just 3-5 Brazil nuts per day can give you your daily dose of selenium. Selenium has an important function as an antioxidant and is involved in supporting the immune system – making it a choice nut in preventing cancer. Brazil nuts have been noted to contain 2,500 times more selenium than any other nut or seed! Brazil nuts, with their high content of organic selenium, are excellent for people with conditions such as Crohn's disease and low thyroid function. They are also excellent for assisting with the excretion of heavy metal mercury out of the body (especially when synergistically combined with chlorophyll rich chlorella and master chelating herb cilantro). This is accomplished by selenium binding to mercury and disallowing it to be reabsorbed before being eliminated by the body. Brazil nuts are also an excellent source of magnesium, thiamine and zinc (essential to digestion and metabolism).
- **Cashews (truly raw & hand cracked)** are a significant source of iron (essential for red blood cell function and enzyme activity), magnesium (promotes energy release and bone growth), phosphorus (builds bones and teeth), zinc (essential to digestion and metabolism) and selenium (promotes continuous antioxidant production that can help combat cancer and other inflammatory conditions). Cashews also contain significant amounts of phytochemicals with antioxidant properties that can protect the body from cancer and heart disease. They also have a lower fat content than most other nuts.

* **Chia Seeds** have long been known as a staple food in the ancient Aztec and Mayan civilizations and are also known to be packed with nutrients that our body vitally needs. Chia seeds (whole, ground or made into a gel) are super rich in omega-3 fatty acids, high in absorbable protein (significantly better than soy and comparable to ground flax), are a great source of soluble and insoluble fiber and are antioxidant rich (more so than blueberries and red wine). Chia seeds also contain an impressive array of vitamins and minerals (such as boron, calcium, magnesium, etc.). They are excellent for athletes, due to their unique characteristics which allow them to increase energy and endurance and hydrate the body. They can actually hold up to ten times their weight in water! Chia seeds are also considered beneficial for diabetics by slowing down the absorption of sugars. Studies have shown that chia seeds can slow down how fast our bodies convert carbohydrates into simple sugars. Eating chia seeds can also help those wanting to lose weight by helping individuals feel fuller and be less hungry between meals (see page 122 for more on chia seeds).
* **Hemp Seeds** are considered the world's most beneficial food! They provide the perfect balance of omega-6 to omega-3 fatty acids and are rich in dietary fiber, natural vitamin E and iron. Hemp seeds are very high in minerals and sulfur-bearing amino acids (helping the liver, nervous system, immune system and more). They are an excellent source of highly digestible plant-based protein – being complete with all 21 amino acids (including the nine essential amino acids that adult bodies cannot produce). Thanks to hemp seeds, we are able to obtain two very important proteins – edestin (which is very similar to the globulin that is present in human blood plasma) and albumin (which helps destroy free radicals). In addition, hemp seeds are a great food source of antioxidants and chlorophyll (which can protect skin from excessive sun exposure). They are truly a nutrient dense superfood (see page 118 for more on hemp seeds).
* **Jungle Peanuts** are a tiger-striped ancient food from the wild Amazonian jungle. They may just be the only true heirloom peanut seed on the planet! Jungle peanuts contain 26% complete protein, higher than any other nut. Jungle peanuts contain all nine essential amino acids, methionine (a major sulfur-bearing amino acid needed for the making of enzymes), arachidonic acid (a unique, yet major brain omega-6 fatty acid and skeletal muscle builder that is typically only found in meat, dairy and eggs) and a whopping 40% of the beautifying and heart-healthy oleic acid (omega-9 fatty acid). Jungle peanuts have been cultivated for thousands of years in remote jungles by indigenous tribes, and have a sweeter flavor and distinctive taste when compared to commercially produced peanuts. Unlike commercial, ground-grown peanuts – which are typically contaminated with a toxic substance produced by molds – jungle peanuts are free from aflatoxins!

- ★ **Macadamia Nuts** are a high energy and heart-healthy food. Like most nuts and seeds, they contain no cholesterol and are the highest food source of healthy monounsaturated fats (containing even more than olive oil). They also contain significant amounts of fiber, broad-spectrum B vitamins and minerals. Macadamia nuts may be one of the highest of all the nuts in fat, but due to the high amount of health-giving monounsaturated fat they contain, they are one of the best nuts at balancing and improving cholesterol levels. They are also very low in carbohydrates.

Please Note: Like all foods, not all nuts and seeds are created equal. Two questions most every raw foodist will ask when it comes to the viability of a nut or seed are: "will it sprout?" and "will it grow?" Without a shadow of a doubt, boiling, roasting or frying will devitalize the nutrient value of all nuts and seeds. What is debatable is the use of temperatures above 118°F, yet still well below the boiling point of water (212°F). Temperatures higher than 118°F will usually degrade and destroy enzymes, certain vitamins, minerals, fatty acids, etc. However, certain nuts and seeds – such as those native to tropical regions – which are carefully and thoughtfully exposed to temperatures higher than 118°F, can and will still sprout and grow.

> **Quick Tip:** If you are serious about your health and want to make certain that you are eating nutrient packed foods that truly live up to all the published literature, research studies and media claims – then I highly suggest purchasing "truly raw," 100% organic nuts and seeds from trusted and reputable sources whenever possible. Many commercial nuts and seeds that are labeled "raw" have still been heat treated at higher than acceptable levels during the hulling (shelling/cracking) or drying process and are not "truly" raw. Some have even been pasteurized or sterilized with the use of high-heat steam or chemical spray methods. For instance, California almonds lost "truly raw" status as of 2007, when the Mandatory Pasteurization Law was passed.

Due to the different fatty acid compositions which nuts and seeds naturally contain, and the fact that different fatty acids have different effects on the body, I always prefer and suggest that a person eat whole nuts and seeds – in their truly raw form – for the majority of their fatty acid needs. This is a whole lot healthier than resorting to processed and refined nut and seed butters and bottled oils. By purchasing fresh, raw nuts and seeds and then processing them yourself in small quantities (and on an as needed basis), the chances of fatty acid oxidation and rancidity are greatly reduced. Once again, this is because when we consume whole nuts and seeds in their most natural and raw form, all their naturally-occurring antioxidants, cofactors, coenzymes, and more (which are needed for the body to properly assimilate them) are protected. Intact nutrients that naturally protect the viability of the food we eat can much more naturally protect the viability of our cells.

> **Quick Tip:** How can you have a different sultry salad dressing or savory dip any day of the week? It's easy! Just add your favorite raw nuts or seeds, a little lemon, lime or raw vinegar, some spring water, a bit of sea salt and your favorite herbs and spices to your blender, and then let it whirl until smooth and creamy.

Food Activism: Making a Political Statement by Voting with Our Dollars

In summation – depending on the particular nut or seed, their fatty acid composition, and the amount of heat or chemicals used during any and all stages of processing, many nutrients may not be as viable, or even worse, may be completely destroyed. As far as I'm concerned, this is not healthy for anyone, and we have the right to know.

To help get around this issue, I only purchase from suppliers who truly care about the integrity of the nut or seed, as well as the process it goes through from Mother Nature to our hands. For instance, the Brazil nuts I purchase are carefully gathered by Indigenous people in a pristine part of the rainforest. Most Brazil nuts are subjected to high heat during the drying process, but the ones I get are never exposed to heat exceeding 120°F. This keeps the oils, protein and original flavor of Brazil nuts pure and uncorrupted. The same goes for the raw cashews I receive from either Bali, Indonesia (1st choice) or Vietnam (2nd choice). They are hand-cracked (shelled by hand) and never roasted. This is very unlike the ones in the grocery store which may claim they're raw, but are actually steamed or fried to remove the shell. Another example are the macadamia nuts which I receive directly from a farm in Hawaii. The nuts are cracked while green and then low-temperature dehydrated at 105°F to preserve the integrity of the nut and the healthy oils within. I could go on – but I think I make my point clear.

Besides, by supporting the Indigenous people, farmers and families who are passionate about their land and care enough to supply us with truly raw, organic, chemical free foods, we are not only supporting their livelihood and protecting their homes and land, we are protecting our wildlife, natural preserves and the rainforest. What better way than this to go green – for real!

Avocado

Want to lose excess weight? Make avocados one of your primary fat sources. A medium Hass avocado fruit contains approximately 30 grams of fat – but the good news is that about 20% of its fats are monounsaturated fats (specifically oleic acid omega-9), which are beneficial for health and will not make you gain weight. Think about it. If you deny your body of fat (especially the healthy essential fats), then it is going to hold on tightly to the fat you already have. That is not all! Avocados are great for lowering cholesterol, regulating blood pressure and are rich in glutathione, the liver's most potent detoxifier and a vital antioxidant that researchers say is important in preventing aging, cancer and heart disease. Like olive oil, avocados high oleic acid content has been shown to prevent breast cancer and prostate cancer in numerous studies. Avocados also contain a considerable amount of folate, which can lower the risk of heart disease and stroke. Want more? Avocados are the best fruit source of vitamin E (an essential fat-soluble vitamin) and lutein (a carotenoid). Lutein is known to protect against macular degeneration and cataracts – two disabling age-related eye diseases.

> **Quick Tip:** Add avocado to every salad for better nutrient absorption. Research has found that certain nutrients are better absorbed in the bloodstream when eaten with a healthy fat source such as avocado. For instance, in one study, individuals who ate their salad with avocado absorbed five times the amount of carotenoids (a group of nutrients that include alpha-carotene, beta-carotene, beta-cryptoxanthin, lutein, zeaxanthin and lycopene) than those who didn't include avocado.

Coconut Oil

Pure, unadulterated coconut oil has been described as the "Healthiest Oil on Earth" and the "World's Only Low-Calorie Fat." Coconut oil, a low-cal fat, you ask? A majority of the general public has been led to believe that coconut oil is unhealthy due to it containing the most saturated fat of all edible oils. Haven't we been told time and time again that saturated fat is the enemy and will only make us fat? Well, from what I continue to discover and decipher on the subject of dietary fats, there's a lot we can gain by learning the actual facts, especially if we care to unveil the real truth behind a multitude of health issues plaguing our society. The stigma that coconut oil has been marked with by being labeled a harmful saturated fat is not only preposterous but utterly untrue. Please read on for the skinny!

I cannot help but notice the large number of people who have been influenced by the negative press and misleading information surrounding fats – especially saturated fats. Some of this I attribute to a lack of understanding in the relationship between food chemistry and our body's chemistry; some I feel is brainwashing and manipulation; and some I blame on downright bad science. For instance, due to erroneous association, pure, natural coconut oil has wrongfully received a bad reputation for many years. In fact, the chemical composition of natural coconut oil is incomparable and differs greatly from saturated animal fats, butter, margarine and polyunsaturated vegetable oils (such as safflower, soybean, corn and canola, to name a few). When we wish to unmask the truth and start carefully analyzing the research, we can begin to learn the difference between "good" and "bad" fats. We learn that certain saturated fats – like the ones found in fresh coconut meat, unpasteurized coconut water and raw coconut butter, cream or oil – are actually vitally important nutrients which are quite necessary for good health. Thankfully, in regards to the saturated fat issue, leading scientists are now recognizing that just as there is "good" cholesterol, there is also "good" saturated fat.

Coconut oil is resistant to rancidity. It is the only oil that is stable enough to resist the effects of heat and still be healthy – even when used in cooking. As we learned in the previous section, unsaturated oils – particularly polyunsaturated oils – are chemically unstable and quite prone to rancidity. Although oxygen, light and even moisture will ignite the rancidity flame, it is actually heat and the heating process that sets the fastest downward spiral into motion.

> *Did you know that according to Dr. Ray Peat, rancidity of polyunsaturated oils (spontaneous oxidation) can occur when they are exposed to oxygen in the body in the same way that rancidity can occur in a bottle of your favorite edible oil?*

Coconut oil is super rich in stable, healthy saturated fatty acids that will not oxidize in the body or produce free radicals. Many of us have been told that unsaturated fats and oils are the healthiest and safest to consume, but this is actually untrue. They have harmful effects which are due to their unstable nature and ability to oxidize rather quickly, leaving them liable to become rancid inside the body – leading to oxidative stress and free radical damage within cells.

In his article, "Unsaturated Vegetable Oils: Toxic," Dr. Ray Peat comments that when unsaturated oils are stored in our tissues – or in the tissues and fats of animals that have eaten a diet containing them – these oils are much warmer and more directly exposed to oxygen than they would be in their seeds. This makes their tendency to oxidize and turn rancid very great. These oxidative processes can damage enzymes and other parts of cells – especially their ability to produce energy. Don't we all seem to need more energy? Isn't that the whole point of eating?

Dr. Ray Peat states that tropical plants live at a temperature that is close to our natural body temperature. Therefore, tropical oils are much more stable and healthful than oils produced in cold climates. However, due to it being much less stable in comparison to coconut oil, Dr. Peat does not recommend palm oil as a food.

Coconut Oil, the Necessary Fat for Human Health

In the past, we have all seen saturated fats get a pretty bad rap, but recent studies are proving that processed and refined polyunsaturated vegetable and seed oils (especially the ones rich in omega-6) are actually the fats to fear. To better put into perspective some of the very detailed and technical information above: when unstable, unsaturated oil is consumed (even worse, cooked prior to consuming) it oxidizes and formulates free radicals in the body that are more toxic than trans-fatty acids. This can lead to an increased risk for heart disease, elevated LDL (bad) cholesterol, liver damage, digestive disorders, weight gain, premature aging, skin diseases, immune dysfunction and cancer.

Coconut oil, on the other hand, has the ability to remains stable, even throughout the cooking process, and will not oxidize or go rancid at high temperatures. Instead, the saturated fatty acids in coconut oil are utilized by the body to protect cell membranes, strengthen the heart muscles, enhance the immune system and boost energy.

Please Note: All the health benefit references on coconut oil are based on studies done with pure, unadulterated versions of coconut oil (natural or virgin coconut oil). Not chemically modified or hydrogenated versions which have been manipulated – making them very unnatural and toxic. Hydrogenation is a commercial processing method used to chemically harden liquid oils of all types. Hydrogenated and partially hydrogenated fats and oils have been known to create trans-fatty acids that are extremely toxic to the body.

> *The saturated fat in a food like raw, virgin coconut oil is a very important building block of every human cell.*

Coconut oil can improve thyroid function and hormone levels. The reversal of hypothyroidism – in those who regularly consume coconut oil – has been closely observed by many researchers. Common symptoms of hypothyroidism include lowered metabolism, cold hands and feet and dry skin. What has been found thus far is that many individuals with this condition are reporting an increase in their basal body temperature with just the consumption of coconut oil. This is very exciting news – but probably not for the medical and pharmaceutical industries, which have become more about big business than true health care.

Studies have already revealed that the medium-chain fatty acids (MCFAs) found in coconut oil can work wonders on a sluggish metabolism, raising thyroid function. When thyroid hormone is present in adequate amounts, the body is capable of enzymatically converting cholesterol (specifically LDL or the "bad" cholesterol) to the vitally important anti-aging steroids and hormones that are necessary to help in the prevention of obesity, heart disease, cancer and many chronic and degenerative diseases.

In several pieces of his work, Dr. Ray Peat suggests that when pure, natural coconut oil is added regularly to a balanced diet, it can lower cholesterol to normal by promoting its conversion into pregnenolone (a precursor to necessary hormones including progesterone). He explains that a decrease in cholesterol is exactly what can be expected when a dietary change raises thyroid function and metabolic rate. He further conveys that when people and animals regularly consume coconut oil, their bodies are lean and remarkably free of heart disease and cancer.

In *Superfoods: The Food and Medicine of the Future,* David Wolfe backs up much of the information stated above. He also makes it a point to zero in on the following findings:

- ★ Coconut oil increases the speed of our thyroid. This not just allows the body to drop excess weight, but allows the body to get rid of accumulated toxins as well.
- ★ Coconut oil helps regulate and support healthy hormone production.
- ★ Coconut oil is a nutritional precursor to the anti-aging hormone compound known as pregnenolone, which is great news for women with hormone imbalances.

Vegetable oils on the other hand, loaded with omega-6 polyunsaturated fatty acids, interfere with the function of the thyroid gland and suppress metabolic rate. They do this by blocking thyroid hormone secretion, damaging the mitochondria of the thyroid cells, decreasing the response of tissues to thyroid hormone and impairing the transport of thyroid hormone on transport proteins. When thyroid hormone is deficient, there are lower levels of the "protective hormones" progesterone and pregnenolone, which in turn can expose the body to increased levels of estrogen and their potentially harmful effects.

In his article, "Unsaturated Vegetable Oils: Toxic," Dr. Ray Peat explains that in the late 1940s, chemical toxins were used to suppress the thyroid function of pigs in order to make them become fat at a much faster rate while consuming less food. When the chemical toxins were found to cause cancer, they turned to corn and soybeans, which were found to have the exact same anti-thyroid effect. Using corn and soybeans also has allowed for the animals to be fattened at a lower cost. Does it now make sense that when the flesh of an animal is chemically similar to the harmful unsaturated fats in their diet, the meat of the animal becomes toxic and equally fattening to the consumer?

When considering the inferior quality of animal products today versus the times of our ancestors, we must realize that this loss in quality is due to the cheap, toxic diets our animals of today are forced to consume. This, by the way, only seems to be getting worse with the increase in genetically modified animal feed (which could someday even include genetically modified grass). Their tissues are so concentrated – or shall I say "saturated" – with toxic levels of omega-6 polyunsaturated vegetable fats from corn and soybeans, that ultimately we end up harming all the systems of our body by consume these animal products. The animals are sickened and diseased, and so we are becoming sick and diseased.

Coconut oil has age-defying power! By keeping our blood vessels firm, yet flexible, we can really improve circulation – thereby improving the overall functioning quality of every bodily system. Many researchers in the field, such as Dr. Bruce Fife, have found that pure, natural coconut oil contains no appreciable levels of cholesterol, no trans-fatty acids and is not hydrogenated. Actually, the quality fats it contains can help normalize cholesterol levels and support the health of our cardiovascular system. According to David Wolfe, the sticky saturated fats that come from eating cooked and pasteurized animal products (such as beef, chicken, cheese, milk, etc.) are what eventually clog up the arteries with calcium-forming organisms. Calcium-forming organisms are what cause calcification (hardening and stiffening of arteries, tissue, bodily fluids, etc.) – and it is the process of calcification happening in our bodies that inevitably becomes the main contributing factor in nearly every chronic inflammatory condition we just so happen to blame on "old age."

In *Superfoods: The Food and Medicine of the Future,* David Wolfe makes another very important point worth mentioning, which I feel coincides with the cruel diet our animals of today are forced to eat. He states that all the factory-farmed animal products (meat, dairy, cheese, etc.) are themselves already contaminated with calcium-forming organisms. So, by consuming these animal products, we are increasing our own calcification rates.

Coconut oil provides some immense health benefits that you simply cannot get from any other food!

Coconut oil is the metabolic fuel for life and can help with weight loss. Yes, that is correct – weight <u>loss</u>! We have all been brainwashed for years to think that by eating fat it will make us fat, especially saturated fat. This may be true for the saturated animal fat of today – due to the sick and unhealthy diets they are forced to eat – but raw, virgin coconut oil is a tropical plant-based saturated fat with a completely unique fatty acid profile unlike any other food. A profile our body can translate into health-giving energy and vitality, with the added benefit of weight loss and long-term weight management.

In his book, *The Healing Miracles of Coconut Oil,* Dr. Bruce Fife states that when it comes to losing excess body fat and keeping it off, the wisest decision we could make would be to replace all the fat we now eat with coconut oil. Research has shown that consuming coconut oil promotes thermogenesis (burning of calories to produce heat). According to Dr. Bruce Fife, coconut oil is the one fat that can rev up metabolism even more than protein; it is the one fat that immediately gets converted into energy much like a carbohydrate. It is also the one fat that can actually encourage the burning of other fats. How is this possible? Haven't we all been told that a fat is a fat and that calories coming from a fat, no matter what, are all the same? Well, once again understanding the relationship between food chemistry and our body's chemistry is the key that unlocks the door to good nutritional science and the true quality of our existence.

It all comes down to the <u>size</u> of the molecule, or in this case, we can say the chain <u>length</u> of the fatty acid. Let's break it down. Literally!

- ★ **Short-chain fatty acids (SCFAs)** and **medium-chain fatty acids (MCFAs)**, like the ones found in coconut oil, are small enough in size to be absorbed directly into the blood via the intestinal capillaries of the gastrointestinal tract. Therefore, they do not require any pancreatic enzymes to break them down, which results in less work on the pancreas.
- ★ Next, SCFAs and MCFAs travel through the portal bloodstream where they are burned in the liver as readily available energy.
- ★ SCFAs and MCFAs are easily digested and absorbed by the body, are very efficient and quick sources of energy and pose the most amazing health-promoting properties.

On the other hand, most every other fat (in the standard American diet of today) is in the form of large molecules called long-chain fatty acids (LCFAs). Both animal fats and processed and refined vegetable oils are composed almost entirely of LCFAs.

LCFAs get digested and broken down more slowly. They also get transported throughout the body quite differently.

- ★ **Long-chain fatty acids (LCFAs)** are larger in size, meaning they are not small enough to be directly released into the bloodstream via intestinal capillaries. This means LCFAs require pancreatic enzymes and bile salts in order to be broken down into smaller molecules before they can be absorbed into the fatty walls of the intestine.
- ★ Next, LCFAs are mixed with cholesterol and protein to form triglyceride-rich lipoproteins called chylomicrons.
- ★ These lipoproteins are sent into the bloodstream where they are deposited directly into our fat cells.
- ★ <u>**For Your Information:**</u> These lipoproteins are also the fats that can end up on our artery walls. We know them as low-density lipoproteins (LDL) or the "bad" cholesterol.
- ★ LCFAs can cause much stress to the digestive tract, pancreas, stomach and gall bladder during the process of digestion. All of which may further result in gallbladder attacks, stomach pain, diarrhea, cramps and bloating.

In *The Healing Miracles of Coconut Oil,* Dr. Bruce Fife also explains that due to coconut oil being so super rich in MCFAs, it is the only naturally low-fat fat. Coconut oil actually yields fewer calories than all other types of dietary fat; approximately 2.56 percent less to be precise. I find this fascinating!

As we just learned above, the smaller size molecules of MCFAs (abundantly found in coconut oil) are not formed into lipoproteins and sent into circulation to be stored as fat. Instead, they are easily digested and burned as immediate energy in much the same way as carbohydrates are utilized for energy. Even proteins! Therefore, as long as we consume the correct form, and in proportions that our body can handle and burn as energy, we will not pack on the pounds.

On the other hand, most all other dietary fat will eventually get deposited directly into our fat cells; where they sit and wait for the need to be removed from storage and burned as energy. Therefore, if we are already overweight, have a sedentary lifestyle and are not physically active, we have no good reason to be consuming many of these other dietary fats. Especially now that we know they are headed straight for our fat cells to be stored, lead to weight gain and unsightly cellulite, and may start sticking to the walls of our arteries.

Thankfully, most of us are not living in times of famine. So then why are we feasting so much? When we over-eat beyond our energy needs, day after day after day – especially on all the toxic-laden fast foods – what is to be expected? Did someone say "gluttons for punishment?" Whether in the form of excess body fat, or one of the many health consequences associated with excess body fat, we are essentially asking for ill-health. We need to stop raising our hand to carry the load of excess baggage – filled with toxins, no less. If we really care about anti-aging and beauty (hopefully as much on the inside as the outside), then we need to start changing the face of our current Western diet. Right now, it is not looking so pretty. It consists almost entirely of processed and refined omega-6 polyunsaturated fatty acids which contain a ton of long-chain fatty acids (and not the healthy ones). The current state of our food system may be shameful, but there's still hope for us yet. Just by making a change in our food choices we can send a powerful message. Not to mention, dramatically improve the quality of our lives. We all have choices. Which will you make? I certainly made mine.

Coconut oil is considered one of the best fuels for healthy brain development and function. Did you know our brain is comprised of mostly saturated fat, and that coconut oil is one of the best fuels for boosting brain development and function? Again, this is due to its richness in MCFAs. MCFAs have the ability to bypass bile metabolism and go directly to the liver where they are converted into ketones. The liver then immediately releases the ketones into the bloodstream where they are transported to the brain and used as fuel. According to Dr. Mary Newport, one of the leading authorities on MCFAs research, ketones can help a heart patient recover from a myocardial infarction. Furthermore, it has been documented that ketones can help effectively shrink cancerous tumors. In addition, ketones appear to be the preferred source of brain food in individuals affected by diabetes or any neurodegenerative condition such as Alzheimer's, Parkinson's, amyotrophic lateral sclerosis (ALS) and multiple sclerosis (MS), to name a few.

Coconut oil increases our absorption of vital nutrients. Did you know that coconut oil can be used for the purpose of enhancing the absorption of calcium as well as magnesium? Healthy saturated fats like the ones found in coconut oil are needed for correct bone development and in order to prevent osteoporosis. A good amount of saturated fat is needed in order for the body to properly utilize calcium. Hence, a low-fat diet with plenty of calcium and calcium supplements is not necessarily going to prevent osteoporosis.

Please Note: According to Dr. Tom Levy, aggressive calcium supplementation is not the answer to restoring the integrity of osteoporotic bones. It appears that much of the calcium we purposely pop down our throats is abnormally getting deposited into our tissues instead. Our blood vessels and joints are literally becoming lined and filled with rock-like deposits of calcium salts. Research published in the *British Medical Journal* states that taking in extra calcium can only marginally reduce the risk of bone fractures (if that), and can do virtually nothing to reduce the risk or reverse actual osteoporosis. A slightly decreased risk in developing a bone fracture is not worth the greater risk of having a fatal heart attack. It is also not worth developing a chronically painful and crippling disease like arthritis.

Coconut oil can also improve the digestion and absorption of fat-soluble vitamins and amino acids. Saturated fats act as a carrier for "fat-soluble" vitamins A, D, E and K. When fat is deliberately removed from our food – or by choice from our diet – many vitamins are also removed and our absorption of vitamins goes way down.

In lectures, interviews and several pieces of his work, David Wolfe has recommended that individuals also consume coconut oil when consuming omega-3 containing oils (such as algae, hemp, chia, flax, etc.). Coconut oil seems to help the body utilize essential fatty acids, such as omega-3, more efficiently. According to research, the antioxidant effects of omega-3 fatty acids are also enhanced, becoming twice as effective when taken with coconut oil.

In other research, it was proven that regular consumption of MCFAs increased the phospholipid and omega-3 fatty acid content in the parietal cortex of the brain. Researchers believe that when MCFA are present, they allow omega-3 fatty acids to be released from fat stores which are then utilized in the brain – where they are most needed to help form solid memory centers.

> **Quick Tip:** I <u>always</u> add coconut oil to my superfood filled smoothies and anytime I am consuming foods rich in omega-3 fatty acids (such as chia seeds/oil, hemp seeds/oil, spirulina, chlorella, marine phytoplankton, etc.). I highly advise you do the same.

Coconut oil is the most readily available food source of lauric acid – the powerful antimicrobial that gives coconut oil its claim to nutritional fame! Did you know lauric acid is a main component of human breast milk and can helps protect children from illness during infancy? Lauric acid has to be one of the most miraculous of all MCFAs. And it just so happens to be that coconut oil is the most abundant of all food sources in both! Nearly 50% of the fatty acid in pure, unadulterated coconut oil is lauric acid, which converts to the fatty acid monolaurin in the body. Numerous studies show that the high lauric acid content of coconut oil can be an extremely powerful anti-microbial agent, effective against a broad range of pathologic bacteria, viruses, fungi, yeasts and protozoa. Capric acid, which comprises approximately another 7% of coconut oils fat content, also stimulates anti-microbial activity. This makes coconut oil an invaluable healing tool for those with chronic infections (like *Candida albicans*) and immune deficiency diseases (such as Lyme disease and Epstein Barr virus). Promising studies have also been done on patients suffering with AIDS. Many people have also reported great relief from digestive disorders, such as Crohn's disease and irritable bowel syndrome (IBS), after adding coconut oil into their daily diet. It can also be a useful tool for those who wish to keep the common cold and flu at bay.

Coconut oil can benefit insulin resistance and diabetes. Unlike carbohydrates – our body's usual source of energy – coconut oil will not raise blood sugar or insulin levels. It is a carbohydrate free source of readily available energy, meaning that it can act as a stabilizer for those with diabetes or hypoglycemia.

Sourcing the Best Coconut Oil

Ultimate Superfoods (USF) Raw Centrifuge Virgin Coconut Oil is my favorite! It is the only coconut oil I will consume and use daily! Most virgin coconut oils on the market go through one of two processes to extract the oil from the coconut. USF Raw Centrifuge Virgin Coconut Oil, on the other hand, is extremely unique. It does not go through either the "quick drying" or "wet-milling" processes that many other coconut oils go through. Instead, they use a centrifugal extraction method to derive the oil from the coconut that requires no heat whatsoever! The end result is oil that tastes out of this world! Furthermore, since their coconut supplier owns the USDA certified organic coconut plantation, they are able to provide coconuts that are harvested at the perfect age. Once the coconuts are de-husked and grated, the fresh coconut meat is cold-pressed (to preserves the living enzymes, lauric acid and all other immune building nutrients), and then carefully filtered. In order to provide a sanitary controlled environment, only stainless-steel equipment is used in their processing plant. Very little human handling is required. What's more, no chemicals or preservatives are ever added. This allows us to enjoy only pure, unadulterated virgin coconut oil.

Please Note: Coconut oil is a colorless to pale brownish-yellow oil. It is tropical oil from a tropical climate that has a melting point ranging from 73°F to 78°F. I recommend storing in a cool, dark place. However, refrigeration is totally unnecessary. In comparison to most oils, coconut oil has a long shelf life of up to three years. This is due to its natural ability to not be affected by fluctuating temperatures. You will notice that when the temperature is warmer in your home, coconut oil will be in a liquid state and clear in color; and when it is cooler or cold in your home, it will be in a more solid state and opaque to white in color. This occurrence is absolutely natural and completely normal. Therefore, please do not worry that there is something off or wrong with your coconut oil.

> **Quick Tip:** As stated earlier, coconut oil is fully saturated with hydrogen atoms and, for this reason, very slow to oxidize. Due to its resistance to rancidity, coconut oil is the safest of all oils to use when the addition of heat is anticipated. In comparison, all unsaturated oils (including commonly used olive oil) have a low tolerance to cooking temperatures and, as a result, can easily turn rancid as soon as they hit the hot heat of a pan or stove. Therefore, if planning to bake, sauté, etc. – coconut oil is the one and only oil to choose.

The uses of coconut oil are endless! I love adding it to my smoothies, dressings, dips and sauce creations, and to help with molding raw desserts and treats. Coconut oil is also amazing for your skin and hair. Feel free to use as a shave gel in the shower, as moisturizer after the shower and to rub into the dry brittle ends of your hair.

Olive Oil

Fat and oil is extremely important to human health – but with all the mass marketed and factory produced oils that suffocate our modern society, how can one guarantee finding high-quality oil that has not been processed in ways that either reduce or ravage its nutritional value? Once again, the answer comes with knowing and understanding the chemical composition of the food and caring enough to preserve its inner integrity. This way, it can be nothing less than beneficial to the body.

Some nutritive properties of olives and olive oil are:

- Rich in **oleic acid** – a monounsaturated omega-9 fatty acid that is very efficient in strengthening cell membrane integrity, boosting the power of memory, optimizing the functioning of the brain and improving the functions of the heart, circulatory system and much more.
- Rich in **vitamins E** and **K.**
- Rich in **calcium.**
- Rich in many natural **polyphenol antioxidants**, such as the ones below.
    - **Oleocanthal:** responsible for giving extra virgin olive oil that peppery bite. Oleocanthal has been found to have anti-inflammatory (relieving headache and arthritis pain) and antioxidant properties.
    - **Tyrosol:** a phenolic antioxidant that protects cells against injury due to oxidation.
    - **Hydroxytyrosol:** a phytochemical believed to be one of the most powerful antioxidants. Its oxygen radical absorbance capacity (ORAC) is noted to be ten times higher than green tea!
    - **Oleuropein:** possesses powerful antioxidant activity and gives extra virgin olive oil its bitter, pungent taste. Oleuropein preparations have been claimed to strengthen the immune system.

- **Squalene:** commonly found in shark liver oil, but also obtained from plant-based sources such as olives. Squalene is the biochemical precursor to the whole family of steroids (e.g., cholesterol and vitamin D). According to studies, squalene is an important part of the Mediterranean diet, for it may slow the growth of certain cancers. It is also used in cosmetics as a natural moisturizer for its ability to penetrate the skin quickly and not leave a greasy feeling to skin and hair.

The Olive Oil Ignominy

Olive oil has been around for more than 5000 years. It was noted to be a valuable medicine in the hands of ancient Greek doctors. In fact, Hippocrates mentions at least 60 different conditions which could be treated with olive oil, including skin conditions such as wounds and burns, gynecological ailments, ear infections and others.

Numerous studies have revealed that extra virgin olive oil can reduce cholesterol, lower blood pressure, inhibit platelet aggregation and lower the incidence of colon, breast and skin cancer. Due to its richness in natural antioxidants (e.g., polyphenols and vitamin E), olive oil is capable of reducing the oxidation of LDL cholesterol, which can dramatically decrease the chance of developing heart disease. These same antioxidants also add to the stability and shelf life of the oil. Olive oil is also commonly used in liver and gallbladder cleansing program to help in the expelling of gallstones.

With the exception of a select few, olive oil is very unique among oils in its nutritional profile. If you recall, olive oil is almost all monounsaturated fat. This means that it may not be as stable as coconut oil, but it is far more stable than the majority of unsaturated oils out there – especially the ones with a higher ratio of polyunsaturated fats. The nutritive properties that olive oil possesses – including its high percentage of powerful antioxidants which naturally outweigh any free radical oxidation potential – is what allows this extraordinary oil to be consumed in its raw, crude, unfiltered state without the need for any refinement. Ahh! But here's the twist. In order for us to gain the same health and protective benefits from free radical damage, the oil must be made in the exact same way the Ancient Greeks made it. We sure aren't getting that off our supermarket shelves.

The nutritional quality of our modern-day olive oil is no more!

Due to increasing demand, the majority of today's olive oil is extracted in factories by continuous centrifuge, where hot water is used to help separate out the oil. The problem with this cheap method of processing is that it substantially reduces the nutritional quality and healing benefits of olive oil. Polyphenol antioxidants are water-soluble; therefore, they are completely destroyed and washed away.

Factory Produced Olive Oil vs Real Authentic Olive Oil

Sad but true, almost all olive oil on the market today is processed in ways that lead to a loss of nutrients essential to living healthfully. In order to truly appreciate real olive oil, one should know how a truly high-quality olive oil is produced. Therefore, I decided to paint a little picture by comparing and contrasting some of the major differences between olive oil produced in our modern-day factories and olive oil produced sustainably and ecologically on small family farms.

Factory produced olive oil uses olives that are machine harvested along with the leaves, twigs and debris from the tree. A machine is used to shake the trees, the olives fall to the ground and they are then swept up into piles. Due to the machine doing all the work, bad olives can easily get overlooked and mixed in with the good ones. Many times, these olives are transported in poorly ventilated containers where they sit for too long in large heaped up piles, often getting moldy. The oil is then extracted by continuous centrifuge with high heat, hot water, perhaps chemical solvents and who knows what else.

Real olive oil production begins on a farm that has never been exposed to chemical pesticides and fertilizers. The olives are hand picked off the trees so as not to damage their delicate skin and pulp. Well aerated containers are used to transport the olives in order to avoid excess heat production and mold from forming. Any leaves and twigs are always removed. Olives are manually sorted, washed in cold water and then dried. Depending on the family farm, the actual pressing or olive oil extraction process can differ. For instance, some olives are diced to an olive mush before being extremely slow pressed at temperatures that never exceed 70°F; others are stone ground (milled with a stone wheel) to form a paste before being hydraulically pressed.

The Main Point: No heat, hot water or solvents are ever used in the process of extracting the oil from the olives.

The Result: A pure and raw, cold-pressed, extra virgin olive oil in which all the beneficial properties, rich flavor and aroma have been preserved.

Factory produced olive oil is filtered. Filtering removes many of the beneficial nutrients and causes the oil to be clear in appearance. This step plays a big part in the shorter shelf life of factory produced olive oil – which is only a few months if we're lucky.

Real olive oil, on the other hand, is not filtered. As a result, real olive oil retains much of its beneficial nutrients and looks cloudy.

The Difference: Real olive oil has a shelf life of two to three years.

When I do splurge on an olive oil, my ultimate favorite is the premium, early harvest, unfiltered, extra virgin olive oil which has been ice pressed within 12 hours of harvest. Rallis Olive Oil is extremely unique. It is pressed in the complete absence of heat. Being that it is ice pressed at a temperature 20-30 times colder than cold-pressed olive oils, Rallis Olive Oil has a nutritive and healing potential unlike any other olive oil on the market. This premium, ice pressed, extra virgin olive oil by Rallis is a true raw superfood. For more information and where to buy, please go to www.rallisoliveoil.com.

Another one of my favorites to splurge on is Extra Virgin Botija Olive Oil. It is carefully cold-pressed and unfiltered, a pledge to the preservation of all the prized enzymes and nutrients it possesses. Many low-quality mass market oils say they are cold-pressed, but temperatures often reach over 200 degrees. This totally degrades, if not destroys, the delicate nutritive qualities of olive oil. Low-quality olive oil can even contain cheap fillers such as highly refined polyunsaturated corn and sunflower oils. The process for extracting Extra Virgin Botija Olive Oil is truly pure and raw. The temperature never exceeds 70°F and is always guaranteed to be 100% pure olive oil from 100% pure olives. When available, this oil can be purchased through reputable raw food suppliers.

One more favorite of mine is a truly pure and raw olive oil by Bariani. The Bariani family has origins deeply rooted in the Northern Italian region of Lombardy. Their olives are organic and sustainably grown and their process is authentic. Bariani Olive Oil is true to the original varieties available in the ancient Mediterranean. It is made with great care and respect. Only the ripest of olives are chosen before being ground and milled with stone wheel presses. This process of extracting oil is the closest to the original techniques developed by the Greeks and Romans thousands of years ago. Bariani is truly one of the best California grown, stone pressed, extra virgin olive oils on the market. Please see www.barianioliveoil.com for more information.

Please Note: When high-grade liquid oil at room temperature is desired, I only suggest using one of the three olive oils listed above.

Will Your Current Olive Oil Pass the Palm Test?

Dribble a few drops of your olive oil into the palm of your hand and simply lick it off your palm. If there is a greasy residue left behind, either heating of the oil occurred during the extraction process or the oil is not purely made from 100% olives.

The term "extra virgin" has no official meaning in the United States; therefore, a label reading "extra virgin" is no guarantee of quality.

Are You Getting the Quality You Deserve or Are You Being Duped?

A high grade of olive oil can be a very healing and nourishing choice of oil for the body. It can be highly alkalizing as well. This is due to the olives being rich in alkalizing minerals such as calcium. However, this is clearly not the case if we are getting olive oil in which the alkalizing minerals (along with everything else) have been destroyed by high heat or processing techniques that put off too much heat; by a refining process or chemicals; or were diluted down with cheap and highly refined fillers.

- ★ A measure for grading olive oil is its level of free fatty acid acidity (FFA). Freshly pressed oils, made carefully from fresh-picked, healthy olives and without the use of excessive heat, normally have a pretty low acidity level of well under 0.5% FFA. "Extra virgin" olive oils normally have less than 0.8% FFA versus just "virgin" olive oils that can have an acidity of up to 3% FFA or higher.
- ★ Buyers beware! Believe it or not, lower quality olive oils can be refined to bring the acidity down in order to be labeled as "extra virgin." Nonetheless, do we really want to be eating refined oil? I think not!

- Some of the most popular Italian oils labeled "extra virgin" may have been diluted and contain up to 20% highly refined hazelnut oil as filler. Some California olive oils may actually contain highly refined corn and sunflower oils as fillers.
- Now what I'm about to say may seem contradictory, but it is only because the majority of manufacturers in the food industry can have a way of manipulating words when it comes to marketing and advertising their product. For this reason, my number one rule is to never believe what the front of the label states. Always turn the bottle around and look at the actual ingredients. Now, you do want the olive oil to be made from 100% pure olives, but you don't want the oil itself to go through a "purifying" process. Very deceiving, I know. If you see an olive oil label that reads "pure," "light" or just plain "olive oil," it almost always means that it has been refined. Oil that is refined can mean any or all of the following: cleaned, filtered, neutralized, bleached or deodorized with solvents such as hexane.

A Few General Tips on Selecting a High-Quality, Authentic Olive Oil

The following tips and suggestions are in accordance to many olive oil experts and connoisseurs:

- For an olive oil to be considered "extra virgin" it first needs to be made from 100% pure organic olives and nothing else.
- It should be truly cold-pressed, unfiltered and have a greenish, slightly cloudy appearance. Therefore, look for it to read "first cold pressed" somewhere on the label.
- Always research your olive oil to make sure chemicals have not been used in the oil extraction and separation process. Refining and the addition of chemicals have an unduly negative effect on oils. They can diminish or completely devastate all the health-giving elements within, as well as cause premature oxidation and rancidity.
- Good quality olive oil should be made from one type of olive, not a mix.
- Please note the dates! There should be two of them. One will state when the oil was produced, the other will state when it expires. At the very least, there should always be an expiration date.
- Only purchase an amount of olive oil that can easily be used prior to expiration. Once opened, be sure to use up within one year (preferably 6-8 months); and always store in a cool, dark place away from light, heat and moisture.
- It may not be an industry requirement, but it is best if the oil is packaged in a dark glass bottle. It will keep fresher longer. The darker glass protects the oil from the damaging effects of light and heat.

> **Quick Tip:** Once opened, you can always transfer a smaller amount into a small dark bottle for daily use. This will keep from constantly exposing a bigger bottle to air or a clear bottle to air and light.

Hemp Seed Oil

The oil extracted from hemp seeds has an amazing essential fatty acid profile. Hemp seed oil can provide us with a healthy plant-based alternative to the animal-based omega-3s most commonly found in fish. This is truly a Godsend, especially since most fish these days are severely contaminated with heavy metals (like mercury), PCBs and other toxins. Fish oil supplements are also no longer considered safe by many. According to an ABC-7 (San Francisco) aired news report in March of 2010, a lawsuit was put into action over cancer-causing contaminants being allowed in fish oil supplements. The lawsuit named eight companies: CVS Pharmacy, General Nutrition (GNC), Now Health Group (NOW Foods), Omega Protein, Pharmavite, Rite Aid, Solgar and Twin Lab. According to the attorney, lab test results showed that some of the products contained 70 times as many PCBs as others. In my opinion, this is slow murder. Even if unsafe levels of contaminants are not detected, can any amount of any contaminant realistically be considered safe if we are taking these supplements on a daily basis? We need to question their accumulative effect. Other drawbacks of fish oil are the following:

- ★ Powerless in its content of antioxidants, fish oil is liable to spoil rather quickly. This is of major concern for the many that opt for fish oil as a way of increasing their intake of two important omega-3 polyunsaturated fatty acids, DHA and EPA. Why? Because now you need a lot more antioxidants on board. Without enough antioxidants in our diet (and how do we determine what "enough" is?), fish oils can oxidize and become rancid in the body – leading to that unhealthy free radical free-for-all we discussed earlier.

Hemp seed oil, on the other hand, is very high in naturally-occurring vitamin E in the form of alpha-, beta-, gamma- and delta-tocopherols, as well as alpha-tocotrienols. These constituents are powerful antioxidants. Because they are found naturally in hemp seeds, they can act as a natural preservative throughout the cold-pressing process, as well as naturally extend shelf life. Even though hemp seed oil is considered the highest plant-based source of health-giving essential fatty acids and offers a great amount of antioxidant protection, please do not forget that it is still predominantly made up of polyunsaturated fats. Hemp seed oil should always be purchased in a dark bottle to protect its vital nutrients from light damage. Additionally, it should always be stored in the refrigerator, where it will remain in a liquid state.

- ★ **Buyers Beware:** Unfortunately, most food retailers have very little knowledge (or just no appreciation) for the storage requirements of highly unsaturated oils. Moreover, many retailers have little or no spare refrigerated space for yet another new product. Ideally, you want to purchase from the refrigerated section; if you do not find it there, I suggest taking a little time to politely educate the store manager and employees on proper storage of this delicate but valuable oil.

Please Note: Please do not ever heat hemp seed oil. Heat will damage all its prized and perfectly balanced essential fatty acids, not to mention all its natural antioxidants and many other nutrients. Instead, use this oil as a condiment, on salads or in a smoothie. It gives a great nutty taste that many find much more palatable than flax seed oil.

> *According to David Wolfe, hemp seed's content of vitamin E is three times higher than flax seed!*

Not only is hemp seed oil richer in antioxidant vitamin E, but it also contains more essential fatty acids than flax seed oil. To boot, it provides them in a ratio of about 3:1, which is considered by most health organizations to be the perfect ratio of omega-6 to omega-3 for the human body. With the exception of chia seeds, hemp seeds are the only plant-based food where this ideal balance occurs. You don't see it in flax seeds, almonds, walnuts or soybeans, to name but a few.

Together, and in the right balance, omega-6 and omega-3 play a crucial role in proper brain function, vision and eye health and normal growth and development.

Not having the ideal balance of omega-6 to omega-3 – from the foods we eat and supplements we take – will lead us to nutritional deficiencies and imbalances which sooner or later can turn into major health issues. This means daily supplementation of the more popularized flax seed oil can potentially create dangerous nutritional imbalances. You may ask how this is possible if flax seed oil is so high in the much-needed omega-3 ALA. It's a case of flax seed oil not being healthfully balanced for the human body. Flax seed oil is tipped a bit too far in the opposite direction with an omega-6 to omega-3 ratio of 1:4. It may take a year or longer, but a nutritional imbalance in our diet will eventually rear its ugly head.

> *Hemp seed's essential fatty acid (EFA) profile is closer to fish oil than any other vegetable or seed oil!*

According to much research, another considerable advantage hemp seed oil has over flax seed oil is its content of the rare direct metabolites of omega-6 and omega-3 called **gamma-linoleic Acid (GLA)** and **stearidonic acid (SDA)**. These same metabolites are found in the oil of fish and are involved in specialized functions of the immune system and in the production of prostaglandin for hormones.

★ GLA is considered a "Super Omega-6," which some studies have shown may help reduce inflammatory related conditions such as Alzheimer's, arthritis, asthma, dry eyes, eczema and psoriasis, to name a few. It may also reduce symptoms of nerve pain in people with diabetic neuropathy, allergy symptoms, breast tenderness, premenstrual syndrome (PMS) and menopausal symptoms such as hot flashes and night sweats. Some studies suggest that GLA may help in the treatment of various human cancers, help to decrease high blood pressure, reduce heart disease and modify lipids to reduce triglycerides. GLA is also believed to help bypass enzymatic blocks in individuals with sluggish metabolisms due to aging, stress and environmental toxicity.

★ GLA can be difficult to obtain from the diet, as it only occurs naturally in a small amount of foods. Under normal circumstances, the body can convert omega-6 linoleic acid (LA) to GLA, yet it has been discovered that there are many factors that can interfere with effective conversion (stress, smoking, alcohol, processed fat/oil and sugar consumption, vitamin and mineral deficiencies [in magnesium, zinc, vitamin C and certain B vitamins] and certain health conditions such as cancer, heart disease, diabetes, thyroid issues, viruses, etc.). Hemp is one of the only plants to contain GLA in a bio-available form. This means the body does not have to rely on converting it. This makes hemp extremely unique and beneficial to those that may be too ill to synthesize GLA from LA.

★ SDA is considered a "Super Omega-3," and, excitingly, offers about five times the potency of the more common essential omega-3 we know as alpha-linolenic acid (ALA). SDA is powerful stuff! According to a study published in Journal of Nutrition (139.1 [2009]: 5-10), the structural benefit of SDA is that it is less unsaturated, meaning that it is less oxidative and much more stable. Can ALA be converted to SDA and then EPA and DHA? Sure. However, the extent of critical fatty acid conversions in the human body appears to be much less efficient and highly influenced by certain behavioral risk factors. The biggest one is poor food choices and the dietary habits of our typical Western diet. According to the research of Dr. Udo Erasmus (author of a considerable number of articles dedicated to the subject of fats and oils) about 95-99% of the population gets less omega-3 than required for good health. One of the main factors that interferes with omega-3 conversion is too much omega-6 in the diet. Omega-6 actually slows down the conversion of omega-3 (please review "Factors that Affect Conversion" on page 74).

★ Apart from sea vegetables, SDA is not typically found in plant-based sources and is rarely found in commonly consumed vegetables, fruits, seeds, nuts or commercial oils. Once again, hemp demonstrates its uniqueness. This makes it highly beneficial to those whose health is compromised and incapable of synthesizing SDA from ALA.

The King of All Oils!

According to Manitoba Harvest, one tablespoon of hemp seed oil will provide you with the following numbers of omega-3-6-9:

★ Omega-3 (ALA): approx. 2.4 grams
★ Omega-3 (SDA): approx. 140 mg
★ Omega-6 (LA): approx. 8 grams
★ Omega-6 (GLA): approx. 420 mg
★ Omega-9 (Oleic Acid): approx. 2 grams

What makes hemp seed oil the king of all oils in my book? Aside from the fact that hemp seed oil is truly unique among all other plant-based oils – being that it contains all of the essential fatty acids, including GLA and SDA – hemp seed oil provides each of the essential fatty acids in the perfect balance for maintaining and improving health. Furthermore, it furnishes us with the following nutrients:

- ★ Antioxidants
- ★ Vitamins A, D, C and E
- ★ Naturally-occurring chlorophyll: known to improve energy, circulation and oxygenation.
- ★ Naturally-occurring plant sterols: shown to reduce total blood cholesterol by an average of 10% and LDL (the "bad" cholesterol) by an average of 13%. These plant sterols are also recognized for protecting against colon, prostate and breast cancer.

Hemp seed oil's health benefits are legendary! Researchers around the world have discovered that it can help boost the body's natural ability to heal by supporting healthy immune system function, by improving essential fatty acid imbalances in the body and by improving cell growth and organ function.

Top Quality Choice Hemp Seed Oil

My favorite source for raw, organic, cold-pressed hemp seed oil is Manitoba Harvest. I really like this company and respect what they stand for – quality, consumer education and sustainability. Feel free to substitute hemp seed oil for any other oil that will not require heat. It has a deliciously nutty flavor that complements just about any dish.

> **Quick Tip:** Be sure to keep hemp seed oil refrigerated. As an additional little side note, when I use hemp seed oil to make a sauce, dip or dressing, I always add at least one teaspoon of coconut oil to assist in the conversion of ALA to EPA and DHA in the body. I suggest doing the same when adding hemp seed oil to smoothies. Always think synergy!

Wrap-Up

I give tremendous thanks to Dr. Ray Peat, Dr. Bruce Fife, David Wolfe, Dr. Udo Erasmus, Dr. Wayne Coates, Mary G. Enig and Dr. Mary Newport for shedding light on the mass confusion and many unexplained mysteries surrounding fats, fatty acids and oils. Their personal research, shared knowledge and support have allowed many to gain a much clearer understanding of dietary fats and their effects on the human body.

An important shift we can all make to improve the overall function of our mind and body is to replace all the highly processed and refined omega-6 polyunsaturated vegetable and seed oils with the following three oils.

- ★ 100% raw, virgin coconut oil: for a plant-based source of cholesterol free saturated fat that has the power to boost metabolism, halt sugar cravings, control weight and support proper immune function.
- ★ 100% raw, extra virgin olive oil (unfiltered preferred): for a healthy source of heart-healthy monounsaturated fat, natural antioxidants and anti-viral properties.
- ★ 100% raw, cold-pressed hemp seed oil: for its proper balance of omega-6 to omega-3 polyunsaturated fats, multitude of anti-inflammatory properties and richness in naturally-occurring antioxidants.

What Is the Take Home Message?

The more stable and less oxidative and stressed our food supply is, the more stable and less oxidative and stressed we will be. We are what we eat, absorb and assimilate – so choose wisely!

CHAPTER 4
DETOXIFICATION IS A LIFESTYLE,
NOT THE LATEST CRAZE

KEEP YOUR HOUSE CLEAN; TAKE THE TRASH OUT!

The human body was designed to self-detoxify from <u>normal</u> amounts of internal toxins it produces on a daily basis. This self-detoxification occurs as a result of the many metabolic processes our body must go through in order to keep us alive, energized and healthy. For instance, our liver, lungs, kidneys and intestines work continuously to clean out every cell, organ and tissue in our body. But what happens when we take these metabolic reactions for granted? Well, let me pose this question. What happens when we become too lazy to throw out the trash that we add to on a daily basis? The garbage bag can't do its job, and either overflows onto the floor or bursts from getting too full. The same goes for our organs. They become enlarged and inflamed and eventually start backing up, spilling toxins into the bloodstream. In other words, the excess ill effects forced upon these individual organs will inevitably spill over and affect other systems of the body.

Let's go a step further. What happens if you leave the putrefying trash and spillage all over the floor? It can start to attract all kinds of critters and bugs, penetrate the floor, get sticky or dried-up and become much harder to clean. Wouldn't it make better sense to routinely take the trash out <u>before</u> it created a ton more work and inadvertently invited a bunch of unwanted guests who started penetrating your space and damaging your house? Well, the same goes for the one body we have that houses our organs. If we want to keep viruses, bacteria, mold, Candida and parasites to a minimum, and want to keep pathological and pre-pathological cells from forming, then the human body must be able to detoxify efficiently and routinely. And if our natural detoxification system is being neglected and overworked on a daily basis (which it no doubt is in today's modern society), then detoxification needs to become more of a lifestyle and conscious effort – not just something we do between bad food binges and long stretches of physical abuse.

Never in the history of our planet have we been more subjected to such an overwhelming amount of toxins at such a frightful and towering rate!

All this external excess in our world today is creating internal havoc on our organs and bodily systems. It seems the more high-tech, commercial and advanced our external world becomes the more stressed, chaotic and less capable our internal terrain becomes. In our effort to <u>live</u> longer, we are in actuality <u>dying</u> longer.

Why Do We Constantly Continue to Complicate What Was Already Made So Simple?

Our body is naturally comfortable with whole food constituents. Not a bunch of synthetics in the form of vitamin/mineral isolates and pharmaceutical drugs. Not foods that have been significantly altered by the negative effects of heat and radiation, genetically modified, literally made and flavored in a laboratory or dangerously altered by an immense number of toxic chemicals and chemical additives. When we eat real food in its purest and most natural and organic state, our body intuitively knows what it must do and how to do it. Whole food nutrients are highly complex structures that provide us with a variety of enzymes, coenzymes, antioxidants, trace elements and activators, as well as many unknown and yet to be discovered naturally-occurring compounds. Only life can create life, which is why synthetics are considered inferior and potentially dangerous. Synthetics are not only life-less, they are not readily recognized by the body and can interfere and upset our body's normal rhythm and function. The potency of whole food or whole food supplements has much more to do with synergy than with actual nutrient levels. It is the combined effect of food constituents working together as a whole rather than the chemical effect of a single part that is of most importance when it comes to enabling the body to do its job. This is what makes familiar and naturally-occurring chemical compounds – found only in whole foods and whole food supplements – much less of an internal stressor; making them much less of a concern for developing any long-term ill effects.

Beware of the Impostors!

Synthetically altered "fake" foods, vitamin and mineral isolates, heavy metals, toxic chemicals and chemical additives, man-made pharmaceutical drugs and man-manipulated herbs are what I call imposters. Imposters are sneaky and sly! Although they may slip under the radar for a while, they are still considered foreign invaders that eventually disrupt our homeostasis and block or natural rhythm and flow. How does this happen? Many <u>unnatural</u> chemical substances closely resemble in structure <u>natural</u> chemicals our body truly needs, meaning they can easily get mistaken for real nutrients or neurotransmitters our body requires. I find it a bit disturbing that this type of invasion can go unnoticed for a good period of time. Why so long? Many of these imposters work as slow-acting poisons with a cumulative effect on the body. Don't forget, our bodies can be quite adaptable and ingenious when it comes to protecting us as best as it can, for as long as it can. But this shouldn't give us the right to abuse our body and push it beyond its limits. Especially once we become aware and conscious of the danger and disruption these imposters can cause. If we continue to downplay, ignore and deny, major imbalances <u>will</u> inevitably set in and become part of the matrix. Before long, our natural abilities and defenses will become weakened and the imposters will take total control, eventually breaking down.

As the old saying goes, "an ounce of prevention is worth a pound of cure." So, before we find ourselves in over our heads, we should want to learn to tune in and listen to our body's cues and internal wisdom. We should want to find faith and trust in our inner intelligence and guidance to do the right thing. Like anything worthwhile, there will be trials and tribulations. If you believe as I believe – that we are here on this earth as students, to not only learn from our mistakes and misfortunes, but to better evaluate ourselves in certain situations and fine-tune what is individually necessary – then precious time and efforts put forth can never be considered a waste of time.

When our minds are open and clear to receive, we can better accept our experiences as stepping stones towards success. Moreover, when we surround ourselves with like-minded individuals, we can learn from each other's experiences and get encouraged to turn what may seem like stubborn stumbling blocks into stepping stones to success. All in all, we must learn to <u>embrace</u> rather than <u>fear</u>. Because in this game we call life, learning to embrace will only help better guide us through what stumps or stops us from moving forward. What's more – it helps us help others to do the same.

> **The standard American diet (aka SAD) hijacks the brain. Not just the one in our head, but the one in our gut.** Did you know the gut functions as a second brain? The gut produces millions of neurotransmitters every minute. Therefore, if we continue to pollute our digestive tract with less than the best food, water and air, it can have a dramatic influence on our mental health (creating anger, anxiety, depression, etc.). Our food and drink choices, along with the materials they're packaged in, may just have a greater effect than we think. Especially when it comes to the choices we make, how well we respond to stress, and how we react in different situations. All the chemicals and plasticizers we absorb can truly influence how well our brain works. If we learn nothing but one thing, it should be that "everything is interconnected."

Stuck in a Rut

Have you ever stopped to think how much our eating revolves around routine, social pressures and emotions rather than the true harmony of our biology? Have you ever heard that our so-called food cravings are actually the body's cry for adequate and balanced nutrition? The body doesn't want pizza, bread and pasta; ice cream, cake and cookies; etc. It wants pure water, active enzymes, phytochemicals, vitamins and minerals. A lifestyle of popping pills, stuffing our faces and filling up our stomachs with toxic foods devoid of micro-nutrients is no different than duct-taping a baby's mouth shut to stop the crying. Do you desire quality of life and longevity? Only health-giving, organic, raw and living, whole foods hold the master key. Once again, this is because whole foods come perfectly packaged with synergistic components, such as mineral activators, co-vitamin helpers, phytochemicals and enzymes, that our brains and bodies need in order to thrive – not just get by.

False Hope in a Bottle

Don't think that you can fill in the blanks by taking a synthetic multivitamin or a bunch of isolates. They may work initially, but when taken long-term they may actually induce side effects that are difficult to identify and correct. The misbalancing of nutrients is no joke. For instance, if a toxic overload is created, it can burden the body and trigger a cascade of new problems. Another issue that many fail to concern themselves with is the contamination of raw materials. Many nutritional products have been either fumigated, irradiated or contain significant pesticide residues – even some labeled organic. Lastly, people need to become more aware of the toxic binders, fillers and flowing agents commonly used in the process of creating tablets and capsules. Consumed over time, these toxic agents can accumulate and create serious toxicity and absorption problems.

Learning to Listen to Our Body's Intuitive & Intelligent Guidance

It is important to keep in mind that each and every one of us is chemically unique and built on a different foundation. Therefore, each and every one of us is dealing with an internal terrain that is distinctively individual. This can make our bodily response to food constituents different from that of friends and even family members. So, practice not fighting it.

When a therapeutic effect is desired, the amount we take in can differ dramatically from what is <u>generally</u> recommended. But as long as it is whole food-based and free of contaminants (such as radiation, heavy metals, pesticides, binders, fillers and "glues"), then this is okay because we are building a new foundation. Once the toxins are out, balance can be restored and immunity can regulate. The next goal is to maintain this level of health. This means "when?" and "how much?" will depend on how one feels. Remember, this is not a fad – this is a lifestyle.

Also, let us not forget that each and every day is undeniably different and can bring a set of spontaneous changes and unpredictable challenges. Where we are in the present moment – physically, emotionally, mentally and spiritually – will predict where we need to go. This means nutritional requirements may need some shifting from day to day, week to week and month to month. Just go with the flow and do whatever it takes to keep centered and on the right path.

Allergies, or Toxic Overload?

An unpleasant feeling or negative response can be due to a number of things; some of which warrant serious attention. Keeping this in mind, never disregard your symptoms or take them too lightly. Unfortunately, conventional medical doctors are trained to treat the symptomology of a condition – not the whole person. This usually leads to the individual feeling all alone in their struggle to figure out the root cause of their problem before it spirals out of control. Personally, I suggest a holistic approach when it comes to addressing the primary causes and triggers of allergy or allergy-like symptoms.

Real food can be chemically complex. So, let's not throw the baby out with the bath water. For instance, many unexplainable symptoms – for which we so desperately want a diagnosis – could simply be a nutritional imbalance gone unnoticed or allowed to get too far. Don't be so quick to blame it on a specific food or food category. More often than not, many symptoms we chalk up and label as food sensitivities or allergies are in fact overlooked nutritional imbalances.

To go one step further, many nutritional imbalances are a direct result of the immense amount of environmental toxins and stressors we are bombarded with on a daily basis. These stressors start out by slowly interfering with the proper functioning of bodily systems until they eventually cause an accumulation of bad bacteria, chemicals, heavy metals, mycotoxins (mold), parasites and viruses. Then when our body is no longer able to absorb what it needs, due to this toxic overload creating such internal devastation, it can become hypersensitive to just about anything – good or bad.

Speaking from my experience as an oncology nurse, it is very possible to become majorly deficient in what we truly need to thrive when we become overburdened with toxins (both known poisons and synthetic forms of natural substances). Sensitivity or allergy-like symptoms could be our body's way of telling us that there is an imbalance somewhere that needs to be evaluated and properly addressed.

Please Note: Toxic overload is also a major concern for those who habitually make food and beverage choices that are fast, fake and foreign; even for those who are asymptomatic and appear to be well. Hmm… food to-go, or shall we call it deficient from the get-go?

> **Quick Tip:** Everyone can benefit from a whole body internal cleansing program from time to time. It is great preventive maintenance for all the major detoxifying organs and supporting systems. For an all-inclusive kit, I highly recommend the Internal Cleansing Kit by Blessed Herbs. For a cleansing and rejuvenating program that can be personalized for your individual needs, I suggest the product line by Premier Research Labs (PRL). Whether you work with a PRL trained practitioner, or put together a detox protocol for yourself, I highly suggest a particular order for opening up your body's primary pathways of elimination and detoxification.
>
> This is the order I generally like to follow: 1) colon and parasite cleanse, 2) kidney cleanse, 3) liver and gallbladder cleanse, 4) blood and lymphatic system cleanse and 5) lung and skin cleanse. Be sure to drink a lot of purified water and organic green juices during this time. I also suggest only eating organic non-starchy vegetables and low-sugar fruits. You may wish to incorporate colonics, enemas or sea salt flushes during this time to make sure you are fully eliminating and not reabsorbing toxins. Always seek the advice of a qualified holistic practitioner before embarking on any type of cleansing and detoxification program.

Symptoms of Detoxification: Nothing to Be Afraid of when It's for the Better!

Sometimes we feel lousy from what we're constantly putting in our body and sometimes we feel lousy from what's coming out. I like to equate detox and cleansing reactions to an exorcism. It's "the expelling of the evil lurking within." Without proper understanding and steady support, the temporary brain fog, headaches, fatigue, irritability, insomnia, chills, nausea, bloating, diarrhea, constipation, skin eruptions, body aches, cold and flu-like symptoms, increase in body odor and/or drastic drop in weight can rattle the faith of even the most sincerely motivated health seeker. But if you are eating as cleanly as possible, as freshly as possible and as balanced as possible, then have no fear, this too shall pass. Think of it this way: when our body finally gets some strong team players – and enough of them to put up a good fight – we are going to feel the effects of battle as our body takes back what the enemy stole. If your health, longevity and quality of life mean anything to you, then you're going to have to "pull yourself up by your boot straps," "get your head in the game" and repeat "it's not over, 'til it's over."

Please Note: It is unlikely that one will experience all of the above detox and cleansing reactions. Some may pull through without any side effects whatsoever. It all depends on the person.

CHELATION & HEAVY METAL DETOXIFICATION: WELLNESS TIPS AND TOOLS TO LIVE BY

There are many highly effective detoxification protocols out there to assist in the natural expelling of toxic metals. But in order for any protocol to be considered truly successful, a few important steps should be taken <u>first</u> before diving right in.

Step One

This is very important! If you are someone with silver (50% mercury by weight) amalgam fillings in your mouth, then I highly suggest the safe removal of these fillings by a well-qualified dentist <u>before</u> attempting to chelate and detoxify this form of inorganic mercury from your body. Deal with the root cause <u>first</u>! If the source of toxicity is known, as with dental amalgams, a protocol for removal should be discussed with a qualified dentist. Always do this prior to any aggressive chelation and intense self-detoxification program. The last thing you want to do is vaporize and mobilize this dangerous neurotoxin found lurking in your mouth at an even greater and faster rate than it already is. Exposure to mercury vapor is known to cause an accumulation of mercury in the brain and spinal cord, as well as the heart, kidneys and endocrine glands. It has been implicated in metal-induced autoimmunity with an emphasis on multiple sclerosis (MS), rheumatoid arthritis (RA) and amyotrophic lateral sclerosis (ALS). It can also cause chronic fatigue, emotional problems (including depression, anxiety and unexplained anger), brain fog and memory problems, muscle twitches and tremors, and a long list of mysterious and unexplainable digestive, endocrine, skin and heart problems (including elevated cholesterol and triglycerides). Scientists have proven that amalgam fillings are emitting mercury vapor 24-hours per day. Just think, every time you brush your teeth, chew gum and foods, drink hot fluids or grind your teeth – you are vaporizing mercury. It is literally penetrating the blood-brain barrier and entering your central nervous system (CNS). The brain and CNS are where mercury can do its most harm. When mercury attacks the nerves, it destroys the myelin sheath that covers and protects them. Think of an exposed/frayed wire.

Please Note: The removal of mercury amalgam fillings is no joke. You cannot just go to any dentist to have this done. You need to go to someone educated in the dangers of mercury; someone with plenty of experience in setting up their environment in the safest manner possible; someone who will avoid unnecessary exposure; and someone trained on how to handle this toxin for the safety of everyone. If this first step is not taken seriously, you risk exposing yourself and others to a large bolus dose of mercury that can make you even more toxic and potentially worsen your symptoms. Avoid setting yourself back on your wellness journey before having the chance to even start. Feel free to type the following link into your web browser in order to find a practitioner in your area that is following a safe amalgam removal protocol: http://quicksilverscientific.com/clinical/practitioner-locator.html

When it comes to detoxifying your body from inorganic mercury (e.g., dental amalgam fillings), I feel it is in your best interest to have a qualified holistic practitioner make certain that all three phases of the human detoxification system are functioning properly. However, if you decide to embark on a self-detoxifying program, I strongly suggest at least having some very specific blood work done. It will provide you with a baseline that can give tremendous insight on what organs of the body need extra TLC before and during detoxification (e.g., intestines, kidneys, liver, and lymph). When it comes to differentiating the two most common forms of mercury, and how well our body is excreting them, not just any lab work will do. I urge you to be proactive and ask your practitioner to order a Mercury Testing Lab Kit from Quick Silver Scientific. You may even be able to order it yourself. At this present time, the Quicksilver Scientific Tri-Test is the only clinical testing suite that measures both the exposures and excretion abilities for each of the two main forms of mercury we are exposed to. The QS Tri-Test utilizes mercury speciation analysis – a patented advanced technology that separates methyl mercury (e.g., that from fish) from inorganic mercury (e.g., that from dental amalgams) and measures each directly. Go to www.quicksilverscientific.com for more information.

Step Two

If you have had all your dental amalgams removed – or if your heavy metal toxicity is not due to dental amalgams, but due to the various other ways we are continuously exposed to heavy metals on a daily basis (environmental exposure, working environment, smoke inhalation, contaminated water, contaminated fish/fish oil supplements, contaminated high fructose corn syrup found in most all processed foods, etc.) – then the next step that is of equal importance, <u>before</u> jumping feet first into any type of chelating protocol, is to make a conscious effort and shift towards a lifestyle free from processed food. By wiping out conventionally grown, processed and refined foods – and eating more organically grown, raw and living vegetarian foods – you can dramatically start decreasing inflammation on major detoxification organs and bodily systems. This step is extremely important in prepping and maintaining your body for the safe removal of toxic metals. The main organs of excretion for heavy metals are as follows: intestines, kidneys, liver, lymph, lungs and skin. If these organs (and the systems they belong to) are sluggish and not excreting at an optimal level, <u>before</u> beginning a heavy metal detoxification protocol, there is a danger of becoming more toxic and experiencing more symptoms of toxicity.

Self-Supporting Your Body's Primary Systems of Detoxification

The glutathione system is the most important of the detoxification systems. It includes glutathione and the enzyme that works with it called glutathione S-transferase (GST). If this system is not functioning optimally, no matter what chelation or heavy metal detoxification protocol you choose, you may end up with more mobilization of toxins than can effectively be eliminated from the body. This can lead to circulating metals (as well as other toxins) getting reabsorbed and deposited back into the body, potenially causing additional symptoms and harm to brain and body tissue. This process is called redistribution (or re-toxification) and is possibly the most dangerous issue related to self-detoxifying heavy metals from the body.

Please Note: Glutathione is not well absorbable when taken by mouth. It typically gets destroyed in the stomach and during the process of digestion. Therefore, I would not waste my time and money buying capsules. Intravenous glutathione and rectal suppositories are the best ways to effectively absorb this vital nutrient and antioxidant. That being said, intravenous infusions can be expensive to procure and time-consuming to say the least. Therefore, I suggest the use of suppositories such as Xeneplex. It is an excellent and effective alternative. These suppositories contain glutathione, which is the "master antioxidant" that both the liver and lungs use to detoxify the body. They also contain coffee extract. Coffee taken rectally (not by mouth) increases the enzyme glutathione S-transferase that "turns on" glutathione. In addition to increasing this important enzyme, coffee taken rectally can dilate blood vessels and bile ducts to help aid in the removal of toxins faster.

Why can't you just drink coffee and get the same effect? It's hard to believe, but drinking coffee and coffee taken rectally have totally different effects on the human body. When coffee is taken orally, there are digestive enzymes and acids in the mouth, stomach and intestines which chemically alter caffeine and other important compounds in the coffee before they ever get a fair chance at reaching the inside of the liver. When taken orally, the caffeine in coffee can be very irritating to the stomach. Once intestinally absorbed into the bloodstream, coffee taken orally acts as a central and peripheral nervous system stimulant. This increase in activation of the sympathetic nervous system (which involves the fight-or-flight stress response) can add a tremendous amount of undue stress to bodily organs, making it counterproductive to the process of detoxification. On the other hand, when caffeine and coffee's other important constituents are allowed to bypasses the stomach and digestive system (via enema or suppository), all the relevant components get delivered directly into the liver (via the rectal veins that comprise the hepatic portal system) undigested, undiluted and fully intact.

Xeneplex suppositories can easily and safely be utilized as part of a total detoxification system. It does a lot more than just support the body in removing heavy metal toxins. As part of a maintenance plan Xeneplex can support the body in removing pesticides, herbicides, fungicides, petrochemicals, plasticizers, pharmaceuticals, solvents, dyes, artificial colors/flavors, aflatoxins, molds and the many other toxic chemicals we are bombarded with on a daily basis through our food, water, air and soil.

There is not one person on this planet who is not exposed to heavy metals and chemicals. Some may be more than others, but we are all exposed. How? We all share the exact same atmosphere. Therefore, when I get asked if I routinely cleanse and detoxify from heavy metals, chemicals and even parasites, my answer is yes, yes and yes!

Last but Not Least

Once dental amalgam fillings have been safely removed, and you have properly prepped your body – by improving your diet, decreasing inflammation and making sure all detoxification pathways are open – then starting yourself on nature's natural chelators can be the next and final step you take for continued detoxification and maintence. I strongly feel that this last step should be an ongoing and everlasting one. Especially if the ultimate goal is to keep your daily exposure to unavoidable stressors (our toxic load) down to a level that is not burdensome and does not cause over exhaustion to organs and bodily systems.

Please Note: It is unrealistic to think we can escape all the stressors in our life. However, by balancing and regulating our body's immunity and keeping our detoxification pathways open, our ability to respond to environmental stressors can greatly improve. By strengthening our adaptability, we can better keep the toxic effects of stress from interfering with our overall well-being.

If the plan is to self-detoxify, I cannot stress enough how important it will be to ensure that you are eating a supportive diet with all the right viable nutrients on a daily basis (e.g., whole food sources of selenium, calcium, magnesium, zinc and iodine). It will also be just as important to consume these foods at the right times and in the right order – especially when the best possible results are desired. For instance, studies have shown that cilantro (coriander or Chinese parsley) is a great detoxifier and capable of mobilizing mercury, cadmium, lead and aluminum in both bones and the central nervous system. However, due to cilantro's ability to mobilize more toxins then it can effectively eliminate from the body, it is highly possible that cilantro – when used alone – will cause redistribution of heavy metals. If cilantro is part of your detox strategy, I highly suggest using it in conjunction with a product that has some substantial binding power. *Chlorella pyrenoidosa* powder and Modifilan capsules (brown seaweed extract) are my top two go-tos.

Please Note: When it comes to heavy metal detoxification, I strongly suggest ramping your way up slowly to the therapeutic recommended daily dosage of chlorella (see page 158 for more on chlorella). If taking both chlorella and cilantro, I would take chlorella <u>first</u> (on an empty stomach) 30 minutes prior to cilantro. When self-detoxifying from the initial load of heavy metals and other toxins stored in our tissues, I also feel it is a good idea to add an additional intestinal toxin-absorbing agent to your regimen. Take the key ingredient found in brown sea algae (aka seaweed), for example. Brown algae is known to be high in a polysaccharide known as alginic acid. Scientific researchers, including a team led by Dr. Tanaka at McGill University, demonstrated that alginic acid has the ability to bind with any heavy metals in the intestines, rendering them indigestible and causing them to be eliminated. Alginic acid is abundant in sea vegetables classified as brown algae or seaweed, and includes kombu, hijiki, arame and wakame.

One brown seaweed product which I have grown to love and highly recommend in large amounts is Modifilan. Modifilan is the purest, most natural concentrated extract of the brown seaweed Laminaria Japonica. It contains life-essential organic iodine, alginates, fucoidan and laminarin. To learn more about these amazing elemental treasures found in the brown seaweed, and how they can help nutritionally balance your bodily systems as they gently detoxify, go to www.modiflan.com.

Another good option is to ingest a quality source of activated charcoal or bentonite clay. I prefer Premier Research Labs Medi-Clay-FX, as it is a rare smectite form of calcium bentonite clay with powerful <u>ad</u>sorptive, as well as <u>ab</u>sorptive detoxification properties. <u>Ad</u>sorption is the process by which substances stick to the <u>outside</u> surface of clay molecule – similar to the way a strip of velcro works. <u>Ab</u>sorption, on the other hand, is the process of drawing substances into the <u>internal</u> molecule structure – similar to the way a sponge absorbs water. Out of seven clay mineral groups, smectite is the only clay group with the ability to <u>ad</u>sorb and <u>ab</u>sorb toxins and other impurities. To boot, it does both at a greater rate than any other clay.

All three of the whole foods described above (chlorella, cilantro and brown seaweed) are not just great in aiding the process of detoxifying heavy metals (and other poisons) from the body; they also improve mineralization, keeping us from becoming malnourished in the process.

> **Quick Tip:** When it comes to viable, whole food nutrition, I find it easy to make a cilantro pesto which synergistically combines foods that contain many necessary and supportive vitamins, minerals, amino acids and omega-3 fatty acids. You will need these on your detoxification and cleansing journey to vital health and longevity anyhow, so why not kill two birds with one stone by having something enjoyable to look forward to in the process? Please see recipe on page 356.

What About I.V. Chelation Therapy?

I.V. chelation is an invasive treatment that can be very expensive, time-consuming and potentially dangerous if the body is not properly prepped and prepared for intense and aggressive detoxification. I know many people who have undergone I.V. chelation therapy and unfortunately ended up worse off than when they started. Why? I assume because they (including the administering practitioner) did not address step one and two above or continue to appropriately support the detoxification pathways (phase I, II and III). As a result, their bodies were not able to keep up with how quickly the metals were being pulled into circulation. So instead of effectively eliminating the toxins, they piled up in their detoxifying organs. Envision a major traffic jam on the freeway. A situation like this can overstress the body right into locking up and shutting down. Personally, I feel there are much safer ways to detoxify. And in the case of heavy metal poisoning, a slow and steady approach with an ongoing maintenance plan in mind is much safer. Remember, if your goal is to be in it for the long haul, there is no such thing as a fast and easy solution. Just stay positive and keep your eye on the prize.

Although I.V. chelation treatments are a very viable option and have their place, they're not right for everyone. I much prefer chelation suppositories. As long as step one and two above have been appropriately addressed, most anyone can feel safe with this method. What's more, it can be done in the privacy of your own home. It is also a lot more affordable. These are important points to consider when keeping up with a maintence schedule that is right and realistic for your personal needs and goals.

> **Quick Tip:** I like Medicardium EDTA chelation suppositories. It is Magnesium Di-Potassium EDTA in a base of cocoa butter. Unlike Di-Sodium EDTA and Calcium Di-Sodium EDTA (which tend to turn off the relaxation response and stimulate the fight-or-flight response), Magnesium Di-Potassium EDTA is proclaimed to have a calming effect on the peripheral nervous system by resetting the autonomic (aka involuntary) part of the nervous system. It does this by taking us out of the sympathetic mode ("fight-or-flight") and into the parasympathetic mode ("rest-and-digest"). In my opinion, calcium free Medicardium suppositories are the preferred method of EDTA chelation for several reasons. Some of which I discuss below.

As we age, the calcium pumps in our cells become less efficient, causing calcium to build up in all the places it does not belong. For instance:

- ★ **Calcium can build up in our soft tissue making us stiff and less flexible.** When calcium builds up in muscle cells, it can cause our muscles to remain in a contracted position. If this happens, we will eventually become stiffer and stiffer, thereby experiencing a dramatic decrease in our flexibility and range of motion. This can lead to an increase in pain and inflammation. A condition called Fibromyalgia is a great example involving this build-up of calcium in the muscles. The ultimate example would be that of rigor mortis after death, in which all the muscles of the body flood with calcium and contract. However, rigor mortis only happens after death.
- ★ **Calcium can build up in our arteries causing arteriosclerosis (hardening of the arteries) and atherosclerosis (the most common type of arteriosclerosis caused by plaque build-up).** Much of this plaque build-up is hard calcium deposits that have infiltrated the lining of the arteries. When calcification of our arteries happens, it makes them less flexible. Less flexible arteries tend to cause an increase in blood pressure and are much more prone to damage and rupture.
- ★ **Calcium can accumulate in the joints, leading to severe joint pain, degeneration of the joint and restricted movement of the joint.**
- ★ **Calcium can accumulate in the kidneys and gallbladder.** A major and contributing factor in the formation of kidney stones and certain types of gallstones (i.e., pigment stones that show up dark brown to black).

Please Note: To help support the body in dissolving kidney stones, gallstones and bile sludge (which, by the way, can help in resolving unexplained and stubborn issues with parasites, Candida, constipation and irritable bowel syndrome), I suggest the use of Glytamins suppositories. Glytamins replaces the dated kidney and liver/gallbladder flushes with amino acids and herbs that naturally support the body as a whole. Unlike liver/gallbladder flushes – which may get rid of stones, but tends to drain the body of bile fluid in the process – Glytamins suppositories administer three very important amino acids: glycine, taurine and phosphatidyl choline. These three amino acids are then delivered directly to the liver where they can get straight to work on detoxifying the causes of bile sludge and stones. The root cause being a deficiency in these three amino acids. When the root cause is not rectified, stones will tend to continuously form – flush after flush.

> **Quick Tip:** When self-detoxifying, I highly suggest the use of Glytamins along with Medicardium and Xeneplex. The combination of these three products synergistically forms a complete detoxification system which can and should be repeated every 4-6 months to obtain optimal health.

- ★ Calcium can even deposit in any of our glands such as the thyroid gland, pituitary gland, prostate gland and mammary glands of the breasts!
- ★ Calcium can pretty much build up anywhere in the body, causing calcification diseases that we typically blame on old age and the aging process.

In Conclusion

Medicardium EDTA chelation suppositories is specially formulated for health benefits that go well beyond the safe and effective removal of toxic heavy metals from the body. Toxic heavy metals include mercury, lead, aluminum, cadmium, nickel, barium, arsenic, uranium, thallium and oxidized iron. Being that Medicardium is calcium free, it may also help to reverse the aging effects of calcium build-up. It does this by supporting the mobilization and removal of toxic calcium from soft tissues and arteries.

The best natural detoxification system is the one you already have: your body's detoxification system. So, don't inadvertently work against your body by unintentionally clogging your body's primary filters. Instead, take it slow and gently work with your body.

To play it safe, I like to combine several different methodologies in an effort to decrease my body's chances of accumulating burdensome heavy metals and other toxins and impurities. These include, but are not limited to, the daily use of chlorella powder, MSM powder and camu camu berry powder (all described further on in this book). As part of my preventative maintenance plan, I will periodically include the use of Medicardium Magnesium Di-Potassium EDTA, Glytamins and Xeneplex suppositories; colon hydrotherapy, coffee enemas and sea salt flushes; dry skin brushing and saunas; as well as rebounding. Daily cardiovascular exercise, stretching and yoga are also extremely valuable to my ability to stay healthfully balanced. I choose to do all of these routinely and on a regular basis as part of my personal preventative maintenance plan. It has made a huge difference in helping me safeguard myself from the ill-effects of life's many unavoidable stressors.

CHAPTER 5
THE BEST OF THE BEST

The following includes SUPERFOOD, SUPERFRUIT and SUPERHERB "must haves" for every SUPERNATURAWL lifestyle.

> *A Superfood is any plant-based, natural food with a nutrient dense profile and health-protecting qualities. It is a food containing a high concentration of multiple constituents such as complex carbohydrates, essential amino acids, essential fatty acids, vitamins, macrominerals, microminerals (trace minerals), phytochemicals (phytonutrients), active enzymes and more!*

There are some powerful plant-based options for all the essential nutrients our bodies crave. We just need to be open to the truth and never, ever compromise on true quality.

One of the questions that people frequently ask me, is "how do you get enough protein?" This is such a great question, and I love addressing it because nobody associates a raw, plant-based diet with someone who can work out every day, has loads of energy and a good amount of muscle tone and definition. Well, like I always say – there's a <u>right</u> and a <u>wrong</u> way to doing everything. This does not exclude a plant-based raw food lifestyle. I'm writing this book with my full intention focused on educating and empowering others to make the best possible decisions based on my years of researching and questioning every painstaking detail. People who know me realize that I'm not someone who can take just anyone's word and be done. I need to evaluate all the variables and weigh out every possible option. I typically need days – weeks – months – and sometimes years of digging before I will say, "yup, this is good." It appears to be embedded in my DNA to be very analytical and detail oriented; which may explain my innate desire to want to learn and understand the physical chemistry and biological chemistry of just about everything out there. This is especially true when it comes to food and nutrients and how they affect the health and function of the human body. Once I embark on a new mission, I'm on a quest for truth. In the end, my only hope is that what I can share helps to inspire and motivate others to become more conscious and self-connected, with a desire to make better nutritional choices.

> *Along with the many superstars which I've already shared (avocados, coconut oil, green leafy vegetables and sea vegetables, to name but a few), the following are THE BEST OF THE BEST. I feel anyone can add and consume these regularly for balanced and complete whole food nutrition.*

HEMP SEEDS

Now I know I covered a great amount of detail about hemp seeds under hemp seed oil, but there is more! For instance, did you know that just one pound of hemp seeds can sustain a human life for two weeks? Moreover, just one tablespoon provides the recommended daily allowance of essential fatty acids (EFAs).

Can you imagine? Just one pound of hemp seeds can provide all the protein, essential fatty acids and dietary fiber necessary for human survival for a whole two weeks. How far would one pound of meat take you? In *Superfoods: The Food and Medicine of the Future,* David Wolfe comments that hemp seeds are packed with 33-37% of pure digestible protein. Hemp seeds are a much more digestible protein than meat, eggs, cheese, human milk, cow's milk and all other high protein food sources. This makes hemp seeds an excellent bio-available protein choice for everyone – from pregnant women, moms and babies; to athletes, bodybuilders and weekend warriors; to anyone suffering from acute or chronic health challenges. These tiny seeds pack a big punch when it comes to your health and nutrition.

★ Hemp seeds come well-equipped with all their original life-force energy, enzymes, phytonutrients, antioxidants, vitamins, major minerals, trace minerals, fiber and even chlorophyll intact!
★ Hemp seeds are considered by many to be one of nature's richest sources of complete and absorbable protein. The protein content in hemp seeds is higher than that found in nuts, other seeds, meats, dairy products, fish and poultry. Just three tablespoons of hemp seeds will provide 10-11 grams of protein. According to David Wolfe, only algae (such as spirulina and marine phytoplankton) exceed hemp seeds in protein content.
★ Hemp seeds are said to contain nearly every single vitamin and mineral needed by the body. According to David Wolfe, hemp excels at absorbing major minerals and trace minerals from the soil. These include phosphorous, potassium, magnesium, sulfur, calcium, iron, manganese, zinc, sodium, silicon, copper, platinum, boron, nickel, germanium, tin, iodine, chromium, silver and lithium.
★ Hemp Seeds are considered a gluten-free and allergen-free food. They can be enjoyed by those unable to tolerate nuts, gluten, soy, corn, dairy, eggs and sugar, as there are no known allergies to hemp seeds.

Hemp Seeds: The Most Complete, Edible & Usable Protein in the Plant Kingdom

Besides being an excellent source of highly digestible plant-based protein – complete with all 21 amino acids (including nine essential amino acids adult bodies cannot produce) – hemp seeds and hemp protein are superior and quality sources of the following amino acids:

★ **Arginine:** known to play an important role in cell division, immune function, the healing of wounds, removing ammonia from the body and the release of hormones. As a precursor to nitric oxide, arginine may also have a role in helping conditions where vasodilation is required such as in chronic hypertension (high blood pressure).
★ **Histidine:** known to maintain healthy tissues in various parts of the body, particularly the myelin sheaths which enclose nerve cells as they ensure the transmission of messages from the brain to the rest of the body. Histidine is also known to be crucial in the production of red and white blood cells.

- **Sulfur-Bearing Amino Acids, Methionine & Cysteine:** both of which are necessary in the production of vital enzymes within the body. In *Conscious Eating*, Dr. Gabriel Cousens refers to cysteine as not only an amino acid, but an antioxidant that is also anti-radiation. According to Dr. Gabriel Cousens, this high-quality sulfur helps to remove free radicals in the body and can protect against radiation (e.g., X-rays and cobalt-60).
- **Branch-Chain Amino Acids (BCAAs), Leucine, Isoleucine & Valine:** known to promote the healing of injured tissues, speed up recovery and protect against muscle tissue breakdown (catabolism) during exercise. BCAAs are important for developing and building muscles. Since they are so crucial for the proper functioning of muscle tissue, hemp protein can be a very popular choice for endurance athletes, body builders and anyone simply looking to maintain lean body mass.
- **Globular Proteins, Edestin & Albumin:** both abundantly found in hemp seeds in a highly digestible form. Unlike the proteins of whey, soy, dairy, peanuts and tree nuts (which are potential allergens), edestin and albumin are considered hypo-allergenic. Being that the protein in hemp seeds closely resembles that of human blood, consuming hemp seeds on a regular basis can provide individuals (young, old and everyone in between) with the necessary raw materials needed for proper immune system function.

> "The best way to insure the body has enough amino acid material to make the globulins is to eat foods high in globulin proteins. Since hemp seed protein is 65% globulin edestin and also includes quantities of albumin, its protein is readily available in a form quite similar to that found in blood plasma. Eating hemp seeds gives the body all the essential amino acids required to maintain health and provides the necessary kinds and amounts of amino acids the body needs to make human serum albumin and serum globulins like the immune enhancing gamma globulins. Eating hemp seeds could aid, if not heal, people suffering from immune deficiency diseases. This conclusion is supported by the fact that hemp seed was used to treat nutritional deficiencies brought on by tuberculosis, a severe nutrition blocking disease that causes the body to waste away." – Czechoslovakia Tubercular Nutritional Study, 1955.

King of the Plant Kingdom!

Compared to other seeds in the plant kingdom that are also complete in their amino acid profile, hemp may not seem all that special; however, what makes hemp seeds so exceptional are their innate balance of these amino acids. They naturally provide them in a ratio that is ideal for the human body. Also unique, is the fact that the protein found in hemp seeds comes in the form of globular proteins – 65% edestin and 35% albumin.

Globular proteins are precursors to some of the most vital chemicals within the human body, such as hormones. Hormones regulate all the body processes. For instance, hormones regulate enzymes, which are organic, biological catalysts that start, promote and speed up biochemical reactions. Hormones also regulate hemoglobin, an iron-protein compound in red blood cells that gives blood its red color and transports oxygen, carbon dioxide and nitric oxide.

- ★ **Edestin** is a high-quality plant globulin protein that is similar to protein found in human blood plasma. This makes edestin perfectly suitable to aid in meeting the body's cellular repair needs – such as DNA repair. Edestin has the unique ability to stimulate the buildup of antibodies against foreign invaders (such as bacteria, viruses and other pathogens, as well as toxins and antigens) as they enter the body. Also, it is a protein that is gentler on the kidneys, making it ideal for anyone suffering from kidney problems or who just wants to avoid kidney issues.
- ★ **Albumin** is a high-quality globulin protein typically found in egg whites and is considered a major free radical scavenger.

Another important point to bring up regarding the protein in hemp seeds is that it is free of trypsin inhibitors, which are known to block protein absorption. Trypsin inhibitors are commonly found in soybeans and soy-based products. In addition, hemp seeds are free of oligosaccharides, which are also found in soybeans and soy products. Oligosaccharides can cause upset stomach, gas and bloating in some individuals.

A significant number of people are becoming allergic to soy products, most likely because most all soy is from genetically engineered crops or grown with the use of chemicals. Hemp, on the other hand, requires no pesticides, herbicides or toxic fertilizers in order to grow and is not a genetically engineered crop. Hemp could be the answer for a much greener planet. With less pollution and fewer toxic chemicals leaching into our food and water supply, we would have much less people becoming overwhelmed by toxins and getting sick.

As a little side note, I've recommended hemp seeds and hemp protein powder for smoothies to a number of individuals and the report back is always that it did not cause bloating or gas like the many soy, whey or other proteins on the market did. My hunch is because this is a highly digestible protein our body loves and thanks us for. Unlike soy, which has super high amounts of phytic acid (the anti-nutrient that prevents us from absorbing minerals), hemp contain no phytic acid whatsoever. This is just another reason to choose hemp as a base for smoothies over soy-based products.

Please Note: Even certain nuts, such as the popularized almond, contain high amounts of phytic acid. Therefore, be sure to soak almonds for at least 8-12 hours before consuming or making into nut mylk.

How to Use Hemp Seeds

The recommended minimum daily intake for adults is about 4-6 tablespoons (more for athletes). For teenagers, anywhere from 2-4 tablespoons is a good start (depending on their size and activity level). For small children, I would start with 1-3 tablespoons.

> **Quick Tip:** I love adding a few tablespoons of hemps seeds to my morning smoothie. I also love mixing a few tablespoons in a small glass mason jar along with raw coconut flakes, bee pollen, cacao beans, goji berries or golden berries and snacking on this powered up blend throughout the day. Just pack it in a small cooler with a spoon and away you go! Due to their higher and more bio-available protein and mineral content, I even find them more filling as a salad seed than your traditional pumpkin, sunflower or sesame seeds. I also love making a fabulous hemp pesto sauce with them that I enjoy over spiralized zucchini and kelp noodles. Please see recipe on page 357.

The Best Source for Quality Hemp Seeds

I consider Manitoba Harvest one of the world's leading hemp food suppliers. They are truly passionate when it comes to nutrition, education, community and sustainability. If you are interested in learning even more about hemp foods, I suggest going to Manitoba Harvest (www.manitobaharvest.com) and checking out the number of articles and studies they have listed under hemp nutrition.

CHIA SEEDS

During the days of the ancient Aztec empire, long before there were phones or the internet, tribes could only communicate via foot messengers. Aztec Indian Warriors would go on 100-mile runs, traveling from one tribe to the next, carrying only chia seeds. Legend has it that these men ran for days on end sustained on as little as one teaspoon full of chia seeds in a 24-hour period – with no other nourishment.

> *Chia: the Mayan word for strength*

Chia *(Salvia hispanica L)* can be traced back over 3000 years to the Central Valley of Mexico. These tiny seeds were used as a staple food by the Mayans, Aztecs and Incas for energy and endurance. Chia seeds are known as the running food, and were also considered a medicine and used for currency. They were prized more highly than gold due to their incredible health enhancing properties. Chia was also noted to be the Aztecs third most important crop, behind only corn and beans. However, once the Spaniards arrived, they banned chia along with many other native crops due to religious and cultural reasons. Lucky for us, this ancient superfood is making a major comeback!

One of the primary benefits of chia is its high concentration of essential fatty acids (EFAs). What's more, it contains these EFAs in a perfectly healthy balance of omega-6 to omega-3 with a ratio of 2:3. This is in total contrast to the imbalanced ratio of 1:4 found in flax seeds. Coming out on top yet again, chia seeds are touted to have the highest content of omega-3 out of all plant-based sources – even more than our highly popularized flax seeds! Chia seeds contain a whopping 64% alpha linolenic acid (ALA) compared to 55% ALA in flax seeds. The other major plus are the higher amounts of antioxidants chia seeds have over flax. The high number of antioxidants in chia seeds act as a natural preservative. They preserve the integrity of all EFAs and other nutritive properties, as well as allow chia to be stored for long periods without the worry of rancidity. On top of all that, guess what? Unlike flax seeds, you do not need to grind them in order to obtain all the EFA benefits these little gems have to offer. The outer shell of chia seeds are easily broken down and completely digestible even when swallowed whole. Therefore, ground or whole, your body can absorb all the goods!

Did you know the human brain is approximately 60 percent fats?

EFAs are super important to the nervous system as they regulate the production of serotonin. Just by adding high-quality EFAs to your diet, you can allow your brain to produce an adequate enough amount of serotonin to keep issues of anxiety, anger and depression in check. All without the need of unnecessary pharmaceuticals!

Chia seeds are unique for many reasons, all of which are beneficial!

- ★ **Chia seeds are the highest plant-based source of omega-3.** Plus, their omega-6 to omega-3 ratio is ideal for heart and brain health. Just by adding chia to your daily diet, you can start to balance out the undesirable ratio found in the standard American diet.
- ★ **Ounce for ounce, chia seeds have eight times more omega-3 than wild Alaskan salmon.** Fish are known to be great sources of omega-3, but they can also contain toxic levels of mercury, along with PCBs and other toxic substances. The use of chia as an omega-3 source can prevent depletion of natural fish stocks. Furthermore, it eliminates the concern of the accumulation of toxin.
- ★ **Chia seeds are a rich source of bio-available protein.** Like hemp seeds, chia seeds are a complete protein. Depending on the source, three tablespoons of chia provides between 6-9 grams of protein (7.5 grams on average).
- ★ **Chia seeds are rich in minerals and B vitamins.**
    - o Chia seeds provide five times the calcium of milk, plus boron, which is a trace mineral that helps transfer calcium into your bones. The calcium in chia will not only support bone health, but parathyroid, kidney and liver function as well.
    - o Chia seeds give us three times more iron than spinach.
    - o Chia seeds have two times the amount of potassium as bananas.
    - o Chia seeds also provide us with vitamins A, B1, B2 and B3 and minerals phosphorus, magnesium, manganese, copper, molybdenum, niacin and zinc.
- ★ **Chia seeds are packed with antioxidant protection!** Chia seeds have been noted to have more antioxidants than red wine. They also provide three times the reported antioxidant strength of blueberries.

- A study by researchers at the University of South Carolina found that **quercetin**, one of the powerful antioxidants found in chia, can significantly boost endurance capacity and maximal oxygen capacity (VO2max) in healthy men and women who haven't had any previous exercise training. Therefore, the fatigue-fighting and anti-inflammatory properties of quercetin, found in chia seeds, may not just benefit the extreme athlete, but anyone battling fatigue and stress on a daily basis.
- **Chlorogenic acid**, another antioxidant found in chia, has been found to inhibit tumor growth and progression. It may also reduce the risk of cardiovascular disease. Chlorogenic acid is also claimed to slow the release of glucose into the bloodstream. This can be extremely helpful in reducing the risk of diabetes. In addition, it has been noted that chlorogenic acid can assist the flow of bile, thereby reducing bile stagnation and promoting gallbladder and liver health.
- **Caffeic acid**, yet another antioxidant found in chia seeds, may be useful in maintaining a healthy immune system, as well as work to reduce the risk of developing colitis, certain cancers, cardiovascular disease and other inflammatory conditions.

★ **Chia is energy enhancing and hydrophilic (meaning, they love water).** Chia seeds can absorb more than ten times their weight in water. This makes chia seeds extremely helpful in keeping electrolytes in check and the body well hydrated for long periods of time. For someone like me, who thrives on some form of physical fitness every day, chia is one of my top superfoods. With chia being one of the most abundant sources of EFAs (especially anti-inflammatory omega-3), a great source of protein and fiber, super high in antioxidants, rich in important minerals and hydrophilic, chia is a true winner in my book for just about anyone! This includes athletes, weightlifters, runners, hikers, bikers, hot yoga enthusiasts, weekend warriors – even those who are sedentary and want to improve their diet to achieve more energy. Who needs highly processed cereals, sugar-filled power drinks, bottled water with synthetic vitamins thrown in, or the dehydrating and adrenal exhausting effects of coffee and Red Bull, when you can add chia seeds to just about anything and get all benefit and no downside!

★ **Chia is gluten-free and has the highest amount of usable fiber of any seed, making it a great choice for keeping your stools and bowel movements regular and your blood sugar and cholesterol in check.**
- Fiber is essential for gastrointestinal health. It promotes normal bowel function and can prevent constipation, hemorrhoids, diverticulosis (the formation of small pouches in the lining of the colon or large intestine) and diverticulitis (when these pouches become inflamed or infected). Eating high fiber foods has even been linked to decreasing the risk of breast, colon, esophageal, mouth, ovarian, pharynx, rectal, stomach and prostate cancers, as a result of their ability to reduce and absorb cancer causing toxins.

Please Note: When it comes to transitioning into a lifestyle of fiber rich raw foods, the massive amounts of fiber and roughage can be a bit of a shock to your intestines; especially when coming off of years of cooked, devitalized and depleted foods that lack adequate fiber and moisture. Please do not become discouraged if you experience some initial stomach upset, gas and bloating. It is completely normal to experience these cleansing symptoms while all the fiber and roughage is internally scrubbing and brushing away old fecal matter and toxic build-up. I like to think of it as boot camp for your entire digestive tract. Soon you will be well adjusted with strong and toned intestinal muscles!

> When facing adversity, I like to remember this quote by Winston Churchill: *"If you are going through hell, keep going."* Meaning, do not stop, keep your eye on the prize and continue ahead until you've made it through. Nothing better describes how we should best respond to difficult situations.

★ Chia seeds are packed with both insoluble and soluble fiber; and both have different but very important duties in the body. **Insoluble fiber** acts like a broom in the gut. It helps to restore the optimal pH of the intestines by keeping food waste moving along, while at the same time dislodging and sweeping out toxins such as acids, parasites and microbes. **Soluble fiber**, on the other hand, acts like a sponge. It can prolong stomach emptying time so that sugar is released and absorbed more slowly; it draws fluid in so that you can feel satiated longer; and it can absorb impurities as it moves through the digestive tract, such as bile acids, cholesterol and other toxins.

Please Note: Be sure to take in plenty of purified, filtered water, raw juicy fruits and vegetables. Fluid is a very important part to this process being successful, as without the fluidity and continuous flow of bowel waste moving out, you can risk constipation and the reabsorption of toxins. Also, when you are able to eliminate waste regularly and efficiently, your colon is free to absorb and assimilate much more nutrients from all your foods.

- Chia seeds possess a special type of fiber that allows the seeds to form a bead of gel on their exterior when exposed to liquid. This gelling action helps to lubricate the colon, absorb toxins for elimination and increase peristalsis. Unlike flax and psyllium, you do not need to grind chia to a powder in order to obtain its nutritive and regulating benefits. In all forms, chia is known to be gentle on the digestive tract while providing a myriad of nutrients at the same time!
- Everyone is told to eat oatmeal for its good amount of fiber and for a healthy heart, but what about chia? One serving of chia, which is only one ounce (2-3 tablespoons), provides a whopping 11 grams of fiber. On the other hand, it takes one-half cup of dry oatmeal to add up to one serving and you're still only getting four grams of fiber. On top of that, oatmeal (whether it be the old-fashioned rolled oats or instant) doesn't even come close when compared to chia and its wealth of nutritive properties. Cheers to chia!

- Besides containing heart-benefiting soluble fiber, we also have the preferred ratio of EFAs and super high content of heart-healthy omega-3 to thank for the cholesterol lowering effects of chia. The research that I have dissected on chia indicates that chia seeds can work just as well as fish oil when it comes to lowering levels of triglycerides and LDL cholesterol, while at the same time helping to raise beneficial HDL cholesterol. You really do get the best of all worlds when you consume chia seeds – lots of fiber, antioxidants and other nutrients, properly balanced EFAs and loads of omega-3 to boot!
- The fiber in chia is not just great at helping to regulate the colon and keeping cholesterol levels in check but may greatly benefit diabetics and anyone trying to control or lose weight as well. This is because the fiber in chia slows down the metabolic conversion of carbohydrates to simple sugars. This helps keep energy levels steady and allows that fuller, more satisfied feeling to last longer.

More Chia Benefits
- ★ Chia is a sustainable and environmentally friendly product.
- ★ The high oil content in the leaves of chia act as an extremely potent insect repellent, eliminating the need to use pesticides to protect the crop.
- ★ Solvent extraction and artificial preservatives are never needed.

How to Use Chia Seeds
A typical serving of chia seeds is approximately 2-3 tablespoon per day for teenagers and adults. For children, I would recommend up to one tablespoon.

> **Quick Tip:** I use these tiny nutritional powerhouses in my smoothies just about daily! Chia seeds are incredibly versatile. Because they are so mild in taste, chia seeds will never dilute, cover up or add to the flavor of any food or recipe. In fact, chia seeds are known to help balance and distribute flavors instead. I find chia seeds particularly great to use in raw food creations when a thicker consistency or more dense texture is desired. For instance, they work fabulously when creating raw jam-like fruit spreads, puddings, superfood breakfast porridges and blended soups. The ability of chia to absorb fluids makes them ideal when looking to mold certain raw desserts such as cakes and pies. You can also use them as a substitute in recipes that call for flax seeds such as dehydrated cracker, cookie and bar. When in doubt, just know that you can throw them into (or onto) just about anything you wish!

A Daily Dose of Chia May Help Keep the Doctor Away
Due to chia being high in heart-healthy omega-3 fatty acids (which are known to decrease blood viscosity and reduce the workload of the heart), you should use caution if you are cur-

rently taking blood pressure lowering supplements/medication, or blood-thinning herbs or pharmaceutical drugs. Always consult a healthcare practitioner before altering any medication regimens on your own. Also, please make sure your healthcare practitioner is aware of what you are eating or taking prior to any surgical procedures.

Please Note: Unless you are going to use chia seeds in a wet recipe, or to absorb excess liquids from added too much water or water rich fruits and vegetables (such as blended drinks, smoothies and soups), then I suggest making a basic chia gel before just consuming them dry. This will allow them to hydrate before they have a chance to steel from the hydration in your colon. Chia gel is super simple and fast to make. All you have to do is place ⅓ C chia seeds to the bottom of a glass jar, add in 16 ounces of purified water, cover and shake until the seeds are well distributed, and then place in the fridge where it will keep for up to two weeks.

> **Quick Tip:** Chia gel is particularly handy for anyone wanting to use chia seeds as an effective natural remedy for gastroesophageal reflux disease (GERD), ulcers, gastritis and irritable bowel syndrome (IBS). With the chia gel already made, you can easily get a few spoonfuls eaten throughout the day. Another great idea is to cold-brew your favorite loose-leaf tea or tisane (or pre-brew and then allow it to cool) and use in place of plain water. This will give your chia gel a nice bit of flavor.

Where to Learn More About Chia Seeds

If you would like to learn more about chia seeds, I highly suggest the book, *Magic of Chia: Revival of an Ancient Wonder Food* by James F. Scheer. Also, Dr. Wayne Coates, who is probably one of the world's leading authorities on chia, has a couple of great books and several research articles published. All his brilliant reads can be found at his website (www.drwaynecoates.com).

CACAO

Thanks to David Wolfe and Shazzie, who literally "wrote the book" on raw chocolate, titled *Naked Chocolate: The Astonishing Truth about the World's Greatest Food,* I will try hard not to get too crazy, but with cacao being my absolute favorite food and ingredient (what I like to call my "sensible vice" in my disciplined life), I will forewarn you; I have a tendency to enjoy talking about it just as much as I enjoy indulging in it.

Before we go any further, I would like to personally thank and acknowledge David Wolfe (co-founder of New Horizon Health and TheBestDayEver.com) for constantly sharing his knowledge and experiences on the topic; Robert Williams for his continuous dedication to sourcing out and bringing only the best quality cacao to the people (and I mean the best in every sense of the word); and everyone else out there who is passionate about this sacred food and truly keeping it real. So, without further ado, I say "let's get down to it!"

Karen A. Di Gloria

> Much of the spark for my extensive research and in-depth search into the nutritional and chemical properties of cacao has been inspired by the passion and enthusiasm behind David Wolfe's sharing of knowledge and groundbreaking information on the topic for several years now. David Wolfe is one of the world's leading authorities on raw food nutrition and nutrition in general. If you are as fascinated as I am by this magical and medicinal food, I highly recommend *Naked Chocolate: The Astonishing Truth about the World's Greatest Food,* by David Wolfe and Shazzie. In addition, I really love *Superfoods: The Food and Medicine of the Future,* as well as *The Latest Word on Superfoods: Raw Chocolate!,* both written by David Wolfe. In my opinion, we cannot learn enough about the properties of raw cacao and the amazing ability it has to balance brain chemistry, elevate mood, increase alertness, focus and so much more!

What Is Cacao?

Cacao beans are the "seeds" or "nuts" of the cacao (chocolate) fruit, which grows on jungle trees native to the tropical rainforest regions of Central and South America. Cacao, otherwise known as Theobroma cacao, literally means "cacao, the food of the gods." According to history, the use of cacao beans goes back well beyond 5,000 years, and was consumed and highly respected by the Native Americans, Aztecs, Olmecs and Mayans.

Did you know that cacao beans were so highly revered by the Aztec and Mayan civilizations that they were used as currency instead of gold? Chocolate also played a special role in royal and religious events. The priests would actually present cacao beans as offerings to the gods and serve chocolate drinks during sacred ceremonies.

Did you also know that it wasn't until cacao spread across Western Europe that everything angelic about chocolate made a change for the worse? Yup, that's right! It was the Europeans who first combined cacao with refined sugar and fattened it with milk. The Native Americans preferred pure, bitter chocolate.

> *The manufacturing of chocolate, as most of us grew up knowing it, generally consists of heating the cacao beans at approximately 250°F – a process that destroys the world's most powerful, antioxidant rich food!*

Pure cacao beans are the food that all scientific studies on chocolate are actually referring to. Not chocolate that has been roasted, sugared up or diluted down with dairy; and certainly not chocolate that has been stripped, cut or altered with chemicals, preservatives, anti-caking and emulsifying agents. That was a "light bulb moment" people! Keep this in mind whenever you see any scientific study hit the mass media. Most likely the study has been done on a food in its pure, unadulterated form and not the over-processed, refined-to-death, synthetic, isolated and chemically manipulated versions. Nor are the studies ever based on knocks-offs. The food industry is notorious for teasing and enticing with knock-offs, so beware.

Cacao vs Cocoa

Although the two terms are related, there is a difference and reason for the different spelling.

- ★ **Cacao** is the term used for beans that are raw and unadulterated.
- ★ **Cocoa** is the term used for beans that are cooked and adulterated.

In other words, cocoa is the processed or refined product of cacao.

Dirty Little Secrets in the Food Industry

Did you know that most conventional milk chocolate bars and candies are only about 10-20% cocoa? Even some of the so-called "better" and more expensive chocolate on the market (sweet, semi-sweet and bitter sweet dark) don't reach 50% cocoa. As a matter of fact, manufacturers of higher quality chocolate candidly argue that mass production produces bad quality chocolate. Some mass-produced chocolate actually contains much less cocoa (as low as 7% in many cases), fats other than cocoa butter (like vegetable oils), and artificial vanilla flavoring – and for what reason – to mask poorly fermented or roasted beans. So, what's making up the other 50% or more of our fake chocolate bars, candies and other chocolate products? The shortened answer is sugar, milk or milk powder, flavoring and in many cases, artificially derived anti-caking agents and cheap emulsifiers.

Most of us are aware that refined sugar causes blood sugar disorders, but are you aware that refined sugars are known to leach important life-sustaining minerals right out of the body, causes dehydration and is one of the most chemically addictive, habit-forming substances known to man?

How many of us grew up with milk chocolate candies, hot chocolate, chocolate ice cream and chocolate covered ice cream bars? Who can forget the fun of pouring chocolate syrup in our milk or blanketing our ice cream with it? Unfortunately, according to European researchers, eating milk chocolate (or milk with your chocolate) will not raise antioxidant levels in the bloodstream. Results suggest that milk and other dairy products somehow discourage the body's ability to absorb the protective antioxidant compounds in chocolate. In other research studies on blueberries and tea (white, green and black), it was concluded that proteins in milk and dairy products, called caseins, are the culprits. It appears that when polyphenol antioxidants bind with milk and dairy proteins, the proteins block all the health-promoting properties of the antioxidants present, rendering them inactive.

What other food combinations can you think of where milk and dairy proteins could be cancelling out the positive effects of antioxidants? Here's my short list: milk or cream with tea or coffee, milk with fruit on morning cereal or oatmeal, milk or yogurt-based fruit smoothies, yogurt or cottage cheese as housing for your fruit, cheese on salads, creamy/cheesy salad dressings, vegetable dips and spreads, cream of tomato soup, cream of broccoli or spinach soup, cheese on just about every tomato-based Italian dish (which I grew up on) or cheese on just about everything imaginable (guilty as charged before my own "light bulb moment"). Hmm... just another reason for why milk doesn't do your body good!

Did you know that most conventional cocoa powders on the market are treated with alkaline salts (such as potassium carbonate, sodium carbonate, sodium hydroxide, etc.), all of which neutralize the naturally-occurring acids and make the powder easier to dissolve in liquids? Are you aware that these are the same alkaline salts used in dishwashing detergents? According to material safety data sheets (MSDS) on these substances, they can be toxic and considered poisonous!

* An MSDS sheet for **potassium carbonate** stated the following – "Ingestion: Ingestion may cause irritation and burns from the mouth to the stomach. Ingesting massive amounts may cause ulcerations, vomiting and death from shock."
* An MSDS sheet for **sodium carbonate** stated the following – "Ingestion: Sodium carbonate is only slightly toxic, but large doses may be corrosive to the gastrointestinal tract where symptoms may include severe abdominal pain, vomiting, diarrhea, collapse and death."
* An MSDS sheet for **sodium hydroxide** stated the following – "Ingestion: Corrosive! Swallowing may cause severe burns of mouth, throat and stomach. Severe scarring of tissue and death may result. Symptoms may include bleeding, vomiting, diarrhea and fall in blood pressure. Damage may appear days after exposure."

Alkalized cocoa powder is used in ice cream, hot cocoa mixes, candies, beverages and chocolate syrups where a full-bodied, smooth, chocolate flavor is desired. But buyers beware – you are being duped and deceived. Unfortunately, while you may think alkalized cocoa powder is more palatable and convenient, the processing that alkalized cocoa powder undergoes substantially reduces or destroys all the antioxidant value. It also devalues a tremendous amount of all the other health-giving properties pure cacao beans are prized for.

Cocoa powder may also contain added starch (e.g. corn starch) to keep it from caking during storage. Corn is everywhere, and in everything! Corn is one of the most genetically modified crops in the U.S., at a whopping 85% GM. Even higher than corn are the following: sugar beets (95% GM), soy (91% GM), cotton (88% GM) and canola (85% GM). People around the world have joined forces to refuse GM foods and crops because of the dangers they present to our health and the future of our food supply. For instance, years ago France and several other European countries banned Monsanto's corn along with many other genetically modified food crops. Great for them! But why are we so far behind? Are we so distracted by illusions, that we have lost touch with what is truly sacred and real? Are we allowing the world's perception of Americans to be fact? Other countries already have us tagged as "naive," "ignorant" and "stupid." And trust me, there's raw data and statistics to prove this statement. I say it's time to wake up and smell the real cacao!

Are you aware that much of our mass-produced chocolate contains another genetically modified crop in the form of soy lecithin? Although there are a few higher quality manufacturers that prefer to exclude this ingredient for purity reasons (and to remain GM free), there are many who don't care what they're adding in just as long as that perfectly smooth texture is achieved. In many cases, lecithin is chemically extracted from soybeans using hexane, a constituent of gasoline. Oh yum, just what I wanted!

Another cheap emulsifying agent that some manufacturers use (such as Hershey and Nestles) is polyglycerol polyricinoleate (PGPR). PGPR is an artificial emulsifier made from castor oil which allows chocolate makers to reduce the amount of cacao butter while maintaining the same mouth feel. PGPR is virtually always paired with lecithin (or some other plastic, viscosity-reducing agent in the mass-production of chocolate making).

> *"Biochemically, love is just like eating large amounts of chocolate."*
> *– John Milton (Al Pacino) in The Devil's Advocate*

According to David Wolfe, raw chocolate straddles the line between a food and a powerful, potent medicine. Cacao beans contain over 1,200 chemically identifiable constituents! This makes cacao the most uniquely complex food on planet earth. But buyer beware – the overall quality, antioxidant and nutritional value of any chocolate, including raw cacao products, greatly depends on place of origin (where it was grown), cacao variety (sub-species) and post-harvesting practices (the fermentation and drying process).

According to ORAC (Oxygen Radical Absorbance Capacity) antioxidant laboratory analysis, raw cacao contains the highest concentration of antioxidants of any known food in the world!

- ★ Polyphenols are a class of antioxidants found in cacao which can also be found in a plentiful array of fresh fruits and vegetables, berries, nuts, seeds, teas, herbs and spices. As a general rule, the deeper and more vibrant the color, the more antioxidant power it will have.
- ★ Cacao is particularly high in a subclass of polyphenols called flavanols (catechins and Proanthocyanidins), which are actually a subclass of flavonoids.
- ★ Scientists theorize that plants naturally produce antioxidants to help them survive harsh growing conditions and to protect them from environmental stresses. Therefore, the same compounds that protect plants can in turn protect us – but only when we eat them as close to their natural state as possible. As nature intended. Antioxidants work by protecting our cells from damaging molecules called free radicals. As we learned earlier on, free radicals are basically unstable oxygen molecules which can negatively trigger changes in normally healthy cells, thereby destroying their positive bodily functions.

> *The ORAC value of a high-quality raw and unsweetened cacao powder is approximately 95,500. The ORAC value of heated and processed cocoa powder is approximately 26,000.*

Our bodies have systems to deal with free radicals, but with increased stress, excessive exercise, poor dietary choices, cigarette smoking, prescription and over-the-counter drug use, alcohol consumption, environmental pollution and other toxic exposures, our bodily systems become overwhelmed. Any combination of the above can lead to early deterioration, degeneration and aging. Now, no one that I've ever known chooses to age earlier; especially if aging means looking and feeling like death warmed over. In fact, most of us would like to dive head first into the fountain of youth. So, what is the best advice I can give for keeping that youthful glow and spring in your step? No, it's not putting your plastic surgeon's number on speed-dial. I guess that's fine if you have a fetish for looking like a plastic doll on the outside, while feeling like hell and looking like a rotted, putrefied zombie on the inside. The answer is also not in the next anti-aging cream manufacturers would love for you to bathe in. What I'm talking about has to do with beautifying yourself from the inside out. You can start by re-charging your antioxidant power. How? By consuming a sufficient amount of fresh fruits and vegetables, raw and living sprouts, low-temperature steeped white and green loose-leaf teas and introducing small amounts of a variety of superfoods such as hemp, chia, goji berries and cacao into your day. Raw cacao has every food beat, and even supersedes the well-known antioxidant superstars such as acai, goji berries and pomegranates. By eating a small amount of quality, organically grown superfoods throughout the day, every day, you wouldn't need a cupboard of isolated synthetic drugs and supplements. Raw chocolate instead of pills – how does it get any better than this?

Raw cacao is the #1 natural food source of magnesium! Magnesium is the most deficient major mineral in the typical Western diet. Did you know that over 80% of Americans are chronically deficient in magnesium? No wonder four million Americans suffer from frequent constipation! Are you aware that approximately $725 million is spent on over-the-counter (OTC) laxative products per year in America? Not only are most Americans not consuming enough fiber and liquids – in the form of water-rich foods and pure, quality drinking water – to counter balance this "royal pain in the butt" of constipation; the majority of Americans are suffering from severe mineral deprivation issues. Even our conventional fruits and vegeta-bles are being grown in mineral deficient soil, so we certainly can't count on these foods to give us enough of what we essentially need to fill in nutritional gaps.

> In his book, *Diet for a New America*, John Robbins states that the U.S. has lost as much as 75% of its mineral rich topsoil in the past 200 years.

Sick and starving soil means sick and starving plants, which then equates to sick and starving animals and people. This is where superfoods come into play. With a variety of superfoods dispersed throughout the day, we don't need to feel like a bunch of grazing cows, waiting for the "mineral quota reached" alarm to ding. There is no doubt that everyone can benefit from adding a lot more greens to their diet; but who has time to eat a pound or more of greens per day? It is a goal worth striving for, but the amount necessary is not realistic for the vast ma-jority. I get pretty darn close, which I'm quite proud of, but it's not as fun and exciting as add-ing and experimenting with superfoods on a daily basis to fill in the gaps.

Cacao has enough magnesium to help reverse various deficiencies. Magnesium is one of the top five essential minerals needed in over 300 biochemical reactions in the body. Magne-sium aids in the body's absorption of calcium and plays a key role in the strength and for-mation of bones and teeth. Magnesium is also vital for maintaining a healthy heart. It pro-motes normal blood pressure, keeps heart rhythms steady and can improve cholesterol. It also helps maintain proper muscle function, as it works to keep muscles properly relaxed and increases flexibility. Research has shown that magnesium can also support a healthy immune system; regulate blood sugar levels; relieve bronchial spasms in the lungs (asthma, chronic bronchitis, etc.); protect hearing from excess noise; improve parathyroid function (calcium regulation in the bloodstream); improve the bio-availability of Vitamin B6; help improve the functioning of the nerves; promote quality sleep; and be instrumental in energy metabolism and protein synthesis.

Cacao contains a high level of iron. Iron exists in every cell of our body and affects our body's ability to deliver oxygen to all its parts. A deficiency of iron may lead to anemia, a condition marked by severe fatigue, shortness of breath, cognitive problems and cold extremities.

Cacao is high in the beautifying mineral sulfur. Sulfur is an amazing mineral with a historical reputation for healing various conditions and alleviating the symptoms of many disorders.

- ★ Sulfur helps to keep hair, fingernails and skin lustrous, strong and healthy. It plays an important role in the production of collagen (the protein found in connective tissue), which helps to improve and maintain skin elasticity. It also helps wounds to heal better and faster.
- ★ Sulfur helps the body rid itself of toxins, which is why it is known as a body detoxifier. It is also known to play a significant role in heavy metal detoxification. Sulfur increases blood circulation, detoxifies the liver, promotes the flow of bile and supports healthy pancreas functioning.
- ★ Sulfur is remarkable at relieving pain and inflammation. From sore and tight muscles after a work-out to joint stiffness due to arthritis, consuming more sulfur-rich foods and supplementing with a clean source of methyl-sulfonyl-methane (aka MSM) can be a tremendous help (see page 152 for more on MSM).
- ★ Increasing your sulfur intake will help to restore the flexibility and permeability of cell walls. This in turn allows water and nutrients to flow into the cell with ease and harmful substances and toxins to flow out.
- ★ Sulfur helps protect the fat layer in the brain and is believed by many to repair the white matter on the end of every nerve in the body, called the myelin sheath. The main function of the myelin sheath is to allow rapid and efficient transmission of impulses along the nerve cells. When this insulating sheath surrounding nerve cells is damaged, nerve impulses slow down or stop. This often happens with autoimmune diseases (such as multiple sclerosis and Guillain-Barre), errors in metabolism and infections. With multiple sclerosis (MS), your immune system destroys the myelin sheath of your central nervous system (brain and spinal cord); while with Guillain-Barre your immune system destroys the myelin sheath of your peripheral nervous system (the nerves outside the brain and spinal cord).
- ★ Sulfur also plays a key role in the metabolism of several important B-complex vitamins, including B1, B5 and biotin.

Cacao is rich in the following important trace minerals:

- ★ **Chromium:** Chromium is essential for the metabolism of carbohydrates and also helps balance blood sugar, which is beneficial for people with diabetes.

- **Manganese:** Research suggests that manganese possesses powerful antioxidant properties which can help combat the damaging effects of free radicals. It plays an important role in the proper growth and maintenance of healthy bones and cartilage, as well as in the formation of synovial fluid, which is known to lubricate joints. Manganese is also known to activate various enzymes in the body required for proper digestion. It allows the body to convert protein and fat into energy, and is involved in blood sugar regulation. Manganese enhances the absorption of B1 and vitamin E and works with all B-complex vitamins to combat anxiety, depression and other nervous system disorders. It improves the function of the thyroid gland and helps maintain a healthy reproductive system.
- **Zinc:** Zinc is involved in thousands of vital enzymatic reactions throughout the body and has a wide range of functions. Zinc is particularly important for healthy skin, boosting immunity and fighting infections. It has been noted that men need more zinc than women due to high concentrations found in the prostate gland and semen. Zinc appears to be more bio-available once we have detoxified our bodies of heavy metals (like cadmium).
- **Copper:** Copper is required to make an enzyme that keeps your arteries from hardening and possibly rupturing. It is required for the synthesis of phospholipids, a class of fats found in the myelin sheath that surrounds and protects the nerves. Copper plays a significant role in bone and connective tissue health. Copper also influences the production of collagen, keeping the skin supple. It has anti-inflammatory properties, benefiting those suffering from arthritic joint pain. It also aids in the absorption of iron, which helps to balance hemoglobin levels in the bloodstream. It can regulate good and bad cholesterol levels, thereby improving and maintaining heart health. Copper is a well-known component of melanin, which pigments the skin, hair and eyes. Copper is vital to the proper functioning of the thyroid gland; especially in the production and absorption of thyroid hormones.

Cacao in its raw form (and raw form only) contains valuable vitamin C. Humans do not synthesize vitamin C; therefore, it must be obtained through the diet. All roasted and processed chocolate contain zero vitamin C. Water-soluble vitamin C is responsible for a multitude of functions throughout the body. Vitamin C is a powerful antioxidant and can protect the body from free radical damage. It stimulates collagen production, which works like netting by holding our cells and organs together. It assists our immune system and can speed the healing of wounds and bruises. Vitamin C also keeps our gums healthy and strong. In summary, vitamin C is essential for proper cell growth, healing and the repair of tissues.

Cacao contains essential omega-6 fatty acids. In contrast to raw cacao, roasted and processed chocolate contains unhealthy, rancid omega-6 fatty acids which can set off the body's inflammatory response when eaten. Once the cacao beans are roasted they are automatically considered "damaged goods" with nothing left to brag about.

Cacao: The Perfect Food for a Happy Mood

How is it that we marvel at the constant advances being made in our world of modern technology and communications – only wanting the latest and greatest TVs, computers and cell phones, and will do anything to keep them operating smoothly – but when it comes to our built-in communication system, we fail to appreciate it, and tend to take it for granted? According to numerous experts, the brain stands as the most underrated organ in the body, yet it controls everything. People compare the inside of a computer to the human brain constantly, but truth be told, there is no technology that can compare to the vast complexity of the human brain.

> *David Wolfe describes cacao as "Nature's Prozac" due to its many mental and emotional amplifying abilities.*

Is It Time to Upgrade?

Next time you think about "upgrading" your tech toys, stop and think about what you do for the precision and performance of your body's very own control center – your brain. You may not be able to trade your brain in for a new one, but you can always "upgrade" your food choices. Sourcing the cleanest and purest raw cacao is one way to start.

Keep Those Synapses Firing!

I refer to cacao as "food with a complexity of pure and utter greatness." So, let's indulge a bit more and try wrapping our minds around the amazing chemical compounds found in this mystifying food.

ANANDAMIDE

Anandamide is also known as the "Bliss Chemical." This is due to its ability to activate inner bliss and tranquility.

> *According to David Wolfe, anandamide has only been found in one edible plant, and (drum roll please) that one edible plant is <u>cacao</u>!*

★ Anandamide is a naturally-occurring chemical messenger. It is produced by the body to help our brains process all sorts of sensations that can affect our mood and overall well-being. Besides making us feel great, anandamide plays a key role in appetite, depression, fertility, memory and pain.
★ Anandamide is defined as an endogenous cannabinoid neurotransmitter. It is naturally synthesized in areas of the brain that are important to the control of movement and cognition, including higher order thinking and cognitive engagement.
★ Outside of the brain, anandamide plays a rather important role in pregnancy. It provides synchronization between embryo and uterus. According to several research studies, a higher plasma anandamide level at ovulation, as well as a significantly lower level during implantation, is required for a successful pregnancy to occur.

- ★ Receptor sites for anandamide have also been found in the lungs. It appears that its function here is to relax the smooth muscle of the bronchioles, thereby improving air exchange and oxygenation.
- ★ Probably the most explored function of anandamide involves our body's natural ability to trigger its release in times of prolonged stress, pain and inflammation.

Have you ever been out for a run – or maybe right in the middle of an intense workout or endurance sport – and all of a sudden you feel extremely happy, exuberant and invincible, as if you were standing on top of the world? For years many have called this phenomenon a "runner's high" (since at least the 70s, from what I've gathered) and attribute it to an "endorphin rush." However, endorphins (for the most part) are much too large to cross the blood-brain barrier and alter your mood and state of mind – at least in the way in which endurance and intense exercisers describe. This little-known fact had many researchers scratching their heads for years, until one day in 2004 when a marathon running neuroscientist, Dr. Arne Dietrich, decided to perform a study involving runners and bicyclists. His findings were quite the "ah-ha" moment. Both runners and bicyclists had 80% more anandamide in their blood after exercise, with the greatest increase among the runners. Since anandamide is a very small fatty acid (definitely small enough to easily cross the blood-brain barrier), the "runner's high" theory finally had more solid, scientific proof.

For me, anandamide is the most logical explanation; therefore, it takes home the gold. This is not to say that endorphins (our body's own natural opiate-like painkillers) don't have a role to play, or that it's not possible that they kick in when the body senses it is being overworked. However, that "in the zone" or "flow" phenomenon that many runners and athletes experience is most likely attributed to the synthesis of anandamide.

Who wouldn't love to be naturally intoxicated with bliss and happiness at any given time?

Do you ever wish that you could just stop time when that exhilarating feeling of euphoria sets in? Have you ever wondered why the height of that sensation doesn't last longer? According to research, that feeling of elation that anandamide rewards us with is rather short-lived due to an enzyme that breaks it down shortly after its release.

Wouldn't we all love to bottle that feeling and make it last as long as possible without the need for psychoactive drugs (legal or illegal) that may have harmful side effects? What about getting it whenever we want, without it having to lead down a destructive path of worsening brain chemical imbalances, dependency and more drugs? We can!

When we finally choose to see the forest instead of just the trees, we realize that no matter how hard we may try (consciously or unconsciously), we cannot, and never will, replicate Mother Nature.

Nature in its rawest form always provides us with all the answers.

In a neuropharmacological research study launched by Dr. Daniele Piomelli and his colleges at the Neurosciences Institute in San Diego, CA (published August 22, 1996, in *Nature*), it was discovered that cacao naturally contains not just anandamide, but two chemical cousins of anandamide: N-oleoylethanolamine and N-linoleoylethanolamine. What are these two anandamide-like compounds? They are naturally-occurring ethanolamide lipids. What do these two structural chemical cousins do? They act as enzyme inhibitors, delaying the natural breakdown of anandamide. What's more, they do this without attaching themselves to the receptor sites themselves. What is the ultimate effect? Anandamide (either our own or that which is found in cacao) remains in the brain longer, making us feel great and rather blissful longer! Heaven really can exist on earth; especially through the consumption of great cacao.

After discovering this, it makes total sense why I've been able to feel so clear-minded and energized, yet still joyfully relaxed and zen-like after drinking one of my post-workout/recovery smoothie concoctions made with raw cacao – and I'm talking for several hours after, mind you! I was intensifying and prolonging my own workout induced anandamide. Ahh! Pure and utter satisfaction!

Anandamide: The Brain's Natural Marijuana

What do moderately intense exercise, eating quality raw chocolate and smoking marijuana have in common? Surprise! It appears that the same cellular receptor sites that are activated by our own naturally produced anandamide (or by cacao consumption) are also activated by Tetrahydrocannabinol (THC) – the active chemical compound found in the leaves and flowers of marijuana plants.

Now, you may be asking yourself the following questions: Why then, does reaching that "runner's high" or getting "blissed out" on chocolate not result in intense munchies? Why would one not get that giddy and euphoric "high" commonly experienced when one smokes marijuana? How can it be that eating chocolate makes you feel "good," with an increased sense of optimism and liberation, but will not make you feel "stoned?"

- ★ First of all, our bodies naturally produce anandamide. It is an endogenous chemical, meaning that it is derived from within the body. Our brain and body already know what it is and what to do with it. Taking this into consideration, when our body absorbs a familiar or well-known substance (like anandamide) from a whole food or herb (as is the case with pure, uncontaminated raw cacao), it also knows what to do with it. How? Foremost, it is a substance the body is familiar with already. What's more, it is delivered along with various other familiar chemical compounds and necessary nutrients that the body requires or must have available in order to induce a positive effect.
- ★ The whole point behind whole food is proper balance. In its most pure and raw form, whole foods can promote or enhance balance and harmony within the brain and body.
- ★ This is not the case with unfamiliar substances, which can create imbalances or potentially worsen an already existing condition. There is no such thing as a "quick-fix" – just an easy cover-up. Remove the rug and the crack in the floor still exists.

> *Whole foods are perfectly packaged "all-in-one kits" that are harmoniously balanced just the way they are!*

★ In contrast, THC is a foreign substance to the human brain and body. It is considered exogenous, meaning, derived from outside the body. When THC is introduced into the body, it can mimic or block actions of our naturally produced neurotransmitters and interfere with normal brain and bodily functions. The same goes for synthetics and isolates. If any chemical compound is not in whole food form, or accompanied by synergistic cofactors, then I wouldn't risk it. There is a reason why natural and whole foods come packaged the way they do; so, let's stop complicating what Mother Nature intended to be simple.

★ Anandamide is a short-lived, fragile molecule which, as we learned, our body naturally tends to break down rather quickly. THC, and more specifically THC's numerous metabolites (which all exert their own effects), hang around for days. Not hours. Days! Once the acute drug effects of THC have worn off, metabolites of THC have a tendency to linger. In fact, they can linger in body fluids and the fatty tissue of organs for up to 90 full days. Metabolites reside in the fat cells of major organs such as the brain, liver and kidneys. It's the buildup of metabolites and their ill-effects that evidently raise the highest health concerns; especially the health of the brain and its cognitive functions.

★ To summarize a few points made by Dr. Piomelli in the previously mentioned study: the ability for our body to regulate and break down anandamide rather quickly makes it much less potent than THC or synthetic cannabinoids. Therefore, anandamide raises no concern for inducing a dramatic and lasting high. Additionally, even if the anandamide in cacao were isolated and could be made in concentrations that compared to THC, the body would still have very different responses to the two.

★ In conclusion, THC may be able to mimic the streamlined 3-dimensional structure of anandamide – allowing THC to bind at the same receptor sites and share (to a certain degree) some of the same and similar pharmacological characteristics – but anandamide and THC are in no way the same. They get handled by our body quite differently, yielding very different health effects.

> **Researcher Christian Felder of the National Institute of Mental Health estimates that a 130-pound person would have to eat the equivalent of 25 pounds of chocolate in one sitting to get anything close to a marijuana-like high.**

In order to better understand (from a general standpoint) how our body relates to familiar substances versus foreign or man-made substances, let's get a bit technical and continue using native anandamide and its imposter, THC, as examples.

- ★ Native neurotransmitters (like anandamide) are released from a pre-synaptic neuron for the sole purpose of sending a message to a post-synaptic neuron. Once neurotransmitter molecules get their message across the synapse (which is accomplished by binding to receptor molecules on the surface of the post-synaptic neuron), they must be quickly and efficiently cleared from the synaptic gap (synapse) in order to prepare for the next message in need of being sent. How do neurotransmitters get cleared from the synapse? They are cleared by dispersing into the extracellular space, meaning, they get reabsorbed and repackaged for future use, often times referred to as reuptake. They also can get broken down metabolically by enzymes.
- ★ The role of anandamide as a pleasure enhancer is rather indirect and limited. Not only is it a fragile chemical messenger that quickly gets broken down by enzymes shortly after its release, it can only bind to cannabinoid receptor sites in regions of the brain where it is already naturally produced. Furthermore, if that pleasurable sensation is to be prolonged, anandamide (either our own or that from cacao consumption) must be actively present and in the same place at the same time as its two anandamide-like cousins. According to Dr. Piomelli's research, cacao appears to be abundantly high in these two chemical cousins. Though, if you recall, these two chemical cousins (from a structural perspective) cannot lock onto cannabinoid receptors. This means we not only get to experience bliss longer by having an abundance of these two chemical cousins present, but that they also cannot hog the cannabinoid receptor sites away from anandamide.
- ★ On the other hand, THC is a rather robust bully of a molecule; when someone smokes marijuana, the THC activates all the cannabinoid receptor sites! Picture being attacked by a swarm of killer bees or a massive home invasion. This is why and how THC can create what Dr. Piomelli describes as a "global high."
- ★ In summary, THC has a tendency of overwhelming the nervous system. This ultimately puts the body in a state that is far from its normal equilibrium. Like so many other foreign chemical substance – including synthetic supplements and drugs – THC can be quite the invader and receptor site hog! This can lead to major problems down the road. So, the next time you're feeling a little down in the dumps, try reaching for the purest of raw cacao. It will have you feeling dazzled and clear, not dazed and confused.

PHENETHYLAMINE

Phenethylamine (PEA) is a natural monoamine alkaloid, or trace amine, that functions as a neuromodulator or neurotransmitter in the central nervous system. PEA is probably one of the more unique neurotransmitters found naturally in cacao. Similar to anandamide, it is believed that introducing whole food sources of PEA into the body can help give a boost to the natural amount in the brain. As a result, mood, energy and metabolism can greatly improve.

- ★ Have you ever been so captivated by a book, movie or activity that you lost track of time and the outside world? This is due to the elevated levels of PEA in the brain allowing that tremendous staying power and ability to remain super focused.
- ★ Chemically similar to amphetamine, PEA is a mild stimulant that the body produces naturally as a byproduct of the amino acid phenylalanine. The PEA found in cacao is sometimes referred to as "Chocolate Amphetamine" due to the subtle changes it can create in heart rate, blood pressure and blood-sugar levels; this usually result in feelings of excitement, increased focus, alertness and contentment. It has been discovered that PEA can improve mood and decrease depression quite similarly to amphetamines, but does not tend to result in the same tolerance or addiction. Again, this is probably due to the fact that we produce PEA naturally in our brains, so our bodies are set up to know how to handle it.
- ★ PEA is rapidly metabolized by the enzyme monoamine oxidase B (MAO-B), which prevents significant concentrations from reaching the brain. Because only small amounts reach the brain, PEA does not contribute to any discernible psychoactive effects. Interestingly, it appears that those suffering from attention-deficit hyperactivity disorder and clinical depression have been found to have abnormally low concentrations of PEA in the brain. On the other hand, producing abnormally high levels of PEA has been associated with the incidence of schizophrenia.
- ★ PEA is also known as the "Love Chemical," as it is naturally produced when we fall in love, find joy and passion and feel pleasure. It can be triggered during sexual arousal, orgasm and other forms of excitement. This is probably how chocolate achieved its label as a natural aphrodisiac food. If you are able to feel the effects from cooked up and diluted down chocolate, just wait until you try cacao in the raw! Need I say more?

Does this answer why so many women seem to prefer chocolate over sex?

Could this also be why chocolate is the #1 food favorite for Valentine's Day and has been for years and years?

- ★ Along with other "happy" brain chemicals, hormones and endorphins, PEA is responsible for the release of well-known norepinephrine and dopamine. All of these collectively and synergistically induce that energized, slightly euphoric, head-over-heels feeling.

> Did you know PEA surges in the brain in response to arousing visual stimuli? Ha! I wonder if this is why we commonly use the phrase "love at first sight?"

TRYPTOPHAN

Tryptophan is an essential amino acid that the body uses to synthesize the proteins it needs. It's well known for its role in the production of nervous system messengers, especially those related to relaxation, restfulness and sleep.

- ★ Cacao happens to be rich in tryptophan. Having the right amount of tryptophan on board can help prevent vitamin B3 (niacin) deficiency, as a small amount of tryptophan is converted into B3 by the liver.
- ★ Tryptophan also functions to serve as a precursor (chemical building block) for the production of serotonin. Serotonin is the primary neurotransmitter in the body that helps regulate appetite, mood, sensory perception, sleep patterns and temperature. Mind you, this list is in no way complete. With each passing day, researchers are discovering more about serotonin. One thing we know for sure is that serotonin plays a big role in our mental and emotional well-being. Without enough serotonin, individuals may experience anxiety, aggression, depression, impulsive behavior, insomnia and possibly even suicidal thoughts.
- ★ Once in the body, tryptophan reacts with broad-spectrum B vitamins (like B6) in the presence of magnesium (already present in raw cacao) to produce serotonin. Therefore, instead of chasing that short-term serotonin quick-fix by binging on high carbohydrate, yet nutrient deficient, chemical-laden foods, I suggest getting your dose through naturally whole foods such as raw cacao. Cacao has a tremendous amount to offer due to its whole food chemical complexity. **FYI:** Raw black walnuts, pumpkin seeds, sesame seeds and sunflower seeds are also good natural sources of tryptophan.

Please Note: I know most people think of turkey when they hear tryptophan. However, according to certain studies, tryptophan is heat sensitive and most likely damaged in many high protein foods that are cooked. The same goes for all the conventional processed and roasted chocolates on the market. If your goal is quality health through whole food nutrition, as it is mine, then if it doesn't say "raw," don't waste your time or money.

MAO Inhibitors

MAO Inhibitors-Monoamine Oxidase Enzyme Inhibitors (MAOIs) act by inhibiting the activity of the enzyme monoamine oxidase, thereby preventing the breakdown of monoamine neurotransmitters and increasing their availability in the brain.

- ★ There are two types of monoamine oxidase: **MAO-A** and **MAO-B**. MAO-A favorably deaminates the neurotransmitters serotonin, melatonin, epinephrine and norepinephrine. In chemistry, deaminate simply means to remove an amine group from a molecule. MAO-B favorably deaminates phenylethylamine (PEA) and trace amines. Dopamine is equally deaminated by both MAO-A and MAO-B.
- ★ MAOIs should not be confused with digestive enzyme inhibitors found in many grains, legumes, nuts and seeds. These rare MAOIs actually produce favorable results when ingested by allowing more serotonin, as well as other important neurotransmitters (mentioned above), to circulate in the brain.
- ★ In addition, due to the content of MAOIs found in cacao, raw cacao consumption appears to work as a natural appetite suppressant.

★ According to clinical tests conducted by Dr. Gabriel Cousens, MAOIs help facilitate youthfulness and rejuvenation. Children tend to have a higher level of neurotransmitters than adults. So how do we get that "kid at heart" feeling back? 100% unadulterated cacao! Now that's what I'm talking about!

THEOBROMINE

Theobromine is a bitter alkaloid of the cacao tree. The Greek roots *theo* ("God") and *brosi* ("food"), means "food of the gods." The suffix *-ine* stands for the alkaloid being a nitrogen-containing compound.

★ Theobromine belongs to the methylxanthine class of chemical compounds (aka methylated xanthines). Other chemical compounds in this class include theophylline and caffeine. Theophylline can be found in cacao but, contrary to popular opinion, is an irrefutably poor source of caffeine. According to the data revealed by David Wolfe, a typical serving of raw cacao beans will yield anywhere from zero caffeine to 1,000 parts per million of caffeine (0%-0.1%). On average, this is less than $1/20$ of the caffeine found in coffee.

★ **Where then does the stimulating effect of chocolate come from?** The answer is none other than theobromine.

How is theobromine different from caffeine? Although theobromine is a chemical relative to caffeine and can exert similar effects, theobromine does not affect the body by stimulating the central nervous system (CNS). Therefore, it is highly unlikely to cause the jitters and tremors that we associate with too much caffeine consumption. Instead, theobromine goes to work on smooth muscle tissue.

★ As a vasodilator, theobromine has a great impact on the cardiovascular system, meaning, it has the ability to increase blood flow to all the vital organs. Being a myocardial stimulant as well as vasodilator, theobromine has the ability to get the heart rate up, while at the same time dilating blood vessels – causing a reduction in blood pressure. Researchers also feel that this decrease in blood pressure may be attributed to the high number of antioxidants (flavanols) found in raw cacao.

Did you know that from 1890-1930, theobromine, the primary bitter alkaloid found in cacao, was used intravenously on heart attack patients in order to revive their hearts?

★ As a bronchodilator, theobromine has the ability to improve breathing quality and enhance the delivery of oxygen to muscles and vital organs. In fact, a 2004 study published by Imperial College London found that theobromine can suppress the vagus nerve which controls coughing even better than codeine, making it an effective cough suppressant. Another interesting fact is that theobromine can be quite helpful in the treatment of asthma. It appears to relax the smooth muscles found in the bronchi.

★ As a diuretic, theobromine goes to work in the kidneys. It can greatly decrease inflammation and edema by increasing capillary fluid filtration. This results in less stress and strain on the heart, lungs, blood vessels, etc.

When our brain receives adequately oxygenated blood, our energy, mental alertness and ability to concentrate can greatly improve. In the right amounts, this is the kind of stimulation that we should be after, as it can benefit the health and productivity of our vital organs.

Understanding what I know now, I prefer getting my stimulatory kick by consuming quality cacao and tea (such as steamed yerba mate or fermented pu-erh), rather than all the coffee and espresso I used to drink. I just make sure to consume them early in the day, otherwise my brain is on, and all I do is think, plan and create, rather than sleep. As much as I love being full of imagination and enthusiasm, I must admit, I also love bedtime and getting a good night of deep sleep.

Another plus raw cacao has over coffee is due to the presence of an additional methyl group theobromine has over caffeine. By having three methyl groups instead of two, the half-life of theobromine is increased. This means its clearance from the body is steady and slow; thereby making the effects of theobromine last longer in the system. This is great news for those who are tired of the energy roller-coaster ride they get from adrenal exhausting coffee, soda and commercial energy drinks – not to mention sugary, starchy and carbohydrate rich foods.

Please Note: If you are highly sensitive to even the most minute amount of caffeine (or its chemical relatives), it may be advisable to either use cacao sparingly or not at all; at least until the underlying issue(s) are addressed and resolved. If it's a concern, yet you desire the bounty of other benefits raw cacao has to offer, I suggest using whole, raw cacao beans or stone-ground, raw cacao paste in place of cacao powder. The bean's fat is still fully present in cacao beans and paste and will allow for a steadier break down, release, absorption and assimilation of the numerous chemical compounds. If you prefer using raw cacao powder (say, in your smoothie), try adding a quality, synergistic fat source, such as coconut oil, Brazil nuts, hemp seeds or chia seeds, to slow down the rate at which it affects your system.

In summary, unlike caffeine, theobromine can give you that increase in energy you desire without making you anxious, nervous or jittery.

> As a Side Note, Dr. Gabriel Cousens (world renowned physician, medical researcher and best-selling author of several books, including *There Is a Cure for Diabetes*) discovered the following during clinical tests performed on healthy individuals: cacao does not elevate blood sugar in the same way as caffeine-containing foods or beverages.
>
> As a matter of fact, Dr. Gabriel Cousens found that cacao has less of an effect on blood sugar than nearly all other foods, and may actually help to improve some blood sugar disorders!

DEMYSTIFYING CHOCOLATE MYTHS

Myth: Chocolate Causes Acne

SO NOT TRUE! Cacao, in and of itself, does not cause or increase acne. However, there are numerous studies which show a link between foods that spike blood sugar levels and acne. Did you know that Candida feeds on sugars, and when an overgrowth of this yeast occurs in the body it can cause acne, eczema and other skin infections? This means that refined sugars added to processed chocolates may be the culprit behind an acne outbreak. <u>Not</u> the cacao itself.

Myth: Chocolate Causes Allergies

NOT LIKELY AT ALL! A recent study showed that only one out of 500 people who thought they were allergic to chocolate actually tested positive. In its true form, allergies to cacao are quite rare. According to today's medical literature, allergies to cacao are virtually non-existent. When an individual says they are allergic to chocolate, it is most likely because they are allergic to one or more other ingredients present within the chocolate-containing food. Most of the chocolate candy and chocolate containing foods commercially available in the marketplace contain small amounts of roasted cacao mixed with a number of additives such as milk, nuts, gluten, corn, soy and caffeine.

Myth: Chocolate Contains Caffeine

LITTLE TO NONE! It is quite common to see references which confuse caffeine and theobromine; but these two chemicals, although similar in structure, have very different properties, effects and origins. Maybe everyone finds it easier to attribute all stimulating-type symptoms to caffeine, but in reality, there is a whole class of chemicals (with fundamentally different effects on the human body) of which caffeine is but one example.

The Biochemist (Apr/May 1993, p 15) did chemical composition tests where they precisely distinguished the difference between caffeine and theobromine. Caffeine was not detected at all in cacao; but they did continuously find up to 1.3% theobromine, 2.20% phenylethylamine, 1.54% tele-methylhistamine and occasionally up to 5.82% serotonin by weight.

Depending on the variety of cacao beans, caffeine can be either extremely low or completely absent. According to the research of David Wolfe, much of the caffeine found in industrialized chocolate products is due to the addition of kola nut or guarana seed. Both kola nut (the original flavoring for cola soft drinks) and guarana seed are stimulants which contain even more caffeine than coffee. In fact, guarana has been noted to contain approximately two times more caffeine than coffee beans. If you are trying to avoid the negative effects of caffeine (e.g., panic attacks, addiction, dehydration, PMS, insomnia, emotional fatigue and adrenal burnout), then I suggest consuming only 100% pure and uncontaminated cacao for your energy fix. Be sure to stay clear of all processed chocolate and chocolate containing products.

As Forest Gump says, "You never know what you're gonna get."

Myth: Chocolate Causes Migraine Headaches

FALSE! Moffet, Swash and Scott studied a group of 25 migraine sufferers, giving them a chocolate sample and a placebo sample (made with carob) two weeks apart. Each individual had to complete a questionnaire regarding their reactions within 48 hours of consuming each sample. Their findings indicated that there was no difference in headache occurrence after either sample. In a second study, the researchers repeated the same procedure with 15 of the 25 individuals, and once again, found no difference in headache occurrence after either sample.

In a totally different study, using a large group of women who suffered from migraine and tension-type headaches, Pittsburgh State University also found no relationship between chocolate consumption and the occurrence of headaches. Results indicated that chocolate was no more likely to trigger a headache than carob. Even among all the women who strongly believed chocolate to be a trigger food.

Myth: Chocolate Makes You Fat

ABSOLUTLY NOT! Cacao does not promote obesity in any way. That being said, all the refined sugar and dairy found in commercial chocolate candy bars and chocolate flavored confections will. Processed cocoa – and the mass-marketed products you find it in – usually contains hydrogenated fats and refined sugars (like sucrose), which can cause a vicious cycle of insulin spikes, overeating and weight gain.

- ★ A low-calorie, yet nutritionally rich and complex food, such as the raw cacao bean, requires more calorie burning energy from the body than the number of calories that will be extracted from cacao itself. This gives cacao a tremendous, natural fat-burning benefit.
- ★ Raw cacao also contains chemical compounds that increase serotonin in the brain. The appetite-suppressing effect of serotonin allows us to feel satiated for longer stretches of time.

Myth: Chocolate Rots Your Teeth

THE COMPLETE OPPOSITE! According to Dr. Arman Sadeghpour and a team of researchers at Tulane University – which included scientists from the University of New Orleans and

Louisiana State University School of Dentistry – cacao consumption can benefit the health of our teeth. The dental benefits of cacao are due, yet again, to its theobromine content. In this study, theobromine was compared to fluoride on the enamel surface of human teeth. Surprisingly, theobromine outshined fluoride on strengthening tooth enamel. Thanks to cacao containing theobromine, Dr. Sadeghpour states that individuals who eat chocolate can actually help their bone tissue. Imagine if we completely cut out the refined sugar that theobromine has to compete against in commercial chocolates and only consumed raw cacao in its purest form. I'd love to see the results of that research study!

Theobromine is also a highly effective antibacterial that can destroy *Streptococci mutans*, the primary organism that causes cavities.

Cacao: a few beans a day could keep the dentist away!

Myth: Chocolate Is Addictive

CACAO ITSELF IS IN NO WAY PHYSICALLY ADDICTIVE! If we're talking about processed chocolate and all its refined sugars and chemical additives, then we may have a good case to back up the physically addictive claims. However, if we are to base this statement strictly on the natural chemical compounds in pure, unadulterated cacao, then there is no supportive evidence.

Let's explain physical addiction. A physical addiction is when you actually become physically dependent on a particular substance; one that produces a chain reaction in the body and can actually induce structural and functional changes in the brain. When a foreign substance is allowed to continuously hog receptor sites – receptor sites that would otherwise be used by neurotransmitters naturally produced in the brain – our body is forced to adapt to what it thinks is extra of what it naturally produces. Can you see how it is possible for an individual to rapidly build a tolerance to higher and higher amounts of a dangerous substance? Individuals who are physically addicted to a substance will usually find themselves needing more and more; chasing after the desired short-term effect and running away from the dreaded withdrawal symptoms.

When a physically addicted individual stops using a substance (e.g., drugs, alcohol or cigarettes), he or she may experience withdrawal symptoms that could include: flu-like symptoms, diarrhea, headaches, mood swings, shaking and generally feeling awful. Withdrawal is the body's way of trying to clean itself of toxic, foreign invaders. Therefore, when an individual is no longer using a substance for its short-term, intended purpose, but is instead using it long-term in order to avoid withdrawal symptoms, then a true physical addiction is safe to assume.

Our relationship with cacao appears to be more psychological or ritualistic in nature than anything else; especially if you are eating the best and purest quality raw cacao. If you are going to have a secret love affair with a food, you might as well make it with only the best quality chocolate money can buy. In study upon study, the findings are evident. The magical, chemical make-up of quality raw cacao can keep your arteries from clogging, your airway from going into spasm, your teeth from rotting, your blood pumping with anti-aging and anti-cancer antioxidants and your brain from developing dementia. Moreover, the side effects – or shall I say side benefits – are feeling energized, focused and happy. What's not to love about this little piece of heaven?

> **Please repeat after me:** I (name) vow to never touch lips with chocolate that has been either nutritionally destroyed by high heat roasting or gas drying, cut with refined and processed sugars or antioxidant suffocating milk, or cheapened with a bunch of caffeinated fillers, chemical additives or unnatural flavorings.

Please Note: It is always in one's best interest to address underlying emotional issues which can cause attachments to foods and activities that have negative consequences. On the other hand, if a certain food or activity is ultimately good for us, consumed or done with respect and in moderation, does not negatively interfere with normal activities of daily living, and is actually creating more good than harm, I say, "why not?"

Real food – food that is not synthetic, laden with toxic chemicals or contaminated with mold – should never cause a physical dependency or create a response that is detrimentally negative.

Myth: Chocolate Is Toxic

CACAO ITSELF IS NOT TOXIC! Quality, quality, quality! This is pivotal people, and it should be the essence of everything. If you are not mindful about your sources you can just as easily end up with contaminated nuts and apples as you can cacao beans. But I don't see certain sectors of the raw food community vilifying those foods.

Every whole food has a different tolerance level to the elements it is subjected to in nature. The conditions of the environment in which they grow (natural or unnatural) can greatly determine whether a food or herb is healthful and beneficial to the body or potentially harmful and detrimental. Additionally, every whole food has its own individual chemical make-up, just as we do. Therefore, having the chemistry of the foods and herbs we plan to ingest thoroughly analyzed may be the wisest action we have available to us. The findings can provide insight on food compatibility and whether or not any preparation or processing is required for proper absorption and assimilation. They can also ensure that the processing methods utilized are gentle enough to never exceed the innate tolerance of our precious foods and herbs. To conclude, any process a food or herb goes through should never create molecular changes that no longer benefit the chemistry of the human body. We cannot (and should not) expect that we can just throw everything through the same process and it will have the same results.

We, as a nation, would not be dealing with a chronic and degenerative health crisis if we didn't rely so heavily on everything being faster, easier and cheaper. There is a solid message to be learned from the following phrases we commonly use, but rarely think long and hard about: "nothing in life worth having comes easy," "pay now or pay later" and "slow and steady wins the race."

The first step in preventing toxic build-up is to eliminate our direct exposure to hazardous chemicals as much as possible from our food, water and air supply. These include, but are not limited to: antibiotics, growth hormones, pesticides, heavy metals, bisphenol A (BPA) and the Teflon and Scotchgard family of perfluorochemicals (PFCs). If our soil, water and air are contaminated, weak and sick, then guess what – SO ARE WE! Sure, true organic, true wild-crafted and true cold-temperature and low-temperature processed foods and herbs which are tested for potency and purity on a regular basis may currently cost more; the reason we should yearn for them for ourselves, our families and our future is not rocket science, though. If we aspire to be well, and wish for our children and future generations to have a strong foundation, then we need to start somewhere. As they say, "Rome wasn't built in a day," and it takes a long time to carry out an important task.

We can thank blind faith and trust placed in government, food manufacturers, pharmaceutical companies and our current healthcare system for the reason we are paying the ultimate price to reverse the damage that has already been done. If we don't wake up and see faster, easier and cheaper for what it really is, we will continue this out of control downward spiral! I'd much rather pay now to keep what is pure, rich and real on the rise, so as to pay less for it later with a healthy body, a wealthy spirit and wise mind to show for it.

Setting the Record Straight

There are no scientific studies that show any detriments to consuming raw cacao. Nonetheless, there are some anecdotal cases of people having a bad reaction. This may be due to the unique chemical make-up of the individual, a contamination issue with the cacao or a low-quality hybridized variety of cacao. For the majority, if the cacao is coming from pristine and native areas, is not contaminated and (preferably) sun-dried, then cacao has the ability to benefit all who consume it.

> *Did you know that from the 16th through the 20th centuries, medical texts reported no less than 100 medicinal uses for cacao?*

Please Note: If your constitution is imbalanced, then depending on the type of imbalance, raw cacao may or may not be suitable. When starting out, I suggest consuming it in small, tolerable quantities. At least until your body reaches a healthful, balanced state again. Cacao has many medicinal properties that can seem magical; due to its nutritional density and chemical complexity, cacao is often combined with other superfoods and superherbs to increase their efficacy. When a powerful synergistic healing effect is what you desire – then cacao is the perfect delivery system for your medicine. For this very reason, cacao should always be treated and eaten with respect.

Finding the Quality Cacao You Deserve!

As with everything else, not all cacao beans are created equal. The quality of cacao beans and raw chocolate products is heavily reliant on the quality of its growing conditions and the processing methods after harvest. I like to choose my cacao the same way I once chose my wine. Have you ever gone out and reluctantly drank some really cheap wine? Even if you couldn't tell how cheap it was by the taste or feel in your mouth, there was no mistaking the cheap wine hangover you had the next day. Well, if the cacao beans are low-quality – or if the cacao paste, powder or butter is processed poorly – then you're probably not going to be so "blissfully happy."

I wonder if all the cacao bashers out there ever considered their source as the culprit for experiencing negative effects. It is highly possible that they were dealing with a contaminated batch (pesticides, mold growth, fat rancidity, high levels of heavy metals, etc.). If this is the case, then the answer is fairly simple: do your research and switch to a reputable source. To me, a reputable source is a company with a long and lengthy track record; a company with a true passion for health-giving foods; a company with extensive knowledge through dedication and industry experience; a company with the integrity to always be able to willfully back their claims. Many times in the past, for example, when I would either purchase a raw chocolate snack while out at the local health food store or a dessert made with raw chocolate while dining at a raw food restaurant, I could tell right away that the quality of the cacao was poor. I would feel like I was pumped up on speed. Sometimes I'd even get a dull headache or loopy feeling and then not sleep well all night. If I didn't know better, I might have assumed this to be true of all sourced cacao. Thankfully, though, I do know better and can tell the difference right off the bat. I would get the same exact feeling every time I ate out at a raw food place that claimed to be organic; only to later find out that just one to a few ingredients were actually organic. What's the point of having only one or a few organic ingredients if the rest getting tossed in the mix are commercially grown with chemical fertilizers and contaminated with pesticides? Thanks, but no thanks! If you're going to advertise yourself as being organic, you owe it to yourself and the consumer to follow that rule 100%. Otherwise your intentions are not true and your motives cannot be taken seriously. You never know when the health of someone may be at serious risk; what they put in their mouth may just be the only thing they can control and rely on to make a valuable difference.

Thankfully, there is one source of cacao I can trust whole-heartedly which is distributed by New Horizon Health. Their cacao grows high in the mountains of Ecuador where the cacao trees are mature and deep rooted in nutrient-rich volcanic soil which is watered naturally by the rain or springs. Each cacao pod is specially selected and handpicked only when ripened and fully grown. The cacao beans are always sun-dried, never gas dried. As a result, the cacao remains 100% raw from start to finish. I want to give a big thank you to Robert Williams for this cacao! Your passion for sourcing only the highest quality and nutrient-rich superfoods on the planet is appreciated more than words can say; and your excellence, honesty and integrity never go unnoticed.

Please Note: When searching for the finest quality cacao with exceptional aroma and flavor intensity, always be sure to look for 100% heirloom Ecuadorian Arriba Nacional. Otherwise, you are taking a chance it may be the CCN51 clone or another low-quality hybrid. Many companies are selling CCN51 as the Arriba Nacional variety due to its high yield potential; but buyers beware, CCN51 and other hybridized cacao varieties are inferior species of cacao. Unlike true Arriba Nacional, which grows wild in a thriving and balanced jungle ecosystem, hybrid cacao varieties are plants with shallow root systems in a non-thriving and imbalanced ecosystem. Without the nutrient drawing power of deep roots in desirable rich soil, the cacao these hybrids yield cannot be saluted as a nutrient-rich superfood; cannot be marveled at for high mineral content; and cannot be prized for providing the complexity of beneficial chemical compounds spoken of above.

ALOE VERA

Aloe vera (*Aloe barbadensis* Miller) or "true aloe" is a stemless or very short-stemmed succulent plant belonging to the lily family. Although the majority of aloe species are native to Africa (commonly found in South Africa's Cape Province, the mountains of tropical Africa and neighboring areas such as Madagascar, the Arabian Peninsula and the islands of Africa), many aloe species are well-adapted to similar climates in other parts of the world. For instance, many species of aloe grow and thrive in the tropical and subtropical locations of South America and the Caribbean.

Aloe vera produces two medicinal substances: gel and latex. Aloe gel is the clear, jelly-like substance found in the inner part of each aloe leaf. Aloe latex comes from just under the skin of the plant and is yellow in color. Despite strong scientific evidence that supports the laxative properties of aloe latex, it is not advised for regular, long-term use. Aloe gel, on the other hand, is a food rich in nutritive substances and can safely be taken on a daily basis as a digestive and general restorative tonic.

Aloe vera is a rich source of over two hundred naturally-occurring nutritional substances, including: amino acids (containing all eight essential amino acids), enzymes, vitamins A, B-complex, C, D and E, macro and trace minerals, antioxidants, plant sterols, polysaccharides and glycoproteins. The synergy of all these biologically active substances working together in the body is what makes aloe vera truly magical. Aloe vera has what it takes to achieve the optimal in restorative and regenerative nutrition for the maximum in anti-aging health.

Legend has it that aloe vera was Cleopatra's beauty secret.

Most people are aware of the many topical uses for aloe gel, as it is extremely effective for a variety of skin conditions. From burns, sunburn, frostbite, insect bites, eczema, dermatitis and psoriasis to open sores and ulcers of the skin, oral herpes (aka cold sores) and genital herpes. Used on hemorrhoids, aloe gel has the amazing power to soothe and cool as it heals. But what about the many curative and nutritional benefits when aloe gel is taken internally? By mouth, aloe gel can treat osteoarthritis, irritable bowel syndrome (IBS), inflammatory bowel diseases (e.g., Crohn's disease and ulcerative colitis), stomach ulcers, cancerous growths and a multitude of other immune-mediated inflammatory diseases. It is also commonly used for allergies, asthma and diabetes, in addition to alleviating some side effects of radiation treatment.

Aloe Vera Benefits:

- ★ Aloe vera taken before meals can help with digestion and with the absorption and assimilation of many nutrients.
- ★ Aloe vera supports the health of mucus membranes everywhere in the body. It also promotes rapid mucus membrane rejuvenation throughout the entire urinary tract and gastrointestinal tract.
- ★ Aloe vera has anti-inflammatory properties which can reduce the pain and inflammation associated with a host of inflammatory conditions (e.g., allergies, arthritis, burns, infections, skin rashes and conditions, stomach and bowel disorders, surgery and ulcerations).
- ★ Aloe vera, coupled with a raw and living foods plant-based diet, can smooth the inner walls of the intestinal tract and help heal growths that can lead to cancer.
- ★ Aloe vera contains polysaccharides known to boost and balance the functioning of the immune system and combat cancer cells.
- ★ Aloe vera has proven effective against viruses, including influenza, herpes, HIV and even the measles virus!
- ★ Aloe vera can increase blood flow to the brain. Aloe vera may preserve memory and enhance cognitive function in adults with neurological disorders (e.g., Alzheimer's disease).

What to Look for in a Quality Aloe Vera Product

100% pure, organic aloe vera (inner leaf gel) is what you want. The inner leaf of the aloe vera plant is where the magic is. It is the gel which contains most all of the health-promoting properties. Despite the hype, please avoid buying aloe vera juice that is diluted with water or contains toxic preservatives such as sodium benzoate. I consume and recommend AloePro by Premier Research Labs. It is made from 100% certified organic aloe vera (inner leaf gel) and the only preservatives added are natural citric acid and grapefruit seed extract. A product labeled "inner leaf" versus "whole leaf" is much gentler on the stomach and digestive system, and should not have a laxative effect. In addition, aloe vera products containing inner leaf gel go through minimal processing. As a result, their effects are similar to consuming the fresh plant gel itself.

How to Use Aloe Vera

If you have access to organically grown aloe vera plants, you may wish to cut and fillet a few of the outside leaves by hand in order to use the inner leaf gel externally and internally. For instance, you can add fresh aloe gel to any fruit and superfood smoothie. 2-4 ounces of aloe gel is a good amount for beginners. Most would probably agree that the bitterness from the inner leaf gel can easily be disguised by fruits and natural sweeteners added to the smoothie.

> **Quick Tip:** If you are not sure how to fillet an aloe leaf, you can simply go to www.youtube.com and type in "how to fillet aloe vera." A number of great YouTube videos will pop up and are available for viewing.

If taking a bottled aloe vera product (like AloePro), I suggest 1-2 tablespoons, 2-4 times per day. When taken right before meals, aloe vera can enhance digestion by stimulating bile production in the liver. For some individuals, aloe vera has proven to be an effective natural sleep aid when taken prior to bed. For special detoxification programs and intensive colon cleansing, up to two ounces of aloe vera (four tablespoons) may be added to two ounces of purified water and taken every two hours (while awake) for one whole day. Please consult with a qualified holistic health practitioner before starting any type of intensive cleansing/detoxification protocol.

Precautions: Aloe vera may cause diarrhea and cramping in some individuals, so please use with caution. Although aloe vera gel is very non-allergenic, a small percentage of individuals may be allergic. Discontinue use if you experience itching of the skin (when applied externally) or swelling of the lips, tongue or face (when ingested internally). Aloe latex (i.e., laxative aloe vera products) should never be consumed by pregnant or lactating women or the elderly. Conversely, the gel of aloe vera may benefit pregnant women (especially those experiencing nausea), lactating mothers (due to its ability to encourage milk production) and the elderly (due to its natural ability to regulate stomach acids and digestion). That being said, I have also read that aloe vera is contraindicated during pregnancy, as it can cause uterine contractions and drops in blood sugar. This may be due to some companies utilizing the "whole leaf" of the aloe vera plant (gel, latex and rind) versus just the "inner leaf" (gel only). Due to conflicting information, I highly recommend consulting with a qualified holistic health professional before using aloe vera externally or internally if you are pregnant or nursing.

MSM

MSM (methyl-sulfonyl-methane) is naturally-occurring organic sulfur. Sulfur is found in the tissues of all plants and animals and is said to be the fourth most abundant mineral in the human body. It is stored in, and used by, virtually every cell in our body with the highest concentrations found in our skin, hair, nails and joints.

After oxygen, water and salt, MSM (sulfur) is considered to be the fourth most needed element in both human and animal nutrition.

Small amounts of MSM can be found in foods such as fresh fruits and vegetables, grains, unpasteurized milk, eggs, meats, poultry and fish. However, because MSM has such a delicate structure, it is easily depleted during even moderate processing. Cooking, drying, smoking and pickling, not to mention irradiating, pasteurizing and long-term storing, can destroy the MSM content of our foods. Therefore, unless we are eating a diet consisting primarily of fresh, raw foods, it is highly unlikely that we are even close to ingesting a sufficient enough amount of MSM to meet our sulfur needs.

Symptoms of sulfur deficiency may include: allergies, sensitivity to pain and inflammation, slow wound healing, brittle hair and nails, digestive disorders, poor circulation, memory loss, improper immune function, acne and other skin issues, premature aging and cellular damage.

> *Hormones, enzymes, antibodies and antioxidants all depend on sulfur.*
>
> *Due to the body utilizing and expending sulfur on a daily basis, this important nutrient must be continually replenished for optimal health, healing and beauty.*

Where Does MSM Come From?

MSM originates in the oceans where microscopic plankton release sulfur compounds into the seawater. It is then quickly converted to DMS (a volatile sulfur compound) and escapes into the atmosphere. In its suspended, gaseous state, DMS reacts with ozone and ultraviolet sunlight to create DMSO and DMSO2 (aka MSM). MSM then returns to the earth through falling rain, where it is collected and concentrated in plants.

How Is MSM Different from DMSO?

DMSO (dimethyl sulfoxide) is a precursor to MSM. Although DMSO and MSM are chemically similar, they are uniquely different.

- ★ DMSO has a very strong smell. A strong garlic-like taste and the smell of garlic, onions or oysters may be present for 24 hours after DMSO use. Most individuals don't notice this odor, though anyone in close proximity may detect it. Other reported side effects of DMSO include the following: itchy skin, nasal congestion, shortness of breath, excess intestinal gas, nausea and headache. Although these side effects are not very common – or even noted to be harmful – they can be annoying and unpleasant. Also, because DMSO is powerfully effective as a solvent, one must be extremely careful when using it. This is especially true for its topical use(s), as it can carry almost anything through the skin and into the bloodstream. This may be excellent for the trans-dermal delivery of beneficial nutrients and herbs, but can be bad and potentially hazardous if impurities (e.g., microorganisms, toxic chemicals and dyes) get transported into the body. Skin must be thoroughly cleaned before applying DMSO. Once applied, allow skin to thoroughly dry before letting anything touch it (bath towel, clothing, etc.).
- ★ MSM, on the other hand, doesn't have the unpleasant smell or taste of DMSO. It also won't give you body odor that leaves you smelling like low tide, garlic or onions. MSM has no known side effects and may be consumed in significant quantities, for long periods of time, by most all individuals.

How Does MSM Work?

MSM functions as an antioxidant in the body. As MSM scavenges free radicals, it protects our DNA (the cell's genetic blueprint) from oxidative damage.

Along with necessary sulfur, MSM donates much needed methyl groups to the body.

- ★ The body's ability to remove toxins through methylation (i.e., binding the toxins to methyl groups and excreting them from the body) is critically important. Why? Because it has been highly theorized that the primary mechanism behind cellular aging and cellular death is the loss of DNA markers called methyl groups. Stress, poor nutrition, lack of exercise, environmental toxins, radiation, cigarette smoking and too much alcohol all contribute to cellular aging and degeneration. Therefore, all these factors also accelerate the loss of methyl groups from DNA.
- ★ Faulty methylation has been linked to heart disease, stroke, neural tube defects, Alzheimer's disease, cancer, impaired detoxification processes in the liver and defective DNA repair.
- ★ Poor methylation can cause homocysteine levels to elevate. Homocysteine is an amino acid that is toxic to the body. According to studies, high homocysteine levels in the blood can damage the lining of the arteries and may cause or contribute to heart disease and stroke.
- ★ Many important biochemical processes (including metabolism of lipids, hormones, neurotransmitters and DNA) all rely on methylation; a process carried out by methyl donors.
    - ○ A methyl donor is simply any substance that can transfer a methyl group (a carbon atom bonded to three hydrogen atoms-CH3) to another substance. Besides MSM, beet powder (betaine), garlic and onions all contain methyl groups. Broad-spectrum B vitamins (B12, B6 and folate) and SAM-e are also considered methyl donors.
- ★ Scientists speculate that adequate methylation of DNA can prevent the expression of harmful genes such as oncogenes (aka cancer genes).
- ★ Methylation is also a crucial step in the detoxification processes within the liver. Hence, it "turns on" detox reactions that can detoxify the body of harmful chemicals.

MSM cleanses the bloodstream and flushes out the waste and toxins that get trapped in our cells. By restoring flexibility and permeability to cell walls, fluids and nutrients can flow freely into the cells, and wastes and toxins can readily flow out.

MSM Benefits:

- ★ MSM provides a bio-available form of organic sulfur, a mineral that is present in every cell of the body. Sulfur plays a key role in liver detoxification and metabolism; the function of joint cartilage; and the keratin of skin, hair and nails.
- ★ MSM enhances the body's ability to absorb nutrients at a cellular level.
- ★ MSM helps the body restore a healthy balance between acidity and alkalinity and works with the liver to secrete bile – an important process.

- ★ MSM helps to regulate the gastrointestinal tract, especially when synchronized with alkaline minerals. MSM combined with an alkaline rich diet can alleviate heartburn, constipation, diarrhea and the burning pain associated with ulcers caused by too much stomach acid.
- ★ MSM detoxifies the body and improves blood circulation. It does this by removing foreign proteins from the bloodstream and working as a free radical scavenger.
- ★ MSM increases energy, alertness and may contribute to mental calmness and the ability to concentrate. This is due to sulfur being required by every cell for the production of energy at the cellular level.
- ★ MSM increases tissue pliability and can promote the repair of damaged skin. When sufficient sulfur is present for new cells, the skin becomes more soft, smooth and supple. This in turn helps in the reduction of wrinkles, age spots, scar tissue and other skin problems (like rosacea). MSM can also promote faster healing from sunburn or wind damage and can help prevent blistering.
- ★ MSM removes inflammation and eases the pain associated with inflammatory disorders such as osteoarthritis, rheumatoid arthritis, nighttime leg cramps, migraine headaches, etc.
- ★ MSM supports healthy muscles and connective tissues (i.e., cartilage, ligaments and tendons). This makes MSM a valuable tool when dealing with arthritic conditions, bursitis, tendonitis, carpal tunnel syndrome, chronic fatigue and fibromyalgia. MSM can also effectively speed the healing of muscles and joints (due to overuse and trauma). Furthermore, it is effective in reducing muscle pain caused by cramps and spasms.
- ★ MSM may provide relief from food, drug and environmental allergies. Although MSM is not a cure for allergies, it can greatly reduce allergy symptoms by allowing allergens to be removed from the body more quickly. MSM coats mucosal surfaces and occupies the binding sites that may have otherwise been invaded by nasty allergens.
- ★ MSM can enhance insulin sensitivity so that the body requires less insulin release. This is because sulfur is a component of insulin. Studies indicate that due to cells becoming more permeable with regular MSM use, blood sugar levels are better balanced and the pancreas is not so overworked.
- ★ MSM can block parasites from attaching themselves to the intestinal lining and robbing our body of vital nutrients. When MSM takes over receptor sites on the mucous membrane, it is much more challenging for parasites to latch on and keep their grip. As a result, parasites can be flushed out before making themselves at home. MSM has been found to be active against giardia, trichomonads, roundworms and pinworms.

What to Look for in a Quality MSM Product

First, MSM should not be confused with sulfa-based drugs, sulfates or sulfites, which are synthetic and have been known to cause allergic and adverse reactions in many individuals.

MSM is not a drug, a medicine or a food additive. It is food! MSM is a safe form of organic sulfur which can be easily absorbed and assimilated by the human body. In its purified form, MSM is an odorless white crystal with a slightly bitter taste.

I take OptiMSM. Compared to the many different brands and forms of MSM in the marketplace, OptiMSM is held to a higher standard of quality:

- ★ OptiMSM is manufactured here in the United States and is the only MSM supported by double-blind clinical research.
- ★ Every batch of OptiMSM is tested by independent laboratories to guarantee the absence of harmful metal and biological contaminants.
- ★ OptiMSM is always guaranteed 99.9% pure methyl-sulfonyl-methane (MSM).
- ★ Last but not least, OptiMSM is comprised of 34% bio-available sulfur. The richest source known to man!

How to Take MSM

For quick absorption and maximum bioavailability, I prefer MSM powder over MSM capsules and tablets. Studies have shown that individuals receive better results when MSM is taken in powder form versus capsule or tablet form. If you must, capsules would probably be the better choice over the majority of tablets found in the marketplace. Due to being compressed, tablets will generally take longer to dissolve in the stomach, making them harder to digest than capsules.

For some individuals (specifically the highly sensitive), MSM (especially at high dosages) may be better tolerated at mealtime. But if you want maximum health benefits, and all that MSM has to offer, I suggest taking it on an empty stomach and with a natural, high-quality, whole food source of vitamin C (see the "Quick Tip" below for further details). Twenty to thirty minutes before meals is sufficient. Due to the increase in energy MSM can provide, MSM is best consumed in the morning or mid-afternoon. Avoid taking MSM prior to bed, as it may interfere with restful sleep.

How Much MSM Should I Take?

An optimum daily dosage of MSM greatly depends on the nature and severity of any deficiency or condition you may be experiencing. Body size and age are also factors to consider. Therefore, the following suggested dosages are intended to serve as general guidelines for adult use only. If you are new to MSM, you may want to start out with a quarter teaspoon (or less), 1-2 times daily for the first few days to a week. A quarter teaspoon is equivalent to approximately one gram (1,000 mg). Each week, you may work your way up until you reach one tablespoon, 1-2 times daily. One tablespoon is equivalent to approximately 12 grams (12,000 mg). This higher dosage will make up for any sulfur deficiency your body may be experiencing. It will also enable your cells and tissues to release toxins that have built up over the years.

Please Note: If at any time, while increasing the dosage of MSM, you experience a strong healing crisis (aka cleansing reaction, detox reaction or Herxheimer reaction), please know that you can always cut back in order to give your body a chance to catch up. Symptoms can range from feeling flu-like to feeling as if you are re-experiencing the effects of drugs or drug-like substance you may have taken in the past. For instance, heavy coffee drinkers or smokers may feel extra jittery or edgy. Symptoms of a healing crisis usually pass within 1-3 days, but on rare occasions may last up to a week or longer. Be sure to always drink lots of purified water when taking MSM; especially when increasing the amount you are taking. For some individuals, MSM may need to be taken for at least 1-2 weeks before desired effects are noticed. Although rare, some may need to give up to two months before positive effects begin to take hold.

For most individuals, a maintenance dosage of MSM will be between 1-3 teaspoons daily, which is equivalent to 4-12 grams (4,000-12,000 mg). Taking MSM in divided doses is recommended but not necessary.

> **Quick Tip:** MSM is better assimilated by the body when taken with a high-quality source of vitamin C. It has been suggested that by synergistically combining MSM with natural sources of vitamin C – such as citrus fruits, camu camu berry, amla berry, acerola berry, etc. – one can boost the building of new cells and enhance the healing process. When cells are more pliable and permeable, they allow fluids to pass through more easily. With an increase in fluid exchange, cellular waste can be washed out and removed, while proper hydration and nutrient absorption is restored.
>
> Internally, this equates to more efficient elimination of toxins and cellular debris – leading to a reduction in inflammation and pain in the short-term and the rebuilding of damaged tendons, ligaments and joint cartilage in the long-term. Externally, this equates to the synthesis of collagen – for smoother, softer and more resilient skin, as well as hair and nails that grow faster, stronger and more flexible (meaning, less brittle with less breakage).
>
> Camu camu berry powder is my #1 choice for a high-quality source of natural vitamin C. I suggest adding a quarter teaspoon (or more) to every dose of MSM powder. You may wish to start with a smaller amount and work your way up (see page 186 for more on camu camu).

Precautions: While many people are allergic or sensitive to sulfa-based drugs, sulfates and sulfites, no similar reactions have ever been reported with MSM. MSM is extremely safe and considered non-toxic and non-allergenic. In fact, it is considered to be as safe as drinking water. Nonetheless, taking amounts greater than your body's ability to absorb and assimilate may result in loose stools. MSM has been researched for many years and has no known contra-indications with pharmaceutical drugs or over-the-counter medications. Although considered very safe, it is recommended that MSM not be used by pregnant or lactating women or by children under the age of two. It is also recommended that individuals taking blood thinners consult with their doctor before using MSM.

MICROALGAE: NATURE'S NATURAL MULTIVITAMINS

> *Research indicates that microalgae are among the very first life forms on planet earth!*

Chlorella

Chlorella is a single-celled, water-grown green algae. Once its cell wall has been effectively broken, chlorella contains readily available chlorophyll. In fact, it contains the highest amount of chlorophyll per gram of any known plant in the world and is renowned for its numerous blood-building and detoxifying properties. Its innate intelligence allows for it to bond with toxic chemicals (like heavy metal mercury) and safely eliminate them from the body.

> *According to research presented by David Wolfe at the Women's Wellness Conference in February 2012, the chlorophyll content in chlorella is 40 times higher than in the best grown wheatgrass in the world. 40 times higher!*

Chlorella's chlorophyll is nearly identical to human hemoglobin (red blood cells). The only difference is that chlorophyll has magnesium at its center and hemoglobin has iron. If you recall, magnesium has many roles in the human body, but the most important is the critical role it plays in the health of our heart. Without the right amount of magnesium, the function of the heart starts to fail; when the heart is in failure, the rest of the body is not far behind.

Chlorella is also prized for its high level of bio-available protein (including impressive amounts of lysine), numerous vitamins and minerals, antioxidants, enzymes, essential fatty acids, dietary fiber, nucleic acids, polysaccharides, Chlorella Growth Factor (CGF) and other beneficial health-giving properties.

Chlorella Benefits:

- ★ Chlorella has the highest known chlorophyll content! Chlorophyll is an amazing phytochemical that can help destroy cancer cells, rebuild damaged nerve tissue, enhance the function of our brains and more.
- ★ Chlorella assists in relieving inflammation.
- ★ Chlorella accelerates the healing process.
- ★ Chlorella enhances the immune system for whole body rejuvenation.
- ★ Chlorella detoxifies the body by binding to all toxic metals (such as mercury, lead, arsenic, cadmium, etc.), as well as environmental toxins (such as dioxin to name but one).
- ★ Chlorella helps protect against radiation. From medical devices and treatments, to nuclear radioactive fallout. Not to mention day-to-day exposure to cell phones, computers, high-voltage power lines, microwaves, televisions and the many other devices that run on electricity.

- ★ Chlorella is the highest-known food source of the nucleic acids RNA and DNA! When we have a sufficient intake of foods rich in DNA and RNA to protect our own cellular nucleic acids, our bodies are able to use nutrients more effectively and get rid of toxins more efficiently. Used regularly, chlorella can assist in the repair of damaged genetic material in human cells. By decreasing the early onset of chronic and degenerative diseases we can dramatically improve the quality of our health and longevity. This makes chlorella one of the top anti-aging superfoods in the world!
- ★ Chlorella promotes cell reproduction, increases hemoglobin levels, guards against heart disease, reduces high blood pressure and decreases cholesterol.
- ★ Chlorella is effective in reducing the symptoms of many types of cancers, AIDS, Alzheimer's, anemia, arthritis, Candida, diabetes, hepatitis, cirrhosis of the liver, multiple sclerosis (MS), pancreatitis, Parkinson's, peptic ulcers, as well as other viral and bacterial infections.
- ★ Chlorella supports the function of the brain and promotes liver health, making it the "great normalizer."
- ★ Chlorella increases reduced glutathione.
- ★ Chlorella causes the beneficial bacteria in our stomach (lactobacillus) to multiply at four times the normal rate; thus, significantly improving digestion and the body's ability to take in nutrients.
- ★ Chlorella contains enzymes, such as chlorophyllase and pepsin, which aid in proper digestion.
- ★ Chlorella contains 60% high-quality protein that is easy to assimilate! This impressive percentage of protein outshines that of meat and fish, which are only approximately 18-30% protein. On top of that, animal protein is much harder on the body to break down.
- ★ Chlorella is extremely rich in vitamins and minerals such as vitamins C, E, B-complex vitamins, folic acid, beta-carotene, calcium, iodine and iron.
- ★ Chlorella supports healthy weight loss.

Only the Very Best Chlorella Will Do!

There are numerous chlorella products on the market; but I choose to stand behind distributors that will only source their chlorella from a very specific company in Taiwan. New Horizon Health and Ultimate Superfoods get their chlorella from the world's largest and oldest producers of *Chlorella pyrenoidosa* – Taiwan Chlorella Manufacturing Company (TCMC). This chlorella is routinely tested for bacteria, heavy metals and radiation, processed raw to ensure nutrient and enzyme vitality and is certified organic. This is the only chlorella on the market that I will personally consume; therefore, it is the only chlorella that I promote and recommend. It is meticulously grown in fresh water, in a well-controlled environment and without the use of chemicals. Unlike some chlorella manufacturers, TCMC's chlorella is never grown in, nor harvested from open waters. If chlorella is not grown or harvested correctly, the chance of inferior environmental elements and pollutants can pose a severe risk to product quality.

Why Chlorella Pyrenoidosa?

Chlorella pyrenoidosa (aka the "King of Chlorellas") is a four billion-year-old strain of green algae and has been utilized for thousands of generations. This makes *Chlorella pyrenoidosa* one of the oldest foods on the face of the earth. There are over 70,000 species of algae on the planet. Some of these are consumable for nutritive benefit and can be highly medicinal; while others are not safe for consumption and can be highly toxic. Out of all the consumable and marketed strains of chlorella in the health food marketplace, there is only one that has been studied the most and the longest – therefore, there is only one backed by years upon years of scientific research from around the globe. This highly regarded strain is *Chlorella pyrenoidosa*. Although there are other great health-promoting strains of chlorella on the market, including *Chlorella vulgaris*, I feel only *Chlorella pyrenoidosa* can truthfully be credited for all chlorella's health benefiting claims. Many times, when we hear and read about the numerous benefits of chlorella and all that it can do, the strain that the information is actually based on is none other than *Chlorella pyrenoidosa*.

When it comes to health and detoxification success, I only want the strain that matches the long list of innumerable benefits backed by decades of scientific research. In addition, I'm only interested in the producers and manufacturers who hold the highest reputation for insuring and delivering strain purity and nutritional integrity. This leads me to my next vital point: "the validity of a product's beneficial claim on your health is only as good as its <u>finished</u> product." As I've mentioned earlier, I do not like to take anybody's word for anything. I want to see the proof for myself. At the present time, there is only one producer and manufacturer of *Chlorella pyrenoidosa* that has gained recognition for utilizing the most effective, yet gentle and organic method of cracking open chlorella's fibrous cell wall. What's more, the cell wall is successfully cracked without disturbing or damaging all its unique nutritional properties and without exposing it to potential contaminants. It is the finished product of this highly valued chlorella strain – manufactured by the largest and most technically advanced chlorella producer in the world – that makes this particular chlorella product one desirable, dependable gem.

What makes *Chlorella pyrenoidosa* a prized strain in the minds of cleansing and detoxification gurus? Ironically, the same reason some distributers and marketers actually pooh-pooh this particular strain: ITS THICK, STRONG and FIBROUS CELL WALL. Go figure! Other producers and manufacturers may boast about *Chlorella vulgaris* as being more digestively tolerable due to it having a thinner cell wall; but when it comes to effectively detoxifying heavy metals and other highly toxic substances from the body, *Chlorella vulgaris* does not measure up. *Chlorella vulgaris* may have a thinner cell wall, but as a result, it also has much lower toxin-absorbing capabilities. Furthermore, it has less protein than *Chlorella pyrenoidosa*.

Guess what gives *Chlorella pyrenoidosa* the unique ability to effectively bind with heavy metals, radiation and other synthetic toxins? It's the thick layers of a special fiber that comprise its cell wall. The unique characteristics of this dietary fiber are found nowhere else in nature. It's what differentiates *Chlorella pyrenoidosa* from all other algae.

And what gives this particular strain the amazing ability to effectively remove these toxins from the body? Once again, the strong layers of toxin-absorbing fiber found in its cell wall. It does more than just bind and soak up toxins. It can effectively expel them from the body without the potential for reabsorbing them back into circulation.

Cracking this particular strain of chlorella's cell wall without hitting obstacles that may have a major impact on the final product can be challenging to say the least. For this reason, I commend Taiwan Chlorella Manufacturing Co (TCMC) for taking on such a challenge. I also applaud them for making it successfully happen. TCMC utilizes a state-of-the-art pressure release method which can crack the cell wall without touching the chlorella cells. This method not only keeps the numerous nutrients within chlorella cells completely intact, but does so without exposing them to potential contaminants. Furthermore, each and every batch of chlorella harvested is tested for purity, nutritional quality and the overall integrity consumers deserve. This is above and beyond standard practice. More often than not, only randomized batches are tested for economical purposes.

According to expert information, TCMC's highly specialized method can actually open the cell walls of 99.9% of the chlorella they produce. This is the highest open-wall rating of any chlorella brand on the market! Why is this relevant? It means better absorption and utilization of chlorella's nutrients. Many companies will claim to have opened the chlorella cell wall (hence, the label "Cracked Cell Wall Chlorella"). However, when placed under strict scrutiny, their methods fell short of their claims. Additionally, many chlorella producers use antiquated methods that "pulverize," "mill" or "crush" the outer fiber shell. These methods significantly decrease chlorella's shelf life. When nutrients scatter and do not remain intact as they should, they become highly susceptible to oxidation and degradation. Another problem with the process of pulverizing, milling or crushing is the potential for chlorella cells to come into contact with impurities such as heavy metal lead.

Quality in, Quality Out

The chlorella I consume and recommend is the only chlorella in the world exported and allowed to be sold in Japan that is not produced in Japan. That tells you something right there. Its superior quality is confirmed by an annual independent analysis by the Japan Food Research Laboratory. Why is this significant? Japan is the only country known to have strict standards and importation controls over heavy metals and bacterial content.

What's more, the digestibility of TCMCs chlorella is confirmed by the Japanese Government's Ministry of Health to be between 76% and 79%. The highest on the market! Wow! This is significantly higher when compared to a competitor's chlorella that was professionally analyzed and determined to be only 40% digestible.

Chlorella Tidbits

Bob McCauley, Certified Nutritional Consultant and Certified Master Herbalist, states that the Japanese consume more chlorella per capita than Americans consume of the highly popularized vitamin C. He also states that whole food chlorella is many times more powerful than any multivitamin or supplement. I find this bit of information interesting and exciting, as when I started consuming more and more microalgae, I intuitively felt these little treasures replacing my need for multivitamin and mineral supplements. They also provide quality plant-based protein, omega-3 fatty acids and so much more!

- ★ One teaspoon (tsp) = two grams
- ★ Best 20-30 minutes before a meal to aid in proper digestion of food and absorption of nutrients.
- ★ Chlorella can be taken at the same time as probiotics and may actually enhance their effects.
- ★ Ideally chlorella should be consumed throughout the day and not before or after caffeinated foods and beverages, as caffeine is known to interfere and disrupt the digestive process.
- ★ Last but not least, please be sure to gradually work your way up to the dosages listed below. This will help allow your body (especially the digestive system) to adapt to its unique fiber and deep cleansing and rejuvenating effects. Remember, chlorella is a whole food and you cannot eat too much!

Recommended Dosage

Chlorella Pyrenoidosa	Recommended Daily Dosage
Maintenance Dosage	4-6 grams per day
Significant Part of the Diet	6-10 grams per day
Immune System Builder	12-14 grams per day
Primary Source of Protein	12-20 grams per day
Healing Purposes & Heavy Metal Detox	20-30+ grams per day

Please Note: When it comes to heavy metal detoxification, do not inadvertently and continuously re-circulate poisons in the body. As I said earlier, if you currently have silver (50% mercury by weight) amalgam fillings, I suggest getting them removed first. The constant vaporization of inorganic mercury from dental amalgams can dramatically compromise and potentially harm your greatest efforts to detoxify successfully.

> To understand more, I highly suggest re-reading "Chelation & Heavy Metal Detoxification: Wellness Tips and Tools to Live By" on page 111.

Generally, it will take 3-6 months from the time one starts consistently taking chlorella for a decrease in heavy metal blood levels to be noticed. Once the initial heavy metal burden starts to decrease, chlorella can more readily begin to mobilize and bind these toxins. By mobilize, I mean pull them from their storage sites (i.e., fat cells and other tissues), and by bind, I mean push them into the intestines where they can safely and efficiently be removed from the body for good.

Please Note: The process of heavy metal detoxification can be slow; and in order for it to be considered safe and effective, it should be slow. I highly suggest staying the course and being patient. Do not get discouraged, as there are numerous side benefits to taking chlorella. More than just the removal of heavy metals (which is monumental in and of itself), adding this gem of a superfood offers enormous health-sustaining gains. Embrace and enjoy the journey back to vitality!

> **Quick Tip:** In addition to the daily use of chlorella, I highly suggest the periodic use of Medicardium, Glytamins and Xeneplex suppositories. This will not only help boost your heavy metal detox potential, but can keep levels within a low to normal range (view pages 111-117 for further info).

Marine Phytoplankton

Marine Phytoplankton (aka marine microalgae) are a microscopic single-cell aquatic plant. These plants are the most abundant vegetation found in the ocean. More than 99% of all sea creatures depend either directly or indirectly on marine phytoplankton for their survival. Certain species of whales enjoy an active and reproductive life for up to 150 years, thanks to marine phytoplankton.

Marine phytoplankton, the world's smallest plant, nourishes the world's largest animal: the majestic blue whale!

Commonly referred to as "The King of the Ocean," the majestic blue whale feeds only on marine phytoplankton and a select species of krill. And what do krill feed on? Marine phytoplankton!

Our Vital Lifeline

Marine phytoplankton are capable of turning water and light energy from the sun into nutrients and oxygen through photosynthesis. With their amazing ability to convert natural elements into essential nutrients, marine phytoplankton are considered to be the foundation of all other life forms on planet earth!

According to NASA, marine phytoplankton is responsible for producing 50-90% of the oxygen found in the air we breathe.

How does so much of our oxygen come from marine algae? With the oceans covering 71% of our planet and land covering only 29%, it's easy to see how the thousands of algae species living in the ocean can contribute so much of the oxygen in our atmosphere. According to the article, "The Most Important Organism?" by Dr. Jack Hall (posted September 12, 2011, on www.ecology.com), we humans need marine algae a whole lot more than they need us. He states that although trees and land plants are very important for providing us and other critters with food and raw materials, the human species could not survive without the oxygen produced by algae. If we continue to pollute our oceans and freshwater systems, we will continue to kill our vital lifeline. This includes microalgae and marine seaweed (sea vegetables like kelp) which are algae that just look like big plants.

It is equally important to remember that our friends, the algae, also absorb a majority of the carbon dioxide in the atmosphere, which helps in maintaining the balance of our ecosystem. Without homeostasis of our external environment, there can be no homeostasis of our internal environment.

Food for Thrival, Not Just Survival

Marine phytoplankton assist in our body's production of cellular energy without any calories and without stimulation. They accomplish this by bypassing the mitochondria (the energy powerhouses of the cell). Nucleotides (such as ATP, ADP, AGP, etc.) found in marine phytoplankton turn directly into energy once in the body. They are the one food that does not take energy from our body (through the process of digestion) in order to make energy. According to David Wolfe, marine phytoplankton's ability to produce quick and effective cellular energy makes them the leader of the pack in the superfood arena! For those who find themselves working endlessly in high-stress environments; getting little to no rest or quality deep sleep; and desiring long-term energy and mental focus without the use of stimulants (which can only offer a short-lived pseudo boost of energy almost always followed by the dreaded crash), then you will most definitely want marine phytoplankton at the very top of your superfood wish list.

From the seriously ill to the extreme athlete, marine phytoplankton may be the most paramount of all inclusions. Whether to an existing health regimen or new one, simply just add them in!

Marine Phytoplankton Benefits:

- ★ Marine phytoplankton contain just about every life-sustaining nutrient known to man! Marine phytoplankton contain all nine essential amino acids the adult body cannot produce; omega-3 (including EPA and DHA) and omega-6 essential fatty acids; nucleic acids (RNA and DNA) and nucleotides; chlorophyll; vitamins A, B1, B2, B3, B5, B6, B12, C and D; major minerals; trace minerals; polysaccharides; as well as carotenoids and other antioxidant pigments not found in many common foods.
- ★ Marine phytoplankton are a safe and highly effective detoxification tool for anyone at any stage! Marine phytoplankton have the ability to facilitate detoxification without demineralization. This is due to their high chlorophyll and energy content and high amount of alkaline minerals (such as calcium, magnesium, sulfur and zinc).
- ★ Marine phytoplankton are an amazing immune system booster, as they have antiviral, antifungal and antibacterial effects.

- Marine phytoplankton enhance memory and mental focus. This is due to phospholipids* and omega-3 fatty acids (like DHA) having the ability to cross the blood-brain barrier, thereby stimulating neurotransmitter production and improving mental clarity. (*Phospholipids are necessary to transport fat-soluble nutrients to all parts of our body).
- Marine phytoplankton improve eyesight as a result of being loaded with antioxidants (such as carotenoids astaxanthin, canthaxanthin and zeaxanthin) and omega-3 fatty acids (like DHA).
- Marine phytoplankton can boost sleep quality and help battle insomnia due to an increase in omega-3 fatty acids and the body becoming re-mineralized.
- Marine phytoplankton gradually stop cravings and normalize blood sugar imbalances, once again, due to the body becoming re-mineralized with high-quality, balanced nutrition.
- Marine phytoplankton improve digestion and support healthy weight loss.
- Marine phytoplankton enhance physical performance and endurance.
- Marine phytoplankton assist in relieving inflammation – meaning a decrease in aches and pains and improved recovery time from overuse or traumatic injuries.
- Marine phytoplankton enhance functions of the heart, lungs, brain, nervous system and immune system (to name a few); thereby improving a host of conditions (acute and chronic) such as circulatory disorders, behavioral problems and auto-immune issues.

Because they naturally contain a rich supply of antioxidants, long-chain omega-3 fatty acids EPA and DHA, as well as phospholipids (which help in the absorption of long-chain omega-3 fatty acids), marine phytoplankton are considered by many to be superior to most all fish oil supplements.

Looking for Quality in Marine Phytoplankton Products

Just like everything else I've been speaking of, when it comes to the quality and sustainability of our health, longevity and vitality, the following are going to be vitally important: the strain, the environment in which they grow, how they are processed, and the nutritional potency and purity of the final product.

- Look for companies utilizing only the single best, most beneficial strain of marine phytoplankton species identified for human consumption. Their claims should be based on extensive nutritional profiles and scientific research.
- Be interested in understanding the production process. Enquire about harvesting details, manufacturing details, transportation details and storage details. Each stage should be premeditated and carefully thought out and then conscientiously and meticulously carried out to the very end.
- In order to make absolutely sure that the final product is always and consistently free from toxic chemicals, environmental contaminants and other impurities, look for companies that have gone above and beyond the definition of "organic" as we know it today.

> ★ Demand raw, bioactive and bio-available products; cold-processed products; and when appropriate, freeze-dried products. Do your best to actively avoid products that have been heat-processed, pasteurized, irradiated or chemically processed. All of which degrade and destroy delicate nutrients.

One product that meets all the above criteria is Ocean's Alive Marine Phytoplankton by Activation Products. According to the distributor, a team of European doctors, microbiologists and botanists spent many years and millions of dollars researching 40,000 species of marine phytoplankton found in our vast oceans. Only four species of marine phytoplankton were found to be beneficial to humans. Based on nutritional profiles, only one species out of the four was found to be super beneficial: single strain *Nannochloropsis gaditana*. Therefore, this was the strain chosen.

As a result of this extensive research, technologically advanced commercial facilities have now been developed and constructed to produce marine phytoplankton in large volume using sophisticated photo-bioreactors (PBRs). PBRs consist of extensive glass tubing interconnected in a horizontal grid, about the size of a football field. A highly controlled environment is created that allows for natural photosynthesis to occur, using only natural sunlight to grow the phytoplankton biomass. Furthermore, purified seawater is utilized to ensure that no other species can contaminate the phytoplankton biomass. Once the phytoplankton biomass reaches maturity, it is harvested directly from the PBR. It is then meticulously placed into a highly sophisticated centrifuge that can spin the water out from around the phytoplankton cells, leaving the valuable life-force energy of the water within the cells completely protected and intact. Prior to bottling, this living phytoplankton biomass is then gently vortexed into a 100% pure and natural concentrated solution of over 90 highly absorbable ocean-derived ionic and trace minerals.

What about its sodium content? No need for concern! It is produced using a natural evaporation process that utilizes the sun and wind to eliminate 93% of the sodium.

The final product is a totally pure and super-charged liquid concentrate of raw and living whole food nutrients that can proudly be called "beyond" organic!

A BIT MORE ON THE PROFOUNDLY POWERFUL CHOSEN STRAIN

Nannochloropsis gaditana is an extremely unique microalgae species. The complexity of its elements and vital nutrients makes this particular strain highly effective in empowering cellular regeneration and healing. It is also the foremost source of omega-3 DHA in the world! But that's not all. *Nannochloropsis gaditana* is also astonishingly rich in omega-3 EPA; which if you didn't know, works in conjunction with DHA to help produce nearly every nutrient our bodies require.

Did you know that researchers at the Harvard School of Public Health determined that omega-3 deficiency causes between 72,000-96,000 preventable deaths each year in the United States alone?

How to Take Marine Phytoplankton

Ocean's Alive Marine Phytoplankton is intensely powerful. A little bit goes a long way! The daily dose will vary depending on your nutritional needs. I suggest a starting point of 2-5 drops (not droppers-full) twice a day. Try and see what works best for you. As your body becomes adjusted, you may work your way up to more drops and even droppers-full, and then adjust up or down whenever you feel the need. For instance, during intense cleanses I usually take an increased dosage of up to 3-4 droppers-full to ensure proper mineralization. On maintenance, I do well with taking five drops, 2-3 times per day.

> **Quick Tip:** I suggest consuming your drops the most direct way you can by dropping under the tongue. This way, it will get absorbed sublingually, bypassing the gastrointestinal tract, which is extremely helpful for those with gut absorption and assimilation problems. Try to hold the drops under your tongue for at least 2-3 minutes before swallowing. If you prefer not to hold them under your tongue, you may wish to take them with a product such as OptiMSM or MegaHydrate. Both are great potentiators and can significantly improve intracellular absorption. You may also wish to drop it in a superfood smoothie or elixir. If doing this, I suggest adding at least a teaspoon of coconut oil. As we learned earlier, consuming plant-based sources of omega-3 fatty acids with coconut oil has been found to potentiate its absorption and utilization in the brain. **FYI:** For the maximum in nutrient absorption and assimilation, along with coconut oil, I always open up 1-2 MegaHydrate capsules and pour the contents in my superfood smoothies and alchemical elixirs. Every time!

Spirulina

Spirulina is a single-celled, freshwater grown, blue-green spiral algae (hence, the name "spirulina"). Its green pigment is obtained from its richness in oxygen-producing chlorophyll and its blue pigment comes from phycocyanin. Phycocyanin is a water-soluble, highly vibrant blue fluorescent protein that has been demonstrated to have strong antioxidant, anti-inflammatory and anti-cancer properties. Its significant radical scavenging properties can help protect our cells, body tissues and organs from the harmful effects of oxidative stress. Blue-green algae are the only substances in the world known to contain phycocyanin, making spirulina a very unique and unprecedented superfood.

Spirulina is considered the most bio-available source of protein in the world! Gram for gram, spirulina contains the highest concentration of protein of any known food. It far surpasses that of any animal-derived protein, including beef. In his book *Superfoods for Optimum Health: Chlorella and Spirulina*, Mike Adams states that the digestive absorbability of each gram of protein in spirulina is four times greater than the same gram of protein in beef. He also states that since spirulina contains three times more protein ounce for ounce, spirulina offers twelve times more digestible protein than beef!

Spirulina is abundantly rich in the essential fatty acid gamma-linolenic acid (GLA). In fact, spirulina is one of the highest sources of GLA on the planet. According to Dr. Gabriel Cousens, only mother's milk is higher. GLA is extremely important for the growth and development of the brain, nervous system and heart. It has been noted that the standard American diet of processed and refined foods contains virtually no GLA. Now take into consideration the fact that many of us as infants have never been breast fed, like me, and I think it's safe to assume that many of us have been deficient in this critically important fatty acid and prostaglandin precursor right from the get-go! Prostaglandins are important hormone-like chemicals that regulate virtually every major body function, including allergies, blood pressure, blood cell stickiness (clotting), fever, fluid retention, as well as other immune system and inflammatory responses. GLA has been known to relieve symptoms of PMS; improve the condition of individuals suffering from multiple sclerosis (MS); decrease high blood pressure, reduce the tendency to clot, improve circulation and relieve the pain associated with circulatory disorders; improve skin conditions (like eczema); and relieve arthritic pain, as well as many other inflammatory conditions.

Spirulina Benefits:

- ★ Spirulina provides an abundant array of nutrients, such as vitamins A (beta-carotene), B1, B2, B6, E and K; 18 amino acids, including all eight essential amino acids, making it a complete source of protein; and chlorophyll, an important phytonutrient, blood builder and purifier. It also contains a multitude of major minerals, trace minerals, antioxidants, essential nucleic acids (RNA and DNA), fatty acids, polysaccharides and enzymes.
- ★ Spirulina contains 25 times more beta-carotene than raw carrots, making spirulina one of the richest sources of natural beta-carotene! Both chemically and physically, natural beta-carotene coming from a whole food source is far superior to synthetic versions found in capsule form and many multivitamin supplements. Natural whole food beta-carotene will always absorb far better into the body and will not build up and become toxic like synthetic forms can. Research has demonstrated that whole foods rich in beta-carotene, like spirulina, have the potential to prevent and even reverse certain types of cancers, as well as effectively shrink tumors, decrease cholesterol and treat wounds.
- ★ Spirulina contains 65-71% protein, the highest in any known food! Spirulina has long been used as a primary protein source by the people of Mexico City. Many Olympic and world champion athletes, fitness enthusiasts and body-builders alike have reported enhanced energy, endurance and performance just by adding spirulina to their regimen and using it during both their training and competitions.
- ★ The sulfur-bearing amino acids found in spirulina can significantly improve the following: detoxification processes and elimination pathways; the functionality of the liver, gallbladder, bile ducts and pancreas; the activity and function of the immune system; the speed of healing and tissue repair; physical strength, flexibility and agility; as well as the radiance of skin complexion and hair.

- Spirulina supports healthy weight loss without the work of muscle wasting. With just four calories per gram, spirulina gives a major protein punch without unwanted fats or an unnecessary intake of excess calories.
- Spirulina is rich in the following antioxidants that help protect our genetic material, DNA and RNA, from the bioaccumulation and damaging effects of toxins and radiation. These antioxidants are extremely important in the prevention of premature death of healthy cells which can contribute to a variety of illnesses, chronic and degenerative diseases, not to mention accelerate the aging process.
  - **Beta-carotene & other carotenoids:** help to promote proper intercellular communication (an important role in the prevention of cancer); protect bodily cells from free radical damage; and enhance normal immune system activity and function.
  - **Chlorophyll:** helps rebuild and renew blood cells; delivers much needed oxygen to all cells and tissues of the body to promote healthy growth and repair; neutralizes pollutants that we breathe in and intake on a daily basis; neutralizes pH levels within the body; assimilates calcium; chelates (binds) heavy metals; reduces bad breath and body odor; and so much more!
  - **Phycocyanin:** helps draw amino acids together for neurotransmitter formation, which can increase mental capacity. Phycocyanin has also been shown to play a major role in stem cell regeneration, especially in bone marrow and blood cells.
  - **Superoxide dismutase (SOD):** has been proven to function as both an antioxidant and anti-inflammatory in the body. Generally, SOD is known as one of the most important health enhancing metabolic enzymes. It also helps our bodies utilize certain important minerals, such as zinc, copper and manganese, all of which are naturally and conveniently found in spirulina. Having a sufficient intake of SOD can be helpful in the treatment of joint disorders, prostate problems, stomach issues, inflammatory bowel syndrome (IBS), burn injuries, along with long-term damage from exposure to smoke and radiation. It is also considered to be an extremely beneficial adjunct to help decrease and even prevent the detrimental side effects of cancer drugs.
  - **Zeaxanthin:** helps protect the eyes from ultra-violet (UV) damage. Furthermore, it helps in the prevention of free radical damage to the retina and lens of the eye, which is commonly seen with cataracts, diabetic retinopathy, glaucoma and macular degeneration.
- Spirulina is a potent source of gamma-linolenic acid (GLA)! As stated above, GLA is important for growth and development (especially of the nervous system) and is found most abundantly in mother's milk. Next to mother's milk, spirulina is the next highest whole food source of GLA – with hemp seeds not far behind.
- Spirulina has 58 times the iron of raw spinach and 28 times that of raw beef liver! It contains more bio-chelated organic iron than any other whole food. Bio-chelated means that the iron will easily be assimilated into the body.

Spirulina Platensis: The Blue-Green Algae of Choice

Personally, I am not a huge fan of *Aphanizomenon flos-aquae* (AFA) blue-green algae from Klamath Lake. After much research, and trying and testing a few major and well-respected brands of blue-green algae over the past ten years, I will now only consume and recommend one strain. That one and only strain of blue-green algae is *Spirulina platensis*. There are two sources I trust whole-heartedly, as they have no problem supplying (upon request) a certificate of analysis that proves nutritional integrity, quality and purity. In addition, the feedback from individuals I have had the pleasure of working with has been nothing less than phenomenal and reassuring. So, whether you or someone you know is dealing with a health crisis, trying to improve athletic performance or just wanting to feel much better, *Spirulina platensis* is the strain of choice in my book.

Unlike some strains of blue-green algae, *Spirulina platensis* has no toxicity risks or harmful side effects whatsoever. I always source my spirulina from New Horizon Health and Ultimate Superfoods. I find their integrity to be impeccable. Plus, their spirulina is always pure, organic and kosher certified; grown and harvested with care and quality in mind; and processed at temperatures that never destroy or devitalize its abundant array of delicate nutrients.

Recommended Dosage

Spirulina Platensis	Recommended Daily Dosage
Maintenance Dosage	4-6 grams per day
Significant Part of the Diet	6-10 grams per day
Immune System Builder	12-14 grams per day
Primary Source of Protein	12-20 grams per day
Healing Purposes & Heavy Metal Detox	20-26+ grams per day

Microalgae in Summary

Chlorella, marine phytoplankton and spirulina are packed with an abundance of nutrients and phytochemicals that can upgrade your health and fight off disease. In all, these three superfoods are effective in helping to reverse a long list of serious ailments. What's more, they are powerful health enhancers and energy boosters that demonstrate phenomenal benefits, even for those who consider themselves in good health! Personally, I find I am at my best when I consume all three, as they all have unique qualities that can be utilized for different purposes. I tend to allow my body and where I am on my wellness path dictate which one I will need to increase or decrease. For instance, when I'm training hard and working out more than two hours per day, I consume, in divided doses, about 3-4 tablespoons of spirulina and two tablespoons of chlorella. When I'm in more of a cleansing and detoxification mode, I tend to reverse my amounts and take 3-4 tablespoons of chlorella and two tablespoons of spirulina throughout the day. When I'm somewhere in the middle (for example, living day to day in maintenance mode), I tend to consume about two heaping tablespoons of each. I advise everyone to gradually work their way up to the dosage that is right for them. Start with one teaspoon, one to several times per day and gradually work your way up to tablespoons (if that is where you should be). If choosing to consume both, I recommend chlorella 20-30 minutes before meals and spirulina with meals. That being said, spirulina may certainly be taken on an empty stomach with great effectiveness.

The most important message I want to convey is to listen to your body. Tune in and learn to recognize what dosage gives you true satiation and sustainability. For me and the lifestyle I live, I run best on 24-36 grams (total) between the two. I also take marine phytoplankton because I am definitely one of those people who run high on the side of being intense and an overachiever. Interestingly, I have found that by keeping my microalgae levels up, I don't feel like raiding the jar of nuts or dried fruit late at night. I feel much more nourished, balanced, light (yet grounded) and energized. Microalgae and other algae, such as sea vegetables, can truly fill in the blanks and do for us what our mineral deficient soil cannot, giving us the minerals that the majority of grocery store bought produce (including organic) no longer contains.

Please Note: Adding microalgae to your diet will certainly upgrade it, but will not justify the continuation of a lifestyle consuming junk, processed and refined foods. Don't get caught fighting an unnecessary uphill battle.

Final Thoughts

Personally, I feel that if everyone took the recommended daily dosage that fit their personal needs of at least two out of the three microalgae detailed above then, without a doubt, we could adequately replace and sufficiently satisfy the false notion of needing synthetic multi-vitamins and minerals. Moreover, I strongly believe that by utilizing microalgae, we can easily abolish the need for all the highly marketed, all-in-one protein powders, meal replacement shakes and protein bars. The vast majority are made of synthetic isolates and a bunch of fillers and fluff – not to mention highly questionable raw material. Protein products, such as these, are great at doing two things: taxing the kidneys and causing constipation. Two issues we should want to avoid like the plague if we want to achieve vibrant health.

SPROUTS: TINY MIGHTIES!

"The sprout releases all of its stored nutrients in a burst of vitality as it attempts to become a full-sized plant." – Dr. Ann Wigmore (aka "the mother of living foods")

My inspiration to start sprouting came after watching the entire 12 lecture DVD series put out by the Hippocrates Health Institute (HHI). The original location for HHI was Boston, MA, where I was born and raised. Now it is located in West Palm Beach, FL, directly across the state from where I live in the Tampa Bay area. Founded in 1956 by Dr. Ann Wigmore, legendary for bringing the healing powers of wheatgrass and raw foods to fruition, HHI has become one of the world's leading natural health institutes. Currently under the leadership of Dr. Brian and Anna Maria Clement, HHI is world renowned for teaching individuals how to embrace a living-foods lifestyle for optimal health. Successfully attaining health and creating longevity is their ultimate goal for everyone who participates. Achievements are obtained through their ability to deliver cutting edge knowledge coupled with a common-sense approach. Thanks to the hundreds of thousands of individuals who have participated in their Life Transformation Program, HHI has acquired well over 50 years of combined clinical research.

I first learned about the Hippocrates Health Institute while living and working in Boston as an R.N. specializing in oncology and hematology. Although totally intrigued, I unfortunately was kept busy in the conventional world of medicine. It wasn't until I moved to Florida that I decided to whole-heartedly make a clean break. I was ready to make it my business (no pun intended) to research and learn everything attainable on healing the human body from the inside out – and how to do it naturally. I had officially cut my ties to conventional medicine, never to turn back!

> *A true "live" food vegetarian diet is rich in vitamins, minerals and proteins. It can supply our bodies with all the necessary oxygen, enzymes, alkalinity and bioelectrical charges vital to cellular health.*

Brief History of HHI

Dr. Ann Wigmore, visionary and humanitarian, along with the brilliant mind of Viktoras Kulvinskas, founded a concept based on the Hippocratic wisdom – "Let Food Be Thy Medicine." Together they created a comprehensive institute in Boston where the focus was on empowerment. They believed that the confidence to transform quality of life came with learning how to draw on inner resources.

Having cured herself of colon cancer using natural methods, Dr. Ann Wigmore is considered a pioneer in the natural health movement. She will go down in history as having started a revolution in the world of raw food nutrition that continues to grow today.

The mission of HHI is to promote self-healing through a living foods lifestyle. Over the decades, Wigmore and Kulvinskas have helped individuals from all walks of life, teaching them how to restore and rejuvenate their own bodies. Today, guests can expect to meet with physicians and health administrators before starting a program to detoxify their systems. Diet, treatment plan and supplementation are all individually-tailored to meet the needs of each participant.

The Hippocrates Health Institute is available to all! From those with major health challenges to those simply wanting to energize their lives and maintain a state of youth, vitality and stamina.

Other Great Healing Institutes

A number of other institutes carry on the great works of Dr. Ann Wigmore by offering educational programs and retreats, home study courses, recipes, books and other resources. They can easily be found through a quick google of her name.

I, personally, had an amazing three-week experience at the Optimal Health Institute (OHI) in Lemon Grove, CA; but I must make you aware, there are no medical personnel available at OHI if this is what your health challenge warrants or what you desire for more individualized programming. If you are looking for a facility that has licensed medical consultants on staff, I recommend the Hippocrates Health Institute in West Palm Beach, FL or Tree of Life Rejuvenation Center located in Patagonia, AZ (see below).

The Tree of Life Rejuvenation Center in Patagonia, AZ is another great healing facility. Dr. Gabriel Cousens is the founder and director of the Tree of Life Rejuvenation Center, and he and his full medical staff have helped thousands of people reclaim their lives by bringing their bodies back into balance. A wide variety of programs targeted toward specific health challenges, such as diabetes, depression and anxiety, are offered. It is my dream to one day attend their 21 Day Transformation Program and the 27 Day Masters Intensive Program.

Ten Great Reasons to Start Sprouting Today!

1. **Availability:** From Argentina to Alaska and January to July, you can enjoy sprouts year-round! Whether you live in a tiny New York City apartment, on a boat in the water, or in a tent in the woods, sprouting is doable and easy for everyone.
2. **Digestibility:** Sprouts are baby plants. According to Dr. Brian Clement, sprouts are noteworthy for being 10-30 times more nutritious than their mature vegetable counterpart. Sprouts have a delicate cell wall which allows them to release live nourishment much more easily. Their nutrients exist in elemental form and their abundance in live enzymes makes them easy to digest; even for those with weak digestive systems and a loss of digestive fire (aka our metabolism, which is responsible for absorbing and assimilating the foods we eat).
3. **Ecology:** You'll no longer depend on airplanes or fuel/oil driven transport to deliver food to you! Also, there is never a need for toxic pesticides, herbicides and fungicides or synthetic fertilizers when you grow them yourself.
4. **Economics:** Sprouting seeds can multiply anywhere from 7-15 times their weight. And at just a few dollars per pound for organic seeds (give or take a few dollars depending on the variety of seed), this yields one whole pound of fresh, spouted, indoor-grown, organic greens for pennies per day!
5. **Freshness:** Sprouts are always fresh and full of life-giving energy, as they can be eaten the same day they are picked! There will be no loss of nutrients from being transported all over the place or from sitting in warehouses or on grocery store shelves.

6. **Meal-Time Easy:** In minutes, you can toss up a sprout salad or roll them up as part of a wrap. Just use a large collard green, lettuce leaf or nori sheet. How about tossing them down your juicer for vibrant vegetable juices and adding them to your smoothies or blended soups for an extra enzymatic kick?
7. **Nutrition:** Sprouts are baby plants in the prime of their life. Compared to mature vegetables, sprouts are in the early stage of their growth and actually contain the highest concentration of digestible energy, bio-available amino acids, essential fatty acids, enzymes, fiber, vitamins, minerals, phytochemicals, RNA, DNA, etc. When compared with their mature plant counterpart, sprouts can yield a nutrient content up to 30 times higher!
8. **Organic:** When you purchase organic seeds and grow them yourself, there is no question of chemical contamination. You can trust their freshness, quality and purity, as you are the grower!
9. **Little Space/Little Time:** There are no excuses! Self-sprouting is easy for the whole family, no matter how young or old. A green thumb and special lighting are not required. No soil even; just water! A concentrated mineral solution is recommended, but not necessary. To grow one pound of sprouts takes only nine inches of space and a couple of minutes out of your day.
10. **Versatility:** Sprouts offer more varieties of salad greens than your grocery store shelves. They include leafy sprouts like the commonly known alfalfa and clover, as well as the unique, tangy and spicy flavors of garlic, onion, mustard, dill, cress, arugula, radish, kale and my all-time favorites, broccoli, fenugreek and sunflower. Other wonderful, fast and easy sprouts are quinoa and certain legume sprouts such as lentil, pea, adzuki and mung bean. Truly, the sky is the limit when it comes to what you can sprout.

> **Quick Tip:** www.sprouthouse.com and www.sproutpeople.org are two great sites to purchase a wide variety of organic sprouting seeds. I also found them to be great resources on sprouting in general (including technique). I've called them for help on several occasions.

Please Note: According to the expert opinion of many naturopaths, grains (whether refined, whole, cooked or sprouted) may not be as healthy for us humans as originally thought. In fact, unless the sole purpose is to grow them to produce grass (such as wheatgrass, oat grass or barley grass), then grains are not recommended as the staple food we previously believed. You may be wondering why – and the answer is actually pretty clear. Grains, in general, are prone to mold growth and mycotoxin contamination. Add to that the increasing issue of gluten intolerance and celiac disease and this newer theory starts to look more like a verifiable truth. Gluten is a protein and potential allergen found in the grains of wheat, barley and rye. Buyers beware, although oats are considered a gluten-free grain, there is evidence of a common cross-contamination problem when it comes to oats being grown and produced in the traditional manner. When tested, most commercially available oats and mainstream oat products contained unacceptable amounts of gluten.

Surprisingly, the grass of wheat, barley and oats do not contain gluten and are not known to trigger gluten intolerance. Additionally, they are prized for their amazing healing properties when juiced fresh. You may also purchase and consume these grasses in a raw, cold-processed powdered form that is both alive and viable in bio-available nutrients. Although I enjoy sprouting, I have not been able to get myself into growing wheatgrass and the like. This doesn't mean that I don't want to benefit from what they have to offer, though. For this reason, I have some favorite greens in powder form that contain all the live-food healing power of fresh grasses. For whole food grass powders (meaning, fiber included), I love Ormus Supergreens by Sunwarrior and Premier Greens Mix by Premier Research Labs. For concentrated juice grass powders, I love Organic Kamut Blend and Organic Barley Green Juice by Purium. Juicing the fresh grass may be "the best," but when that is not an option (or just plain inconvenient), any of these particular powders runs a close second and requires no time at all except the stir of your spoon.

Shedding Some Light on the "Mother of ALL Grains"

Wait a minute! Didn't I just say grains are not recommended? Ahh, but there is one exception (and only one) – quinoa! Why? Quinoa is actually not a grain. Let me explain. Confusingly, the agricultural term "grain" is based only on the appearance of a food product; so, quinoa has been misidentified and tagged with names like quinoa grain, super grain and pseudo cereal on a lot of commercial packaging, as well as in articles and advertisements. I guess as the saying goes, "if it looks like a duck, walks like a duck and quacks like a duck, it must be a duck!" Botanically speaking though, quinoa is not a grain at all, it's a seed. It belongs to the same family as spinach, Swiss chard and beets and is much more closely related to these crops than cereal crops (such as wheat or rice). This makes quinoa not only gluten-free, but grain-free as well. Because it looks and cooks and tastes like a grain, it is by far the best replacement for all those difficult to digest grains and cereals. Furthermore, quinoa will not feed systemic fungal infection (like Candida) or bacterial infections within the body.

Quinoa, an ancient grain-like "seed" (or shall we say "pseudo grain"), has been cultivated in Peru, Chile and Bolivia for over 5,000 years. It has long been a staple food for the native Indians and has sustained the indigenous people of the Andes mountain range for over thousands of years. According to the literature, even today quinoa is still a staple food grown by farmers at higher elevations throughout most of South America. For the people of these regions, quinoa is a valuable source of high-quality protein (approximately 16-23%).

Quinoa provides more amino acids, enzymes, vitamins, minerals, fiber, antioxidants and phytonutrients than all other "actual" grains. In fact, due to its outstanding nutritional profile, the ancient Incas called quinoa the "mother grain" and revered it as a sacred super-crop. Quinoa was also once considered "the gold of the Incas," as it was traditional for the Inca leader to plant the first quinoa seed using a solid gold shovel each year at planting time. Quinoa also was used to sustain the Inca armies, who could march for days eating "war balls" of quinoa and fat. This is probably why quinoa is labeled so often as a superfood.

Raw Sprouted Quinoa Benefits:

- ★ Quinoa (especially in its raw and sprouted form) contains all nine essential amino acids the adult body cannot produce, making it a complete protein. This makes quinoa another great option for vegans, vegetarians, followers of the Paleolithic diet and anyone who desires to eat less animal protein.
- ★ Quinoa is especially rich in lysine – the amino acid that is essential for healthy tissue growth and repair. It also provides an impressive quantity of methionine and cystine: the two-principle sulfur-containing amino acids.
- ★ Quinoa has more calcium than milk! It is also rich in the minerals potassium, phosphorus, magnesium and iron and contains a good amount of the trace minerals manganese, copper and zinc. When raw and sprouted (not processed and cooked), quinoa can also provide us with a quality source of vitamins B1, B2, B6, B9 (aka folic acid), C and E.
- ★ Quinoa acts as a prebiotic. This means it can stimulate the growth and activity of good bacteria in the gut, which is very beneficial to overall health.
- ★ Quinoa is a rich source of dietary fiber. Its fiber is also considered quite easy to digest. Consuming quinoa on a regular basis is a wonderful way to ensure that you are receiving a valuable source of fiber which will help ease elimination and tone your colon.

Please Note: Much of the packaged quinoa found in your typical grocery store has been processed to remove the bitter sheath, which means it will not fully sprout. Be certain to buy only organic quinoa that is of sprouting quality. Also, be sure to thoroughly rinse before the soaking and repeated rinsing and draining cycles required for sprouting. This will ensure the neutralization of phytic acid and other potential enzyme inhibitors. It will also ensure that the bitter, soapy saponins, as well as any traces of dirt and debris, have been successfully removed.

> **Quick Tip:** I just recently found out about a company called TruRoots. They specialize in sprouted products, including sprouted quinoa, which are then gently, low-temperature air-dried using eco-friendly solar energy at temperatures that preserve all the enzymes, vitamins and minerals. Sprouting (aka germinating) is a time-tested process that breaks down all the complex carbohydrates and proteins and converts them into simpler forms. This makes sprouted quinoa not only much easier to digest but much more readily absorbed by the body. I consider this concept by TruRoots an ingenious one to say the least! They have managed to harmonize ancient wisdom with modern science; while keeping it agriculturally sustainable, organic and raw. I foresee this product being great for the modern-day health seeker – those who are on the go but determined to thrive on nothing less than the absolute best.
>
> Simply add this sprouted quinoa straight into your raw creations such as tabouli salad and other quinoa salad recipes. It can also be rehydrated and used as a substitute for cereal, couscous or rice. Go ahead and add to raw blended soups. For a new twist on the old and mundane dehydrated flax-based crackers, feel free to add some sprouted quinoa to the mix. Use as-is or ground into a flour to make delicious raw cookies and protein bars. For more information and where to buy, go to www.truroots.com.

What About Sprouting Legumes?

When it comes to legumes (beans, peas, lentils, soybeans, peanuts, etc.), I stay away from certain varieties. Unfortunately, they tend to contain a large amount of natural toxins and enzyme inhibitors. For instance, sprouting soybeans and the larger red and black kidney beans is not at all recommended due to the substantial amount of toxins and enzyme inhibitors still present after sprouting. However, I do like to sprout and eat a small to moderate amount of some of the smaller sized legumes such as lentils, peas, adzuki and mung beans. In addition, I prefer to consume certain legumes, such as garbanzo beans, in a fermented form like chickpea miso. Fermentation can dramatically enhance the nutritional quality and digestibility of legumes.

FYI: I love garbanzo beans, but I find garbanzos to be one of the tougher varieties of beans to sprout in Florida without running into some sort of mold issue. Cooler and drier climates (or times of the year) will most likely not have the same negative effect on certain sprouts that tropical climates do. I suggest experimenting during the cooler and drier months with certain beans such as garbanzos. It may also be worth checking the relative humidity of your home.

Cooking vs Sprouting Legumes

The problem with legumes is not so much with legumes in and among themselves; but rather with the way in which they are traditionally prepared, which usually involves cooking for long periods of time. This is especially relevant when we consider the immense number of people who consume them this way as their prime source of dietary protein and fiber. Sure, cooking legumes may effectively reduce the amount of anti-nutrients and make them "relatively" digestible when compared to their dry state; but with the large amount of cooking we put them through, we also lose all the enzymes and a large majority of essential nutrients and required cofactors in the process.

I strongly believe that the best way to consume a variety of legumes is sprouted. By sprouting legumes instead of cooking them, specifically the smaller varieties mentioned above, we not only neutralize many of the natural toxins effectively and efficiently, but we gain an infinite number of other benefits not possibly obtained when cooked to death. Basically, sprouting brings us the best of all worlds: neutralization of anti-nutrients, living enzymes, essential amino acids, essential fatty acids, vitamins, minerals and the increased ability to properly digest, absorb and assimilate it all!

Summing Up Legume Sprouting

Legumes – like grains, nuts and seeds – have anti-nutritional factors, meaning, they contain natural toxins (like enzyme inhibitors) that are naturally produced by plants to defend themselves against various threats like bacteria, fungi, insects and predators. When legumes are cooked, which is the way most individuals consume them, some toxins will neutralize; but cooking also denatures the amino acids (proteins) and destroys many of the other vital nutrients, including water-soluble vitamins. A better method of neutralizing natural toxins, such as phytic acid and other enzyme inhibitors, is to mitigate the germination process by soaking and sprouting. By sprouting, rather than cooking, we not only neutralize many of the natural toxins much more effectively, we unlock and awaken all the vital nutrients of these sleeping beauties. Remember, only from life force energy can we truly gain more life force energy for ourselves!

General Sprouting Benefits:

- ★ Sprouting transforms various seeds from an acid forming food to a more alkaline forming food.
- ★ Sprouting increases enzyme levels dramatically. This is beneficial for enhanced and proper digestion.
- ★ Sprouting converts fats into essential fatty acids.
- ★ Sprouting transforms dense vegetable proteins into simpler amino acids for easier digestion, absorption and assimilation.
- ★ Sprouting increases water-soluble vitamin C and certain broad-spectrum B vitamins.
- ★ Sprouting greatly increases carotenoids.
- ★ Sprouting causes minerals to chelate (merge with protein molecules) in a way that increase their function.

Seeds are tiny, yet jam-packed storehouses of super-powered nutrients that are just waiting for the right temperature and right amount of moisture to start the germination process. Germination is simply the birth and growth of a baby plant. It's what I like to call "the spark that ignites the flame of life!" Take the common sunflower seed, for example. It may only measure about a quarter of an inch long, but it contains the blueprint necessary to provide the development of a six-foot plant.

Sprouts are enzymatic and fully alive when you eat them. They are one of nature's most prized, raw and living superfoods. With just a little TLC, sprouts can easily nourish the world. Seeds are inexpensive and easily available to everyone and ready to grow anywhere and at any time!

> Dr. Gabriel Cousens, a highly regarded medical researcher and internationally-known sprout expert, wrote the following on sprouts in an article titled "A Healthy Perspective of Sprouts" (retrieved from www.newfrontier.com): *"They contain a rainforest of undiscovered and known good health characteristics such as antioxidants, anti-carcinogens, live enzymes, high levels of vitamins, nucleic acids, pacifierans (plant 'antibiotics'), auxones (beneficial plant hormones) and other factors."*

Choosing the Best Sprouter

Trust me when I tell you, I have run the gamut on sprouters. My findings were that certain seeds sprouted well, but living in a humid environment like Florida, even with air-conditioning, can pose some challenges. For instance: mold issues and not always yielding the desired amount.

From Amateur to Sprouting Pro!

Before getting to the sprouter that I absolutely love and adore, I will go through some of my painstaking experiences with other sprouters on the market.

- ★ I absolutely did not like using the hemp bag for sprouting. I couldn't always see what was going on inside the bag and after several days of anxiously waiting, I certainly was not happy if all I harvested was small, wimpy, limp sprouts. In addition, I found it didn't always prevent mold from growing even though it was made from a mold-resistant natural material. And once you have a little mold growing, the whole batch must go.
- ★ I also am not fond of using the jar method. It certainly works, but I found it to be much too much work for the small amount of sprouts it would yield. I like a good amount of sprouts on my salad, which most would consider fit for a family of five. Therefore, this didn't work for me. On top of that, although he never complained, I know my partner, at the time, didn't always appreciate the kitchen looking like a science lab with upside down, slanted and draining mason glass jars everywhere.
- ★ I also tried a terra cotta sprouter. It may have been very pretty, but that's about it. I say don't bother! The terra cotta sprouter wasted more of my time in cleaning than anything else. The tiny, itty-bitty holes got clogged with seeds every single time; and then I would have to use a needle to poke them out. After a couple of weeks of doing this, I was just about ready to stick the needle in my eye! This was certainly not worth the effort of the snack sized amount of sprouts it produced.

Now for What I Do Like; Saving the Best for Last!

- ★ For beginners, I really like the Sprout Master 8x10 trays. If I learned anything from my amateur sprouting days, I learned that no matter what you want to sprout, trays are the way to go.
- ★ I also didn't mind the Easy Sprout sprouter for certain sprouts, such as quinoa and certain salad mixes that included lentils and beans, but did not care for it when it came to leafy sprouts. Again, trays are the best. The Easy Sprout sprouter is great for sprouting while traveling or camping, but the Spout Master trays are a much better option. If you're going to put in the time and effort, you might as well get enough sprouts to last a few days with the ability to stagger and rotate.
- ★ The best brand sprouter by far is the EasyGreen MikroFarm Automatic Sprouter! I learned about this machine during my three week stay at the Optimal Health Institute (OHI), and it was love at first sight. I love it so much that I have more than one. You can find it online for approximately $229.00. If you look carefully, you can find sites that will offer bonuses. For instance, Discount Juicers and the Sprout House has offered one large tray (which I find useful for growing sunflower sprouts, thick bean sprouts and wheatgrass) in addition to the five rectangular cartridges included with your regular purchase. Discount Juicers also has a great automatic sprouter comparison chart that can be accessed at the bottom of their information page for the Easy-Green Automatic Sprouting Machine. I find their chart to be accurate.

Here are just a few points that make the EasyGreen MikroFarm worth buying if you truly desire the freshest organic greens available, loaded with bio-available nutrients, for just pennies a day!

- ★ Has a large growing area. Its rectangular shape allows the ability to easily transfer rectangular cartridges and trays from machine to fridge for the storage of fully grown and uneaten sprouts.
- ★ Grows all sprouts hydroponically using water only. Including grass! This means no soil is necessary to grow sunflower sprouts and wheatgrass. But if you desire the use of soil, you can still do this as well without damaging the machine.
- ★ Requires no presoaking of seeds. You can place dry seeds directly into the tray or cartridges, and the machine will automatically do all the work of soaking, rinsing, misting, oxygenating and draining for you.
- ★ Creates no mold or rotting of seeds. The EasyGreen MikroFarm uses a patented technology that both mists and oxygenates the seeds simultaneously. By cooling the seed's water and air – and oxygenating the seeds and water at the same time – you can harvest sprouts much quicker without running into the issues with mold you would with other methods. Even in Florida, with its hot and humid weather several months out of the year, I can still get the best sprouts year-round!

- ★ Does not re-circulate water that contains toxins and inhibitors, defeating the whole purpose of using fresh and clean water for fresh and clean sprouts. Many other automatic sprouters re-circulate the water, but with the EasyGreen MikroFarm, all used water is drained out of the machine, using only fresh water from the built-in water reservoir for irrigation. This is very important when one considers the fact that sprouts are approximately 80% water.
- ★ Allows the addition of minerals in the form of liquid kelp or sea water solutions to the built-in water reservoir. For aesthetic reasons, I prefer the clear sea water solutions over liquid kelp. The kelp solutions I tried always ended up temporarily discoloring the inside of the machine. It does clean rather easily, but it takes pulling the machine apart a bit if you want to thoroughly clean the inside of the water reservoir.
- ★ To learn more about the EasyGreen MikroFarm, and why I consider it to be the preferred method for sprouting, go to www.easygreen.com. For the best price (including bonuses), as well as unbiased information, I suggest the following distributors: www.discountjuicers.com, www.sprouthouse.com or www.amazon.com. Green thumb not required!

WORLD-WIDE SUPERFRUITS: BEST BANGIN' BERRIES!

Most would agree that out of all the edible fruits on earth, berries are among the absolute best. As a group, berries are prized for being amazingly high in antioxidants, and as we know, antioxidants help protect us against inflammation and free radical damage. Certain berries, such as blackberries and raspberries, are known for their richness in dietary fiber. Blueberries contain powerful phytochemicals, such as anthocyanin, which is the pigment that gives blueberries their blue-violet color. Cranberries are rich in polyphenols and can combat urinary tract infections by preventing *Escherichia coli* bacteria from sticking to cells in the urinary tract. Raspberries contain cancer-fighting phytochemicals such as ellagic, coumaric and ferulic acid. Strawberries surprisingly contain more vitamin C in a one-cup serving than one orange and are particularly high in folic acid, to boot!

All the above are among my commonly known favorites, but what about my exotic favorites? Goji berries and golden berries are two highly regarded berries that carry one heck of a nutritional punch in little but mighty packages. Unless I'm fasting, I don't go one day without having a least one small handful.

Goji Berries

Ron Teeguarden, one of the foremost herbalists in America and a professional practitioner and teacher of the holistic Asian health arts since 1971, states that goji is classified as a "superior tonic" – a class of herbs that people should take on an ongoing basis to preserve youth and to promote general well-being. According to Teeguarden, this classification can be found in China's first herbal encyclopedia written in the 1st century B.C.

In Chinese medicine, goji berries are used to rejuvenate. By harmonizing and nourishing the adrenals, kidneys and liver, a person's "life force" can be restored.

Goji berries are considered a superfruit due to their super high content of antioxidants. Based on the ORAC chart of fruits, vegetables and essential oils, goji berries can contain anywhere from five to ten times the amount of antioxidants found in blueberries.

> *"Taking in goji berry regularly may regulate the flow of vital energy and strengthen the physique, which can lead to longevity."* – The physician's handbook, Ben Cao Gang Mu, recorded during the Ming Dynasty (1368-1644 A.D.)

Goji Berry Benefits:

- ★ Goji berries are one of the highest antioxidant containing foods on the planet.
- ★ Goji berries provide the complete spectrum of antioxidant carotenoids, including beta-carotene (way more than carrots), lutein and zeaxanthin.
  - o Carotenoids are known to support healthy vision and protect the eyes against age-related conditions such as macular degeneration, cataracts, diabetic retinopathy and loss of sight.
  - o Beta-carotene helps support immunity by enhancing the function of the thymus gland, facilitating communication between immune cells and by making the stimulatory action of interferon on the immune system more powerful.
- ★ Goji berries are considered an adaptogenic food.

WHAT IS AN ADAPTOGEN?

An adaptogen is a medicinal plant that has proven to be effective in helping the body "adapt" or "adjust" to the stresses and strains of daily living.

Adaptogens have a unique capability of normalizing bodily functions and balancing bodily systems. This ability to promote homeostasis is one of the most important qualities of an adaptogen.

In cases of hypoactivity (deficiency/low function), adaptogens will strengthen and increase function. If there is hyperactivity (excessive function), adaptogens will gently reduce and normalize functioning.

- ★ Goji berries are a complete protein source and provide a total of 19 different amino acids, including the essential amino acid tryptophan: a biochemical precursor that promotes healthy serotonin production and niacin (B3) synthesis. They also contain the essential amino acid phenylalanine: an important neurotransmitter precursor for healthy adrenal function and thyroid support. **FYI:** It is very rare for a fruit to contain all eight essential amino acids and be such a great overall protein source.

- Goji berries are also a rich source of l-arginine and l-glutamine: two amino acids that work together to boost human growth hormone (HGH) levels. Growth hormone plays an important role in anti-aging, as it promotes healthy bone density and lean muscle mass. It also plays three different roles in metabolism. It increases the rate of protein synthesis, promotes the breakdown of fat and accelerates the rate at which the liver releases glucose into the blood.
    - Goji berries are the only food known to help stimulate the human body's pituitary and pineal glands to produce more human growth hormone (HGH) naturally!
    - HGH is considered the master hormone that drives growth and development. By increasing HGH, one naturally enhances testosterone production, making goji berries perhaps the world's greatest anti-aging superfood for both men and women.
- Goji berries contain 21 or more trace minerals (the most powerful ones being calcium, potassium, iron, zinc, copper, germanium, selenium and phosphorus) as well as vitamin B1, B2 and B6 and even vitamin E, typically not found in fruits. Germanium (rarely found in food) and selenium are even used in a number of clinical trials involving cancer patients.
    - Some proponents say that organic germanium stimulates the body's production of interferon, a naturally-occurring anti-cancer agent. Other advocates claim that germanium helps the immune system by boosting the activity of natural killer cells, a type of white blood cell that attacks invading microbes. All in all, germanium has proven efficacy when it comes to boosting the immune system and reducing tumor size in certain types of cancers (colon, prostate, breast, lung, ovarian and cervical cancers). Germanium has also shown positive results with rheumatoid arthritis and rheumatism.
- Goji berries provide nine milligrams or more of blood-building iron per 100 grams (approximately two to three handfuls).
- Goji berries contain high levels of long-chain sugars called polysaccharides.
    - Polysaccharides are exceptional sources of essential sugars necessary for proper immune function and intercellular communication, meaning, they can help protect cells from genetic mutation.
    - The polysaccharides found in goji berries stimulate interleukin-2 and gamma-interferon, which are anti-inflammatory and immune system enhancers.
- Goji berries help our bodies produce choline, an essential nutrient required by the body for a number of important processes, including liver protection, cell membrane structure and maintaining neurotransmitter functioning.
    - Choline is a building block for the neurotransmitter acetylcholine. Research indicates that choline has a positive effect on memory and the ability to learn.
    - Although research on the benefits of choline continues, studies indicate adequate choline intake is associated with preventing or resolving a number of conditions and diseases, including Alzheimer's disease, dementia, depression and memory loss.

- o In other medical studies, choline has proven to be helpful in lowering homocysteine levels in the blood. High levels of homocysteine (typically seen in meat eaters) may increase the risk of atherosclerosis (hardening and narrowing of the arteries) as well as increase the risk of myocardial infarctions (heart attacks), strokes and blood clots.
★ Goji berries contain betaine, a phytochemical known to help reduce the toxic amino acid homocysteine in the blood (especially effective when taken with sources of folic acid, B6 and B12). Betaine also helps keep the liver functioning at its best. The donation of methyl groups by betaine is very important to proper liver function, cellular replication and detoxification reactions.
★ Last but not least, goji berries can increase our natural production of superoxide dismutase (SOD), our built-in defense against free radical attack and aging.

Overall, it's the unique synergy of phytochemicals, polysaccharides, amino acids, essential fatty acids, vitamins, minerals and trace minerals – all found together in raw and medicinal quality goji berries – that gives these berries the capacity to enhance one's longevity, strength, stamina and sexual function; boost the immune system, heart and brain function; and improve eyesight and sleep quality.

When looking to purchase goji berries, make sure they have been sourced from the pristine area of Ningxia Province in China, where people have grown goji berries wild for centuries. I will only purchase goji berries from New Horizon Health or Ultimate Superfoods. They are lab tested for 400 different chemicals used in agriculture and processing, as well as sulfites. They are also considered more organic than those labeled so in the market. Importantly, these goji berries have won awards from the China Medical Promotion Committee and are Green Food certified.

> Of the eighty different species of goji berries worldwide, only one comes from Ningxia Province in China – *Lycium barbarum*. This variety has by far the highest levels of immune-stimulating polysaccharides of all the goji berry species.
>
> Moreover, *Lycium barbarum* is the only Chinese Lycium species accepted by the Chinese Pharmacopeia.

The taste of goji berries is hard to describe. Some say they taste like a cross between a cranberry and a cherry, while others say they taste somewhat like a raspberry or plum. Enjoy goji berries in trail mixes, topped on salad or blended into your favorite smoothies. They also jazz up a cup of loose-leaf tea if you drop 10-15 in your cup. Then you can eat the rehydrated goji berries as a snack once you're finished your tea. I particularly love goji berries in my morning smoothie or added to a nice cup of green tea.

Golden Berries

Golden berries *(Physalis peruviana)*, also known as Incan berries and Cape gooseberries, are an annual herb indigenous to many parts of tropical South America, including the Amazon. These plump and succulent yellow berries are related to the tomatillo. They are even protected by papery husks similar to tomatillos. They are about the size of a marble and when dried, resemble a tart and tangy raisin. Golden berries have a deliciously exotic citrus flavor and are extremely nutritious. They are a great source of bioflavonoids and carotenoids, as well as phosphorous, pectin, dietary fiber, vitamin B1, B2, B6, B12 and vitamin C. Like goji berries, golden berries are exceptionally high in protein (approximately 16%) for a fruit. In fact, golden berries are even higher in protein than goji berries.

> According to a study, published February 18, 2010 in *BMC Cancer,* Golden berry-derived 4beta-Hydroxywithanolide (4betaHWE) can inhibit the growth of human cancer cells through DNA damage, apoptosis (cell death) and G2/M arrest. In other words, 4betaHWE, a special compound found in golden berries, has the potential to work as a chemotherapeutic agent against lung cancer.
>
> That is exciting news! So, along with a balanced, raw plant-based diet, eat more golden berries for a natural approach to lung cell health and as a way to help prevent the onset of lung cancer.

Golden Berry Benefits:

- ★ Golden berries are high in carotenoids, vitamins B1, B2, B6, B12 and vitamin C, along with phosphorous and vitamin P (bioflavonoids).
    - Carotenoids are naturally-occurring fat-soluble pigments known to aid in keeping eyes, skin and mucous membranes moist. They are also considered potent antioxidants which neutralize free radicals in the body.
    - B-complex vitamins are water-soluble and are prized for helping with the activation of our metabolism; improving memory and energy; reducing stress and fatigue; relieving symptoms of PMS; and reducing the risk of heart disease.
    - Vitamin C is a water-soluble vitamin highly renowned for its potent antioxidant capabilities. In fact, vitamin C is required by more than 300 metabolic functions in the body, including tissue growth, adrenal gland function, healthy gums, metabolism, etc.
    - Phosphorus is the second most abundant mineral in the body and must work together with calcium to aid in bone health. Increasing phosphorus levels in the diet is useful in the strengthening of our bones and teeth and in the maintenance of tooth enamel and healthy gums. Phosphorus is also used in the metabolism where energy is released as a result of burning fat stored in the body.
    - Vitamin P (bioflavonoids) has antioxidants and contains anti-inflammatory, anti-sclerotic, antiviral, anti-histamine and anti-carcinogenic components.
- ★ Golden berries are high in protein, which is very unusual for any kind of fruit. This is great information for many who make fruit a major part of their diet. Our bodies require protein to rebuild and make repairs throughout the body.
- ★ Golden berries are categorized as an adaptogenic food capable of reducing the body's stress level, much like goji berries.

- ★ Golden berries are one fruit that can actually benefit individuals with diabetes. Being that golden berries are high in pectin, they may keep blood sugar levels within optimal range.
- ★ Golden berries have laxative qualities due to their high amount of pectin. Dietary fiber and pectin supports the intestinal tract, which can in turn ensure healthy bowel movements and regularity.

When purchasing, go for raw, wild-crafted and carefully sun-dried golden berries. I like golden berries sourced directly from families in Peru who harvest using only sustainable methods which have been used for generations. Golden berries also should be free from heavy metals, chemicals and pesticides, which is why I trust New Horizon Health and Ultimate Superfoods.

Golden berries can be used in a wide variety of raw food recipes, including smoothies, pies, cookies, energy bars and trail mixes.

Camu Camu

Camu camu *(Myciaria dubia)*, a bush native to the South American rainforest, grows in the black water rivers of the Amazon jungle of Peru. The camu camu berry is an amazing superfruit that is said to contain more vitamin C than any other known fruit in the world! It is estimated to have 30-60 times more vitamin C than oranges in its fresh state, delivering up to 600 times more vitamin C in its low-temperature dried, powdered form. It is also an excellent source of beta-carotene, calcium, phosphorus, potassium, iron, amino acids (such as serine, valine and leucine), thiamine (B1), riboflavin (B2), niacin (B3) and bioflavonoids. Since all these necessary cofactors can be found fully intact in the camu camu berry, our bodies are able to make full use of the immune-supportive vitamin C that it provides and get right to work. No pre-assembly required! What do I mean by this? Your body doesn't have to steal from other areas in order to assemble the proper enzymes, amino acids, minerals, etc., in order for the vitamin C to work properly. This is so unlike the chemically isolated, extracted or man-made forms of vitamin C (aka ascorbic acid) we find in most supplements and prepackaged fortified foods. Do not be fooled! Synthetic ascorbic acid is not the same as natural and whole food sources of vitamin C and does not perform the same in the body.

> According to Dr. Robert Marshall, every 500 mg of isolated ascorbic acid we consume causes us to lose up to 50 mg of precious bone calcium.

The best way for us to obtain the ultimate in antioxidant power from camu camu berries is in a low-temperature dried form that is raw and certified organic with no additives or fillers. If the powder is anything other than a beautiful bright coppery orange/brown color, I would not recommend it. A dull tan or beige color tells me that the processing method used to dry and powder the berries was not optimal, and it may have been allowed to oxidize. Personally, I will only go with the raw, organic camu camu berry powder sourced from the experts at New Horizon Health or Ultimate Superfoods.

The Indigenous Amazonian people carefully hand-pick the camu camu berries while they're in season and then dry and powder them. This process turns the purplish-red, cherry-like fruit to a copperish orange/brown color. It is believed that by consuming camu camu berries one can help ward off the common cold, influenza and other viral diseases, as well as various health conditions such as asthma, edema and heart disease. It is also known to support strong collagen, tendons and ligaments; decrease inflammation; and help deal with stress, anxiety and depression. It has been traditionally used as a medicinal herb for improving the function of the brain, eyes, heart, lungs, liver and skin.

> Some of the extraordinary medicinal properties of this Amazon rainforest fruit are described by Dr. Gary Null, an internationally known nutritionist, researcher, health science expert and activist. In discussing the holistic treatment of depression, he lists 19 plants containing chemical compounds with anti-depressant properties. In order of potency, camu camu is listed second in effectiveness.
>
> When it comes to plants with medicinal effectiveness against the herpes virus, camu camu takes the highest honors as most potent.

Camu Camu Benefits:

- ★ Camu camu beats out rosehips, acerola, oranges and lemons in its vitamin C content.
- ★ Camu camu provides immune system support.
- ★ Camu camu helps ward off viral infection.
- ★ Camu camu helps protect the brain from neurodegenerative disorders, for instance, dementia and Alzheimer's disease.
- ★ Camu camu helps maintain emotional stability and clarity of mind during times of stress.
- ★ Camu camu reduces the risk of heart disease.
- ★ Camu camu improves respiratory function.
- ★ Camu camu enhances liver function; thereby preventing the likelihood of liver disease.
- ★ Camu camu provides anti-mutagenic properties.
- ★ Camu camu helps maintain healthy eyesight.
- ★ Camu camu can help reduce inflammation.
- ★ Camu camu supports healthy collagen, tendons and ligaments.
- ★ Camu camu can improve the health of skin, hair and nails.

How to Use Camu Camu Berry Powder

The delicious and tangy taste of camu camu berry powder can be added to smoothies, loose-leaf iced teas, lemonade elixirs, as well as dessert recipes. It also can be combined with other superfood products, such as OptiMSM and AloePro, for increased health benefits.

> **Quick Tips:** Add ¼-1 teaspoon of camu camu berry powder to juices, smoothies, desserts or drinking water. Dosage may be increased over time. Remember, it is always best when larger quantities can be divided up throughout the day.
>
> Enhance vitamin C absorption by combining with MSM powder or aloe vera inner leaf.
>
> Combine with spirulina or chlorella powder to help boost mental clarity.
>
> Increase iron absorption by blending a small amount in with raw, organic cacao paste, powder, beans or nibs when making a chocolate smoothie or treat.

Baobab Fruit

Baobab may be a newer kid on the superfruit block to us in the West, but it has been providing exceptional nutrition and sustenance to the indigenous people of Madagascar for ages. The baobab tree *(Adansonia digitata)* goes by many nicknames: the "monkey bread tree," the "cream of tartar tree" and the "tree of life;" but nothing sounds more bizarrely interesting than the "upside down tree." This is due to the striking silhouette the baobab tree forms at sundown, giving the appearance of the tree being uprooted and stood on end.

Baobab fruit looks like large, elongated, velvety-green coconuts. Inside their shells are a number of seeds, all embedded in a whitish, powdery pulp. The tangy dried fruit pulp found on the inside actually dehydrates naturally, <u>without</u> the need for processing via heat extraction or freeze-drying. I find this uniquely amazing! The flavor is described as caramel pear with a hint of grapefruit. Whenever I make smoothies and raw ice cream with baobab, it tends to remind me of my yogurt loving days. I would eat frozen yogurt and make yogurt smoothies almost daily. To me, it offers that same sort of sweet-tart flavor and creamy smoothness.

The precious natural powder of the baobab fruit provides all eight essential amino acids; essential fatty acids; vitamins B1, B2, B3, B6 and vitamin C; the minerals calcium, phosphorus, iron, potassium, sodium, magnesium, zinc and manganese; and so much more! With all this vital nutrition, you can see how the exotic fruit of the sacred baobab tree can easily be revered as a superfood for all to enjoy!

Baobab Fruit Benefits:

- ★ Baobab provides 15 times more vitamin C than pomegranates, six times more potassium than bananas, three times more calcium than milk, three times more iron than spinach, as well as three times the antioxidants found in blueberries. In fact, baobab has an ORAC value very similar to that of goji berries.
- ★ Baobab is exceptionally rich in pectin, making it perfect for thickening and bringing flavors together in recipes.

- Baobab is considered an effective prebiotic as well as a probiotic. Studies have shown that the water-soluble portion of the fruit pulp has stimulating effects on the proliferation of bifidobacteria, a strain of beneficial bacteria normally found in a healthy gut.
- Baobab is high in fiber (insoluble and soluble), known to be beneficial to intestinal health, weight management and heart health.
- Baobab can enhance calcium absorption due to its high vitamin C content and array of minerals.
- Baobab is considered a low glycemic food.
- Baobab can help reduce inflammatory conditions due to its fantastic antioxidant and anti-inflammatory properties.
- Baobab may help stave off fungal infections.

SOUTH AMERICAN SUPERHERBS

From the magnificent mountainous highlands to the lush rainforest lowlands, Peru (a country in western South America) is home to many popular superfoods and superherbs which we normally see in powdered or encapsulated form. A few of my favorites have already been mentioned or discussed in prior sections. These include lucuma (page 41), quinoa (page 175) and camu camu berry (page 186). Here, I will address some additional treasured Peruvian favorites of mine. I am excited to also get into a few time-honored herbs that hail from other superb South American countries. For those who are interested, I tend to use maca and yerba mate regularly, while cat's claw, pau d'arco and chanca piedra I tend to use more sporadically, on occasion or as needed.

> *The use of herbs is a long-established way to strengthen and balance the body, as well as treat disease. That being said, herbs can still have side effects and may interact with other herbs, supplements or medications. Always consult with a qualified holistic practitioner, well versed in herbalism, before you start taking any herb.*

Maca

Maca *(Lepidium peruvianum)* is a root vegetable grown throughout the mountainous regions of Peru, high up in the Andes. Its natural growing altitude can reach heights as high as 14,000 feet above sea level. Maca belongs to the cruciferous family of plants, and, although slightly larger, resembles a radish.

Maca is abundant in many essential vitamins, major minerals, trace minerals, fatty acids, amino acids and plant sterols.

Maca is thought to be particularly beneficial for those wanting to bring balance into their day by bringing homeostasis into their body. It is also great for those leading an active lifestyle and is a favorite among those involved in extreme sports. Maca is often called the "Peruvian ginseng."

Maca is a superfood/superherb with an outstanding ability to increase energy, endurance, stamina and strength, as well as one's libido. Like many other superfoods, superfruits and superherbs, maca is considered a powerful adaptogen. If you recall, rather than addressing a specific symptom, adaptogens are used to improve the overall adaptability of the whole body to diverse and challenging situations and stress. Adaptogens have the ability to balance and stabilize bodily systems (such as the cardiovascular system, endocrine system, lymphatic system, nervous system, etc.) and provide more energy when deemed necessary. If the body is not in need of energy intensification, adaptogens (like maca) have the intelligence to not over-stimulate. Adaptogens can also give the immune system a boost and increase the body's overall vitality.

Peruvian research has found that maca can improve mood and memory, increase oxygen in the blood, support the function of neurotransmitters, and boost libido as well as fertility!

Maca Benefits

- ★ Maca is rich in vitamins B1, B2, C and E; the major minerals calcium, magnesium, phosphorous, potassium, sodium, sulfur and iron; and contains several trace minerals such as copper, iodine, manganese, selenium and zinc, as well as bismuth, tin and silica.
- ★ Maca (as a root crop) contains five times more protein and four times more fiber than a potato.
- ★ Maca contains nearly 20 amino acids and seven out of the eight essential amino acids. This makes maca a rich and bio-available source of protein.
- ★ Maca can enhance thyroid function, improve adrenal function, and can help support healthy hormone production.
- ★ Maca is an abundant source of plant sterols, including campesterols, ergosterol, brassicasterol, ergostadienol and sitosterol. These sterols make maca a powerful treatment aid when it comes to naturally balancing hormonal irregularities in both men and women. For instance, these plant sterols may help control the growth of prostatic cells in men – thereby improving prostate health and decreasing the risk of prostate cancer. For women approaching menopause, and who would like to avoid hormone replacement therapy (HRT), these same plant sterols can be a godsend. Many women have reported benefits in a very short period of time; some in as little as a week. All this without the risks and side effects associated with HRT!
- ★ Maca is powerful in its ability to increase energy, endurance, stamina and physical strength and can greatly improve blood oxygenation.
- ★ Maca, as an effective adaptogen, can adequately balance and stabilize a number of bodily systems such as the cardiovascular system, endocrine (hormonal) system and nervous system, to name few.
- ★ Maca has the capacity to activate endocrine glands; thereby boosting energy, vitality and libido.
- ★ Maca is considered to have natural aphrodisiac qualities and is often referred to as natures natural Viagra!

★ Maca may also help to improve the following in many individuals: antioxidant activity, anemia, breast milk production (in women when taken after childbirth), chronic fatigue, depression, memory, glucose tolerance (in both diabetics and non-diabetics), fertility, menopause symptoms (such as hot flashes, vaginal dryness and low sex drive), menstrual symptoms and disorders, andropause symptoms (such as erectile dysfunction, premature ejaculation and loss of sex drive), stress, tension, tuberculosis and more.

How to Consume Maca

The best way to consume maca is 100% organic and in its raw powdered form. Maca has a flavor that is somewhat malty, yet mildly sweet and with a cruciferous/radish-like spiciness. Maca is also a great emulsifier and may be used to draw two different ingredients smoothly together.

Maca may be used in smoothies, nut mylks, loose-leaf teas and tisanes, and just about any natural elixir drink you can creatively concoct. Maca is also a great addition to desserts and sweet treats. Maca has a loving relationship with raw cacao and mesquite and is amazing when blended with these two ingredients in your favorite raw treats and superfood smoothies.

Maca is non-toxic and has no adverse pharmacological effects – even at high dosages. Knowing this is great, but as with everything else, starting out small and working your way up is highly recommended. Maca is a powerful superfood/superherb and should be consumed with respect. Start with one teaspoon and see how you feel after a few days to a week. Slowly increase your dosage until you feel a noticeable difference. Depending on the desired effect one is after (physical energy, mental focus, libido, hormone balance, etc.), the dosage will differ from person to person.

> **Quick Tip:** Try synergistically combining maca with coconut oil to improve the potential of natural hormone production; specifically, pregnenolone, which is a precursor to all the other steroid hormones, including adrenal as well as reproductive hormones.

Maca Dosage & Usage Schedule

For many adults, the ideal therapeutic amount of maca is 1-2 heaping tablespoons per day. You can always take even more if you desire, but again, I suggest gradually increasing over time. Keep reassessing and increase or decrease as needed. As with any medicinal herb, it is recommended that you take a week off during every month of continual use or 1-2 days off per week. For instance, you may wish to take Sundays or full weekends off.

Precautions: If you are taking thyroid medication, the use of maca may accelerate its effects. If you do happen to notice overactive effects with the use of maca, ask your practitioner to check the function of your thyroid via blood tests (six panel test kit for better accuracy). It has been noted that many women have been able to reduce their thyroid medication and some have even been able to stop it altogether!

Cat's Claw

Uncaria tomentosa (aka Cat's Claw in English and Una de Gato in Spanish) is a woody vine which gets its name from the plant's small, hook-like thorns that resemble the claws of a cat. It is considered one of the most powerful botanicals of the Amazonian Peruvian rainforest and has been used medicinally by the indigenous people of South and Central America for hundreds, perhaps thousands of years.

Due to more and more studies starting to surface (since it started to be used by North Americans in the 1970s), the popularity of cat's claw in the United States has progressively grown. As an herbal remedy, cat's claw is used to treat a broad spectrum of health issues, especially those associated with the immune and digestive system. Dr. Brent Davis (chiropractic physician and herbal therapist) has worked with cat's claw for a number of years, and, due to its remarkable and proven ability to cleanse the entire digestive tract, he refers to this herb as "the opener of the way." Thanks to the immense amount of clinical research Dr. Brent Davis has compiled on approximately 150 patients, cat's claw can now officially be credited for the successful treatment of a wide variety of stomach and intestinal ailments: Crohn's disease, colitis, diverticulitis, fistulas, gastritis, hemorrhoids, leaky gut syndrome, parasites, ulcers and more.

As a result of ongoing research being conducted in facilities all over the world (Peru, Austria, Germany, England, Hungary and Italy), it is becoming more and more evident that cat's claw may be beneficial in the treatment of allergies, arthritis, bursitis, cancer, chronic fatigue syndrome, chronic pain, rheumatism, genital herpes and herpes zoster, lupus, systemic Candida, PMS and menstrual cycle irregularities, poisoning from environmental toxins, ulcers, numerous intestinal disorders and even HIV and AIDS.

> In *Healthy and Natural Journal* (Issue 1, October, 1994, pp. 64-65), Dr. Schwontkowski stated that cat's claw is the most powerful immune enhancing herb of all the herbs native to the rainforest of Peru. In her article, titled "Herbal Treasures from the Amazon Part 1," she mentions that preliminary studies suggested that cat's claw had the ability to stop viral infections in the early stages; help chemically sensitive individuals; increase emotional stability (even in the midst of extreme stress); fight infections in individuals suffering from AIDS; and decrease the visible size of certain skin tumors and cysts within two weeks.
>
> Dr. Schwontkowski also reported that cat's claw had been linked with the remission of brain and other tumors, as well as with providing relief from chemotherapy side-effects.
>
> Dr. Schwontkowski currently holds five degrees in health: D.C. (Doctorate in Chiropractic Medicine), B.S. and M.S. in Nutrition, a Master's in Herbology and B.S. in Human Biology.

Cat's Claw Benefits:

- ★ Cat's claw contains powerful alkaloids, tannins, glycosides and several other phytochemicals. Research suggests that these unique alkaloids (found in the bark and roots) can help increase white blood cell activity. This is useful in helping to fight off viral, bacterial and fungal infections, in addition to other microorganisms which can lead to disease.
- ★ Cat's claw may be beneficial to war veterans and their families due to its powerful anti-viral properties and ability to detoxify radiation and chemical toxins from the body.
- ★ Cat's claw promotes the healing of wounds.
- ★ Cat's claw may be used to treat high blood pressure.
- ★ Cat's claw can rid the body of excess fluid.
- ★ Cat's claw can reduce pain and inflammation in a host of conditions. Some of which include arthritis, rheumatism, gout, bursitis and bone pain.
- ★ Cat's claw has anti-tumor and anti-cancer qualities which may work to inhibit healthy cells from becoming cancerous cells.
- ★ Cat's claw has the profound ability to clean the intestinal walls, getting rid of deep-seated infections and built-up toxic debris. In turn, this allows the body to better absorb nutrients, thereby helping to correct nutritional imbalances created by digestive blockages.

How to Take Cat's Claw

Cat's claw may be taken as tea or extract. If you choose to consume cat's claw as a tea, I suggest purchasing the raw, dried and organic or wild-crafted tea-cut form (not powdered). Place one tablespoon in 24-32 ounces of hot water (not boiling) and steep for at least 30 minutes. I like using a glass French press to steep most of my teas, but a simple tea strainer will work just as well. Personally, I'm not too fond of the taste of drinking cat's claw alone. However, when I blend it with pau d'arco and yerba mate, I find it to be much more enjoyable. I also like to squeeze a bit of lemon in the mix, which I've learned helps to extract more of the unique alkaloids from the bark. If you decide to blend cat's claw with other teas, I suggest using one-part cat's claw to two parts pau d'arco, and then, if you wish, you can add a bit of yerba mate for fun.

Capsules of cat's claw are also available, which is the way I prefer to take it most of the time. My favorite product is Cat's Claw Immune by Premier Research Labs. This formula is a synergistic blend of cat's claw, along with a few other powerful phytonutrients, for the superior support of the immune and lymphatic systems.

Precautions: Cat's claw has historically been used to help prevent pregnancies and induce abortion. Therefore, women who are pregnant or trying to get pregnant should avoid the use of this herb. It is also not recommended for lactating women. Children less than three years of age should not take cat's claw. Cat's claw may interact with anticoagulants (aka blood-thinners), diuretics, estrogens or progestins (including birth control pills), and antihypertensive (blood pressure) medications. Cat's claw is contraindicated (meaning, not recommended) for at least one week prior to surgery. Due to its ability to stimulate the immune system, cat's claw is contraindicated before or following any organ or bone marrow transplant or skin graft procedure. Please consult a qualified healthcare and holistic practitioner before use. Medication adjustments and monitoring may be necessary.

Pau D'Arco

Pau d'arco (aka lapacho and taheebo) is probably one of the best known, yet least understood herbs coming out of the Amazonian rainforest. Pau d'arco *(Tabebuia avellandedae* and *Tabebuia impetiginosa)* is the inner bark of a broadleaf evergreen which has been used medicinally by the traditional healers of Argentina, Brazil, Peru and in other South American countries where it grows. Its medicinal uses date back centuries to the Indian tribes of South America, as well as the ancient Incas and Aztecs. As a tea, pau d'arco was used to purify the blood, reduce fevers and treat rheumatism, ulcers and inflammatory conditions of the intestinal tract (especially the colon). Topically, it was utilized to treat many skin conditions, including eczema, hemorrhoids, psoriasis, skin cancers, snakebites and wounds.

> Pau d'arco is given to cancer and leukemia patients in Argentina to protect the liver and kidneys from chemotherapy damage. And get this, it is given for <u>free</u> by their government. Other South American hospitals use it alongside radiation and chemotherapy to help treat cancer, reduce pain and decrease the risk of hair loss and immune dysfunction.

Pau d'arco owes its medicinal benefits to the many chemical compounds found within its bark. Research has found it to have potent anti-fungal properties in laboratory studies, which appear to work better than common prescription anti-fungal drugs. Its anti-fungal properties are so strong, that the bark never molds or mildews after being cut down. From the wettest of conditions to the driest, pau d'arco trees stand tall.

Pau d'arco is also believed to fight bacterial, viral and parasitic infections.

As a strong anti-inflammatory, pau d'arco can relieve pain from arthritis, cystitis and cancer, to name but a few.

Pau D'Arco Benefits:

- Pau d'arco possesses natural anti-cancer substances. The discovery of lapachol (one of the many, main chemical components of pau d'arco) has been thoroughly researched and found to exhibit powerful anti-tumor and anti-cancer activities (especially with certain blood and skin cancers). Lapachol is believed to inhibit the growth of tumor cells by preventing them from metabolizing oxygen.

    Please Note: Use of the whole bark (as in loose tea-cut pau d'arco) is recommended and typically much safer than isolated/extracted lapachol. In high amounts, lapachol, by itself, can contribute to serious side effects such as bleeding, nausea and vomiting.

- Pau d'arco protects the liver by helping to neutralize toxins and poisons typically detoxified by the liver. This in turn may help reduce the appearance of liver spots (aka age spots).
- Pau d'arco is extremely effective in treating fungal and yeast infections – especially those caused by Candida albicans overgrowth in the intestines. When Candida spreads and invades other areas of the body, it is considered systemic candidiasis and can cause oral thrush, canker sores, vaginal yeast infections, jock itch, diaper rash, urinary tract infections and athlete's foot.
- Pau d'arco enhances immune system function, our best defense against viruses like the flu, herpes and hepatitis.
- Pau d'arco contains the alkaloid tecomine, which has been found to be effective in reducing blood pressure, balancing blood sugar levels and reducing insulin dependence in diabetic individuals.
- Pau d'arco possesses powerful blood building and purifying factors and may be used to increase hemoglobin content, as well as the number of red blood cells.
    - As a blood builder, pau d'arco is capable of aiding in the treatment of leukemia and pernicious anemia.
    - As a blood purifier pau d'arco has been used successfully to treat many blood toxicity conditions such as acne, dermatitis, eczema and psoriasis.

With its wide array of medicinal uses, pau d'arco is considered a powerfully effective natural antibiotic. It is capable of combating the likes of bacteria, viruses, parasites, Candida and even cancer – without destroying the normal (good) bacterial flora and wiping out the immune system.

How to Use Pau D'Arco

One of the best ways to ingest pau d'arco is in tea form. I suggest purchasing pau d'arco (tea-cut) that is raw, dried and organic or wild-crafted. Capsules are also available, but have been noted to not be as effective as the tea. Place three tablespoons in 24-32 ounces of hot water (not boiling) and steep for at least 30 minutes. I use a glass French press to steep, but a simple tea strainer will work just as well.

Folk wisdom suggests that pau d'arco be routinely combined with yerba mate. According to the indigenous peoples of South America, who have had centuries of experience with the use of this herb, pau d'arco works best when taken with yerba mate. Apparently, yerba mate has an activating effect on the actions of pau d'arco. Yerba mate, of course, imparts a good deal of medicinal action itself (see page 197 for more on yerba mate).

> **Quick Tip:** If I'm brewing just a cup or less of pau d'arco and yerba mate, I like using the South American "bombilla," a bamboo or stainless-steel straw with a filter on one end. When amounts larger than one cup are desired, then a glass coffee press works really well.

Precautions: Due to its ability to thin the blood, pau d'arco may be contraindicated with the use of prescription blood thinners, over-the-counter drugs and other herbals that do the same. Always consult a qualified healthcare and holistic practitioner before beginning to take new herbs.

Chanca Piedra

Chanca piedra *(Phyllanthus niruri)* is an annual herb indigenous to the Amazonian rainforest and other tropical areas throughout the world. Renowned for its medicinal properties since Incan times, chanca piedra has become increasingly popular worldwide as a powerful herbal remedy. With a name that literally means "stone breaker" or "shatter stone," this beneficial herb has successfully been used for centuries to break up kidney, bladder and gall stones. It also has anti-spasmodic qualities, which can help to relax the urinary tract and the cystic and bile ducts; thereby assisting the body in the expelling of foreign particles much more easily. Chanca piedra is also known to help minimize calcification within the body and reduce the formations of obstructions in the digestive tract. It is believed that this herb can increase the production of bile, aiding in digestion and elimination.

> Dr. Wolfram Weimann of Nuremburg, Germany reviewed 100 cases involving the use of chanca piedra as an herbal remedy for kidney and gall stones. He discovered that chanca piedra successfully removed the stones in 94 out of the 100 cases.

Chanca piedra is used to treat a wide variety of conditions in Brazil, Peru and elsewhere. Although it is primarily used to treat stones of the kidney, bladder and gall bladder, it has also traditionally been used to treat acne, asthma, colds, the flu, diabetes and indigestion. Additionally, it is effective against inflammatory conditions of the intestinal tract (including the cause of constipation), bladder infections, urinary tract infections (UTI) and more.

Chanca Piedra Benefits:

★ Chanca piedra is renowned for its ability to break down and remove kidney stones. It can also be used to prevent kidney stones from forming in the first place.

- ★ Chanca piedra can reduce pain and inflammation in both acute and chronic conditions.
- ★ Chanca piedra supports kidney and bladder, as well as gall bladder and liver health.
- ★ Chanca piedra possesses anti-diuretic properties.
- ★ Chanca piedra can reduce blood pressure and cholesterol levels.
- ★ Chanca piedra assists in the reduction of blood sugar levels.
- ★ Chanca piedra provides protection against viruses, including hepatitis B (HBV), tuberculosis (TB) and HIV.
- ★ Chanca piedra shows promise as a supportive herb for cancer with its ability to prevent cellular mutations.

How to Take Chanca Piedra

Look for 100% organic chanca piedra (tea cut). Place one tablespoon in 24-32 ounces of hot water (not boiling) and steep for at least 20 minutes. Use a glass French press. A simple tea strainer will work as well. If you are preparing this tea to treat kidney problems (e.g., kidney stones), it is suggested to drink one cup, 2-3 times throughout the day.

Precautions: Chanca piedra may increase the effects of diabetic, diuretic and high blood pressure (hypertension) medications. Please consult a qualified healthcare professional before use, as monitoring and drug modification may be necessary. Chanca piedra may also be contraindicated for women who are pregnant, lactating or wish to become pregnant, so please check with your practitioner first.

Yerba Mate

Yerba mate *(Ilex paraguayensis)* is a small shrub related to the holly family and is native to several South American countries (such as Argentina, Brazil, Paraguay and Uruguay). In some areas of South America, yerba mate is considered a national drink. Sipping yerba mate among friends, through a metal filter-straw (known as a "bombilla") in a shared hollow gourd, is how the natives traditionally enjoy it.

According to Dr. Daniel Mowery, Director of Mountainwest Institute of Herbal Sciences located in Salt Lake City, Utah, a group of scientists from the Pasteur Institute and the Paris Scientific Society concluded that yerba mate contains "practically all of the vitamins necessary to sustain life." They focused especially on pantothenic acid (vitamin B5), commenting that it is "rare to find a plant with so much of this significant and vital nutrient...It is indeed difficult to find a plant in any area of the world equal to Mate in nutritional value."

Yerba mate contains an impressive 24 vitamins and minerals, 15 amino acids and 11 polyphenols. Polyphenols are a group of powerful phytochemicals that act as antioxidants. Here's an interesting fact: yerba mate is touted to have more antioxidants than green tea! The long list of nutrients that yerba mate contains includes: carotene, vitamin B-complex (including B1, B2, B3 and B5), vitamins C and E, calcium, magnesium, phosphorus, potassium, sodium, sulfur, trace amounts of iron, manganese, selenium, silica and zinc, and chlorophyll, choline, flavanols, hydrochloric acid, inositol (sometimes referred to as vitamin B8) and saponins.

> Yerba mate, often called the "Drink of the Gods," is found to contain 196 volatile (aka active) chemical compounds. Of those, 144 are also found in green tea.

Yerba mate contains three xanthines: caffeine (called mateine by some), theobromine and theophylline. All three are alkaloids that are commonly used for their mild stimulating effects, while simultaneously being able to relax and open blood vessels and respiratory bronchioles. Compared with coffee, which tends to target the CNS and cause that not so pleasant jittery feeling, yerba mate works on the muscle tissue. It appears to have a relaxing effect on the smooth muscle tissue of the body, yet a stimulating effect on the cardiac muscle. This is most likely due to the combined effects of all three xanthines. They not only all work together, but they work in harmony with all the other nutrients as well. Coffee, on the other hand, has a high amount of caffeine, low theophylline content and zero theobromine. It is not very well balanced. You may recall theobromine is the main active constituent found in cacao (see page 142 for a review).

Yerba Mate Benefits:

- ★ Yerba mate induces mental clarity, alertness and acuity. And it does so without the negative side effects of jitters and increased nervousness. Yerba mate has never been found to be habit forming like many drinks containing caffeine.
- ★ Yerba mate, incredibly, does not interfere with sleep. In fact, the use of yerba mate may improve sleep cycles by increasing rapid eye movement (REM) sleep, as well as the time spent in deep sleep (delta sleep). Many people report that they require less sleep and feel more relaxed when using yerba mate because their sleep is deeper.
- ★ Yerba mate contains the largest antioxidant and polyphenol content among tea-based and non-tea-based drinks according to a study published in the Comprehensive Reviews in Food Science and Food Safety.
- ★ Yerba mate can improve digestion by repairing damaged or diseased gastrointestinal tissues. This in turn helps resolve constipation issues, both acute and chronic.
- ★ Yerba mate can help improve detoxification by stimulating the release of excess water weight, increasing bowel transit time and opening the respiratory passageways.
- ★ Yerba mate has been touted as a treatment and preventive for cardiovascular ailments of all kinds. This is most likely due to its ability to increase cellular oxygen levels in the body thanks to its wondrous nutritional profile.
- ★ Yerba mate leaves contain very special phytochemicals called saponins. Saponins are glycoside compounds often referred to as a "natural detergent" because of the foam they produce. Saponins have been found to stimulate the immune system and protect the body against a host of diseases.

- Dietary saponins have been found to possess cholesterol-lowering properties. One of the most prominent research programs, led by Dr. Rene Malinow at the Oregon Regional Primate Center, proved that saponins can decrease body cholesterol by binding with cholesterol and preventing its reabsorption back into the system. The ability of saponins to excrete cholesterol from the body is similar to many cholesterol-lowering drugs. This makes the dietary use of saponins a promising treatment for individuals with a high cholesterol ratio.
- Studies done at the University of Toronto have indicated that dietary sources of saponins can help inhibit – and may even kill – human cancer cells. They may also have the ability to do this without killing normal cells in the process (unlike the many cancer-fighting drugs currently used in conventional medicine). So far, it has been noted that saponins are particularly effective against blood and lung cancers.
- Dr. A.V. Rao, professor and researcher at the University of Toronto, as well as his colleagues, believe that saponins hold exciting prospects in the prevention of colon cancer.
    - According to Dr. Rao, cancer cells have a different membrane structure with more cholesterol-like compounds. And since saponins are able to bind cholesterol, they have a natural affinity for cancer cell membranes.
    - Research has shown that saponins have the ability to bind bile acids. When primary bile acids get metabolized by bacteria in the large intestine, they turn into secondary bile acids. Secondary bile acids can damage intestinal cells, possibly setting in motion the events that lead to cancer. "By binding up bile acids and reducing the amount that can be transformed into a toxic version, saponins may help lower cancer risk," says Dr. Rao.

    Please Note: Bile formation and excretion is an essential and normal function involved in the process of digestion. Bile not only breaks down fats and increases the absorption of fat-soluble vitamins in the small intestine, but is a very powerful antioxidant which helps to remove toxins from the liver. Unfortunately, with the increase in processed and refined fats, especially pro-inflammatory omega-6 fats (as found in our standard American diet), things can quickly become unbalanced, increasing our risk of cardiovascular and gastrointestinal tract diseases, to name just two areas of concern.

- Saponins are known to have immune-stimulating effects within the plants that contain them. Now, research is discovering that these same effects can indeed be transferred to the human body upon ingestion. Scientists have long been well aware of the important role that saponins play in protecting the immunity of plants, and now they are taking a closer look at how dietary saponins can help humans fight fungal infections, microbes and viruses. Saponins have long been used medicinally as natural antibiotics, and when administered with vaccines, they can not only help the body fight off infections, but make the vaccine more effective.

  Please Note: Although I am not a proponent of vaccines, I wanted to at least make mention of this finding.

- ★ Yerba mate can aid in weight loss by acting as a natural appetite suppressant.
- ★ Yerba mate contains natural thermogenic properties, meaning, it encourages the body to burn calories (especially from fat) by increasing the basal metabolic rate.
- ★ Yerba mate may help lessen the severity and incidence of allergies. Clinical evidence suggests that yerba mate stimulates the adrenal glands to produce corticosteroids, which may prove to be helpful for those who suffer with seasonal hay fever symptoms (and the like).
- ★ Yerba mate can improve lung function. This can benefit athletes, as it promotes optimal breathing and better tissue oxygenation.

As a whole-body tonic herb, yerba mate can stimulate a depressed or weakened nervous system, yet calm an overexcited one. When stress throws our body out of balance (whether it is from anxiety, environmental factors or poor nutrition), one can count on the bi-directional properties of yerba mate to restore homeostasis, while at the same time, not over stimulating any one system. Furthermore, yerba mate has no known addictive qualities and will not cause jitters. For this last reason alone, yerba mate can be an excellent coffee substitute.

How to Enjoy Yerba Mate

Personally, I drink and suggest an organic and un-smoked loose-leaf yerba mate. Un-smoked (aka steamed) varieties of yerba mate, consumed at much lower than boiling temperatures, have not been noted to have the same negative effects most commonly associated with commercially smoked varieties, consumed at high temperatures. While yerba mate has been reported to have anti-cancer benefits, a study published in the July 2003 issue of the medical journal *Head and Neck* reported that drinking yerba mate may increase the risk of developing certain cancers of the upper intestinal tract (such as in the mouth, throat and esophagus).

Please Note: It has been suggested by many experts, who are considered exceptionally knowledgeable in their fields, that the increased risk for developing mouth, throat and esophageal cancer most likely has more to do with one or more of the following: the commercial drying process of the plant material (which involves smoke from the burning of wood); boiling water used in the steeping of the smoked plant material; or the drinking of this beverage at too hot a temperature through a metal straw.

After drinking several varieties of yerba mate over the past ten years, I really love and appreciate the yerba mate by Eco Teas. Eco Teas is an organic and fair-trade company. Their yerba mate is from an organic, family farm in northeastern Argentina. It is dried with a unique smoke-free drying process that is known to retain all the herb's nutritive benefits and provide a clean and smooth flavor. Extra time is taken to remove all the stems and powder, which guaranties the most nutritious and energizing product possible.

When this drink is prepared traditionally, the dry leaves are placed in a gourd called a "mate." Then, a small amount of cold water is added to moisten the leaves and protect the nutrients and flavor. Next, water at 159-169°F (never boiling) is added until all the leaves are thoroughly immersed. Rather than removing the leaves, I prefer to sip my yerba mate through a stainless-steel filter-straw called a "bombilla." This special straw strains the leaves at the bottom and prevents the leaves from going up the inside of the straw. As you finish drinking your first brew (aka steep), you may add more water for multiple infusions. Depending on the amount of time you choose to steep, you may be able to get 3-5 infusions from the same leaves. There are an infinite number of ways to enjoy yerba mate. Depending on your ailment, dosage recommendations and steep times, the number of cups per day can vary. I usually use two tablespoons per 8-12 ounces of water and steep for about five minutes. With this, I can usually get about three good infusions. I also enjoy blending my yerba mate with other herbs. The sky is the limit, so play and enjoy!

Ayurvedic Superherbs

Ayurveda (aka ayurvedic medicine) stands for "the knowledge for long life." It is a 7,000-year-old system of traditional medicine native to India. Ayurveda considers sickness an imbalance in the body that can be resolved by restoring equilibrium rather than treating symptoms.

Shilajit

Shilajit is considered the king herb of Ayurveda. Possessing many almost magical attributes, shilajit is found predominately in the Himalayas – the verdant, mountainous region bordering India, China, Tibet and parts of Central Asia. Shilajit is composed of organic plant material, thought to have been compressed by rock for thousands of years. Shilajit is neither a plant nor animal substance, but a mineral pitch that oozes from the rocks of the Himalayas when the mountains become warm in the summer months. Generally speaking, shilajit is a concentrate of ancient plant matter. It is the ancient life force energy, of once flourishing trees and plants, perfectly preserved upon their return back to earth.

Shilajit means "conqueror of mountains and destroyer of weakness" and is considered one of the greatest rejuvenators and adaptogens of all time. It contains at least 85 minerals in ionic form, as well as trace minerals, ultra trace minerals, humic and fulvic acid, and some other very important phytonutrients. Due to the minerals being in ionic form (and naturally-occurring, of course), our body will easily and completely be able to absorb and assimilate them. The humic and fulvic acid in shilajit is also in its most natural and pure form. Both humic and fulvic acid are naturally-occurring organic compounds created by Mother Earth and can be found in perfectly mineralized nutrient-rich soil.

Want to find the fountain of you? Shilajit is considered to have unparalleled powers when it comes to arresting and reversing the aging process. For many centuries, Indian Yogis kept the existence and use of shilajit a close-guarded secret. They considered it the nectar of longevity. In Sanskrit, the literal meaning of shilajit is "rock like." This means shilajit has the power to make our body as strong as a rock, allowing it to withstand the ravages of age. To this day, it is not uncommon to see Indian Yogis in the Himalayas living to be 100 years of age and having the stamina and body structure of an adolescent. According to Indian Yogis and ancient Indian scriptures, shilajit is not only capable of preserving youthfulness; it can heal the mind and body of virtually any ailment.

Shilajit Benefits:

- ★ Shilajit has the power to amplify the bioavailability and action of other herbs when taken together.
- ★ Shilajit works as a nutrient carrier, as it helps to deliver and drive vitamins, minerals and phytochemicals deep into the cells and tissues of the body.
- ★ Shilajit promotes the movement of minerals – especially calcium, phosphorous and magnesium – into muscle tissue and bone.
- ★ Shilajit is a great cleanser and detoxifier. Its huge, high-valence surface area has the ability to collect deep-seated toxic debris and free radicals and eliminate them from the body.
- ★ Shilajit helps to improve memory, mental vigor and our ability to handle stress. Ayurvedic uses of shilajit as a nerve tonic have proven the anti-anxiety properties (aka anti-stress effects) of shilajit.
- ★ Shilajit possesses anti-inflammatory characteristics, which justifies its use in many acute and chronic pain conditions.
- ★ Shilajit combats osteoarthritis by promoting strong bones and can help heal damaged nerve and muscle tissue. Shilajit is well known for its usefulness in reducing recovery time in muscle, bone and nerve related injuries.
- ★ Shilajit tones and protects the urinary tract and acts as a mild diuretic. Shilajit is often used in kidney disease and various other urinary tract problems. It appears to be effective in relieving pain and burning upon urination and urinary incontinence (often times due to an enlarged prostate and stones in the kidneys, ureters, bladder or urethra).

  Please Note: Although shilajit can be used in the treatment of kidney stones, one must use caution if their stones are a result of uric acid. Uric acid is a natural by-product of the metabolism of purine. Foods highest in purines consist of meat and poultry (especially organ meats), including the gravies made from them; shellfish and seafood (such as anchovies, cod, herring, haddock, mackerel and especially sardines); and foods made from a significant amount of brewers and baker's yeast (such as beer and sweetbread).

- ★ Shilajit can dissolve calcium crystals and safely eliminate them from the body. Calcium belongs in our bones, but not in our soft tissues, joints and brains. When we eat acidic foods and beverages, breathe polluted air, and endure excessive amounts of stress, calcium can leach from our bones (in order to neutralize the acid condition created) and get diverted to other parts of the body where it doesn't belong. This eventually causes hardening of these body parts (aka calcification). Depending on the body part affected, calcification can lead to myocardial infarctions, strokes, benign and malignant tumors, clogged lymph nodes and detoxification pathways, debilitating disorders of the joints and spine, as well as kidney stones that can lead to kidney disease and even kidney failure.
- ★ Shilajit offers anti-ulcerative properties. Thanks to its active constituents, such as fulvic acid, shilajit can be successfully used in the treatment of peptic ulcers. According to studies, shilajit has been proven to increase carbohydrate/protein ratio, decrease the gastric ulcer index, and create a greater mucus barrier that prevents ulcer growth.
- ★ Shilajit provides powerful blood sugar regulating properties. According to extensive research, conducted at the Institute of Medial Sciences in India by Dr. Salil K. Bhattacharya, the presence of humic and fulvic acid is responsible for the anti-diabetic activity of shilajit. It appears that fulvic acid can successfully eradicate free radical damage to pancreatic islet B cells, which is a leading known cause of diabetes.
- ★ Shilajit purifies the blood, improves the functioning of the pancreas and strengthens the digestive process.
- ★ Shilajit is an all in one natural remedy for treating general, as well as sexual weakness. In women, shilajit can improve blood flow to reproductive organs (including external genitalia), increase vaginal secretions and boost interest in sex. In men, shilajit can decrease the incidence of erectile dysfunction, weak erections, premature ejaculation and low sperm count.
- ★ Shilajit is capable of bolstering the immune system and reducing chronic fatigue.

What to Look for in a Quality Shilajit Product

The best shilajit will be native to the natural habitat of the Himalayan mountain range and harvested at over 15,000 feet in elevation. Being that shilajit is derived from vegetation-rich mountainous regions unspoiled by man, the exposure to chemicals, fertilizers and pesticides should never be a concern.

Of all the varieties of shilajit, the pale-brown to blackish-brown variety is the one most commonly used in traditional ayurvedic medicine. It is prized for having the most therapeutic effects.

In ancient ayurvedic texts, two types of drying methods of shilajit are mentioned. The first is a sun-drying process and the second involves fire. The sun-drying method may be a slower process, but is the one that is most preferred. This is because fire-drying (or any method that involves high heat) increases the destruction and evaporation of the many amazing properties and attributes associated with shilajit.

Please Note: If shilajit is not filtered and properly processed, it can contain unwanted substances. Please know your source. Always go with a shilajit that has never been exposed to high temperatures during the cleansing and drying process. Personally, I prefer a cold-water extracted shilajit. This assures me of the potency of all the organic and ionic dietary minerals, trace minerals and ultra trace minerals. Why is this so important? Well, because the magic of shilajit lies in its outstanding mineral content.

How to Use Shilajit

Shilajit makes a great addition to teas, tisanes and elixir concoctions. Add a tad of raw honey or agave for sweetness, along with a little drizzle of raw coconut oil for synergy, and you have one fantabulicious beverage! I also like adding shilajit to my smoothies for a bit of depth, and absolutely love blending it into just about any raw chocolate creation with a dash or two of whole ground vanilla bean powder. Shilajit is quite earthy in flavor, with an almost coffee-like taste and aroma when added to warm water. You may enjoy adding shilajit to the many herbal teas already discussed (such as yerba mate, pau d'arco, cat's claw and chanca piedra). As mentioned above, shilajit pairs deliciously well with raw cacao, offering a mocha-like experience when done right. I also like combining it with mucuna pruriens, another ayurvedic phenomenon (page 204). You can even combine equal parts of MSM and shilajit to purified water for deeper cellular penetration and cleansing ability. Just be sure to start out small and work your way up to about one tablespoon of each.

Recommended Dosage: Start with a ½-1 teaspoon of shilajit, 1-2 times per day, working your way up to more, as desired and tolerated.

Precautions: Avoid Shilajit if you are prone to having high uric acid levels that result in the formation of uric acid type kidney stones or gout attacks. Gout is a type of painful arthritic condition (often called gouty arthritis) that occurs when too much uric acid builds up in the blood and then forms uric acid crystals in the joints.

Mucuna Pruriens

Mucuna pruriens (aka velvet bean) is a tropical legume which can be found in Africa, India and the West Indies (Caribbean). It is an amazing adaptogenic herb that has been used successfully for thousands of years in ayurvedic medicine to treat a number of nervous system disorders (including Parkinson's disease), as well as low libido in both sexes and infertility in men. Mucuna pruriens contains a high concentration of an amino acid called levodopa (L-dopa) which, once in the bloodstream, is able to cross the blood brain barrier and covert to the vital neurotransmitter dopamine.

> *Did you know that over 250,000 worldwide research papers exist on L-Dopa alone, making it one of the worlds most widely researched amino acids?*

Dopamine controls the release of human growth hormone (HGH) which is extremely important for the repair and rejuvenation of aging cells. Unlike synthetic hormone injections, the L-dopa in Mucuna pruriens supports the body's ability to stimulate the pituitary gland to increase its production and natural release of HGH. Dopamine also regulates a number of other brain and bodily functions including attention, learning, behavior, cognition, emotions, mood, motivation, pleasurable reward, voluntary movement, sleep, energy levels, sex drive, cholesterol production and tolerance to pain.

> According to a double blind clinical and pharmacological study published in the *Journal of Neurology, Neurosurgery & Psychiatry* back in December 2004 (volume 75, issue 12), mucuna pruriens seed powder, at a dosage of 30 grams, proved to be safer and more effective in controlling Parkinson's disease than the pharmaceutical drugs Levodopa and Carbidopa. It was suggested that the vast array of other chemical constituents that accompany the natural source of L-dopa in mucuna pruriens may play a key role in its success over conventional L-dopa preparations. This is phenomenal and promising news for the long-term management of Parkinson's disease.

Mucuna Pruriens Benefits:

- ★ Mucuna pruriens helps tonify and balance the nervous system, reproductive system and immune system.
- ★ Mucuna pruriens can raise brain dopamine levels. It appears to be quite useful for those with attention deficit hyperactivity disorder (ADHD), depression sufferers and individuals in the recovery phases of addiction.
- ★ Mucuna pruriens can dramatically improve one's mood and sense of well-being.
- ★ Mucuna pruriens helps to boost energy levels.
- ★ Mucuna pruriens stimulates healthy hormone production via the pituitary gland. Known for its amazing ability to boost testosterone, mucuna pruriens can be used safely and regularly to enhance libido and sexual performance in both men and women.
- ★ Mucuna pruriens promotes the increase of lean muscle mass.
- ★ Mucuna pruriens may assist in the reduction of body fat.
- ★ Mucuna pruriens may reduce the appearance of cellulite and wrinkles.
- ★ Mucuna pruriens helps to enhance the appearance and texture of the skin.
- ★ Mucuna pruriens can increase bone density and improve bone health. Regular use of this herb may help prevent and overcome osteoporosis.
- ★ Mucuna pruriens can optimize sleep quality and promote a deeper state of sleep.

How to Take Mucuna Pruriens

Start out by always looking for a cold-water extracted product in powdered form. With powder, you can easily add it to warm water alone, making a warm tisane, or add it to one of your favorite teas. I love adding it to my yerba mate and shilajit concoctions. I also love making chocolates and chocolate elixir drinks with both mucuna pruriens and shilajit added to them. One of my favorite drinks I call Mind Altering Mochaccino (page 466). It is alchemically amazing!

> **Quick Tip:** Adding a little coconut oil to any of the above can be used to enhance mucuna pruriens' effects further and increase the absorption of certain nutrients. This goes for any and all herbal elixirs and smoothie creations that involve the use of superfoods and superherbs.

Suggested Dosages

If you are looking to use this herb for treating the effects of Parkinson's disease, 30 grams is the suggested dosage according to clinical data. Always consult with a knowledgeable healthcare practitioner, well versed in Ayurveda, before starting mucuna pruriens for the management or reversal of any disorder or disease.

Please Note: Since comparisons are not available, it is difficult to know which extract potency is best for the various conditions mucuna pruriens is known to benefit. Therefore, please view the following as information for experimental purposes only.

In weighing out the mucuna pruriens extract that I use (which happens to be 15.8% L-dopa), I found that 30 grams equates to four tablespoons. This means four tablespoons of this particular mucuna pruriens extract would be the suggested dosage for treating the effects of Parkinson's disease. If you are looking to benefit from its aphrodisiac effect, at least 15 grams is suggested. This equates to two tablespoons of the cold-water extracted powder. Again, due to the unique differences of each individual, as well as variances in extract potency, the dosage suggested for this particular desired effect can only be viewed as a general estimation. More or less may be needed.

Please Note: If you are new to this herb, start out with a small amount (half teaspoon or less) and work your way up to larger amounts (one teaspoon or more). I generally like 1-2 tablespoons per day – sometimes all at once, sometimes divided into two doses.

Precautions: Avoid mucuna pruriens if you are pregnant or nursing. Avoid if you are on monoamine oxidase inhibitor drugs (MAOI's). Schizophrenics and bipolar sufferers who are taking any drug or drugs (especially those that influence the function of neurotransmitters) should also not use mucuna pruriens. Again, be sure to always consult with a qualified healthcare professional, well versed in ayurvedic herbal medicine, before altering or stopping the use of prescription drugs.

Ashwagandha

Ashwagandha (*Withania somnifera*) is a nightshade and belongs to the same family as the tomato. It is a plump and flourishing shrub found extensively in the dry regions of India, northern Africa and the Middle East. That being said, today ashwagandha can be found growing in more mild climates, including the United States. The root of ashwagandha is the part most widely used for its adaptogenic medicinal properties, and is probably the most famous restorative herb that comes to us from ancient Ayurveda. In Sanskrit, ashwagandha means the smell or sweat of a horse, indicating that this herb imparts the strength and vigor of a horse.

The major chemical constituents of ashwagandha root are steroidal alkaloids and steroidal lactones, both of which are part of a class of naturally-occurring chemical compounds called withanolides. In 1970, research showed withanolides to be similar to our own body's steroid hormones. In other words, ashwagandha and its withanolides serve as important hormone precursors that can convert into human physiologic hormones as needed.

In numerous studies, ashwagandha exhibits anti-stress properties and is touted by many to be an adaptogenic, immune tonic superherb. In fact, due to its uses for generalized weakness, stress and anxiety, as well as its effectiveness in improving energy, muscle power and stamina, ashwagandha is frequently referred to as the "Indian ginseng." With the body's improved ability to resist many forms of stress due to taking this herb, energy can be used more productively. As an end result, this can only improve one's overall health and well-being.

> In one of the most complete human clinical trials to date, participants subjectively reported an increase in energy, a reduction in fatigue, better sleep quality and a heightened sense of well-being. Measurable improvements from participants were also noted. Some of which included a reduction in cortisol levels (up to 26%), a decrease in fasting blood sugar level and an improvement in lipid profiles. It appears from this study that ashwagandha may be able to successfully address many physical, as well as psychological issues that plague our society today.

Traditionally, ashwagandha has been prescribed to help people strengthen their immune system after an illness or increase memory and focus in old age. Many modern studies find it to be effective in reducing inflammation, increasing cognitive function and invigorating the body. The most promising research indicates that ashwagandha and its withanolides could regenerate nerve cells. This is great news for individuals suffering with memory disorders, including dementia and Alzheimer's.

Ashwagandha Benefits:

★ Ashwagandha can help in the reduction of stress, anxiety and depression without causing drowsiness.

- ★ Ashwagandha has antispasmodic properties and may be used as a mild muscle relaxant. In traditional ayurvedic medicine, ashwagandha is commonly used as a uterine sedative during childbirth. It may also be used to dilate the bronchioles and facilitate breathing in asthma suffers.
- ★ Ashwagandha has a cooling and calming effect on the brain and is commonly used for treating insomnia.
- ★ Ashwagandha increases the oxygen carrying capacity of red blood cells. A better oxygen supply will always result in better brain and organ function.
- ★ Ashwagandha can enhance energy, thus increasing one's endurance, quickness (aka reaction time) and physical and mental stamina. This makes ashwagandha a great contender for athletes and those involved in high performance sports.
- ★ Ashwagandha is a natural aphrodisiac and may successfully be used to enhance the libido of both men and women.
- ★ Ashwagandha shows great promise as an antioxidant. In one study, ashwagandha exhibited free radical scavenging activity similar to superoxide dismutase (SOD).
- ★ Ashwagandha offers anti-inflammatory benefits and has proven to be an effective aid for individuals suffering from rheumatoid arthritis, gout, etc.
- ★ Ashwagandha can boost the immune system, as it has the capacity to trigger white blood cells to produce more lymphocytes.
- ★ Ashwagandha may benefit people at risk for certain neuronal and memory conditions, including epilepsy, Parkinson's and Alzheimer's disease.
- ★ Ashwagandha is a natural diuretic and is helpful in the treatment of kidney and urinary disorders.
- ★ Ashwagandha is a trusted herbal remedy for women in menopause and may be utilized as a safe and natural alternative to hormone replacement therapy. It helps combat fatigue, anxiety and brain fog and may even help elevate hot flashes.

How to Use Ashwagandha

Start out by looking for a cold-water extracted product in powdered form. I always choose and suggest powder over capsules. Powder allows for increased versatility and dosage control without the worry of additives, fillers and flowing agents most commonly found in capsules.

According to the Beth Israel Deaconess Medical Center (BIDMC) in Boston, MA, the traditional dose of ashwagandha is 1-2 grams (approximately ½-1 teaspoon) taken one to three times daily. This equates to 1-6 grams (approximately 1-3 teaspoons) total per day.

You can easily make a tea with pure ashwagandha extract powder. Add 1-2 grams (approximately ½-1 teaspoon) to just below boiling water and steep for up to 15 minutes. This can be repeated up to three times in a 24-hour period. You may also add it to one of your favorite teas or combine it with other ayurvedic herbs. For instance, you can combine it with equal amounts of shilajit, mucuna pruriens, and tribulus terrestris (another ayurvedic herb known for its beneficial steroidal saponins). I love adding these ayurvedic gems to my experimental liquid elixirs and smoothie concoctions, as well as to all my chocolate creations.

> **Quick Tip:** To induce relaxation for a restful night's sleep, try brewing up a dose of ashwagandha right before bed.

Please Note: Depending on the desired therapeutic effect one is after, the uniqueness and individuality of each person, as well as the subtle variances in extract potency, the dosages suggested above may need to be adjusted up or down. If you are new to this herb, then start out with a small amount (half teaspoon or less, 1-3 times daily) and work your way up to larger amounts (one teaspoon or more, 1-3 times daily). Always consult with a knowledgeable healthcare practitioner well versed in Ayurveda before considering the use of ashwagandha. This is especially important when it comes to the management or reversal of any disorder or disease.

Precautions: Due to its mild anti-depressant effect, one should avoid the simultaneous usage of ashwagandha with alcohol, anti-anxiety or anti-depressant medications – or any other form of sedative for that matter. If you are prone to ulcers, it may be advisable to avoid ashwagandha, as it can irritate the gastrointestinal tract and may cause diarrhea, nausea or abdominal pain. Avoid this herb for at least two weeks prior to any surgery, as it may increase the effects of anesthesia or other central nervous system suppressant(s) given. Avoid ashwagandha during pregnancy. Use caution if you are currently on any thyroid medications or diabetic medications, as ashwagandha may increase their effects. Due to its strong ability to boost one's immune system, it may be best to avoid using ashwagandha if you have been diagnosed with an auto-immune condition (such as lupus, multiple sclerosis, rheumatoid arthritis, etc.).

Turmeric

If there is one herb that everyone should get to know and start using, it is turmeric. There is virtually nothing that this single herb can't help when it comes to healing the human body.

Turmeric (*Curcuma longa*) is a tuberous rhizome with a tough brown skin and bright yellow-orange flesh. It is a tropical perennial plant related to the ginger family and is native to South and Southeast Asia. Turmeric is one of the most valued herbs of the East and has long been used medicinally as a potent antioxidant and powerful anti-inflammatory in both Ayurveda and traditional Chinese medicine. It is a good source of vitamin B6, iron, manganese, potassium and fiber and has been found to be the fourth highest antioxidant rich herb.

Ayurvedic practitioners call turmeric the "golden spice of life," as it has a broad spectrum of actions and beneficial effects. Therapeutically, turmeric primarily works on the skin, heart, liver and lungs and can be used for the prevention and treatment of anemia, arthritis, benign and cancerous tumors, diabetes, digestion of fats and proteins, food poisoning, gallstones, gastrointestinal upsets (including acid reflux, bloating and gas), menstrual irregularities, parasitic microorganisms (including bacteria, viruses and worms), poor circulation, staph infections and external ulcers and wounds.

It's no wonder that turmeric is earning quite a name for itself in Western households and in the Western world of medicine; its versatile actions and uses are virtually endless! Interestingly, the same compounds in turmeric that prevent food from spoilage (due to their antioxidative, anti-mutagenic and anti-microbial properties) are also known to protect the living tissue of our bodies from degeneration. This is most likely why turmeric can be used to protect us from such a variety of diseases, while at the same time positively affecting our life span. The active chemical compounds in turmeric are curcuminoids, with curcumin being the principle curcuminoid found and studied in Western medicine.

Curcumin is currently prized for its action as a free radical scavenger and anti-inflammatory analgesic. In fact, the effectiveness of curcumin has been found to be comparable to pharmaceutical NSAIDs (nonsteroidal anti-inflammatory drugs), but without the toxic side effects. Its anti-inflammatory properties are beneficial in the treatment of arthritis (both rheumatoid and osteoarthritis) and in injuries, trauma and stiffness from both being under active and over active. It also exhibits anti-tumor properties, as well as liver protection and rejuvenation properties and much, much more. I totally look forward to all the research underway. It will help to scientifically prove what the ancient people of India have known for centuries.

> In India, where turmeric is widely used as both a food spice and medicinal herb, the prevalence of four common U.S. cancers (breast, colon, lung and prostate) is ten times lower!
>
> "We have not found a single cancer on which curcumin does not work," states Dr. Bharat Aggarwal, who conducts cancer research at the Jawaharlal Nehru Centre for Advanced Scientific Research in Bangalore, India.

Turmeric Benefits:

- ★ Turmeric reduces inflammation and inhibits oxidative stress in the body.
- ★ Turmeric is well known for its blood purifying properties. Turmeric helps to dissolve blood clots; stimulate the formation of new blood tissue; and can restore circulation and blood flow to all vital organs (including the brain). By improving blood and oxygen flow to the brain, inflammation can greatly be reduced, helping our bodies better protect themselves against diseases such as dementia, Alzheimer's and Parkinson's.
- ★ Turmeric may help reduce the risk of heart disease. Research shows that the antioxidative properties of turmeric can help in the prevention of fat and cholesterol oxidation – both of which are known to be damaging to blood vessels and a leading cause of myocardial infarctions and strokes. In addition, turmeric is naturally rich in one of our very important heart-healthy vitamins: pyridoxine (B6).
- ★ Turmeric can help boost the primary liver detoxification enzyme known as glutathione S-transferase (GST), thereby allowing our bodies to naturally detoxify the liver of harmful toxins, including alcohol.
- ★ Turmeric supports healthy liver and gallbladder function. Turmeric stimulates the gallbladder to increase bile flow, which is required for the proper digestion of fats and considered an intestinal lubricant. As well as stimulating bile flow, turmeric increases the output of the pancreas, which means an increase in digestive enzyme production.

- ★ Turmeric strengthens and improves the entire digestive tract by increasing healthy intestinal flora. Turmeric has been found to enhance digestive and absorptive functions by promoting proper metabolism (correcting both excesses and deficiencies) and improving the elimination of waste and toxins. Evidence suggests that the curcumin found in turmeric can be beneficial for those suffering with Crohn's.
- ★ Turmeric and its curcumin may be used to fight cancer in several different ways:
    - o They can neutralize those substances and conditions known to cause cancer.
    - o They can directly help a cell retain its integrity if threatened by cancer causing substances.
    - o They can decrease the likelihood of cancerous cell formation or growth by completely blocking the formation of cancer causing enzymes. This is pivotal, as cancer causing enzymes are required for the replication of cancer cells.
    - o Although turmeric and its curcumin are best used as a preventative – well before cancer has a chance to grow – research is emerging on how they can destroy cancerous tumors, specifically in the beginning phases of disease.
- ★ Turmeric can protect against harmful environmental chemicals, thereby helping to prevent or lower (at the very least) the incidence of childhood leukemia. Researchers believe that the lower level of childhood leukemia in Asia may be directly linked to their high usage of turmeric.
- ★ Turmeric can help reduce inflammatory skin conditions, such as psoriasis and eczema, and may even prevent and treat malignant melanoma (a more serious form of skin cancer).
- ★ Turmeric's action as an antioxidant supports the respiratory system by protecting the lungs from pollution and toxins. According to one study, turmeric may also protect smokers from some of the adverse effects of nicotine. In the study, researchers observed the positive effects of curcumin and its ability to block nicotine from activating cancer cells.
- ★ Turmeric shows promise for being highly protective against neurodegenerative diseases. In India, the prevalence of neurological disease is very low. Studies have shown that turmeric and its curcumin can block or slow the progression of neurological diseases such as Alzheimer's, dementia and multiple sclerosis (MS).

What to Look for in a Quality Turmeric Product

Most people associate turmeric with authentic Indian cuisine and dishes infused with curry and garam masala spice blends. As we just learned though, the benefits and uses of turmeric go well and way beyond.

What's the difference between a typical turmeric powder found at the grocery store and turmeric root extract in powder or encapsulated form? If your goal is to use turmeric for medicinal and therapeutic purposes, I suggest looking for quality, organic, cold-water extracted turmeric root powder with a curcumin concentration of at least 95%. Turmeric with a concentration of 95% (or more) will ensure that you are getting the maximum percentage of curcumin (the active ingredient responsible for the majority of turmeric's discovered health benefits). Turmeric extract may be more expensive than turmeric spice, but the difference in quality and what you will gain from it is unparalleled. Most turmeric powders found in the grocery store are only about 3-5% curcumin. This is fine for culinary purposes, but not when you are going for a dramatic shift in health.

To understand the difference, let's do a little math: 500 mg of a typical grocery store quality turmeric powder, providing 5% curcumin, will only give you 25 mg of curcumin. Whereas 500 mg of turmeric extract powder, providing 95% curcumin gives you a whopping 475 mg of curcumin. That is 19 times more!

What about taking isolated curcumin instead of turmeric extract? Again, there are other properties in turmeric that I (as well as the experts) believe need to be present in order for it to do the best job it can do. The following is a direct quote taken from Dr. Weil's Q & A Library (published April 28, 2011): *"I frequently recommend turmeric supplements, and I believe whole turmeric is more effective than isolated curcumin for inflammatory disorders, including arthritis, tendonitis and autoimmune conditions."*

For those not keen on the peppery, warm and bitter flavor of turmeric, and who would rather not put it in everything they eat or drink for its desired effects, there are turmeric root capsules. My favorite is by Premier Research Labs. Each capsule is guaranteed to be 500 mg of the finest, organic, grade 10, Indian turmeric – and absolutely nothing else. It makes no sense to buy turmeric that has been irradiated, potentially contaminated, and nullified with cheap binders, fillers and glues.

How to Take Turmeric

Depending on the therapeutic effect one is after, the dosage of turmeric will vary. Keeping that in mind, the recommended dosage for an anti-inflammatory effect is between 400-600 mg, three times per day (1,200-1,800 mg total). If you are new to turmeric but decide to go straight for the gold with a powdered extract of at least 95% curcumin, then I suggest starting out small (quarter teaspoon or less, 1-3 times daily). As your body adapts to its potency, you can gradually work your way up (half teaspoon or more, 1-3 times daily).

> **Quick Tip:** Take turmeric with foods containing some fat (like coconut), as it will be much better absorbed. For even better absorption and bioavailability, you may wish to take it with a small amount (up to an eighth of a teaspoon) of black pepper extract (piperine). Though, please beware, not enough human studies have been done to determine the side effects of chronic supplementation with piperine. In addition, piperine may inhibit a number of enzymes responsible for metabolizing certain pharmaceutical drugs and nutritional substances. Until further information is available, I suggest taking piperine five days on and two days off, as well as taking one full week off each month. It is quite likely that small amounts could provide health benefits, while larger amounts could be toxic and damaging to the liver and other organs.
>
> Taking the above information into consideration, I would refrain from taking supplements that contain both turmeric (curcumin) and black pepper (piperine) together. It would be better to purchase these items separately and then use together accordingly, as well as sporadically. **FYI:** In my own experience with turmeric, it can work well enough on its own when taken correctly and with foods containing high-quality fats. Therefore, unless there is a very specific reason for taking piperine (e.g., vitiligo signs and symptoms), then I don't believe piperine is necessary for everyone.

Precautions: Even though turmeric is considered one of the safest herbs, over consumption and improper usage can lead to a few undesirable side effects. For instance, over consumption of turmeric may lead to gastrointestinal problems such as stomach upset, nausea, diarrhea or ulcers. Due to its uterine stimulating effect, it should not be used during pregnancy. Due to its anti-clotting properties, avoid turmeric for at least two weeks prior to surgery. For the same reason, turmeric may intensify the effects of blood thinning agents; therefore, turmeric may also be contraindicated while taking anti-coagulant or anti-platelet medications. Use with caution if you are diabetic and on diabetic medication, as turmeric has hypoglycemic properties, meaning, it has the potential to lower your blood glucose levels even further. If you have gallstones, obstructed bile ducts or suffer from liver or gallbladder disease, consult with a qualified healthcare practitioner before starting to take turmeric. It is also advised that individuals prone to kidney stones either not take turmeric at all (due to it containing oxalic acid), or at the very least, limit the amount of turmeric consumed and make sure to drink plenty of water.

The Amazing World of Ayurveda

Now I know I only covered four ayurvedic herbs in detail – which just so happen to be my absolute favorites for regular use – but there is an entire arsenal out there to explore. Another collection of my favorites are listed below. I tend to utilize the following on occasion or as needed. Although there are even more amazing ayurvedic herbs to choose from, I suggest starting with the four previously mentioned and graduating to the 12 acknowledged below. These 12 are my honorable mention picks, totally worth doing a bit more homework on.

- ★ **Amla Berry:** A potent, whole food source vitamin C.
- ★ **Bacopa (Brahmi) Monnieri:** Rich in antioxidants and known as a brain tonic for helping to promote mental alertness, cognitive ability and memory retention without over-stimulating.
- ★ **Chamomile:** A gentle sleep aid and mild relaxant.
- ★ **Cissus Quadrangularis:** A natural analgesic, with specific bone fracture healing properties and cortisol blocker characteristics.
- ★ **Green Coffee Bean:** An antioxidant and weight loss promoter.
- ★ **Guggul:** Known to help lower cholesterol levels and protect against the development of arteriosclerosis, otherwise known as hardening of the arteries.
- ★ **Holy basil:** An adaptogenic superherb.
- ★ **Mangosteen:** An antioxidant, anti-inflammatory and immune booster.
- ★ **Neem:** An instant anti-microbial.
- ★ **Noni:** An immune enhancer and whole-body rejuvenator.
- ★ **Tribulus Terrestris:** An aphrodisiac and performance enhancer.
- ★ **Valerian:** A potent, powerful, safe and effective herb for the nervous system; often used as a sedative, antispasmodic, anticonvulsant and in the treatment of migraine headaches.

Please Note: Always look for organic, cold-water extracted herbs, preferably in powdered form. New Horizon Health and Ultimate Superfoods are the top two sources I recommend when working with single ayurvedic herbs in powder form. When capsules are desired, I like working with single herbal encapsulations and synergistic herbal blends by Premier Research Labs.

CHINESE SUPERHERBS

> *Traditional Chinese medicine (TCM) is an ancient medical system that has been practiced for more than 5,000 years. Practitioners believe that there is a life force (aka energy) that moves through everyone known as qi (pronounced "chee"). For yin and yang to be in balance and for the human body to be healthy, an individual must have ample qi that can freely flow throughout the body without any blockages.*

Gynostemma

Gynostemma (*Gynostemma pentaphyllum*) is a hardy, climbing five-leafed vine, indigenous to China, Japan, Korea and Vietnam. It belongs to the cucumber, gourd and melon family, but does not bear any fruit itself. In China, gynostemma is called jiaogulan, which means "twisting-vine-orchid."

Gynostemma is considered one of the most preferred herbs in all of Asia. In fact, due to its health-giving properties, protective qualities and anti-aging effects, the locals who cultivate and consume gynostemma look upon it as the "immortality herb." It is also honored as a "miracle tea" or "magical grass." Ancient Chinese legend states that those who consume gynostemma on a regular basis live longer than those who do not.

The grandness of gynostemma arises from its broad spectrum of adaptogenic properties. Japanese studies signify that gynostemma possesses "double-directional" activity on the central nervous system. This simply means that gynostemma has the innate intelligence to calm when one is overexcited and stressed and gently stimulate when one is tired and fatigued. It also has the ability to restore balance and equilibrium to many other systems of the body, including the cardiovascular system, digestive system, immune system, reproductive system and respiratory system.

The active chemical compounds responsible for gynostemma's amazing adaptogenic attributes are its saponins (aka gypenosides). According to Dr. Tsunematsu Takemoto, a Japanese scientist whose specialty was herbal medicine research, more than 80 saponins exist in gynostemma. This is 3-4 times the number of saponins found in ginseng. Some recent research claims there are more than 100 different gypenosides in gynostemma. Whatever the actual highest number is, gynostemma has earned a noteworthy reputation for containing the widest range of saponins out of all the plants in nature. It also contains an array of amino acids, vitamins, the minerals calcium, iron, magnesium, manganese, phosphorus, potassium, selenium, zinc and more!

Gynostemma Benefits:

- ★ Gynostemma can boost the body's natural resistance to stress by gently restoring internal homeostasis. When left unchecked, stress can lead to a host of issues: from anxiety and depression; to anger, rage and fury; to acute and chronic illnesses of all types (emotional, mental, and physical). Known as one of the best adaptogens in traditional Chinese medicine, gynostemma can bring the entire body back into balance and strengthen the adaptive capacity of those who consume it regularly.
- ★ Gynostemma is a powerful source of antioxidants. According to research, gynostemma can actually stimulate the body's own production of antioxidants, which is much more effective than trying to get enough through ingestion alone.
- ★ Gynostemma's ability to increase superoxide dismutase (SOD) makes it a popular anti-aging herb for longevity. SOD is a powerful antioxidant that is very helpful in preventing oxidation damage from harmful free radicals.
- ★ Gynostemma can invigorate and upregulate the immune system by assisting the liver and enhancing white blood cell production and activity (including lymphocytes and natural killer cells) in those who are deficient.
- ★ Gynostemma can help rev up the body's metabolism, regulate blood sugar levels and remove harmful blood fats. By harmonizing the symphony of body chemistry, one can achieve healthy metabolic functioning. Whether one wants to lose weight by reducing excess body fat, gain weight by building lean muscle mass, or simply maintain a healthy weight – consuming gynostemma proves to be beneficial!

- ★ Gynostemma is not categorized as a laxative, but can promote regular bowel movements and waste elimination. Gynostemma assists the intestines in the removal of harmful toxins and waste material that may otherwise become impacted and reabsorbed back into circulation.
- ★ Gynostemma's saponins (gypenosides) can increase cardiovascular health in a multitude of ways.
    - o They can lower high blood pressure and improve the overall functioning of the cardiovascular system by increasing coronary blood flow and decreasing vascular resistance.
    - o They can cause the lining of the blood vessels to release nitric oxide, thereby resulting in vasodilatation and more efficient blood flow.
    - o They can prevent myocardial infarctions (heart attacks) due to their strong anti-oxidative and anti-inflammatory effects.
    - o They can decrease the risk of heart attacks and strokes by naturally thinning the blood, as well as effectively mitigating the build-up of plaque in blood vessel walls.
    - o They can significantly reduce bad cholesterol and excessive triglycerides floating in the bloodstream. Although both cholesterol and triglycerides are essential for human life, too much of either one (due mostly to poor dietary choices) is unhealthy and can lead to coronary heart disease. **FYI:** Cholesterol is necessary for building and maintaining cell membranes and making several essential hormones. In addition, triglycerides provide much of the energy needed for the proper function of many different bodily tissues. The goal is to maintain a "healthy" level of each.
- ★ Gynostemma supports respiratory health. In China, gynostemma is commonly used to treat chronic bronchitis, cough and the overproduction of sputum (phlegm).

How to Enjoy Gynostemma

One of the easiest and most popular ways to prepare gynostemma is to steep and drink it as a tea. Gynostemma can either be steeped alone or combined with other medicinal and tonic herbs in order to enhance their beneficial effects. I love using this tea as a base for many different liquid elixir concoctions. For instance, I almost always combine it with schizandra berries and will often brew it with a quality, loose-leaf green tea (such as Japanese gyokuro or sencha), white tea (such as silver needles or white peony) or yerba mate (my ultimate favorite). As far as the taste, I find it to be a natural balance of both bitter and sweet.

Use 1-2 teaspoon for every eight ounces of water and steep for about 3-10 minutes. The steep time will vary depending on what you combine the gynostemma with and how strong you like it. For instance, I steep my mixture for about ten minutes (or longer) with 1-2 teaspoons of schizandra berries and 3-4 teaspoons of yerba mate, but only about three minutes with 1-2 teaspoons of green tea and about five minutes with 3-4 teaspoons of white silver needle tea. When finished drinking your first cup, you may add more water for multiple infusions. Depending on your steep time, you may be able to get another 1-3 infusions from the same leaves.

As for where to purchase gynostemma, I only order my tea directly from Jiaogulan (www.jiaogulan.com). Their tea is always fresh and is grown organically in an area with ideal environmental conditions for growing healthy herbs. Their gynostemma is grown in the highlands of Thailand, a region recognized for its abundant rainfall, fertile soil and pristine air.

Precautions: Women who are pregnant are advised to avoid gynostemma; with little information available, it is also not recommended while breast-feeding. With that being said, gynostemma is considered one of the safest herbs in traditional Chinese medicine. As of this writing, the only side effects currently attributed to gynostemma are possible nausea and increase in the number of bowel movements. Due to its blood-thinning properties, gynostemma may increase the risk of easy bruising and bleeding – especially if taken at the same time as aspirin or other prescription drugs or herbs known to thin blood. Gynostemma may also counteract the effects of drugs used to prevent organ transplant rejection. Always notify your doctor of any herbs you are taking or plan to take, as they may interfere with the plans of an upcoming medical or surgical procedure.

Schizandra Berries

Schizandra berries are the dried ripe fruit of *Schizandra chinensis* – a woody vine native to the forests of northern China and the Russian Far East. *Schizandra chinensis* literally means "five flavor fruit," as it possesses all five of the classical "tastes" (sour, bitter, sweet, spicy and salty). This is super significant and stupendously symbolic in traditional Chinese medicine because of the beliefs that:

1. Sourness acts on the liver and gallbladder and can absorb, consolidate and astringe. Sour flavor is often used to treat a chronic cough, halt diarrhea and reduce sweating. It can also be used to slow or even stop bleeding.
2. Bitterness acts on the heart and small intestine and can clear away heat, dry out dampness and purge toxic substances. Bitter flavor is often used to treat a productive (wet) cough. It can promote lowering effects such as urination and bowel movements.
3. Sweetness acts on the stomach and spleen and can moisten, nourish, harmonize and tonify. It is often used to improve mood, as well as alleviate tension, spasms and pain. Sweet flavor is much more bland and neutral; therefore, it is often used to work on weak digestive systems and to help with deficiency syndromes.
4. Spiciness (or pungent) acts on the lungs and large intestine and can ignite digestive fire, moisten dryness and promote qi (the flow of energy). It also assists in the circulation of blood and bodily fluids. Spicy flavor is primarily used for stimulating metabolism and promoting distribution.
5. Saltiness acts on the kidneys and bladder and can dissolve blockages, alleviate stagnation and detoxify while replenishing. Salty flavor is often used to resolve constipation and to soften hardened tissue and nodules found in muscles and organs.

When taking a holistic approach to health and healing, it is very important that we consume all five flavors in a balanced fashion. In traditional Chinese medicine, as well as Ayurveda, one is encouraged to never skip any flavor; otherwise imbalances can occur due to certain organs not being nurtured and properly nourished. Being that schizandra berries possess all five flavors, as well as the essence of all five elemental energies (wood, fire, earth, metal and water), it is no wonder that this herb is treasured as a superior tonic/herb for its ability to extend energy, vitality and life.

> *"The Taoists especially revered schizandra. Schizandra was my teacher's, Sung Jin Park's, favorite herb. This is because Schizandra tonifies all 3 treasures, enters all 12 meridians and nurtures all 5 elements. Master Park considered it to be the quintessential herbal substance."*
> *– Ron Teagarden*

Schizandra Berry Benefits:

- ★ Schizandra contains a host of active ingredient known to heighten one's health. These include phytonutrients such as plant sterols (stigmasterol and beta-sitosterol) and lignans; essential oils; vitamins A, C and E; the minerals chromium, magnesium, phosphorus and silica; as well as essential fatty acids and antioxidants.
- ★ Schizandra is highly regarded as the top herb in traditional Chinese medicine for balancing the body. In fact, schizandra berry is a scientifically-classified adaptogen and is effective at bringing the body back into systematic balance by regulating many bodily functions.
- ★ Schizandra, as an adaptogen, aids the body in adapting to stress. It works by balancing stress hormones and regulating organ function (adrenal glands, etc.) during times of mental, emotional and physical stress. It can also be very beneficial in building our tolerance to environmental stressors. The most significant effects are noted with regular, long-term use. **FYI:** According to Ron Teeguarden, the "cultivation" period for building the three treasures of life in the body (aka jing, qi and shen) is believed to take about 100 days of consecutive use. That being said, one is likely to notice many positive changes in how they look and feel long before the initial 100-day period has run its course.
- ★ Schizandra is a widely used herb for brain and central nervous system health. It can be used to enhance alertness, enrich memory, increase attention and concentration and sharpen one's focus. Unlike caffeine containing substances, schizandra berry will not promote headaches, jitters or nervousness.
- ★ Schizandra will not cause sleepiness. Although, when bedtime arrives, its action on the brain can result in deeper, more restful and satisfying sleep.
- ★ Schizandra can increase physical stamina and reduce recovery time from physical exertion.
- ★ Schizandra is a brilliant, beautifying herb. Due to its ability to help the skin retain moisture and maintain suppleness, schizandra berry is widely known and used for protecting the skin from sun, wind and cold weather damage.

* Schizandra has been shown to have detoxifying, regenerating and rejuvenating properties when it comes to protecting the health of the liver; thanks to its effectiveness in boosting both phase I detoxification (the binding and clearing of toxins from the liver into the bloodstream), as well as phase II (the complete clearance of activated toxins from the body).

  Please Note: It is worth comprehending the distinct difference between these two critical stages of liver detoxification. When an individual is in phase I, for instance, the detoxifying substance goes into the liver and binds with toxins and then releases them from the liver into the bloodstream. This is great, but without the proper functioning of phase II, these same toxins can be reabsorbed and cause an individual to experience a "cleansing reaction" (aka "healing crisis"). Schizandra's primary liver protecting and immune modulating constituents are its lignans (schizandrin, deoxyschizandrin, gomisins and pregomisin).

* Schizandra is famed for acting as an aphrodisiac, especially when used on a regular basis. As an astringent herb, schizandra berry can increase arousal fluids to the sex organs of both men and women. In men it can bolster the production of semen and increase sexual stamina and endurance. In women it is known to increase vaginal lubrication during intercourse and enhance circulation and genital sensitivity.
* Schizandra is capable of dilating the blood vessels. This can prove to be helpful in lowering blood pressure, improving circulation and maintaining the overall functioning of the cardiovascular system.
* Schizandra may be used to soothe respiratory conditions such as asthma (asthmatic coughing and wheezing) and chronic dry cough. It may also help rid the body of excess phlegm by acting as a lung expectorant.

How to Utilize Schizandra Berries

Schizandra may be purchased as whole dried berries, powder or as an herbal extraction. I like using the whole dried schizandra berries for making herbal elixirs. I often add about one tablespoon to my gynostemma concoctions and to my morning yerba mate. If you prefer powder, I suggest starting with one teaspoon (or less), 1-3 times per day. Schizandra (whole or powdered) can be easily used alone, blended with other herbals or added to a tea of your choice (such as a quality green or white tea). Powdered schizandra may even be added to smoothies or raw food desserts for that synergy factor and tangy edge.

When purchasing organic schizandra berries (whole or powdered), I recommend ordering through Mountain Rose Herbs (www.mountainroseherbs.com). If you would prefer to take this herb in extract form, then I highly suggest the Goji and Schizandra Drops by Ron Teagarden's Dragon Herbs. Made with Fingerprint Identical Transfer Technology (FITT), I find this product highly superior to any other product of its kind on the market. According to information published by the company, Dragon Herb's FITT is a proprietary process that utilizes mechanical forces to break raw materials down to a micron level. The entire process is performed at a low to moderate temperature that never exceeds 40 degrees C (104°F).

This eliminates the drawbacks of heated extractions and greatly preserves all the valuable components of the herb.

Precautions: Due to its ability to increase stomach acids, avoid schizandra berry if you have gastroesophageal reflex disease (GERD) or peptic ulcers. For this same reason, schizandra may cause gastric disturbances in some individuals; therefore, be sure to use with caution and adjust dosage as needed. Schizandra is contraindicated in women who are pregnant, as it can cause uterine contractions that may result in miscarriage. Although the reasoning is unclear, experts agree that schizandra should not be taken by individuals who suffer from epilepsy. In addition, it is highly advisable to avoid schizandra if you have high brain (intracranial) pressure due to diseases or conditions that create abnormally high pressure within the skull. This includes brain tumor, hemorrhagic stroke or hydrocephalus, as well as the swelling of brain tissue due to encephalitis or a traumatic head injury. Please be sure to always consult with a knowledgeable healthcare professional well versed in Chinese tonic herbalism before taking Schizandra for the management or reversal of any disorder or disease.

Ginseng

Asian ginseng (*Panax ginseng*) has to be one of the most legendary and treasured herbs utilized in traditional Chinese medicine. According to scientific research, ginseng is an adaptogenic herb possessing stimulating and regulatory properties to both the central nervous system (CNS) and endocrine system. It can help a person adapt to life's daily stressors, as well as boost endurance, physical performance and resilience under stressful circumstances and traumatic events. Although ginseng contains many active ingredients, the most important are its saponins called ginsenosides. As we learned above, saponins are important to adaptability improvement, and ginsenosides in particular are believed to be instrumental in building muscle tissue and improving strength and endurance. This is what makes ginseng quite popular among athletes.

It should be noted that there are many varieties of ginseng. However, authentic and high-quality ginseng belongs to the Panax genus. If you are after the favorable effects of ginsenosides, then you must look for "Panax" in the botanical/genus name. Panax means "all-heal" in Greek, which translates to "panacea" or "cure-all" in English.

In addition to saponins (ginsenosides), ginseng contains dietary fiber; vitamins B1, B2, B3, B5 and C; and the minerals calcium, magnesium, potassium, phosphorous, iron and zinc. It is also noted to possess potent anti-inflammatory, antioxidant and anti-cancer properties.

Asian Ginseng vs American Ginseng

Asian ginseng (*Panax ginseng*) grows wild in China, Korea and Japan, while American ginseng (*Panax quinquefolius*) is native to the rich, moist woodlands of North America. Asian ginseng is considered a yang tonic herb, as it is known to be warm to hot in nature. This is in contrast to America ginseng, which is considered a yin tonic herb and known to be cool in nature.

<u>Asian</u> ginseng and its warming properties are more suited for individuals who tend toward having the following characteristics: lack of energy and motivation, low physical stamina, low mental acuity and staying power, low basal body temperature and metabolism, poor circulation, cold extremities, passive temperament, etc.

- ★ Asian ginseng helps strengthen the lungs, spleen and stomach.
- ★ Asian ginseng is commonly used to enhance energy and accelerate the healing and recovery process.
- ★ Asian ginseng may be effective in the treatment of male erectile dysfunction.

<u>American</u> ginseng and its cooling properties are more suited for individuals who tend toward having the following characteristics: highly energetic and hyperactivity, high blood pressure, high rate of metabolism, aggressive behavior, ruddy skin complexion, hot and fiery temperament, etc.

- ★ American ginseng helps strengthen the lungs, heart and kidneys.
- ★ American ginseng may be useful in treating menopausal hot flashes, night sweats, hot hands and feet, nervousness, anxiety and insomnia.
- ★ American ginseng can be used as an alternative to hormone replacement therapy in women who have reached or passed menopause.

Both Asian & American Ginseng Benefits:

- ★ Both Asian and American ginsengs are touted as general health tonics and immune system modulators.
- ★ Both Asian and American ginsengs are used for regulating blood sugar levels in individuals with diabetes.
- ★ Both Asian and American ginsengs are used as adaptogens. They can help individuals cope more effectively with stress by improving energy at the cellular level. In fact, adaptogens are known to have a restorative effect on mitochondria (the powerhouses of our cells).
- ★ Both Asian and American ginsengs are used for enhancing energy and amplifying alertness and diligence.

What to Look for in a Quality Ginseng Product

Due to the wide varieties of ginseng on the market, I strongly recommend that any and all ginseng products be purchased from acclaimed and respected suppliers. This will ensure that one obtains only the highest quality ginseng; a ginseng that I describe as being naturally grown and prepared with the best of intentions and purest form of integrity. According to Ron Teagarden, recognized as a leader in Chinese tonic herbalism, one must beware of low-grade ginseng products, as they are often made from immature roots that have an imbalanced chemistry. Cheaply grown and cultivated ginseng has, unfortunately, been known to increase tension, cause headaches and even increases blood pressure. Mature and high-quality ginseng, on the other hand, grown in pristine environments and without the use of chemicals, has never caused or contributed to negative side effects. Therefore, do your research and build a good rapport with your source(s) before purchasing.

Since I've already done my investigative work, I highly recommend Ron Teagarden's Dragon Herbs and George Lamoureux's Jing Herbs when it comes to learning which ginseng is right for you and purchasing a quality product. I also really like Ginseng-FX by Premier Research Labs. This ginseng is unique, in that it has been made fully bio-available due to a breakthrough fermentation process. This is great news for individuals with chronic health issues, as research shows that only about 33% of people in general, 8% of people with cancer and 4% of diabetics can actually absorb ginseng's super-powered nutrients. In addition, this product contains the most ancient and recognized species of ginseng, otherwise known as Korean, red Panax ginseng. It is the primary species used in scientific studies to explore ginseng's health-giving properties.

How to Use Ginseng

Ginseng dosage will vary depending on what you are looking to use it for. For instance, clinical studies have successfully used as little as a 100 mg for the prevention of colds and flus and as much as 4,500 mg (in divided doses) for memory loss and Alzheimer's.

- ★ If looking to take Asian ginseng as an adaptogen (meaning, to increase your resistance to stress), as well as for overall energy balance, well-being and immune support, studies suggest a daily dosage of about 200 mg. If you find yourself feeling tired and run-down more often than not, start with about 200-250 mg per day and increase to one gram (1,000 mg), three times per day as needed.
- ★ According to studies, 200 mg of Asian ginseng can assist in the management of type 2 diabetes (aka non-insulin dependent diabetes). In other studies that used American ginseng, the dosage was three grams (3000 mg). With type 2 diabetes, it is recommended that ginseng be taken no more than two hours before a meal; otherwise blood sugar levels may become too low.
- ★ For erectile dysfunction (ED), up to one gram (1,000 mg) of Asian ginseng taken three times per day is recommended. Try for at least a month before deciding if it helps or not.
- ★ For improving memory, it is recommended to start with one gram (1,000 mg) three times per day. It is highly suggested to try for at least three months before deciding whether ginseng will work or not. **FYI:** There are many stages of Alzheimer's. Ginseng may work on some stages of the disease, but not work on all of them. Please be sure to always consult with a knowledgeable healthcare practitioner, well versed in Chinese tonic herbalism, before starting ginseng for the management or reversal of any disorder or disease.

Please Note: Although ginseng is considered a tonic herb (which typically means an herb that is safe to consume on a daily basis), I still think it is a good idea to take a break from the habitual and regular use of ginseng. I suggest taking weekends off or one full week off for every one month of consistent use.

Precautions: Due to its regulatory effect on blood sugar, ginseng may increase the effectiveness of insulin and other pharmaceutical drugs or herbs known to lower blood sugar levels. Asian ginseng in particular may interact with anticoagulants and other drugs or herbs known to act as blood thinners. Use caution if you are currently on any immunosuppressant drugs (such as cyclosporine or prednisone). Be very cautious if you are taking certain antidepressants (like MAOIs). Due to ginseng having an estrogen-like effect, women who are pregnant or breastfeeding should refrain from using it; unless advised otherwise by a healthcare practitioner. Both Asian and American ginsengs have a stimulatory effect and may cause nervousness or sleeplessness when taken in high doses. Although ginseng is considered a relatively safe herb for the majority of individuals, it can occasionally cause side effects. This is more specifically directed toward those who are highly sensitive (or consider themselves allergic) to stimulants. Before starting on ginseng or drastically changing your current regimen, it is highly advisable to first consult with a qualified healthcare professional well versed in Chinese tonic herbs.

Medicinal Mushrooms

When most people think of mushrooms, they think of the popular portabella mushroom or common white cap mushroom used in cooking. Some may recollect being told to beware of picking poisonous mushrooms, while others may reminisce about their days tripping on psychedelic mushrooms. But what about the hundreds of species of mushrooms found to possess superior nutrition and medicinal properties?

Exotic Asian mushrooms (such as shiitake, maitake, etc.) have more than triple the number of vitamins and minerals as portabellas. In fact, their nutrient concentrations are so high that they reach therapeutic dosages when it comes to enhancing health and vitality, preventing a host of illnesses and halting the progression of certain diseases.

> Medicinal mushrooms are mushrooms that are used or studied as potential treatments for diseases. Research indicates that medicinal mushrooms may have powerful anticancer, antiviral, antibacterial, anti-parasitic, anti-inflammatory, anti-hyperglycemic, liver-protective and cardio-protective activities.

The concept of a "medicinal mushroom" is far from new. In fact, mushrooms have been used medicinally as far back in history as we can go in writing. For thousands of years, the Chinese (as well as other cultures) have traditionally used mushrooms as medicine to promote health and longevity.

There are approximately 700 species of mushrooms that can be consumed as nutritious food!

Although the general medicinal benefit of mushrooms is to restore balance and function to the immune system, various mushrooms have varying degrees of specific benefits. The following is just a taste of what medicinal quality mushrooms have to offer: the promotion of immune function and immune system balance; decreasing the risk of cancer and in some instances, assisting in the eradication of cancer all together; reducing inflammation; fighting allergies; helping balance blood sugar levels; boosting cardiovascular health; and warding off bacteria, viruses and mold. That's right! Although fungi themselves, medicinal mushrooms are not known to cause or contribute to Candida, yeast, mold or fungus within the body. In fact, certain medicinal mushrooms, such as cordyceps and reishi, can actually help treat these insidious infections. According to Paul Stamets, a dedicated mycologist for over 30 years, there's an abundance of scientific literature referencing how the metabolites of mushrooms actually produce natural antibiotics that can combat Candida overgrowth.

Polysaccharides (specifically beta-glucans) are at the heart of medicinal mushroom benefits and are said to awaken the immune system. Beta-glucans are currently known as "biological response modifiers." Research has proven that beta-glucans possess the ability to stimulate macrophages, natural killer cells (NK cells), T cells and immune system cytokines.

- **Macrophages** are a type of white blood cell that ingests foreign invaders in the body, such as infectious microorganisms. They can be found in the liver, spleen and connective tissues of the body.
- **NK cells** are small lymphocytes that originate in the bone marrow. They are part of our first line of defense against cancer cells and virus-infected cells.
- **T cells** are a type of white blood cell that is of key importance to the immune system and is at the core of adaptive immunity. They protect our bodies against disease by eliminating cancerous cells, as well as cells infected with viruses and bacteria.
- **Cytokines** are small proteins that serve as molecular messengers between cells. The body produces different types of cytokines, which include: interleukins, lymphokines and cell signal molecules (such as tumor necrosis factor and the interferons), all of which trigger inflammation and respond to infections.

What to Look for in a Quality Medicinal Mushroom Product

It appears that combining several types of medicinal mushrooms in a formula creates the most superlative synergistic immune response and most powerful therapeutic punch. This is because each species brings its own unique combination which can then activate a broad spectrum of receptor sites in the immune system. For this reason, I believe everyone can benefit from Host Defense MyCommunity by Fungi Perfecti. As a natural preventative against a multitude of life's daily stressors, I do not go one day without taking this magical mushroom blend at least once or twice per day. MyCommunity is the powerful 17 species host defense formula created by Paul Stamets. It is considered by many, including naturopathic physicians and herbalists, to be the most comprehensive formula for supporting natural immunity.

> In the article titled "Beta-Glucan Analysis and the Seven Pillars of Immunity," posted February 21, 2012 on www.fungi.com, Paul Stamets states the following: "The immune system is activated multifactorially by many components in mushrooms. Beta-glucans are just one. Other constituents include, but are not limited to, alpha-glucans, ergothioneines, antioxidants, anti-inflammatory sterols, lipids, glycosides and mycoflavonoids – many of which work synergistically to optimize health. The efficacy of a multi-constituent approach has been positively confirmed in the scientific literature."
>
> Paul Stamets then goes on to list the seven primary constituent classes (aka "pillars") of immune benefits from medicinal quality mushrooms. The seven pillars are as follows:
>
> 1. **Polysaccharides:** possess immune modulating properties (e.g., alpha and beta-glucans)
> 2. **Glycoproteins:** possess immune modulating properties (e.g., PSK)
> 3. **Triterpenes:** sterols (e.g., sistosterols, stigmasterols and campesterols)
> 4. **Lipids:** cholesterol modulating
> 5. **Proteins (enzymes):** antioxidants
> 6. **Cyathane Derivatives:** possess potent stimulating activity for nerve-growth factor (NGF) synthesis (e.g., erinacines and hericiones)
> 7. Secondary metabolites

Host Defense MyCommunity provides the following 17 medicinal mushrooms: Royal Sun Blazei, Cordyceps, Enokitake, Amadou, Agarikon, Artist Conk, Reishi, Oregon Polypore, Maitake, Lion's Mane, Chaga, Shiitake, Mesima, Birch Polypore, Zhu Ling, Split Gill Polypore and Turkey Tail. This product is my first choice for broad-range protection. When a more targeted approach is desired, I suggest the use of Host Defense MyCommunity in conjunction with the medicinal mushroom(s) shown to have the most activity against the specific disorder or disease you are striving to address.

Organic, Organic, Organic! All mushrooms by Fungi Perfecti are grown at their very own certified organic farm situated at the base of the Olympic Peninsula – the large arm of land in Western Washington State that lies across Puget Sound from Seattle. Because of this location, clean air and pristine water is always in abundance. As a result, Fungi Perfecti has increased their sales to certain Asian markets where an increase in pollution has been on the rise and environmental contamination is a major concern.

Along with the entire Host Defense line by Fungi Perfecti, I am also in love with the two mushroom extracts by SurThrival (e.g., Reishi and Chaga single liquid extracts). Similarly, I am highly impressed with a couple of the more unique mushroom products by Dragon Herbs (e.g., Reishi Spore Oil, Duanwood Reishi and Wild Siberian Chaga), as well as Jing Herbs (e.g., Ye Sheng Reishi Mushroom capsules and STR-12 powder).

When it comes to knowledge, passion and dedication to quality and safety, I whole-heartedly trust the medicinal mushroom products by the following individuals: Paul Stamets (Fungi

Perfecti), Ron Teagarden (Dragon Herbs), George Lamoureux (Jing Herbs), David Wolfe (New Horizon Health), Daniel Vitalis (SurThrival) and Dr. Robert Marshall (Premier Research Labs). Their commitment to honesty and integrity is truly and utterly admirable!

I cannot possibly give all the medicinal mushrooms in the entire mushroom kingdom the justice each and every one deserves in just a few words. For this reason, I choose to leave all the intricate details and important attributes of each medicinal mushroom entirely up to the experts. To learn more about medicinal mushrooms and all their miraculous health benefits, I highly suggest reading the following books. Any and all will make a great addition to your new-found health and longevity library!

- ★ *MycoMedicinals: An informational Treatise on Mushrooms* by Paul Stamets and C. Dusty Wu Yao
- ★ *Mycelium Running: How Mushrooms Can Help Save the World* by Paul Stamets
- ★ *The Fungal Pharmacy: The Complete Guide to Medicinal Mushrooms and Lichens of North America* by Robert Rogers and Solomon P. Wasser
- ★ *Sugars That Heal: The New Healing Science of Glyconutrients* by Emil I. Mondoa and Mindy Kitei
- ★ *Chaga: King of the Medicinal Mushrooms* by David Wolfe

How to Take Medicinal Mushrooms

As already stated, my #1 choice for preventing and potentially reversing a number of immune system disorders is Host Defense MyCommunity. Although this product is available in both capsule and liquid extract form, I prefer the liquid extract and suggest taking one full dropperful, twice daily. For broad-spectrum immune modulating and powerful anti-oxidant, anti-microbial, anti-mutagenic and anti-cancer properties, I additionally like to take chaga and reishi.

> *Out of all tree mushrooms in the mushroom kingdom, chaga is considered to be "the king" and reishi "the queen."*

When targeting a localized disorder and organ-specific disease, I highly recommend utilizing Host Defense MyCommunity along with the particular medicinal mushroom(s) found to have a targeted therapeutic effect against the disorder and disease in question. Please consult with a qualified healthcare professional well versed in the activities and properties of each medicinal mushroom before attempting to manage and reverse any specific disorder or disease on your own. Dosage can depend on several factors and, for this reason, would be best determined by a practitioner with medicinal mushroom expertise.

Please Note: In both of his books listed above (*MycoMedicinals* and *Mycelium Running*), Paul Stamets provides a cross-index of mushrooms and their targeted therapeutic effects. In addition, he graciously provides a table which lists mushrooms and their activity against specific cancers.

> **Quick Tip:** Capsules or liquid extracts may be taken on an empty stomach and added to your favorite hot or cold beverage when mixed with a small amount of water. You may also synergistically blend any medicinal mushroom into your favorite superfood smoothie, herbal elixir or raw chocolate concoction.

The Charm of Traditional Chinese Herbalism

I have barely skimmed the surface when it comes to all that traditional Chinese medicine has to offer, but I have at least described my top favorites, which I feel can benefit just about anyone. If you are as fascinated as I am with this ancient healing art, then I suggest diving in deeper. Other natural treasures you may want to explore include:

- **Astragalus:** A potent tonic herb used to strengthen the body as a whole and improve immune response and metabolic function.
- **Deer Velvet Antler:** Contains a powerful blend of naturally-occurring insulin-like growth factors which are involved in every cellular function in the human body. It is also revered for its regenerative, reparative, rejuvenative and revitalizing properties.

  Please Note: due to antler and placenta products containing growth factors, avoid if you suffer from benign growths and malignant tumors until the underlying cause has been rectified and eradicated.

- **Dong Quai/Chinese Angelica:** Used in the treatment of menopause, menstrual cramps and PMS symptoms.
- **Eucommia:** Helps athletes, people who exercise and the elderly maintain structural integrity of skeletal and muscle tissue. It improves flexibility and stability.
- **Ginkgo Biloba:** Improves blood flow and oxygenation to the brain, thereby enhancing memory and slowing mental decline. It is often used to treat peripheral vascular disease.
- **He Shou Wu/Fo-Ti Root:** Restores and nourishes the root energy of the body. Prized for its ability to prevent premature aging and enhance longevity and youthfulness. It is also often used to promote the growth of hair and reduce or reverse premature graying.
- **Pine Pollen:** Nature's answer to natural testosterone and all its benefits for both men and women. It is traditionally used as a health restorative, anti-aging nutrient and longevity tonic.
- **Rehmannia:** Used to restore energy and vitality; strengthen the liver, kidney, adrenal glands and heart; and to treat a variety of ailments such as anemia, constipation, diabetes and urinary tract problems.
- **Rhodiola:** A potent adaptogen used to strengthen the nervous system; help support concentration and memory; and improve physical strength, endurance and sexual vitality.

- **Royal Jelly:** An effective anti-aging tonic with an amazing array of master nutrients necessary to sustain life, promote longevity and youthfulness, increase energy and strength, along with vigor and vitality. It helps to naturally regulate and balance hormones.
- **Tongkat Ali:** A male sexual tonic and libido enhancer.
- **Uva-ursi:** Used to treat kidney and urinary tract problems such as UTIs.

Please Note: Always look for single Chinese herbs and Chinese tonic herbal formulas comprised of only the <u>highest</u> quality raw ingredients. Organically grown and wild-crafted is what everyone should strive for in their quest for the absolute best.

When it comes to unique and classic Chinese herbal formulations, I recommend Dragon Herbs and Jing Herbs. Please read their "quality control" and "quality assurance" pages on their websites to better understand what true quality means and how their raw materials differ from the majority of other herbal companies in the American marketplace.

STRIKING A BALANCE

Many people ask why I drink "hot" teas and "warm" herbal elixirs if I'm a "raw" vegetarian. My answer is "I eat my foods raw and drink my teas and tisanes hot in order to obtain the maximum amount of medicinal benefits that each food and herb has to offer." It is more about my desire to understand and acquire the optimal in nutritional science. By doing so, the best from all possible worlds becomes attainable.

Take into consideration the given information: when one decides to look deep enough at the chemical composition of most foods, it becomes clear that by over processing and cooking we devalue and destroy most all the vital nutrients within that food. On the other hand, there are many majestic plants, herbs and roots which are hardy and fibrous, and the only way to unleash their miraculous adaptogenic or medicinal powers is to extract them via hot water or alcohol extraction.

Conforming to a healthy lifestyle should not be based on radicalism, but instead on rationalism.

If you find yourself interested in the many superior and medicinal herbs used in traditional Chinese medicine (TCM), then you will most certainly discover the following to be true. Many prized and popular Chinese herbs are in actuality roots (such as astragalus, he shou wu, ginseng, etc.). Therefore, in order to absorb and assimilate their active ingredients, we must break down their strong cell walls prior to consuming. When careful and attentive processing techniques are applied the <u>true</u> essence of their healing powers can be relished by all.

CHAPTER 6
TOOLS OF THE TRADE

THE RAW NECESSITIES

Before we get into recipes, let's go over the most valuable kitchen tools and pieces of equipment you will need for setting up your raw food kitchen.

Please Note: Glass, stainless-steel and bamboo are the best materials for coming into contact with food. If you do choose plastic, please be sure to store all food and liquids in BPA free plastic or food grade plastics only. Look to purchase plastics with the following label and number: HDPE (#2), LDPE (#4) or PP (#5).

The Necessary Kitchen Gear

- **2 Cutting Boards** (preferably bamboo): One for garlic and onions and another for fruits and vegetables.
- **Knives** (stainless-steel and ceramic)
- **Blender:** Blendtec (1st choice) or Vitamix (2nd choice), which can be utilized for making almost everything. Nutribullet for simpler, smaller and more personal uses.
- **Food Processor:** Cuisinart or KitchenAid (one mini 4 C capacity for small amounts and one larger 8 C plus capacity for large amounts).
- **Salad Spinner(s):** Zyliss (4-6 servings)
- **Mixing Bowls** (stainless-steel and glass sets)
- **Glass Containers with Lids:** Various sizes of wide mouth mason jars (e.g., pint, quart and half gallon) for storing nuts, seeds, powders, bulk superfoods, etc. In addition, Pyrex and Anchor Hocking bowls w/lids are great for basic refrigerated food storage.
- **Colanders & Strainers:** small and large
- **Measuring Cups & Spoons** (stainless-steel and glass)
- **Strong/Firm Spatulas** (silicone): slim and regular sizes
- **Whisks** (stainless-steel): small and large
- **Citrus Squeezer** (stainless-steel)
- **Garlic Press** (stainless-steel): Great for pressing pieces of ginger root as well.
- **Vegetable Swivel Peeler**
- **Spirooli Spiral 3-in-1 Slicer:** A must have for fast and easy spiralized veggie noodles, ribbon sliced veggies and for thinly shredded veggies.
- **Cake & Muffin Pans** (silicone): Great for molding raw desserts. Non-stick silicone makes popping out your raw treats a snap (view page 368 for more info).
- **Sprouter** (manual): Sprout Master 8x10 trays

Advanced & Optional Kitchen Gear

- **Juicer:** Green Star Elite GSE-500 Juicer (1st choice) or Heavy Duty Commercial Champion Juicer (2nd choice)
- **Dehydrator:** Excalibur 3900 Deluxe Non-Timer Series 9 Tray Food Dehydrator (or 3926T 9 Tray w/ 26 Hour Timer) or Sedona Digitally Controlled Food Dehydrator (SD-9000) by Tribest
- **Sprouter** (automatic): EasyGreen MikroFarm Automatic Sprouter
- **Squeeze Handle Dishers** (stainless-steel): These make for easy scooping when making dehydrated cookies, burger patties, nut/seed balls, etc. A 1-1 ½ oz is great for cookies and macaroons; a 2-2 ½ oz size is perfect for falafel and nut/seed balls; and a 3-4 oz size is a good size for burgers and mini pizza crusts.
- **Milk Frother** (stainless-steel): Aerolatte brand is the one I like and can be used to break down clumpy powders (like xylitol) in liquids.

When to Use Which Blender

A Blendtec or Vitamix is ideal for making just about everything. Why? Because they can break down almost anything – but there is a small catch. With the Blendtec or Vitamix, you need at least eight ounces of liquid in order to cover the blade; this is so the job gets done as "smoothly" as possible. Blenders are meant to work with liquids. They are not food processors. Therefore, when making creations in a blender that are meant to be spoon-thick, I suggest making an amount that justifies the inclusion of at least eight ounces of water.

The Blendtec or Vitamix can easily get utilized daily (and maybe even more than once a day); especially since either of the two are "the best" on the market for making smoothies and raw soups that call for water rich fruits, bulky vegetables and a good amount of other ingredients as well. Both are also outstanding at making smooth and creamy nut/seed cheezes, crèmes, sauces and dressings. Again, just be sure to make enough so your blender has the right amount of liquid to do its job, and do it well.

Blendtec & Vitamix Tips:

- Always add wet and soft ingredients before adding dry and solid ingredients. This will give both of these blenders something to work with in order to do what they do best, which is to create a vortex within the pitcher that pulls the ingredients downward and toward the blade faster and more efficiently.
- Make sure the blender has at least eight ounces of liquid ingredients in total to work with (water, oil, lemon juice, raw agave, etc.), especially when the majority of the other ingredients are dry and solid (nuts, seeds, powders, etc.).
- Due to both the Blendtec and Vitamix being high volume capacity blenders, aim to yield at least 12-16 ounces of a finished product. Having too little ingredients and liquid can cause the ingredients to bounce up and around too much rather than being efficiently pulled down toward the blade. With the Blendtec and Vitamix, more is actually better for the smoothest and creamiest of creations.

- ★ To avoid cavitation issues, which is when an air pocket develops around the cutting path of the blade, please pay attention to the following tips: have the right ratio of liquid (wet) to solid (dry) ingredients; always start at a slower speed (ramping it up a little at a time); and place cold temperature and frozen foods in last (ideally after at least one blending cycle with all the other ingredients).

    Please Note: The ratio of wet to dry ingredients will vary depending on the individual characteristics of each ingredient. Be prepared to test run certain recipes and creations.

- ★ If and when cavitation occurs, simply stop the machine and do one or more of the following as needed: add more liquid, manually release air pocket with a spatula and/or vary speed until ingredients are back into the blending vortex.
- ★ If planning to blend with the addition of warm to hot liquids, I suggest keeping a hand on the blender lid for security. The build-up of pressure from the steam can blow the cover right off. You also want to make sure to never fill your blender more than half way with a warm or hot liquid.

In contrast to the Blendtec and Vitamix, the Nutribullet is ideal for concocting single serving nutrient extracted smoothies and personal elixir drinks. I also prefer the Nutribullet for blending together ingredients with warm liquids, like tea, as the twist on extractor blade acts like a cover, decreasing the chance of an accident. That said, I highly advise against ever using hot or boiling liquids – and for more than just blender explosion reasons (see page 478 for more info).

The Nutribullet comes with two blades: an extractor blade and a milling blade. With the milling blade, the Nutribullet can replace any need for a coffee grinder and can handle much larger quantities, to boot. It is great for grinding all kinds of dry nuts, seeds, herbs and spices. With the extractor blade, the Nutribullet makes whipping up just 1-2 servings of something special an easy task (such as a savory dressing for a salad or a sweet crème for a small dessert). Due to its unique design and smaller size, the Nutribullet does not seem to require as much liquid in order to keep the ingredients close to the blade. I find this to be perfect for making smaller quantities of all those thicker textured recipes. What's more, it does an amazing job at smoothing and creaming (as good as the Blendtec or Vitamix) – and with smaller quantities. For instance, I have made half batches of dips, sauces and dressings, where I have only added about 4-6 oz of liquid (or less), and each and every time they have come out super smooth and creamy.

If you have not yet invested in a Nutribullet, I would seriously consider doing so; especially if you are someone who plans on making smaller quantities of certain recipes. Having both the Blendtec and Vitamix myself, I really didn't think I could possibly have much use for the Nutribullet, but boy was I wrong. I was also pleasantly surprised at the amount of power it has! I have noticed that what can be a bit of a challenge for the Blendtec or Vitamix (mainly small quantities) is absolutely perfect for the Nutribullet. If it is possible to own a Blendtec or Vitamix, along with the Nutribullet, this would be ideal. Money well spent!

When to Use a Food Processor over a Blender

As already mentioned, a blender is designed to work with liquids. It is what you use when you desire a really smooth and creamy consistency. A food processor, on the other hand, doesn't require liquids. It is what you use when you desire an appliance that can give you a number of different cutting styles. Think of your food processor as your helping hand (or hands) in the kitchen. Depending on the model, you will be able to chop (with the S-shaped blade), slice, grate and more. If you like evenly chopped and fine shredded veggies, a food processor is a must. What would normally take you 30 minutes (or longer) will only take 30-60 seconds with a food processor.

One last thing I would like to mention is that both a blender and a food processor will puree quickly and easily. The main difference between the two is that a blender makes a smooth puree and a food processor (with its pulse feature) can make a chunky puree.

Kitchen Measurements & Equivalent Conversion Charts

The following charts are handy to have whenever you find yourself trying to decipher what is what in the kitchen. A great idea would be to copy these charts and slip them into a plastic sleeve for easy access. If you have the ability to laminate, that's even better! **FYI:** The following are based off of the U.S. Food and Drug Administration (USFDA) requirements for measurements.

Must-Know Kitchen Abbreviations

Recipe Abbreviations		Quickies	
Cup = C	Pound = lb	1 TBS = 3 tsp	1 C = ½ lb
Fluid = fl	Quart = qt	4 TBS = ¼ C	1 lb = 16 oz
Gallon = gal	Square = sq	2 TBS = 1 fl oz	16 oz = 2 C
Ounce = oz	Tablespoon = TBS	1 fl oz = 30 ml	1 kg = 2.2 lb
Package = pkg	Teaspoon = tsp	8 fl oz = 1 C	
Pint = pt			

Small Volume Liquid Measurements

Tablespoons	Cups	Fluid Ounces/ Milliliters
1 TBS	3 tsp	½ fl oz = 15 ml
2 TBS	⅛ C	1 fl oz = 30 ml
4 TBS	¼ C	2 fl oz = 60 ml
5 TBS + 2 tsp	⅓ C	2 ½ fl oz + = 80 ml

| 8 TBS | ½ C | 4 fl oz = 120 ml |

Tablespoons	Cups	Fluid Ounces/ Milliliters
10 TBS + 4 tsp	⅔ C	5 fl oz + = 160 ml
12 TBS	¾ C	6 fl oz = 180 ml
16 TBS	1 C	8 fl oz = 240 ml

Large Volume Liquid Measurements

Cups	Fluid Ounces	Pints/Quarts/Gallons
1 C	8 fl oz	½ pt
2 C	16 fl oz	1 pt = ½ qt
3 C	24 fl oz	1 ½ pt
4 C	32 fl oz	2 pt = 1 qt
8 C	64 fl oz	2 qt = ½ gal
16 C	128 fl oz	4 qt = 1 gal

Dry Measurements

Cup		Tablespoon		Teaspoon		Milliliter
1 C	=	16 TBS	=	48 tsp	=	240 ml
¾ C	=	12 TBS	=	36 tsp	=	180 ml
⅔ C	=	10 TBS + 4 tsp	=	34 tsp	=	160 ml
½ C	=	8 TBS	=	24 tsp	=	120 ml
⅓ C	=	5 TBS + 2 tsp	=	17 tsp	=	80 ml
¼ C	=	4 TBS	=	12 tsp	=	60 ml
⅛ C	=	2 TBS	=	6 tsp	=	30 ml
1/16 C	=	1 TBS	=	3 tsp	=	15 ml

Dash, Pinch or Smidgen = less than ⅛ tsp

Please Note: Measurements are rounded up.

Tips of the Trade: What You Need to Know

Tip #1: Substituting Sweeteners

All sweeteners listed in the recipes that follow may be replaced with another choice. Please see tips below for when an alternative is desired.

Please Note: Honey, sun-dried cane juice crystals, coconut crystals and xylitol can be used similarly to regular granulated or powdered cane sugar. Therefore, feel free to exchange in equal amounts and adjust as needed. Agave and stevia taste sweeter than cane sugar, so be prepared to make adjustments with these two. Depending on the recipe, you may also have to make adjustments to the amount of fluid you add. For instance, an <u>increase</u> in fluid may be needed when using a <u>dry</u> sweetener (e.g., sun-dried cane juice crystals or xylitol) instead of a <u>wet</u> sweetener, and a <u>decrease</u> in fluid may be needed when using a <u>wet</u> sweetener (e.g., raw agave or honey) instead of a <u>dry</u> sweetener. Please read on for a better understanding.

Substituting Raw Honey for Agave

Due to the distinct and sometimes strong flavor of certain varieties of honey, I suggest replacing agave with honey in equal quantities. More honey can always be added for more sweetness if desired.

Substituting Raw Agave for Honey

Despite having a low glycemic index (GI), raw agave is definitely sweeter to the taste than honey and most other traditional sweeteners; therefore, you may wish to decrease the amount of agave by about an eighth (or more), and add more as needed.

Substituting a Dry Sweetener Similar in Sweetness to Regular Sugar for Agave

If you decide to use sun-dried cane juice crystals, coconut crystals or xylitol – instead of agave – increase your dry sweetener by about a quarter of the amount called for in the recipe. For instance, if a recipe calls for ½ C raw agave, but you want to use sun-dried cane juice crystals instead, you will want to replace the ½ C of agave with about ⅔ C sun-dried cane juice crystals to start. Then taste and evaluate the need for more.

Substituting a Dry Sweetener for a Wet Sweetener in a Wet Recipe

When choosing a dry sweetener to replace raw agave or honey in a wet recipe (one with a high fluid content), you may or may not need to increase the fluid. Evaluate as you go and add a little at a time.

Substituting a Dry Sweetener for a Wet Sweetener in a Dry Recipe

On the other hand, for a dry recipe it will all depend on the other ingredients. I suggest adding up to ¼ C of water (or more), but start with 1 TBS at a time (4 TBS = ¼ C). Continue to add until desired texture is reached.

Substituting a Wet Sweetener for a Dry Sweetener in a Wet Recipe

When choosing agave or honey to replace any dry sweetener in a wet recipe (one with high fluid content), I suggest decreasing the amount of fluid called for by at least ¼ C. Remember, you can always add more; if you add too much at once, you cannot take it out.

Substituting a Wet Sweetener for a Dry Sweetener in a Dry Recipe

On the other hand, for a dry recipe it will all depend on the other ingredients and desired texture. For instance, if using a wet sweetener instead of a dry sweetener in a dessert recipe, and it becomes too wet or sticky to hold and mold, you may wish to add a small amount of a neutral tasting dry ingredient such as chia. This will help to bind and make molding much easier.

Substituting Green Leaf Stevia for Sweeteners

Although I prefer to use xylitol as a low glycemic option in most recipes (especially dessert recipes), if you choose to substitute green leaf stevia (powder or whole leaf) for any of the above sweeteners, please use these basic conversion guidelines to help you out a bit. To allow for more freedom, I've given a range. It is always better to start small and add a bit more at a time – especially since a little stevia can go a long way. Adding the right amount will balance flavors and offer a subtle amount of sweetness, but adding too much can turn the recipe and give it a bitter taste.

- ★ 1-2 TBS sweetener = ⅛-¼ tsp green leaf stevia powder or ½-1 tsp whole leaf
- ★ ¼-½ C sweetener = ½-1 tsp green leaf stevia powder or 1 ½ tsp-1 TBS whole leaf

> **Quick Tip:** To help prevent the bitter aftertaste of stevia in recipes that will require more than 1-2 TBS of a traditional sweetener, I suggest using ½-¾ xylitol with ½-¼ stevia. I find this works especially well with recipes that call for ¼ C or more of sweetener.

For the most part, I reserve stevia for those times when there's that slight bitter edge that needs to be taken care of. For instance, it works great for taking the bitter edge off a green smoothie with kale, an elixir drink with reishi mushroom and certain herbal teas. It also works great for balancing soup recipes and tomatoey recipes. Just add a pinch at a time until the flavors are balanced to your liking. Personally, I like to think of stevia as a finisher ingredient rather than a main ingredient.

Tip #2: Substituting Oils

Any oil listed may be replaced with chia, hemp, olive or coconut oil.

Please Note: When adding coconut oil, make it the very last thing that goes into your blender, as it can congeal and stick to the sides of your blender when it hits anything cold. In order to measure coconut oil with better ease and accuracy, I suggest running the bottle under warm water or placing it in a basin filled with warm water. This will liquefy enough coconut oil in the bottle for easy pouring.

Tip #3: Substituting Lemon Juice & Vinegars

Lemon juice, coconut vinegar or apple cider vinegar may all be used interchangeably depending on availability and preference. The only exception would be lime juice, as I feel it brings out unique flavor characteristics one is usually after in certain ethnic recipes (such as Thai, Mexican, Japanese, etc.).

Please Note: If limes are unavailable, the next best option would be to use lemons. When the flavor of lime is what you desire, you can add a tad of lime peel essential oil along with fresh lemon juice. For instance, if you have fresh lemons on hand (but no limes) I suggest adding 1 drop lime peel essential oil plus 1 TBS of lemon juice for every 1 TBS of lime juice you are substituting.

If you have neither lemons nor limes, I suggest adding 2-3 drop of lime peel essential oil for every 1 TBS of lime juice you are substituting (more or less to taste). **FYI:** Lime peel essential oil can be purchased through Mountain Rose Herbs (view pages 240-241 for more info).

Substituting Lemons for Limes or Limes for Lemons

Half a lime, juiced, equals about 1 TBS of lime juice. Therefore, one whole lime, juiced, equals about 2 TBS of lime juice. Due to lemons varying a bit more in size, I have found one lemon can yield anywhere from 3-4 TBS of juice.

Substituting Coconut Vinegar or Apple Cider Vinegar for Lemon Juice

The general rule of thumb to follow is: 1 TBS of vinegar = 2 TBS lemon juice. I don't always follow this rule when using small amounts, such as a single teaspoon or tablespoons full. That being said, it doesn't hurt to start out with what is generally advised. So, go ahead and use half the amount of vinegar to start, give it a taste, and then feel free to add more if more zing is needed. To me, this half the amount rule makes more sense when using larger amounts. For instance, if a ½ C lemon juice is called for, but I want to use vinegar instead, I will cut the amount of vinegar down to ¼-⅓ C. Then I taste before determining the need for more.

Tip #4: Herbs & Spices

Herbs and spices (especially cayenne and sea salt) may be increased or decreased to your desired taste.

Please Note: Unless otherwise noted (like for juice recipes) most all my food recipes call for herbs in their dried form. Therefore, if you would prefer to use fresh herbs at any time, feel free to use this general rule as a guideline when substituting fresh herbs for dry herbs: 1 TBS of chopped fresh herbs = 1 tsp of dried herbs.

Tip #5: Rehydrating Sun-dried Tomatoes

To rehydrate sun-dried tomatoes, place sun-dried tomatoes in a glass bowl or mason jar and add just enough room temperature to slightly warm water to just cover them. Let soak for 30-45 minutes or until softened. You may also soak overnight by letting the sun-dried tomatoes sit in room temperature water on your countertop until ready to use the following day (which is the method I use and much prefer). Any remainder can be stored in the refrigerator (in its soak water) and used within the week for other dishes. For example, any leftover can simply be sliced and tossed onto a salad. Even the soak water can be used to replace water in a wet recipe like salad dressing.

Tip #6: Rehydrating Dried Mushrooms

To rehydrate dried mushrooms, place dried mushrooms in a glass bowl or mason jar and add just enough warm water to just cover them. Let soak for 30-45 minutes or until softened. If using a bowl, you may need to place a cover over them to keep them from floating. You may also soak dried mushrooms overnight by letting them sit on your countertop in room temperature water until the following day. I find that by not having to soak in warm to hot water, the mushrooms retain much more of their rich flavor. Once softened, squeeze the excess water out prior to slicing. Any remainder can be stored in the refrigerator and used within the week for other dishes. Rehydrated mushrooms are also delicious tossed into a salad.

Please Note: My favorite source for whole dried or powered mushrooms (such as chaga and shiitake) is Mountain Rose Herbs. **FYI:** I use herbs from Mountain Rose Herbs and Starwest Botanicals for culinary purposes only and not for therapeutic and medicinal usage. To review my recommendations for medicinal quality mushrooms, please see page 223.

Tip #7: Rehydrating Seaweed

To rehydrate arame seaweed – place arame in a glass bowl and add just enough room temperature to slightly warm water to just cover it. Let soak for 10-15 minutes. Drain and prepare according to recipe. Whole leaf sea vegetables that are dense and thick will need to be soaked overnight. However, whole leaf dulse does not need to be soaked at all. Dulse can be used straight out of the bag or slightly moistened. The less the more delicate seaweeds soak, the more minerals they retain for us to benefit from.

Please Note: Straight dulse, nori and wakame flakes, as well as sea vegetable powders, can be ordered through Mountain Rose Herbs. Starwest Botanical also carries a few good options (like kelp flakes). Main Coast Sea Vegetables is a quality brand among local natural grocers. Their Triple Blend Flakes and Applewood Smoked Dulse are a must have when available!

Tip #8: Consistency Is the Key

For recipes that call for the addition of water, I suggest always starting with just below the specified amount of purified water called for, and then slowly add more to the consistency you desire. For a thicker consistency (like with soups), you will want to add less water; for a thinner consistency, you will need to add more.

Tip #9: *More Is Not Always Better*

Remember, you can always add more of just about any ingredient, but if you add too much, you can't take it away. It's worth the extra couple of seconds it takes to taste test before you go on. Always start with a small amount, increase in small increments, and then make note of what tickles your fancy!

CHAPTER 7
RAWLICIOUS RECIPES

BLENDING HERBS & SPICES

Preparing your own spice blends is super fun and easy and can be quite cost effective in the long run. Additionally, it allows you to investigate the quality and take control of each raw material prior to blending. A few areas I like to pay attention to include place of origin (where it grows), growing and harvesting conditions (including whether it is grown organically or wild-crafted) and post-harvesting practices (such as the drying and preservation process). When blending yourself, you can also guarantee that there will be no undesirable preservatives or anti-caking/flowing agents added.

Another great reason for home-blending herbs and spices is to eliminate the low-quality, unripe pepper and refined salt varieties from the equation. I will always choose and recommend the use of cayenne (a ripe, red fruit), and occasionally certain other chili peppers over black pepper (a cooked, dried unripe fruit). Plus, everybody has a different preference and tolerance for pepper and salt, and this will give you the opportunity to control the amount in a recipe and allow for that personalized touch to individual dishes.

> In the *Pakistan Journal of Nutrition* (3.4 [2004] 244-249), I learned that the pretreatment of black and white pepper *(Piper guineense)* involves steeping in boiling water for up to 20 minutes, surface disinfecting with a 2% formaldehyde solution and washing. These pretreatment methods are apparently necessary in order to reduce the load of coliforms, yeast, mold and certain other species of bacteria commonly found in fresh untreated black and white pepper samples. According to this same study, "The microflora associated with the untreated fresh pepper samples included species of *Staphylococcus, Micrococcus, Bacillus, Serratia, E. coli, Aspergillus, Fusarium, Itersonilia, Botrydiplodia, Penicillium, Mucor, Candida* and *Brettanomyces.*"
>
> After reading this study, I was not only displeased to learn about the high microbial loads found in this particular species of black and white pepper, but I was totally turned off to discover the use of formaldehyde in the treatment process. With further investigation, I found that this was common practice.

When it comes to choosing a salt that is "high-grade" in every sense of the term, I can be very particular. I would much prefer to purchase only the highest quality salt (and have to house-blend my own spices) than trust in the quality of the salt found in most premade spice blends on the market. With salt varieties, I'm especially interested in place of origin, methods of harvesting and the drying and grinding process. What you can expect to get (but don't have to accept) in most store-bought varieties and blends is a cheap grade of salt that is less than healthy and totally not mineral rich. Although there are a few wonderful and amazing solar-dried sea salts out there, my favorite is Premier Pink Salt by Premier Research Labs.

My favorite rock salt is a raw, stone-ground Himalayan crystal salt. Whether it is sea salt or rock salt, neither should have been exposed to metal during the grinding process. Exposure to metal can cause undesirable levels of nickel. A high-quality sea salt or rock salt (like the ones I speak of) will have gone through the least amount of processing. As a result, these extraordinary salts contain 84 major minerals and trace minerals, giving them the ability to restore and maintain proper electrolyte balance inside and outside the cells of our body.

> *Salt is essential for life, without it we die. Therefore, we should want to consume a salt that has the power to contribute to good health – not take it away.*

One more reason I enjoy formulating my own spice blends is because I often use a couple of blends in specific recipes where ginger is not always necessary, but would traditionally be included in a pre-made spice blend (such as my pumpkin pie blend in dessert recipes or my curry blend in dishes where I would like to infuse the taste of lemongrass instead). By having the freedom to not add ginger to a blend that traditionally has it, it allows for the addition of fresh ginger or the use of ginger essential oil instead. The same goes for any other herb or spice. Sometimes you may want it in the mix, sometimes you may not. Sometimes you may wish to add a spice fresh, or use a little less or a little more. When you home-blend your own, the choice is yours!

Asafoetida (aka hing) is a widely used spice in India; especially in Vishnu temples and yoga ashrams where onions and garlic are strictly prohibited. By itself, I find asafoetida to have a strong garlicky/onion-like smell, but once blended into recipes and dishes, the sent goes undetected. Furthermore, asafoetida will never leave you with bad breath.

Asafoetida is ideal for raw food recipes. It is easily one of my favorite spices. Asafoetida is perfect when one desires the depth and savory flavors of onions and garlic, but not the lingering aftertaste or overpowering odor. A tiny bit of asafoetida goes a long way, so be sure not to use in the same way you would onion or garlic powder.

Asafoetida is also great for individuals who are sensitive to onions and garlic and their somewhat irritating effects. What's more, asafoetida is well known as a digestive aid. Regular use has also been known to help those who have problems with asthma and bronchitis.

The best source for high-quality asafoetida is Starwest Botanicals. Many other sources will use gum arabic, wheat and rice flour in the blend. It appears to never be sold straight due to its potency. Starwest Botanicals only blends their asafoetida with natural fenugreek, another fabulous and complimentary spice that is also highly regarded and often used in Indian cuisine.

When it comes to common culinary dried herbs and spices, I trust Mountain Rose Herbs and Starwest Botanicals. They have a great selection of organically grown and wild-crafted herbs and spices which are dried at low temperatures to preserve their nutritional integrity. I also love their selection of essential oils; some of which are safe for internal use and can make a great addition to soups, dressings and pâtés – as well as certain desserts such as ice creams and chocolates. A few of my favorite essential oils for internal use include the following: ginger, lavender, lemon, lime peel, sweet orange and peppermint.

Precautions: It is highly advisable to not take essential oils internally unless working with an expert or qualified practitioner. This is especially true for ones that are not therapeutic quality. Always look for essential oil to be 100% pure and steam distilled. Citrus essential oils should always be cold-pressed. I highly advise against ingesting essential oils that are labeled absolutes or resins. Unlike those that have been steam distilled or cold-pressed, absolutes and resins have most likely been extracted using solvents and other substances that are not considered suitable for therapeutic use.

Please Note: If you choose to forego making your own blends, I highly recommend finding an alternative blend from either Mountain Rose Herbs (www.mountainroseherbs.com) or Starwest Botanicals (www.starwest-botanicals.com).

THE RAWKIN' SPICE BLENDS

Italian Blend

- ★ ¼ C basil
- ★ ¼ C summer savory
- ★ ¼ C oregano
- ★ 2 TBS sage
- ★ 2 TBS rosemary

Mediterranean Blend

- ★ 6 TBS summer savory
- ★ 4 TBS thyme
- ★ 4 TBS oregano
- ★ 4 TBS sage
- ★ 4 TBS rosemary

Optional Addition

- ★ 2 TBS paprika

Poultry Blend

- ★ ¼ C rosemary
- ★ ¼ C sage
- ★ ¼ C thyme

Optional Addition

- ★ 1-2 TBS paprika

Pumpkin Pie Blend

- ★ ¼ C cinnamon
- ★ 1 TBS nutmeg
- ★ 2 tsp ground cloves

Optional Addition

- ★ 1 TBS ginger

Apple Pie Blend

- ★ ¼ C cinnamon
- ★ 2 TBS nutmeg
- ★ 1 TBS ground cloves
- ★ 1 TBS cardamom

Curry Blend

- ★ 6 TBS coriander
- ★ 6 TBS cumin
- ★ 6 TBS turmeric
- ★ 4 TBS ground brown (or yellow) mustard seeds
- ★ 2 TBS cayenne
- ★ 1 TBS cardamom
- ★ 1 TBS ground cloves
- ★ 1 TBS cinnamon

Optional Addition

- ★ 1 TBS ginger

Spicy Infusion Blend

- ★ 4 TBS summer savory
- ★ 2 TBS ground brown (or yellow) mustard seeds
- ★ 1 TBS cumin
- ★ 1 TBS curry blend (see above)

Optional Addition

- ★ ¼ tsp asafoetida powder (aka hing) for onion and garlic flavor

Garam Masala Blend

- ★ 6 TBS coriander
- ★ 3 TBS cumin
- ★ 1 TBS cardamom

- ½ TBS cinnamon
- ½ TBS ground cloves

Taco Blend
- 4 TBS cayenne
- 2 TBS cumin
- 2 TBS paprika
- 2 TBS oregano
- 2 TBS cilantro
- ¼ tsp green leaf stevia powder (or 1 tsp whole leaf)

Optional Addition

- ¼ tsp asafoetida powder (aka hing) for onion and garlic flavor

Chili Blend
- 4 TBS cumin
- 2 TBS paprika
- 2 TBS cayenne

Optional Addition

- ¼ tsp asafoetida powder (aka hing) for onion and garlic flavor

Asian Blend
- ¼ C ground cloves
- ¼ C ground fennel seeds
- ¼ C coriander
- ¼ C cinnamon
- ¼ C cayenne
- ¼ C paprika
- 1 TBS ground anise seeds

Moroccan Blend
- ¼ C cinnamon
- 2 TBS nutmeg
- 1 TBS ground cloves
- 1 TBS cardamom
- 1 TBS ginger
- 1 TBS cayenne

Creole Blend

- 3 TBS paprika
- 1 TBS oregano
- 1 TBS thyme
- 1 TBS basil
- 1 TBS cayenne

Optional Addition

- ¼ tsp asafoetida powder (aka hing) for onion and garlic flavor

Cajun Blend

- 3 TBS paprika
- 1 TBS oregano
- 1 TBS thyme
- 1 TBS basil
- 1 TBS cayenne
- 1 TBS coriander

Optional Addition

- ¼ tsp asafoetida powder (aka hing) for onion and garlic flavor

ALL-DAY BREAKFAST FOODS

What better way to start your day than with a superfood filled smoothie! How about a protein packed parfait, a bowl of supercharged cereal, or some "grawnola?" Nutritional experts refer to breakfast as the most important meal of the day. Numerous studies have proven that people who skip breakfast are much more likely to experience concentration and mental focus problems, as well as metabolism troubles and weight gain issues. So then why do so many people choose to skip breakfast entirely? Or maybe even worse, go to the other extreme by consuming highly processed and carb-heavy foods that will only make them sleepy and sluggish?

The word "breakfast" literally means to break your fast. It is something every single one of us experiences each new day after our bodies have undergone a mini-fast during the night.

Not all carbohydrates are created equal. Sugary and starchy foods, such as boxed cereals, bagels, muffins, pancakes, waffles and toast, are so not the breakfast foods of champions. We should never fuel our bodies and brains with highly processed and refined carbohydrate foods (such as the ones just mentioned). Not at breakfast, lunch, dinner or anytime in-between.

Ponder this...if you knew that dumping sugar into your gas tank could destroy the engine of your car, would you do it? Nah, I didn't think so. So, if you wouldn't pour sugar into your gas tank – especially since sugar is known to plague the life of your vehicle when it gets sucked into the fuel lines and starts clogging up all the vital parts of your engine's fuel system – then why would you continue to gobble up any form of this substance on a daily basis yourself? Just as sugar is not the fuel your car needs, it is also not what your body needs. If this doesn't stop and make you think, then how about the fact that sugar feeds yeast, fungus, bacteria, viruses, parasites and cancer cells, just by its acidifying nature? We certainly don't need an overgrowth of any of these in our body.

Instead of choosing processed and refined carbohydrate foods, which are notorious for aggravating health conditions rather than appeasing them, how about choosing natural carbohydrate foods in the form of whole, raw fruits and vegetables?

Did you know that blending whole fruits and veggies into smoothies provides a predigested supply of nutrients? That's right, blending breaks down fibrous foods into tiny functional pieces, making them easier on the digestive tract to absorb and assimilate. For this reason alone, smoothies allow for a lot more nutrient absorption – and with extreme ease and convenience to boot! What's more, it makes getting in a ton of superfoods convenient as well. I actually sometimes prefer making jam-packed superfood smoothies a few times per day rather than sit-down meals that requires a lot of chewing. Smoothies loaded up with superfoods can not only efficiently refuel your entire system after an intense workout, but they can sustain you throughout a busy work day.

> Due to the majority of the food we buy at the grocery store being cultivated versus wild, I feel superfoods are an absolute must for everyone. If we are to achieve our nutritional needs the way God intended, we need to be filling in the blanks with foods that are super rich in bio-available nutrients. So instead of dumping tons of money on synthetics at the drug or vitamin store, load up on superfoods, superfruits and superherbs that can give your body what it craves in a form it knows exactly how to digest, absorb and assimilate.

Quick Smoothie Tips:

When making smoothies with frozen fruit, I suggest adding the frozen fruit last; preferably during the last one or two blending cycles. Blend your fresh fruit along with all dry ingredients and water first, and then add frozen fruit and blend again until completely broken down and smooth. I find this order allows for all the ingredients to get broken down without clumping up into a frozen ball.

> **Please Note:** Depending on the blender you have, I recommend starting at a slow speed and then ramping it up to as high as you need to go. For instance, Blendtec blenders have programmable keys that are great for this. On the model I have, I use "fresh Juice" (50 sec) first; especially when I am adding a lot of leafy greens. Then I choose "frozen fruit" (40 sec) for right after I add frozen fruit. Sometimes these two cycles are enough; but if you are making double or adding lots of extras, you may need to blend for another cycle or two. This is when I like using a short cycle such as "sauces, dips" (23 sec). You may also use the pulse key for times when you want to blend a bit extra toward the end, but don't necessarily need a cycle.
>
> **Make sure to always secure your lid before starting your blender!**
>
> If you are using a Vitamix, keep the dial low (#1) and then ramp up to high (#10) until fresh and dry ingredients are broken down and moving freely. Then add frozen fruit and slowly ramp up the dial from low to high again. At this point, you may want to flip the extra switch on the left side from low to high for a short while. Make sure to always flip the switch back down to the low position and turn the dial all the way back down to #1 before shutting off. This will make certain that all your buttons are in the right position before you blend again. Otherwise, you risk having quite a mess, with foods all the way up the sides of the pitcher and into the lid. Not pretty!

Have you ever noticed that the majority of smoothie recipes out there always seem to call for bananas? Yes, I understand bananas give a good amount of natural sweetness and the perfect amount of creaminess, but what if you are like me and not fond of bananas? Whether you dislike something about their flavor, texture, high glycemic index, or the fact that they are a highly hybridized fruit, please know that there are other fruits, besides bananas, that can provide a rich and creamy texture.

> **Please Note:** My favorite whole fruit replacements for bananas are pears and mangos. Apples, peaches and papaya are also great options. Just remember the following tip: the less watery the fruit, the creamier the smoothie. You may also add nut/seed butter or coconut oil to add creaminess to your smoothie concoctions. There are also many superfood powders that do an amazing job of adding thickness and creaminess. I feel the best ones are lucuma, baobab and maca. I also love Tocotriene Ultra by Premier Research Labs. Want more creaminess, how about hemp seeds? Want more thickness, add chia seeds. Learn to get chemistry creative with your concoctions!
>
> If you like bananas, but are not too keen on how hybridized the common grocery store brands of today are (including organic), then I highly suggest stocking up on vine-ripened banana flakes or powder. New Horizon Health offers highly mineralized, heirloom banana products that are made from the sweet fruit of sun-ripened Ecuadorian red bananas. To maintain the maximum amount of nutrients, their banana flakes and powder are always air dried (never heat dried). In fact, because the flakes and powder contain only about 3% water, the nutrients are much more concentrated. What's more, additives and preservatives are never added!

When it comes to making raw vegetarian smoothies, nuts and seeds are your dairy replacements (milk, yogurt, etc.). I like adding whole nuts and seeds (fiber and all) to my superfood smoothies; because of this, none of my recipes call for the additional work of preparing nut or seed mylks (aka milks). Nut/seed mylks are fine for pouring over your cereal concoctions, or for when you desire drinking them straight up, but the pre-making and straining involved is totally unnecessary for smoothies. This is especially true when using a high-speed blender. If a thinner consistency is desired, just add a bit more water. It's that simple.

> **Please Note:** If you insist on pre-making nut and seed mylks, then I suggest consuming them within 72 hours of the time they are made. You wouldn't want all the essential fatty acids to oxidize before you had the chance to benefit from them. For this reason alone, I highly recommend making your own rather than buying the already oxidized ones sitting in a box on grocery store shelves.
>
> Commercial nut/seed milks may have the convenience factor going for them, but that's about all. They are certainly not as economical as making your own. And more importantly, commercial nut/seed milks can't hold a candle to fresh homemade batches when it comes to nutrient density values. There is absolutely no comparison. You also have no control over the quality of the nuts or seeds used; have no clue how they've been processed into their milky form; or any idea how much the processing method affected the end product.
>
> From my understanding, most commercial nut/seed milks include additives, low-quality processed oils and stabilizer. In cases like this, it doesn't make a bit of difference if the nuts or seeds used to make the product were even raw or organic. Why? The end product is tainted.

Although I give suggestions as to the nuts and seeds to use in various smoothie recipes, please remember that you can substitute with any nut or seed you wish. You may also cut the number of nuts or seeds called for (adding just enough for creaminess) and add a plant-based protein booster. In my opinion, the best quality protein powders on the market are raw hemp protein (by Manitoba Harvest) and two Sunwarrior protein products (Classic Protein [natural], made from sprouted brown rice and Warrior Blend [natural], made from pea, hemp and cranberry protein). Remember to always be adventurous with your creations and have fun varying your concoctions with every chance you get.

> **Please Note:** Everyone always asks me what I use in my smoothies (which I will share later), but when it comes to the creamy base, hemp seeds are my personal favorite. I absolutely love the fact that you do not need to presoak them in order to benefit from their significant amount of protein and minerals. They're already sprouted! I also love adding chia seeds to my daily smoothie concoctions. Chia is loaded with plant-based essential omega-3 fatty acids. Chia also provides a healthy amount of dietary fiber, antioxidants, minerals and protein to boot.
>
> Superfood hemp seeds and chia seeds are my smoothie staples. To me, they give the biggest nutritional bang for their buck. A couple of times per week I may add or replace hemp seeds for selenium rich Brazil nuts. All other nuts and seeds I tend to reserve for special occasion drinks, desserts and treats. So, there you have it!
>
> To gain a greater appreciation for the two super seeds mentioned above and all the ways you can healthfully benefit from them, please refer back to "The Best of the Best" on page 118.

Personally, I prefer to purchase raw, sprouted almonds. This means they have already been conveniently soaked and dehydrated. If you choose to buy regular (unsprouted) raw almonds, I highly suggest soaking, draining and rinsing them ahead of time to increase their digestibility, meaning, the absorption and assimilation of their vital nutrients. Store in an airtight glass jar in the fridge and be sure to consume within one week. Dehydrating is not necessary for smoothie use.

> **Please Note:** If you have a dehydrator, you may wish to dry your soaked almonds in order to bring back their crunchy texture. Soaked and dehydrated almonds have a wonderful sweet taste and make a great crunchy snack. However, the dehydration step is not necessary if planning to only use for smoothies or other wet recipes.
>
> If there are any nuts or seeds more suitable to purchase already sprouted, it is almonds. Firstly, almonds take the longest to completely dry (about 32-48 hr). Secondly, by the time they finish drying, I often times find them growing a whitish-gray fuzzy mold on the inside. I've never encountered this with any other nut or seed. If I had to guess why this happens to almonds, I'd say it must be due to the excess moisture that inevitably gets trapped between their two halves during the soaking process, and also how long it takes for them to dry. When it comes to almonds, I definitely have more confidence in the raw conscious companies working with commercial grade dehydrators, and have no problem leaving the sprouting and dehydrating up to them.

What about the addition of sweeteners? It is (and should be) totally up to you. Due to all the natural sweetness of fruit, you may choose to forgo the addition of extra sweetness all together, or choose to do what I do and add a pinch or two of green leaf stevia. By using green leaf stevia (whole leaf or powder form), you not only benefit from a sweet taste that is zero in calories and zero on the glycemic index (GI), you benefit from its digestive properties as well.

> **Please Note:** Stevia is believed to provide antibacterial, antifungal, antiseptic and antioxidant properties. It can help prevent and benefit those with gingivitis. It can also soothe the stomach and help to benefit those who suffer with heartburn and gastrointestinal issues. It has also been stated that stevia can help stimulate calcium absorption in the body. Just remember, a little stevia goes a long way; therefore, you may not need more than a pinch or two for a single smoothie.
>
> Review "Sweet Flavor for Your Creations, Being Sweet Savvy with Nature's Best" (page 34) for other natural sweetener options that make my best of the best list.

Although I lump all my superfood smoothie recipes under "Rawk Star Smoothies," they are technically subdivided into two categories: Fruit Smoothies (which are primarily fruit-based) and Green Smoothies (which are a combination of greens and fruit). Just remember, you can always add greens to any fruit-based smoothie if you would like.

> **Please Note:** If you are looking to add some leafy greens to your fruit smoothie, but are a bit concerned about altering the taste, add a milder green such as baby spinach or baby kale. I also will sometimes choose to use a little romaine, green leaf or red leaf lettuce (up to 3 C, packed). These are some great options and even go undetected in many cacao-based smoothies.
>
> My next favorite greens to add are a bit on the bitter side, so I usually reserve these for smoothies I intend to be green with envy. For instance: 2-3 collard or lacinato kale leaves (stems removed), 2-3 C packed endive or escarole, 1-2 C packed arugula or ½-1 C packed watercress.

RAWK STAR SMOOTHIES

When is a smoothie more appropriate than juicing? Let me first start out by stating that juicing and blending are both beneficial to our overall health. What makes them different is the way in which their nutrients are delivered, meaning, how quickly these nutrients are digested, absorbed and assimilated.

Because blending whole fruits and vegetables retains the skin and pulp, which is where we find the majority of vital nutrients and cancer fighting properties, I believe blending can be more beneficial than juicing for overall well-being and long-term health. The presence of the fiber in a blended fruit or vegetable smoothie means it will not just be more filling than a juice but will also keep much longer than a juice without losing a lot of its nutritional value. Although I still advise consuming smoothies as fresh as possible, they will not oxidize anywhere near as quickly as juice. A smoothie can typically be stored in an airtight glass jar in your refrigerator for 24-32 hours. You will just need to give it a quick shake or stir when the water separates.

Although fiber is not considered to be a nutrient, it is a very important and necessary component of nutrition and health. Dietary fiber is essential for the proper elimination of waste and toxins from the digestive system. When toxins build up in the colon, it is fiber that cleans them out before they have a chance to be reabsorbed into the bloodstream. Having fiber present can also help stabilize blood sugar levels by slowing the release of sugars into the bloodstream. This is a very important consideration for diabetics. The slower and steadier nutrients get delivered into the bloodstream, the less chance there is of experiencing blood sugar spikes. Fiber is also known to reduce bad cholesterol (LDL) and can help prevent a number of diseases such a cardiovascular disease and colon cancer.

Please Note: My preference for blending is not meant to devalue the tremendous benefits of juicing in any way (especially chlorophyll-rich green juices), but in the long run, I strongly believe that whole fruits and vegetables, grown as nature intended, should be the staples that make up the bulk of what you consume. For my answer on when juicing may be more appropriate, please see page 283.

FRUIT SMOOTHIES

> **Recipe Note & Quick Tip:** Always add coconut oil last and preferably after one blending cycle. This will help prevent it from sticking to the sides of the pitcher and solidifying.

Pow-Wow Cacao Smoothie

Chop fruit into small chunks, place in <u>high-speed blender</u> along with all other ingredients, and then blend until smooth:

- ★ 1 banana (or pear)
- ★ 6-8 Brazil nuts
- ★ 3 TBS cacao powder
- ★ 1-2 TBS maca powder (optional)
- ★ 1 TBS mesquite powder
- ★ 1 dash whole ground vanilla bean powder
- ★ Sweetener of choice, to taste (optional)
- ★ 1 TBS coconut oil (liquefied)
- ★ 8 oz purified, filtered water (more as desired for thinner consistency)

Add frozen fruit (and ice cubes, if desired), and then blend again until well broken down and smooth:

- ★ ½ C frozen mango

Optional Additions & Boosters

- ★ Add 1 dash of cinnamon or Pumpkin Pie Blend prior to blending.
- ★ Add 1 pinch of cayenne prior to blending.
- ★ Add 2-3 TBS of goji berries prior to blending.
- ★ Add 2-3 tsp spirulina prior to blending.
- ★ Pulse in 1-2 TBS of cacao beans (or nibs) during the last cycle for a little texture.
- ★ Stir in some bee pollen after blending.

> **Recipe Notes & Quick Tips:** To benefit from the potent antioxidant properties of whole vanilla, try whole ground vanilla bean powder in place of vanilla flavoring or extract. The authentic and aromatic flavor of whole ground vanilla is unsurpassed and will enhance the taste of almost any food or beverage. Ultimate Superfoods provides raw, wild-crafted vanilla bean products that are harvested from the flower by hand and naturally cured in the sun for days. Their dark Tahitian vanilla is grown on the islands of the South Pacific. Tahitian vanilla is much more rare than Madagascar vanilla.

Orange Screamsicle Smoothie

Chop fruit into small chunks, place in high-speed blender along with all other ingredients, and then blend until smooth:

- ★ 1 banana (or pear)
- ★ 1 orange (peeled & seeded)
- ★ 3 TBS hemp seeds
- ★ 3 TBS goji berries
- ★ Sweetener of choice, to taste (optional)
- ★ 1 TBS coconut oil (liquefied)
- ★ 8 oz purified, filtered water (more as desired for thinner consistency)

Optional Additions & Boosters

- ★ Add 1-3 tsp Sunwarrior Ormus Greens prior to blending.
- ★ Stir in some bee pollen after blending.

Choco-Cherry Smoothie

Chop fruit into small chunks, place in high-speed blender along with all other ingredients, and then blend until smooth:

- ★ 1 pear (or banana)
- ★ ¼ C pecans
- ★ 3 TBS cacao powder
- ★ 1-2 TBS maca powder (optional)
- ★ 1 TBS mesquite powder
- ★ 1 dash whole ground vanilla bean powder
- ★ Sweetener of choice, to taste (optional)
- ★ 1 TBS coconut oil (liquefied)
- ★ 8 oz purified, filtered water (more as desired for thinner consistency)

Add frozen fruit (and ice cubes, if desired), and then blend again until well broken down and smooth:

- ★ ½ C frozen pitted cherries

Optional Variations, Additions & Boosters

- ★ Substitute ¼ C cashews, ¼ C walnuts or 3 TBS hemp seeds for the pecans.
- ★ Add 1 dash of cinnamon or Pumpkin Pie Blend prior to blending.
- ★ Add 2-3 TBS of sun-dried mulberries prior to blending.
- ★ Add 2-3 tsp spirulina prior to blending.
- ★ Pulse in 1-2 TBS of cacao beans (or nibs) during the last cycle for a little texture.
- ★ Stir in some bee pollen after blending.

Choco-Mint Smoothie

Chop fruit into small chunks, place in <u>high-speed blender</u> along with all other ingredients, and then blend until smooth:

- ★ 1 pear (or apple)
- ★ 3 TBS hemp seeds
- ★ 3 TBS cacao powder
- ★ 2-3 tsp spirulina
- ★ 6-8 fresh mint leaves (or 3-4 drops peppermint or spearmint essential oil)
- ★ Sweetener of choice, to taste (optional)
- ★ 1 TBS coconut oil (liquefied)
- ★ 8 oz purified, filtered water (more as desired for thinner consistency)

Add frozen fruit (and ice cubes, if desired), and then blend again until well broken down and smooth:

- ★ 1 frozen banana

Optional Variations & Boosters

- ★ Substitute banana for the pear or apple, making it 2 bananas total for smoothie.
- ★ If avoiding bananas, substitute ½ C frozen peaches or mango for the frozen banana.
- ★ Add 1-3 tsp Sunwarrior Ormus Greens prior to blending.
- ★ Pulse in 1-2 TBS of cacao beans (or nibs) during the last cycle for a little texture.
- ★ Stir in some bee pollen after blending.

Chunky Monkey Smoothie

Chop fruit into small chunks, place in <u>high-speed blender</u> along with all other ingredients, and then blend until smooth:

- ★ 1 banana
- ★ ¼ C walnuts
- ★ 2 TBS lucuma powder
- ★ 1 TBS mesquite powder
- ★ 1 dash whole ground vanilla bean powder
- ★ 1 pinch cinnamon or Pumpkin Pie Blend

- ★ Sweetener of choice, to taste (optional)
- ★ 1 TBS coconut oil (liquefied)
- ★ 8 oz purified, filtered water (more as desired for thinner consistency)

Add frozen fruit (and ice cubes, if desired), blend again until well broken down and smooth and then add cacao beans (or nibs) and pulse until well dispersed:

- ★ 1 frozen banana
- ★ 2-3 TBS cacao beans or nibs

Optional Variations & Boosters

- ★ If avoiding bananas, substitute a pear for one of the bananas and ½ C frozen peaches or mango for the other banana.
- ★ Stir in some additional cacao beans or nibs, coconut flakes and/or bee pollen after blending.

> **Where do you get your protein?** There is no shortage of protein in the life of a raw vegetarian. Hemp seeds and chai seeds are both packed with protein (offering 9-10 grams of protein in every 3 TBS). They are also both bio-available and a complete source of protein, to boot! With 1.2 grams of protein per tsp, bee pollen contains more protein than beef, eggs or cheese of equal weight. At 1.9 grams, avocados are a quality source of protein (more than cow's milk). For being fruits, even golden and goji berries provide a substantial amount of protein (about 3-4 grams of protein per ¼ C each). Want more? Look what you can get just by adding one or more of the following to your superfood smoothie: 4 TBS of hemp protein powder provides a whopping 15-20 grams of additional protein; 1 scoop of Sunwarrior protein gives a colossal 17 grams of added protein; and just 1 TBS of spirulina awards an amazing 10-11 grams of added protein.

Banana Split Smoothie

Chop fruit into small chunks, place in <u>high-speed blender</u> along with all other ingredients, and then blend until smooth:

- ★ 1 banana
- ★ 3 TBS hemp seeds
- ★ 2 TBS lucuma powder
- ★ 1 TBS baobab powder
- ★ 1 dash whole ground vanilla bean powder
- ★ Sweetener of choice, to taste (optional)
- ★ 1 TBS coconut oil (liquefied)
- ★ 8 oz purified, filtered water (more as desired for thinner consistency)

Add frozen fruit (and ice cubes, if desired), blend again until well broken down and smooth and then add cacao beans (or nibs) and pulse until well dispersed:

- ½ C packed, frozen strawberries
- 2-3 TBS cacao beans or nibs

Optional Variations & Boosters

- If avoiding bananas, use pear instead.
- Substitute ¼ C almonds, cashews or walnuts for hemp seeds.
- Substitute ½ C frozen cherries for strawberries.
- Stir in some additional cacao beans or nibs, coconut flakes and/or bee pollen after blending.

Almond Joy Smoothie

Chop fruit into small chunks, place in high-speed blender along with all other ingredients, and then blend until smooth:

- 1 pear (or apple)
- ¼ C almonds
- 3 TBS cacao powder
- 2 TBS coconut flakes
- 1 TBS lucuma powder (or baobab)
- 1 dash whole ground vanilla bean powder
- Sweetener of choice, to taste (optional)
- 1 TBS coconut oil (liquefied)
- 8 oz purified, filtered water (more as desired for thinner consistency)

Add frozen fruit (and ice cubes, if desired), and then blend again until well broken down and smooth:

- ½ C frozen mango

Optional Additions & Boosters

- Add 1 dash of cinnamon or Pumpkin Pie Blend prior to blending.
- Pulse in 1-2 TBS of cacao beans (or nibs) during the last cycle for a little texture.
- Stir in some coconut flakes after blending.

Strawberries & Crème Smoothie

Chop fruit into small chunks, place in high-speed blender along with all other ingredients, and then blend until smooth:

- 1 apple (or pear)
- 3 TBS hemp seeds
- 3 TBS goji berries
- 1 TBS baobab powder
- 1 dash whole ground vanilla bean powder

- ★ Sweetener of choice, to taste (optional)
- ★ 1 TBS coconut oil (liquefied)
- ★ 8 oz purified, filtered water (more as desired for thinner consistency)

Add frozen fruit (and ice cubes, if desired), and then blend again until well broken down and smooth:

- ★ ½ C packed, frozen strawberries

Optional Additions & Boosters

- ★ Add 1 dash of cinnamon or Apple Pie Blend prior to blending.
- ★ Add 1-3 tsp of Sunwarrior Ormus Greens prior to blending.
- ★ Stir in some cacao beans or nibs, coconut flakes and/or bee pollen after blending for a little texture.

Blastin' Berry Smoothie

Chop fruit into small chunks, place in <u>high-speed blender</u> along with all other ingredients, and then blend until smooth:

- ★ 1 pear (or apple)
- ★ 3 TBS hemp seeds
- ★ 3 TBS sun-dried mulberries
- ★ 1 TBS lucuma powder
- ★ 1 dash whole ground vanilla bean powder
- ★ Sweetener of choice, to taste (optional)
- ★ 1 TBS coconut oil (liquefied)
- ★ 8 oz purified, filtered water (more as desired for thinner consistency)

Add frozen fruit (and ice cubes, if desired), and then blend again until well broken down and smooth:

- ★ ½ C frozen mixed berries (or berries of choice)

Optional Variations, Additions & Boosters

- ★ Substitute ¼ C almonds or 6-8 Brazil nuts for hemp seeds.
- ★ Add 1 dash of cinnamon or Pumpkin Pie Blend prior to blending.
- ★ Add 2-3 tsp spirulina prior to blending.
- ★ Stir in some cacao beans or nibs, coconut flakes and/or bee pollen after blending for a little texture.

Inflammation Soother Smoothie

Chop fruit into small chunks, place in <u>high-speed blender</u> along with all other ingredients, and then blend until smooth:

- ★ 1 pear
- ★ 3 TBS hemp seeds
- ★ 3 TBS golden berries
- ★ 1 tsp turmeric extract powder (95% curcumin)
- ★ 1 dash Pumpkin Pie Blend
- ★ 1 dash whole ground vanilla bean powder
- ★ Sweetener of choice, to taste (optional)
- ★ 1 TBS coconut oil (liquefied)
- ★ 8 oz purified, filtered water (more as desired for thinner consistency)

Add frozen fruit (and ice cubes, if desired), and then blend again until well broken down and smooth:

- ★ ½ C frozen mango (or peaches)

Optional Variations, Additions & Boosters

- ★ Substitute ½ C cranberries (fresh or frozen) for frozen mango or peaches.
- ★ Add ½-1-inch piece ginger root (or 1-2 drops ginger essential oil).
- ★ Stir in coconut flakes and/or bee pollen after blending for a little texture.

Get your buzz on with bee pollen! Bee pollen is often referred to as nature's most perfect food, as it contains nearly every element required for sustaining life. Some people may have an allergic reaction, but truth be told, bee pollen can actually help allergy sufferers. If you have never had bee pollen before, I suggest starting out with a small amount (as little as a ¼ tsp or less). If you do not respond negatively, feel free to work your way up to more and more. If you do have an allergic-type reaction, you can either back down (to as little as one pellet, working your way up slowly as tolerated) or stop entirely.

Bee pollen provides over 22 amino acids, every vitamin known to man (with an extraordinary presence of B vitamins), 28 different minerals and trace minerals, 11 enzymes and co-enzymes, bioflavonoids, phytosterols, omega-3 fatty acids, carbohydrates, carotenoids, globulins, lecithin, quercetin, rutin, hormones, as well as other biologically active compounds.

Bee pollen has been noted to increase energy, endurance, stamina, speed, muscle growth, as well as strengthen the immune system and more! So, what are you waiting for? Stir some in!

GREEN SMOOTHIES

Apple-Avocado Green Smoothie

Chop fruit into small chunks, place in <u>high-speed blender</u> along with all other ingredients, and then blend until smooth:

- ★ 1 apple

- ½ avocado (peeled & pitted)
- 2 C packed baby spinach
- 2 collard leaves (stems removed)
- 2-3 tsp spirulina
- 1 dash Apple Pie Blend
- Sweetener of choice, to taste (optional)
- 8 oz purified, filtered water (more as desired for thinner consistency)

Optional Variations, Additions & Boosters

- Substitute kale leaves or additional spinach for collard leaves.
- Add ½-1-inch piece ginger root (or 1-2 drops ginger essential oil).
- Add 1-2 tsp (or more) of a superfood green powder.
- Add 1 dash of whole ground vanilla bean powder.
- Stir in some bee pollen after blending.

> **Recipe Notes & Quick Tips:** Try adding up to ½ cucumber and 1-2 celery stalks to any green smoothie for a new twist that is both refreshing and hydrating. Cucumbers have an extraordinary amount of water that is naturally purified; this makes their water content much better in quality than ordinary water. They are also mineral rich, making them ideal for combating dehydration. Like cucumber, celery is also extremely high in naturally purified water and minerals. Just a few celery stalks per day can replenish our body's levels of calcium, magnesium, potassium and sodium.

Pear-Avocado Green Smoothie

Chop fruit into small chunks, place in <u>high-speed blender</u> along with all other ingredients, and then blend until smooth:

- 1 pear
- ½ avocado (peeled & pitted)
- 2 C packed baby spinach
- 2 lacinato kale leaves (stems removed)
- 2-3 tsp spirulina
- 1 dash Pumpkin Pie Blend
- Sweetener of choice, to taste (optional)
- 8 oz purified, filtered water (more as desired for thinner consistency)

Optional Variations, Additions & Boosters

- Substitute collard leaves or additional spinach for kale leaves.
- Add ½-1-inch piece ginger root (or 1-2 drops ginger essential oil).
- Add 1-2 tsp (or more) of a superfood green powder.
- Add 1 dash of whole ground vanilla bean powder.

- ★ Stir in some bee pollen after blending.

Orange-Banana Green Smoothie

Chop fruit into small chunks, place in <u>high-speed blender</u> along with all other ingredients, and then blend until smooth:

- ★ 1 orange
- ★ 1 banana
- ★ 2 TBS hemp seeds
- ★ 1 TBS chia seeds
- ★ 2 C packed baby spinach
- ★ 2 lacinato kale leaves (stems removed)
- ★ 2-3 tsp spirulina
- ★ 1 dash cinnamon or Pumpkin Pie Blend
- ★ Sweetener of choice, to taste (optional)
- ★ 1 TBS coconut oil (liquefied)
- ★ 8 oz purified, filtered water (more as desired for thinner consistency)

Optional Variations, Additions & Boosters

- ★ Substitute collard leaves or additional spinach for kale leaves.
- ★ Add 1-2 tsp (or more) of a superfood green powder.
- ★ Add 1 dash of whole ground vanilla bean powder.
- ★ Sprinkle and stir in some bee pollen after blending.

Pear-Mango Green Smoothie

Chop fruit into small chunks, place in <u>high-speed blender</u> along with all other ingredients, and then blend until smooth:

- ★ 1 pear
- ★ 3 TBS hemp seeds
- ★ 1 scoop Warrior Blend (natural)
- ★ 2 C packed baby spinach
- ★ 2 collard leaves (stems removed)
- ★ 2-3 tsp spirulina
- ★ 1 dash Pumpkin Pie Blend
- ★ Sweetener of choice, to taste (optional)
- ★ 1 TBS coconut oil (liquefied)
- ★ 8 oz purified, filtered water (more as desired for thinner consistency)

Add frozen fruit (and ice cubes, if desired), and then blend again until well broken down and smooth:

- ★ ½ C frozen mango

Optional Variations, Additions & Boosters

- ★ Substitute kale leaves or additional spinach for collard leaves.
- ★ Use Sunwarrior Classic Protein (natural) instead of Warrior Blend.
- ★ For a **Pear-Peach Green Smoothie**, substitute frozen peaches for mango.
- ★ Add 1-2 tsp (or more) of a superfood green powder.
- ★ Add 1 dash of whole ground vanilla bean powder.
- ★ Stir in some bee pollen after blending.

Apple-Berry Green Smoothie

Chop fruit into small chunks, place in <u>high-speed blender</u> along with all other ingredients, and then blend until smooth:

- ★ 1 apple
- ★ 3 TBS hemp seeds
- ★ 2 TBS hemp protein powder
- ★ 2 C packed baby spinach
- ★ 2 collard leaves (stems removed)
- ★ 2-3 tsp spirulina
- ★ 1 dash Apple Pie Blend
- ★ Sweetener of choice, to taste (optional)
- ★ 1 TBS coconut oil (liquefied)
- ★ 8 oz purified, filtered water (more as desired for thinner consistency)

Add frozen fruit (and ice cubes, if desired), and then blend again until well broken down and smooth:

- ★ ½ C packed, frozen strawberries or ½ C frozen wild blueberries or mixed berries

Optional Variations, Additions & Boosters

- ★ Substitute kale leaves or additional spinach for collard leaves.
- ★ Add 1-2 tsp (or more) of a superfood green powder.
- ★ Add 1 dash of whole ground vanilla bean powder.
- ★ Stir in some bee pollen after blending.

Banana-Mango Green Smoothie

Chop fruit into small chunks, place in <u>high-speed blender</u> along with all other ingredients, and then blend until smooth:

- ★ 1 banana
- ★ 3 TBS unhulled tan sesame seeds or raw sesame tahini
- ★ 2 C packed baby spinach
- ★ 2 collard leaves (stems removed)
- ★ 2-3 tsp spirulina

- ★ 1 dash cinnamon or Pumpkin Pie Blend
- ★ Sweetener of choice, to taste (optional)
- ★ 1 TBS coconut oil (liquefied)
- ★ 8 oz purified, filtered water (more as desired for thinner consistency)

Add frozen fruit (and ice cubes, if desired) and then blend again until well broken down and smooth:

- ★ ½ C frozen mango

Optional Variations, Additions & Boosters

- ★ Substitute kale leaves or additional spinach for collard leaves.
- ★ Substitute 3-4 TBS of TruRoots sprouted quinoa or one scoop Sunwarrior protein for sesame seeds or raw sesame tahini.
- ★ Add 1-2 tsp (or more) of a superfood green powder.
- ★ Add 1 dash of whole ground vanilla bean powder.
- ★ Stir in some bee pollen after blending.

KAREN'S SUPERFOOD SPOONABLE SMOOTHIES

So thick, you eat them with a spoon!

Okay. You asked for it. What does Karen put in her daily superfood smoothie(s)? Let me first pre-warn you, I tend to power-up my smoothies with a lot of superfoods. For example, my morning smoothie is so satisfying that it gets me through breakfast and lunch. It not only refuels me after an intense workout routine, it carries me straight through to dinner. For me, the thicker and richer the smoothie, the closer I am to heaven.

The following are my four personal staple smoothie recipes, along with how I like to change them up from time to time. Feel free to alter as you wish and put your own personal spin on each.

"Brain on Bliss" Cacao Spoonable

Chop fruit into small chunks, place in <u>high-speed blender</u> along with all other ingredients, and then blend until smooth:

- ★ 1 pear (or apple)
- ★ 3 TBS goji berries
- ★ 3 TBS cacao powder
- ★ 2-3 squares cacao paste
- ★ 2 TBS hemp seeds
- ★ 2 TBS black sesame seeds or black sesame tahini
- ★ 1 TBS chia seeds or ¼ C chia seed gel (see page 127 for recipe)

- ★ 1 TBS spirulina
- ★ 2 TBS maca powder
- ★ 1 TBS mesquite powder
- ★ 1 TBS vine-ripened banana powder
- ★ 1 tsp shilajit
- ★ 1 tsp green leaf stevia (whole leaf)
- ★ ½ tsp whole ground vanilla bean powder
- ★ ¼ tsp Pumpkin or Apple Pie Blend
- ★ ¼ tsp Premier Carnosine (Premier Research Labs)
- ★ 3-5 drops D3 Serum (Premier Research Labs)
- ★ 1 dropper full of Chaga Mushroom Extract (Surthrival) or 2 opened capsules (contents only) of Siberian Chaga (Dragon Herbs)
- ★ 3-6 opened capsules (contents only) of C from Nature (Purium)
- ★ 1-2 opened capsules (contents only) of MegaHydrate
- ★ 1 TBS coconut oil (liquefied)
- ★ 8-12 oz purified, filtered water (more as desired for thinner consistency)

Add frozen fruit (and ice cubes, if desired), and then blend again until well broken down and smooth:

- ★ ½ C frozen mango

Variations, Additions & Boosters

- ★ If cacao paste is unavailable, add 1 additional TBS of cacao powder and coconut oil.
- ★ Stir in 1-2 TBS of bee pollen and/or cacao beans after blending.

Super Sunwarrior Spoonable

Chop fruit into small chunks, place in <u>high-speed blender</u> along with all other ingredients, and then blend until smooth:

- ★ 1 pear (or apple)
- ★ 3 TBS goji berries
- ★ 1 scoop Sunwarrior Classic Protein (natural)
- ★ 2 TBS hemp seeds
- ★ 1 TBS chia seeds or ¼ C chia seed gel (see page 127 for recipe)
- ★ 1 TBS spirulina
- ★ 2 TBS maca powder
- ★ 1 TBS mesquite powder
- ★ 1 TBS baobab powder
- ★ 1-2 TBS Premier Greens Mix (Premier Research Labs)
- ★ 1 TBS Tocotriene Ultra (Premier Research Labs)
- ★ 2 large handfuls of greens (baby spinach, endive, escarole, romaine, etc.)
- ★ ½ tsp whole ground vanilla bean powder
- ★ ½ tsp green leaf stevia (whole leaf)

- ¼ tsp Pumpkin Pie Blend (or Apple Pie Blend)
- ¼ tsp Premier Carnosine (Premier Research Labs)
- 3-5 drops D3 Serum (Premier Research Labs)
- 1 dropper full Reishi Mushroom Extract (Surthrival) or Duanwood Reishi (Dragon Herbs)
- 3-6 opened capsules (contents only) of C from Nature (Purium)
- 1-2 opened capsules (contents only) of MegaHydrate
- 1 TBS coconut oil (liquefied)
- 8-12 oz purified, filtered water (more as desired for thinner consistency)

Add frozen fruit (and ice cubes, if desired), and then blend again until well broken down and smooth:

- ½ C frozen mixed berries

Variations, Additions & Boosters

- Substitute Warrior Blend (natural) for Sunwarrior Classic Protein.
- Substitute Organic Kamut Blend (Purium), Organic Barley Grass Juice (Purium) or Ormus Greens (Sunwarrior) for Premier Greens Mix. **Note:** Decrease or remove stevia when using Ormus Greens.
- Stir in 1-2 TBS of bee pollen and/or cacao beans after blending.

> **Carnosine: fountain of youth in a bottle!** One of the most popular anti-aging substances currently in use is carnosine. It is a natural di-peptide consisting of the amino acids beta-alanine and L-histidine. Carnosine is naturally and abundantly found in nerve and muscle cells and helps extend the life of key building block cells such as DNA, lipids and proteins. It is stated to be the most effective glycation fighter that the body naturally produces. It is a powerful antioxidant, helps to prevent the cross-linking of sugars and proteins and helps to slow the aging process and prevent free radical damage. Carnosine is not a drug, vitamin or mineral and does not react with any drugs. We are born with high levels of carnosine, but unfortunately it decreases with age. What's great is that we can replace carnosine naturally with just a ¼-½ tsp (500-1,000mg) daily.

Muscle Mania Spoonable

Chop fruit into small chunks, place in high-speed blender along with all other ingredients, and then blend until smooth:

- 1 apple (or pear)
- 3 TBS golden berries
- 1 scoop Warrior Blend (natural)
- 2 TBS hemp seeds
- 1 TBS chia seeds or ¼ C chia seed gel (see page 127 for recipe)
- 1 TBS spirulina

- ★ 2 TBS maca powder
- ★ 1 TBS mesquite powder
- ★ 1 TBS lucuma powder
- ★ 1-2 TBS Premier Greens Mix (Premier Research Labs)
- ★ 1 TBS Tocotriene Ultra (Premier Research Labs)
- ★ 2-3 large handfuls of greens (baby spinach, endive, escarole, romaine, etc.)
- ★ ½ tsp whole ground vanilla bean powder
- ★ ½ tsp green leaf stevia (whole leaf)
- ★ ¼ tsp Pumpkin Pie Blend (or Apple Pie Blend)
- ★ ¼ tsp Premier Carnosine (Premier Research Labs)
- ★ 3-5 drops D3 Serum (Premier Research Labs)
- ★ 1 dropper full Reishi Mushroom Extract (Surthrival) or CordyChi (Host Defense)
- ★ 3-6 opened capsules (contents only) of C from Nature (Purium)
- ★ 1-2 opened capsules (contents only) of MegaHydrate
- ★ 1 TBS coconut oil (liquefied)
- ★ 8-12 oz purified, filtered water (more as desired for thinner consistency)

Add frozen fruit (and ice cubes, if desired), and then blend again until well broken down and smooth:

- ★ ½ C packed, frozen strawberries (or 1 C frozen wild blueberries)

Variations, Additions & Boosters

- ★ Substitute Sunwarrior Classic Protein (natural) for Warrior Blend.
- ★ Substitute Organic Kamut Blend (Purium), Organic Barley Grass Juice (Purium) or Ormus Greens (Sunwarrior) for Premier Greens Mix. **Note:** Decrease or remove stevia when using Ormus Greens.
- ★ Stir in 1-2 TBS of bee pollen and/or cacao beans after blending.

What is Tocotriene Ultra? Tocotriene Ultra by Premier Research Labs (PRL) is often called the "Super Nutrient Formula of Champions." It is a super nutrient formula featuring the whole vitamin E complex, stabilized rice bran, stabilized rice protein and FOS. PRL only use the "first run," most nutrient-dense rice bran with the highest antioxidant concentration (not the poorer, more oxidized, refined grades of rice bran with low nutrient levels). Current research shows that stabilized rice bran contains 100+ different antioxidants (all naturally occurring). Among the most powerful are oryzanols, tocopherols and tocotrienols. Tocotrienols have recently been shown to have 6,000 times greater antioxidant activity than vitamin E. They are also rich in broad-spectrum B vitamins, CoQ10, alpha lipoic acid, essential amino acids, essential fatty acids, enzymes, phospholipids, polysaccharides, squalene and more!

Power Pumpin' Spoonable

Chop fruit into small chunks, place in <u>high-speed blender</u> along with all other ingredients, and then blend until smooth:

- ★ 1 apple (or pear)
- ★ 3 TBS golden berries
- ★ 3 TBS hemp protein powder
- ★ 2 TBS hemp seeds
- ★ 1 TBS chia seeds or ¼ C chia seed gel (see page 127 for recipe)
- ★ 1 TBS spirulina
- ★ 2 TBS maca powder
- ★ 1 TBS mesquite powder
- ★ 1 TBS vine-ripened banana powder
- ★ 1-2 TBS Ormus Greens (Sunwarrior)
- ★ 1 TBS Tocotriene Ultra (Premier Research Labs)
- ★ 2-3 large handfuls of greens (baby spinach, endive, escarole, romaine, etc.)
- ★ ½ tsp whole ground vanilla bean powder
- ★ ¼ tsp green leaf stevia (whole leaf)
- ★ ¼ tsp Premier Carnosine (Premier Research Labs)
- ★ 3-4 drops D3 Serum (Premier Research Labs)
- ★ 1 dropper full Chaga Mushroom Extract (Surthrival) or 2 opened capsules (contents only) of Siberian Chaga (Dragon Herbs)
- ★ 3-6 opened capsules (contents only) of C from Nature (Purium)
- ★ 1-2 opened capsules (contents only) of MegaHydrate
- ★ 1 TBS coconut oil (liquefied)
- ★ 10-12 oz purified, filtered water (more as desired for thinner consistency)

Add frozen fruit (and ice cubes, if desired), and then blend again until well broken down and smooth:

- ★ 1 C frozen mango

Variations, Additions & Boosters

- ★ Substitute ¼ C TruRoots sprouted quinoa or a scoop of Sunwarrior protein for the hemp protein.
- ★ Substitute Premier Greens Mix, Organic Kamut Blend (Purium) or Organic Barley Grass Juice (Purium) for Ormus Greens (Sunwarrior). **Note:** You may want to increase stevia when using green powders that do not already include it.
- ★ Stir in 1-2 TBS of bee pollen and/or cacao beans after blending.

> **Recipe Notes & Quick Tips:** I almost always use maca in my daytime smoothie (except on weekends or the one week per month I take off from it). I feel it keeps my physical energy and stamina at an even keel. Cacao does the same thing, but also for my mental energy and focus.
>
> If you are making a smoothie at night, you may not want to add maca or cacao – unless, of course, you are trying to open your internal energy centers at that time.
>
> At night is the time to add more greens. Leafy greens can have a relaxing and calming effect on the body. They will not make you tired, but they can help prepare your body for a better night sleep. This is why it is always considered ideal to start your day with some fruit and end it with greens.

RAW PRANA PARFAITS

By definition, a parfait is a dessert made by alternating layers of various ingredients. Parfaits usually include something creamy and something fruity or sweet. When made with the right ingredients, a parfait can even act as a complete breakfast. This is especially true when they contain raw plant-based protein, essential fats, healthy carbohydrates, and are packed with vitamins, minerals and enzymes. Because parfaits are lusciously layered, they are amazingly appealing to the eye. What a great way to get kids to eat healthier without them even knowing!

Quick Parfait Tips:

With the exception of Brazil nuts, hazelnuts, macadamia nuts, pine nuts, pistachio nuts, and chia, flax and hemp seeds, you may wish to soak, drain, rinse and strain the following nuts and seeds in preparation for parfait making: almonds, jungle peanuts, pecans, walnuts and pumpkin, sesame and sunflower seeds. Although this is optional, it can really help to improve digestibility and nutrient absorption. If you happen to have a dehydrator, you may wish to dehydrate your soaked nuts and seeds at 105-115°F until fully dry and crunchy, and then store them in an airtight, glass container in a cool, dark place.

> **Please Note:** If you choose not to dehydrate nuts that have been soaked, be sure to drain well, rinse well, strain well, and then store in an airtight container in the fridge. I suggest consuming within one week. To review "The Science Behind the Soak," "General Soaking Schedule for Nuts & Seeds" and other great tips, please refer to page 26.

Although I like suggesting the use of fresh, seasonal, organic fruit whenever possible, there is nothing wrong with using organic frozen fruit. In fact, I sometimes prefer using frozen fruit, especially berries, cherries and mangos.

> **Please Note:** I also give some yummy raw fruit jam recipes under this section that can be made from fresh, frozen and dried fruit. They are perfect as dessert plate scapers, layered in parfaits, topped on raw cheeze cake, brownies and even raw ice cream. You may even want to use them as a dip for sliced fruit or as a spread for flax or chia crackers along with some nut or seed butter. Yum! Nut butter and jam sandwiches!
>
> Raw fruit preserves are delish spread on chocolate chia crackers with hemp butter and topped with coconut flakes, cacao nibs and bee pollen. Check out "Decadent Desserts & Sweet Treats" (page 366) and "Dehydrated Pizza Crusts, Craks & Chips" (page 435) for more dessert and dehydrated cracker ideas.

Feel free to serve your beautifully layered parfaits in wine goblets, martini glasses, or even shot glasses for special occasions. Otherwise, you may serve them in traditional parfait or sundae glasses. They even look nice served in small mason jars.

For all the following recipes, please refer to the instructions at the very end, where I give simple layering ideas for your "pretty as a picture" parfaits!

Nut-Berry Parfait

Sweet Crème Layer

Place the following ingredients in <u>high-speed blender</u> and blend until smooth and creamy:

- ★ 1 C cashews (or macadamia nuts)
- ★ ¼ tsp whole ground vanilla bean powder
- ★ ¼ tsp Pumpkin Pie Blend (optional)
- ★ 1 dash sea salt
- ★ 2 TBS raw honey or agave
- ★ 2 TBS lemon juice
- ★ 2-4 oz purified, filtered water (as needed)

Nut/Seed Layer

Mix the following ingredients together in a bowl or coarsely pulse-chop them together in a <u>food processor</u> (being sure not to over process into flour):

- ★ 1 C almonds
- ★ 1 C walnuts
- ★ ½ C pumpkin seeds
- ★ ½ C sunflower seeds

Optional Additions

- ★ Add 1 C in total using the following superfruits: goji berries, golden berries, mulberries, Hunza golden raisins or other dried fruit of choice.

- ★ Add ½ C in total using the following superfoods: cacao nibs, bee pollen and/or coconut flakes.

Berry Layer

Use any one of the following fresh, organic berries in your parfait. You may also combine any of your favorites. If fresh berries are unavailable, feel free to use defrosted berries:

- ★ Blackberries
- ★ Blueberries
- ★ Raspberries
- ★ Strawberries (sliced)

Optional Variations

- ★ Instead of fresh fruit, you may use a raw fruit jam (see pages 268-269 for raw fruit jam recipe ideas).

Instructions:

1. In parfait glasses (or other glasses of choice), place a small amount of nut/seed mixture.
2. Top nuts/seeds with a thin layer of sweet crème.
3. Top sweet crème with a few tablespoons of fresh berries of choice.
4. Top fresh berries with a thin layer of sweet crème.
5. Repeat 1-4 (nuts/seeds, crème, berries and crème) and then top last sweet crème layer with a sprinkle of nut/seed mixture.

Raw Berry Jam

Place the following ingredients in high-speed blender (or food processor) and blend (or process) until well combined and smooth:

- ★ 2 C packed berries (fresh or defrosted). Fresh strawberries, raspberries or blackberries work the best. You may also choose frozen mixed berries which have blueberries incorporated.
- ★ 2-3 TBS chia seeds
- ★ 2 TBS raw agave (or to taste)
- ★ 1 TBS lemon juice
- ★ 1 dash sea salt
- ★ 1 pinch cinnamon (optional)
- ★ 2 oz purified, filtered water

Raw Apricot Jam

Place the following ingredients in high-speed blender (or food processor) and blend (or process) until well combined and smooth:

- ★ 2 C packed, dried Turkish apricots (presoaked for 10-15 minutes & then drained)
- ★ 1-2 TBS raw agave (optional)
- ★ 1 TBS lemon juice
- ★ 1 dash sea salt
- ★ 1 pinch cinnamon (optional)
- ★ 4 oz purified, filtered water

Raw Fig Jam

Place the following ingredients in <u>high-speed blender</u> (or <u>food processor</u>) and blend (or process) until well combined and smooth:

- ★ 2 C packed, dried Turkish figs or black mission figs (presoaked for 10-15 minutes & then drained)
- ★ 1-2 TBS raw agave (optional)
- ★ 1 TBS lemon juice
- ★ 1 dash sea salt
- ★ 1 pinch cinnamon (optional)
- ★ 4 oz purified, filtered water

> **Recipe Notes & Quick Tips:** Use the recipe guidelines to make other raw fruit jams. Just pick your favorite fresh or dried fruits and give them a whirl. Plus, always feel free to add any sweetener of choice, to taste (if needed). It doesn't have to be agave.
>
> Once made, be sure to transfer to an airtight, glass mason jar and store in the coldest part of your refrigerator. I suggest using smaller sized (wide mouth) mason jars so you can have less open at a time. This will allow for a larger amount of the jam to stay fresher longer. You may also want to consider keeping one jar in the fridge (that you will use within 3-5 days) and store the rest in the freezer for future use.

"Just Peachy" Parfait

Sweet Crème Layer

Place the following ingredients in <u>high-speed blender</u> and blend until smooth and creamy:

- ★ 1 C macadamia nuts (or cashews)
- ★ ½ C packed Turkish apricots (presoaked for 5-10 minutes & then drained)
- ★ ¼ tsp whole ground vanilla bean powder
- ★ ¼ tsp Pumpkin Pie Blend
- ★ 1 dash sea salt
- ★ 1-2 TBS coconut vinegar
- ★ 6-8 oz purified, filtered water (as needed)

Nut/Seed Layer

Use the following ratios as a guide and then pulse-chop in a food-processor to create a well-combined, course-ground sprinkle (being sure to not over process into flour):

- 1 C almonds
- 1 C walnuts
- ⅓ C pumpkin seeds
- ⅓ C sunflower seeds
- ⅓ C coconut flakes

Peach Layer

Slice and dice fresh organic peaches (about ½-¾ C per parfait depending on size of serving ware). If fresh peaches are unavailable, feel free to use defrosted frozen peaches:

- Peaches

Instructions:

1. In parfait glasses (or other glasses of choice), place a small amount of nut/seed mixture.
2. Top nuts/seeds with a thin layer of sweet crème.
3. Top sweet crème with a layer of fresh sliced (or diced) peaches.
4. Top fresh peaches with a thin layer of sweet crème.
5. Repeat 1-4 and then top last sweet crème layer with a sprinkle of nut/seed mixture.

Kiwi-Pineapple Parfait

Sweet Crème Layer

Place the following ingredients in high-speed blender and blend until smooth and creamy:

- 1 C macadamia nuts (or cashews)
- ½ C packed strawberries (fresh or frozen)
- ¼ tsp whole ground vanilla bean powder
- 1 dash sea salt
- 2 TBS raw honey or agave
- 2 TBS lemon juice (or lime juice)
- 2-4 oz purified, filtered water (as needed)

Nut Layer

Use the following ratios as a guideline and then pulse-chop in a food-processor to create a well-combined, course-ground sprinkle (being sure to not over process into flour):

- 1 ¼ C almonds

- ★ 1 ¼ C Brazil nut (or macadamia nuts)
- ★ ½ C coconut flakes

Kiwi-pineapple layer

Slice and dice fresh organic kiwi and pineapple (enough for each serving to have a least a ¼ C mixture of the two):

- ★ Kiwi (peeled)
- ★ Pineapple (peeled & cored)

Instructions:

1. In parfait glasses (or other glasses of choice), place a small amount of nut mixture.
2. Top nuts with a thin layer of sweet crème.
3. Top sweet crème with a layer of fresh kiwi-pineapple mixture.
4. Top kiwi-pineapple layer with a thin layer of sweet crème.
5. Repeat 1-4 and then top last sweet crème layer with a sprinkle of nut mixture.

Optional Variations

- ★ Substitute mangos for the pineapple and you have a **Kiwi-Mango Parfait.**
- ★ Substitute papayas for the pineapple and you have a **Kiwi-Papaya Parfait.**

Pumpkin Spiced Cranberry Parfait

Sweet Crème Layer

Place the following ingredients in <u>high-speed blender</u> and blend until smooth and creamy:

- ★ 1 C cashews
- ★ ¼ tsp whole ground vanilla bean powder
- ★ 1 dash sea salt
- ★ 2 TBS raw agave
- ★ 2 TBS lemon juice
- ★ 2-4 oz purified, filtered water (as needed)

Pumpkin Spiced Layer

Chop sweet potatoes into small chunks, place in <u>high-speed blender</u> along with all other ingredients, and then blend until smooth:

- ★ 2 sweet potatoes (peeled)
- ★ ½ C Turkish apricots (presoaked for 5-10 minutes & then drained)
- ★ ½ tsp Pumpkin Pie Blend
- ★ 1 dash sea salt
- ★ 2 TBS raw agave (or to taste)

- ★ 2 TBS coconut oil (liquefied)
- ★ 4-6 oz purified, filtered water (more only as needed for blending)

Cranberry Layer

Place the following ingredients in a <u>food processor</u> and process until well combined (somewhere between chunky cranberry sauce and pureed):

- ★ 1 C cranberries (fresh or defrosted)
- ★ ¼ C raw agave

Instructions:

1. In parfait glasses (or other glasses of choice), place a layer of pecan pieces. You may also add a sprinkle of cacao nibs to the layer if you wish.
2. Top pecan pieces with a layer of pumpkin spiced sweet potato mixture.
3. Top pumpkin spiced layer with a layer of sweetened cranberry mixture.
4. Top cranberry layer with a layer of sweet crème.
5. Repeat 1-4 and then top last sweet crème layer with pecan pieces and optional cacao nibs.

> **Please Note:** Raw sweet potatoes contain trypsin inhibitors, which can block the digestive breakdown of proteins. Natural enzyme inhibitors may or may not be fully neutralized during the blending and/or low-temperature dehydrating process. In order to get the most out of all the foods we choose to eat, I highly recommend practicing a food rotation plan that includes proper food combining on a regular basis. Learning the basics of food combining – as well as getting into the habit of rotating your food – can protect against nutritional toxicities and deficiencies. (Please refer to **Appendix D** for more on food combining.)

CEREAL OF CHAMPIONS

Raw cereals made with nuts and seeds are a great grain-free and gluten-free way to start your day. Loaded with pure, concentrated nutrients like energy-enhancing antioxidants, bio-available protein and essential fatty acids, you can see how these combinations truly make the cereals of champions! Give kids one taste and you may never have to make a trip down the cereal aisle again. What's more, a nourishing bowl of raw cereal can have their mental focus and concentration soaring in the classroom.

Quick Cereal Tips:

With the exception of Brazil nuts, hazelnuts, macadamia nuts, pine nuts, pistachio nuts, and chia, flax and hemp seeds, you may wish to soak, drain, rinse and strain the following nuts and seeds in preparation for cereal making: almonds, jungle peanuts, pecans, walnuts and pumpkin, sesame and sunflower seeds. Although this is optional, it can really help to improve digestibility and nutrient absorption. If you happen to have a dehydrator, you may wish to dehydrate your soaked nuts and seeds at 105-115°F until fully dry and crunchy, and then store them in an airtight, glass container in a cool, dark place.

> **Please Note:** For cereals, I sometimes enjoy dehydrating certain nuts and seeds and leaving others wet (especially since they are going to be saturated in a nut or seed mylk anyhow). For instance, you can keep walnuts or pecans moist, and dehydrate pumpkin and sunflower seeds. Just be sure to always drain the water they have been soaking in and give them a thorough rinsing. Always store wet nuts and seeds in an airtight container in your refrigerator and consume within one week. To review "The Science Behind the Soak," "General Soaking Schedule for Nuts & Seeds" and other great tips, please refer to page 26.

What about milk? I'm not at all a fan of cow's milk or soy milk and, although there might be a place for raw and organic goat's milk, I highly advise getting to know your source and building a relationship with them first. With that said, my safest answer for all (infants to the elderly) is going to be homemade nut or seed mylks. I highly suggest making your own from scratch (with high-quality, organic, raw nuts and seeds) versus buying commercial nut and seed milks. Truth be told, nut and seed mylk recipes are some of the easiest to tackle. The small amount of invested time will truly pay off in a big way. You also truly do feel a sense of pride whenever you can create something from scratch. More importantly, you are making valuable use of quality and wholesome ingredients which will only benefit you and your family.

> **Please Note:** Homemade nut/seed mylks are not only tastier, naturally sweeter and fresher than commercial nut/seed milks bought in a store, but they are healthier (no cheap emulsifiers, flavorings, preservatives or stabilizers), much richer in vital nutrients (not oxidized nutrients) and much more economical in the long run.
>
> I am not one to strain my nut/seed mylks. I prefer to just shake, use and consume them straight (fiber and all). But for those who do prefer straining their mylks, you may either use a nut mylk bag or, better yet, a coffee brewer/press such as those made by Bodum. I find nut mylk bags to be messy and a pain in the butt! Therefore, my solution is to have a few coffee presses around that can be used for various purposes (none of which involve coffee). Coffee presses have a mesh strainer which is finer than most of the tea presses on the market, which is why I prefer and recommend them for brewing loose-leaf teas and herbal tisanes, as well as for straining nut/seed mylks in a snap.

Raw Nuts N' Berries Cereal

Use the following ratios as a guide and feel free to mix any nuts and seeds you like. It is truly a matter of personal preference. You may also add dried fruits and/or superfoods to this mix as well (see optional additions below).

Nut & Seed Cereal Blend

Mix the following ingredients together in a bowl or coarsely pulse-chop them together in a food processor (being sure not to over process into flour):

- ¼ C almonds
- ¼ C walnuts
- ¼ C pumpkin seeds
- ¼ C sunflower seeds

Optional Additions

- Add ¼ C in total of: goji berries, golden berries, mulberries, Hunza golden raisins or other dried fruit of choice.
- Add 1-2 TBS Sunwarrior protein and/or maca powder for an extra boost of energy.
- Add 1-2 TBS of superfoods (cacao nibs, bee pollen and/or coconut flakes).

Fruit Blend

Top nut and seed blend with fresh, organic berries of choice:

- Blackberries
- Blueberries
- Raspberries
- Strawberries (sliced)

Pour your favorite nut or seed mylk creation over the fresh fruit and raw cereal blend and enjoy (see pages 275-277 for nut/seed mylk recipe ideas).

> **What are mulberries?** Raw, sun-dried mulberries are treasured for their high levels of antioxidants and their rich supply of protein, iron, vitamin C, dietary fiber and calcium. High levels of the potent antioxidant resveratrol (the anti-aging nutrient normally found in grapes and red wine) make mulberries a fabulous food for fighting cellular damage caused by free radicals.
>
> Mulberries also contain anthocyanin. Anthocyanins act as powerful antioxidants and can support good cardiovascular health and a strong immune system. What's more, mulberries have a unique protein content of three grams per ounce. This puts them right up there with goji and golden berries!
>
> Mulberries are scrumptiously sweet and have a flavor resembling that of fig. They are chewy with a slight crunch and make a delicious addition to trail mixes, grawnola, raw desserts, cereals and smoothies.

Go-To Nut Mylk

Place the following ingredients in <u>high-speed blender</u> and blend for 1-2 minutes, until smooth:

- ★ 1 C raw nuts of choice; almonds, Brazil nuts or cashews are the best
- ★ ¼ tsp whole ground vanilla bean (or to taste)
- ★ 1 dash sea salt (or to taste)
- ★ 1 pinch cinnamon, Pumpkin or Apple Pie Blend (optional or to taste)
- ★ Up to ¼ C raw agave or other natural sweetener of choice
- ★ 1-2 TBS coconut oil (liquefied)
- ★ 32 oz of purified, filtered water

Optional Additions & Boosters

- ★ Add up to ½ C of raw cacao powder for **Chocolate Mylk**. May also add 1-2 TBS (or to taste) of maca, mesquite and/or lucuma power.

Go-To Seed Mylk

Place the following ingredients in <u>high-speed blender</u> and blend for 1-2 minutes until smooth:

- ★ 1 C raw seeds of choice; hemp seeds or unhulled tan sesame seeds are the best. Using unhulled sesame seeds will ensure the maximum amount of calcium that can be obtained.
- ★ ¼ tsp whole ground vanilla bean (or to taste)
- ★ 1 dash sea salt (or to taste)
- ★ 1 pinch cinnamon, Pumpkin or Apple Pie Blend (optional or to taste)
- ★ Up to ¼ C raw agave or other natural sweetener of choice
- ★ 1-2 TBS coconut oil (liquefied)
- ★ 32 oz of purified, filtered water

Optional Variations, Additions & Boosters

- ★ Use raw honey in the place of agave, which is delicious in sesame mylk.
- ★ Add up to ½ C of raw cacao powder for **Chocolate Mylk**. May also add 1-2 TBS (or to taste) of maca, mesquite and/or lucuma powder.

Coconut Mylk (short cut)

Place the following ingredients in <u>high-speed blender</u> and blend for 1-2 minutes, until smooth:

- ★ 1 C raw coconut flakes
- ★ ¼ tsp whole ground vanilla bean (or to taste)
- ★ 1 dash sea salt (or to taste)
- ★ Up to ¼ C raw agave or other natural sweetener of choice
- ★ 1-2 TBS coconut oil (liquefied)
- ★ 24 oz purified, filtered water

Strawberry Mylk

Place the following ingredients in <u>high-speed blender</u> and blend for 1-2 minutes, until smooth:

- ★ 2 C packed, frozen strawberries
- ★ 1 C hemp seeds
- ★ ¼ C chia seeds
- ★ ¼ tsp whole ground vanilla bean (or to taste)
- ★ 1 dash sea salt (or to taste)
- ★ 1 pinch cinnamon (optional)
- ★ Up to ¼ C raw agave or other natural sweetener of choice
- ★ 32 oz of purified, filtered water

Optional Additions & Boosters

- ★ Add 1-2 TBS (or to taste) of maca, mesquite and/or lucuma powder.

Hazelnut Chocolate Mylk

Place the following ingredients in <u>high-speed blender</u> and blend for 1-2 minutes, until smooth:

- ★ 1 C hazelnuts
- ★ ½ C raw cacao powder
- ★ ¼ tsp whole ground vanilla bean (or to taste)
- ★ 1 dash sea salt (or to taste)
- ★ 1 pinch Pumpkin Pie Blend (or to taste)
- ★ Up to ¼ C raw agave or other natural sweetener of choice
- ★ 1-2 TBS coconut oil (liquefied)
- ★ 32 oz of purified, filtered water

Optional Additions & Boosters

- ★ Add 1-2 TBS (or to taste) of maca, mesquite and/or lucuma powder.

> **Recipe Notes & Quick Tips:** If you like a richer, creamier and thicker mylk, then you may decrease the amount of water down to about 24 oz in total.
>
> Certain mylks will need little to no sweetener (e.g., almond and cashew mylk), whereas others may require a bit more (e.g., sesame seed mylk). Before adding more sweetener, try adding a pinch or two more of sea salt.
>
> Although I only give raw agave as an example for sweetener, the choice is totally up to your personal preference and needs. Feel free to add as much or as little as you want. You may also choose to combine two in order to cut down on the glycemic index (GI) of one.

To review some basic conversion guidelines when substituting a sweetener for green leaf stevia, please refer to page 235.

Apple Cinnamon Cereal

Nut & Seed Cereal Blend

Mix the following ingredients together in a bowl or coarsely pulse-chop them together in a <u>food processor</u> (being sure not to over process into flour):

- ★ ¼ C almonds
- ★ ¼ C walnuts
- ★ ¼ C pumpkin seeds
- ★ ¼ C sunflower seeds

Optional Additions

- ★ Add 1-2 TBS Sunwarrior protein and/or maca powder for an extra boost of energy.
- ★ Add 1-2 TBS of superfoods (bee pollen, cacao nibs, coconut flakes and/or goji berries).

Fruit & Spice Blend

Top nut and seed blend with the following fruits:

- ★ 1-2 apples (coarsely chopped)
- ★ ¼ C Hunza golden raisins (or currants)
- ★ 1 dash cinnamon or Apple Pie Blend (or to taste)

Optional Variations & Additions

- ★ Replace apple(s) with pear(s) and you have a **Spiced Pear Cereal**.
- ★ Substitute pecans for almonds or walnuts.
- ★ Add fresh banana, blueberries, figs or mulberries.

Pour your favorite nut or seed mylk creation over fruit and raw cereal blend and enjoy!

What are Hunza golden raisins? Hunza raisins are not just golden in color, but golden for your health. They are from the pristine, mountainous Hunza region of Pakistan where they grow 6,000-9,000 feet above sea level and are irrigated by mineral rich glacial melt waters from high altitudes.

Hunza raisins have got to be the tastiest raisins on the planet. They are naturally sweet to the taste and good for you too! Does it get much better than that? Once you've gone gold with Hunza golden raisins, I highly doubt you will ever desire a darker variety again.

Banana-Blueberry Cereal

Nut & Seed Cereal Blend

Mix the following ingredients together in a bowl or coarsely pulse-chop them together in a food processor (being sure not to over process):

- ★ ¼ C almonds
- ★ ¼ C walnuts
- ★ ¼ C pumpkin seeds
- ★ ¼ C sunflower seeds

Optional Additions

- ★ Add 1-2 TBS Sunwarrior protein and/or maca powder for an extra boost of energy.

- Add 1-2 TBS of superfoods (bee pollen, cacao nibs, coconut flakes, goji berries and/or golden berries).

Fruit Blend

Top nut and seed blend with the following fruits:

- 1 small banana (sliced)
- ¼ C wild blueberries (fresh or defrosted)
- ¼ C sun-dried mulberries
- 1 dash cinnamon (or to taste)

Optional Variations

- Substitute pecans for almonds or walnuts.
- Substitute currants, Hunza golden raisins, Turkish apricots, Turkish figs or jackfruit for sun-dried mulberries.

Pour your favorite nut or seed mylk creation over fruit and raw cereal blend and enjoy!

> **What is jackfruit?** Jackfruit is the largest tree-borne fruit in the world and is native to Southeast Asia. It's an instant source of energy and loaded with vitamins, minerals and dietary fiber. The many health benefits of jackfruit include: helping to strengthen the immune system, eliminating cancer-causing free radicals, preventing ulcers and constipation, maintaining healthy vision and skin, lowering high blood pressure, controlling asthma, preventing anemia and more!
>
> Dried Jackfruit is still relatively unknown in the Western marketplace, but once you try it you will never forget its unique and exotic sweet taste. The taste of jackfruit is without a doubt tropical, as its flavor is a combination of banana, mango and pineapple. In its dried state, jackfruit resembles fruit leather and is a favorite among children, teens and adults alike.

CRUNCH CHEWY GRAWNOLA

If there's one great reason to invest in a dehydrator, it's for making homemade grawnola! Grawnola (sticky or crunchy) makes an awesome and yummy snack that anyone can enjoy day or night. You can enjoy it as a cereal by breaking it up and pouring your favorite homemade nut or seed mylk over it; you can eat it as is for an energy enhancing snack when you're on the go; or you can score a sheet of it right before placing it in the dehydrator for when you want grawnola bars.

Your homemade grawnola will also make a great addition to parfaits. Just replace the parfait's nut/seed layer with grawnola and you have another recipe variation that you can enjoy as a breakfast, snack or even dessert.

Making your own grawnola is great fun that even kids can easily take part in. It is also so much more economical than store-bought granola, not to mention a lot healthier as well. No stabilizers, preservatives and other unnatural additives to worry about. Plus, you get to control the sweetener by choosing what and how much you want. So, shall we get started?

Quick Grawnola Tips:

With the exception of Brazil nuts, hazelnuts, macadamia nuts, pine nuts, pistachio nuts, and chia, flax and hemp seeds, you may wish to soak, drain, rinse and strain the following nuts and seeds in preparation for grawnola making: almonds, jungle peanuts, pecans, walnuts and pumpkin, sesame and sunflower seeds. Although this is optional, it can really help to improve digestibility and nutrient absorption.

> **Please Note:** To review "The Science Behind the Soak," "General Soaking Schedule for Nuts & Seeds" and other great tips, please refer to page 26.

When making grawnola, please know that you are free to choose whichever nuts and seeds you desire. You do not need to use the nuts I've chosen in my Go-To Grawnola recipe.

> **Please Note:** I like to use 2 C nuts and 2 C seeds in total, but you may use whatever ratios you want (e.g., 4 C seeds, 4 C nuts, 3 C seeds and 1 C nuts, etc.). I also like to choose nuts that I don't have to soak. For one, it makes it easier to chop them up in the food processor without the worry of turning them to mush. It also saves some time, which can be nice. That being said, walnuts and pecans are great to use for grawnola. You can choose to use 2 C walnuts, 2 C pecans or 1 C of each. Then be sure to <u>slightly</u> pulse-chop only to avoid having them process to a paste. If they do get over processed, don't fret. Your grawnola will still taste fabulous regardless. You just won't have the same variation in texture.

If you don't want to dehydrate your grawnola, that's okay too! All you have to do is add some chia to the mix (which will act as a binder and absorb any excess moisture). Then you can roll into balls or logs before letting them firm up in the fridge.

Go-To Grawnola (dehydrator needed)

Choose Your Nuts

Choose ONE of the following nuts below for your grawnola; coarsely chop in a <u>food processor</u> (which means to pulse-chop into small-medium pieces, but not into a flour); transfer to a large mixing bowl:

- ★ 2 C almonds
- ★ 2 C Brazil nuts

Choose Your Seeds

Choose ONE of the following seeds below for your grawnola and add to mixing bowl with your nuts:

- ★ 2 C pumpkin seeds
- ★ 2 C sunflower seeds
- ★ 1 C pumpkin seeds & 1 C sunflower seeds

Now add the following <u>dry</u> ingredients to mixing bowl and toss until well combined:

- ★ 1 C coconut flakes
- ★ 1 tsp Apple or Pumpkin Pie Blend
- ★ ½ tsp whole ground vanilla bean
- ★ ¼ tsp sea salt

Optional Additions & Boosters

- ★ Add up to ½ C in total using the following: goji berries, golden berries, mulberries and/or cacao nibs.
- ★ Add one (½ C total) out of the following four: ½ C hemp seeds, ¼ C hemp seeds & ¼ C chia seeds, ¼ chia seeds & ¼ C Sunwarrior protein or ¼ C hemp seeds & ¼ C Sunwarrior protein.
- ★ Add up to ¼ C in total using the following: baobab, lucuma, maca and/or mesquite.

Choose Your <u>Dried</u> Fruit

Choose ONE dried fruit for your grawnola, place in <u>food processor</u>, and then before processing add your choice of fresh fruit (see below):

- ★ 1 C packed Turkish apricots (presoaked for 10-15 minutes & then drained)
- ★ 1 C packed currants (presoaked for 5-10 minutes & then drained)
- ★ 1 C packed Turkish figs (presoaked for 10-15 minutes & then drained)
- ★ 1 C packed jackfruit (presoaked for 10-15 minutes & then drained)
- ★ 1 C packed Hunza golden raisins (presoaked for 5-10 minutes & then drained)

Choose Your <u>Fresh</u> Fruit

Choose ONE fresh fruit for your grawnola, coarsely chop, and then add chopped pieces to soaked dried fruit already in <u>food processor</u>. Process both fresh and dried fruit into a paste:

- ★ 1 apple (chopped)
- ★ 1 pear (chopped)
- ★ 1 orange (peeled, seeded & segmented)

Add just enough water to thoroughly break down into a smooth paste (about ¼-½ C), then transfer fruit paste into mixing bowl with all the above ingredients. Toss until thoroughly combined.

Now add the following <u>wet</u> ingredients to mixing bowl and toss until well combined:

- ★ ¼ C raw agave or other natural sweetener of choice

- ¼ C coconut oil (liquefied)
- Purified, filtered water as needed. Only add water if mixture is too dry from the addition of superfood boosters (e.g., chia seeds and powders). Mixture should be thick and stiff enough for a spoon to stand straight up in, yet still moist enough to stir.

Grawnola Instructions:

1. Once all ingredients have been mixed together and well combined, transfer roughly 4 C of grawnola mixture to dehydrator sheeted trays.
2. Spread mixture evenly across sheeted tray using a spatula to a thickness of about ¼ inch.
3. Repeat steps 1 and 2 until all the mixture is used up.
4. Using the tips of your fingers (as if you were striking piano keys) make indentations across and down the grawnola mixture.
5. Dehydrate at 115°F for about eight hours (or overnight), and then flip over onto a regular mesh dehydrator tray without a sheet (see box below).
6. Continue dehydrating for another 12-24 hours or until dry and crunchy all the way through. Be sure to check the middle, as the middle is usually the last to completely dry.
7. Once completely dry, break your grawnola apart into whatever size chunks you desire.
8. Store in airtight glass mason jars in your fridge, where it should keep for up to one month. You may also store a portion in your freezer where it will keep for up to six months. If you wish, leave a small portion that you plan to eat within a few days in the dehydrator to keep it warm and on the crunchy side. Just decrease the temperature down to 100-105°F.

Please Note: Depending on the fruits you choose and the amount of pectin they contain, certain batches will come out chewier and others crunchier. If you like your grawnola crunchier, just dehydrate longer. You can also place refrigerated grawnola (which will naturally become chewier) back into the dehydrator to bring back some crunchy texture.

How to flip like a dehydrating pro: When it's time to flip, take a mesh tray without a sheet; lay it topside down evenly and directly over the tray with grawnola on it; hold the sides firmly (but without squeezing too tight) and quickly flip over. Now just slowly peel the dehydrator sheet from the grawnola and pop the new tray back into the dehydrator for the remainder of the time.

For Grawnola Bars:

- Follow the same instructions as given above, but add more mixture to your dehydrated sheeted trays so that you can spread evenly and to a thickness of about ½ inch (rather than ¼ inch).

- ★ Now you will want to use your spatula (or the back end of a butter knife) to score them into the size bars you want (rectangles, squares, etc.). Be sure to do this while the mixture is still wet, which will make your bars easier to break apart once they are fully dry.
- ★ Due to the added thickness when making bars, you will most likely need to dehydrate longer until they have reached the chewiness or crunchiness you desire.

JUBILANT JUICES

When is juicing more appropriate than blending? First, let me reiterate that both juicing and blending are beneficial to our health. What makes them different is the way in which their nutrients are delivered. Fresh raw juices do not contain fiber; therefore, the concentrated nutrients can be absorbed rather quickly, high in the digestive tract, with little to no digestion required.

Although I tend to favor blending over juicing when it comes to a technique of choice for long-term, daily use, there are times when I feel juicing can take precedence over blending. For instance, certain health conditions can make it very difficult to process the fiber that naturally exists in our many fruits and vegetables, and juicing helps eliminate this issue. There are also times when doing a short-term juice fast can really help kick-start the cleansing and healing process. It can also help wipe the slate clean of addictive food cravings.

One of the main advantages that juicing has over blending is that it requires little to no digestion. This means that nutrients hit the bloodstream and are absorbed and assimilated on contact. By processing the fiber out, the digestive system is allowed to rest. This is an important consideration for individuals who are dealing with severe nutritional deficiencies and have highly sensitive digestive systems. I believe juicing can greatly benefit those who suffer with conditions such as celiac, Crohn's, colitis, diverticulosis, diverticulitis and leaky gut; especially during acute and severe attacks.

In addition, fresh, raw juices allow for a much greater amount of leafy greens to be taken in at once. When properly extracted and consumed within 15-20 minutes, green juices provide the cells of our body with a tremendous amount of readily available chlorophyll, minerals, vitamins and living enzymes.

Please Note: I highly advise always drinking your juices as fresh as possible and within 20 minutes tops. This will ensure that you get the most out of all the living enzymes and nutrients before your juice naturally oxidizes.

What about juicing and blood sugar spikes? Due to the hybridization of our many modern-day fruits, the fact that hybridized foods (in general) have an increased sugar content, and that when we juice fruits (and certain vegetables such as carrots) we remove their fiber content and cause a rapid delivery of sugar into the bloodstream, I highly recommend green vegetable-based juices over fruit-based juices. Oftentimes when we begin to juice, we lean towards the sweeter taste of fruits, carrots and beets. This is okay for a short while when coming off of McDonalds; but as our taste buds change as we cleanse, we should ideally be aiming for juices that offer a much lower content in sugar. Otherwise, we could be spiking our blood sugar levels too high, which will only exacerbate (or may even create) a sugar related health condition such as cancer, Candida or diabetes.

With that being said, fruitier juices are a great way to start the day and can be a great way to kick off the beginning of a juice fast. This is because fruits are known to be very cleansing to the body, while greens are known to be more detoxifying. Therefore, as the day goes on (lunch, snack, dinner, etc.) and as you progress in your juice fast, I recommend decreasing the amount of sweet foods and increasing the amount of greens.

How should one go about doing a juice fast? Short-term juice fasts usually last 3-5 days, which is what I suggest for anyone new to fasting. Once you are accustomed to fasting, you may try fasting on juices and green superfood powders for up to 21-28 days. When you are done, just be sure to break you fast slowly with light superfood smoothies and simple leafy green salads. Not breaking a fast the right way is the #1 reason why most individuals fail at fasting. When breaking a fast (especially one lasting longer than 3 days), you must remember that your body's digestive system has been slowed down dramatically. Think of your digestive system like you would a sleeping bear that has gone into hibernation. I recommend the break-the-fast period last at least half the amount of time as your actual fasting period. Therefore, if you fasted for 21 days, you should eat clean and simple raw foods for at least 11 days. If you fasted for eight days, then your break-the-fast period should last at least four days. Gradually bring in dense/oily proteins (such as avocado, nuts, seeds, etc.), and whatever you do, do not wake the sleeping bear by succumbing to processed foods and foods such as burgers, pizza and pastries. The last thing you want to do is shock your system after fasting. This can cause great danger to your physical health.

Please Note: If you suffer from a sugar related health condition (such as cancer, Candida or diabetes), you may want to avoid, or at least limit, the juicing of all sweet fruits and high starch vegetables. I suggest sticking with low starch vegetables and greens. For diabetics and non-diabetics who experience fluctuations in their blood sugar levels, blending may be a much better option than juicing. At least until the body becomes self-adjusted. Be kind to yourself and ease into it.

Precautions: Before deciding to embark on any type of juice fast or fasting protocol, I highly recommend consulting with a qualified holistic practitioner; especially if you are currently on any medications.

Quick Juicing Tips:
- ★ Always choose organically grown produce that is locally grown whenever possible.
- ★ For optimum results, plan to drink juices on an empty stomach (30 minutes before a meal or 2-3 hours after a meal). Wheatgrass should be taken on an empty stomach at least 60-90 minutes before eating. I suggest drinking your juices in the morning on an empty stomach 30 minutes before eating anything else. It is the best time for cleansing and detoxifying all the vital organs of the body.
- ★ Prior to juicing, be sure to wash all produce well using a natural veggie wash or a 3% food grade hydrogen peroxide (H2O2) solution.

- Remove and toss any wilted parts of a vegetable.
- Unless noted otherwise, I highly suggest keeping the skin intact on all organic fruits and veggies. The skin is where the majority of the magic is!
- While in the process of physically juicing your produce, it is best to alternate between leafy greens, the softer produce and the more solid/fibrous produce (e.g., kale leaf, piece of carrot, romaine lettuce and then piece of cucumber). This will offer better leafy green juice extraction, as well as allow for the juices of the softer produce to completely flush out of the juicer. To avoid tough celery strings getting caught up around the gears (or clogging the screen), I advise waiting until the end to plunge your celery stalks down.
- When juicing greens with smaller leaves (e.g., parsley, cilantro, watercress, etc.), I like to wrap them in a bigger leaf going down the chute (e.g., collard or romaine leaf). You can also roll them into a ball and then use your plunger or harder veggies (such as carrots and celery stalks) to push them down.
- I suggest making approximately 16-24 oz at a time (adding more or less produce as needed).
- Stir and drink immediately for the best beneficial effects of all the living enzymes, nutrients and oxygen (within 15-20 minutes is ideal).
- Savor each mouthful before swallowing, as digestion begins in the mouth.
- Above all, enjoy!

"It's Alive!" Juices

Go-To Juice

This is a great and simple juice all by itself. It also serves as the perfect base for most all of my green juice creations (give or take a couple of celery stalks). Celery and cucumber are both high in water content, making them perfect for juicing together or along with other fruits and vegetables.

- 4-6 celery stalks
- 1 whole cucumber (with skin)

Optional Addition

- ½ lemon

> **Juicing Notes:** Slice ½-¾ of lemon rind off if desired (to decrease bitterness), but leave the majority of the white pith.

Superfood Boosters: Because this juice is so simple, I love adding 1-3 tsp (or more) of green powders or a dropperful or two of marine phytoplankton. My favorite powders to alternate between are Organic Kamut Blend, Organic Barley Green Juice, spirulina and chlorella.

> Celery contains a healthy amount of natural sodium, which is needed to produce hydrochloric acid (HCL). Increasing our ability to produce HCL naturally is important for the efficient breakdown of food in the stomach and absorption of vital nutrients.
>
> Cucumbers have a reputation for being the best kidney cleanser, as they help to clean the kidneys and bladder of debris and stones. In addition, cucumbers are rich in silica, which is essential if we desire to have a clear, glowing complexion and healthy connective tissues (such as muscles, tendons, ligaments, cartilage and bone).

Go-To Juice + Add-ons

Create your very own green juice with the following additions and options. By alternating your choice of greens and choice for sweet, you can have a different juice every day of the week! Use the amounts I give as a guideline, so please don't be afraid to add a little less or a little more.

- ★ 3-4 celery stalks
- ★ 1 cucumber (with skin)
- ★ Leafy greens (feel free to combine or alternate any of the following greens): 2 C packed, curly red or green kale, lacinato kale, red or green Swiss chard, red or green dandelion, collard leaves, baby spinach, mixed baby greens, endive lettuce, escarole lettuce, red or green leaf lettuce, romaine lettuce and/or any other leafy green you desire.
- ★ Optional leafy green herb boosters: 1 C packed parsley, cilantro, arugula, watercress, etc.

Sweet Additions (choose ONE of the following options)

- ★ 1 whole bell pepper (red, orange or yellow), 1 whole granny smith apple (seeded), 2-3 carrots (tops removed) or ½ beet
- ★ Combination of 1-2 carrots and ¼-½ a beet

Optional Additions

- ★ ½-1-inch piece ginger root and/or turmeric root
- ★ 1-2 garlic cloves

> **Juicing Notes:** The skin of ginger or turmeric root can be peeled off or kept intact. I prefer keeping it intact. Just make sure to scrub the skin thoroughly.
>
> Due to the majority of vitamin C being just under the skin of apples, I also recommend juicing apples with the skin intact. Granny smith is my 1st choice, but any variety will do with the exception of red or golden delicious apples. From what I've gathered, red and golden delicious apples are two of the most hybridized of all apple varieties and, as a result, two of the least nutritious.

HEALING FROM THE INSIDE OUT!

Ulcer Eliminator

- ½ head cabbage (green or purple)
- 2 celery stalks
- 1 apple (seeded) or 2 carrots (tops removed)

Optional Addition

- ½ inch piece ginger root

> **Juicing Notes:** Drink 3-4 times per day until ulcer is completely healed.

Colon Cleanser Juice #1

- 4 kale leaves
- 2 C packed baby spinach, mixed baby greens and/or arugula
- 1 cucumber
- 4 celery stalks
- 2 granny smith apples (seeded)
- 1 jalapeno (or other hot pepper)
- ½ lemon

Optional Addition

- 1-2 garlic cloves

Colon Cleanser Juice #2

- 4 collard leaves
- 1 head Boston bibb lettuce (or green leaf)
- 1 cucumber
- 4 bok choy stalks (with greens)
- 1 granny smith apple (seeded)

- 1 pear
- 1-inch piece ginger root
- ½ lemon

Optional Addition

- 1-2 garlic cloves

Ultimate Green Hulk Detoxifier

- 1 cucumber
- 4 celery stalks
- 2 C packed baby spinach
- 1 C packed parsley

Superfood Boosters: This juice is already a pretty powerful and potent detoxifier. If you dare, add one shot of wheatgrass juice or 1-3 tsp of Organic Kamut Blend.

Kidney Cleanser Juice #1

- 3-4 medium 1 ½ inch slices of watermelon (including the skin, rind & seeds)

Optional Additions

- ¼-½ inch piece ginger root
- ½ lemon

Kidney Cleanser Juice #2

- 3-4 medium 1 ½ inch slices of watermelon (including the skin, rind & seeds)
- Few sprigs of mint (peppermint or spearmint)
- ½ lemon

> **Juicing Notes:** About 95% of all the nutrients in watermelon are found in the skin and rind, making approximately 5% found in the fruit flesh. Watermelon skin has chlorophyll, the rind has minerals, and the seeds are commonly known to be cleansing to the kidneys. It has been noted that individuals who suffer from kidney stones and consume all parts of a watermelon can actually dissolve their bigger stones into smaller stones (which will appear more like sand), making them much easier to eliminate from the body.
>
> ★ When juicing whole watermelon, be sure to always use organic watermelon with seeds.
> ★ Wash the outside thoroughly before slicing.
> ★ I suggest drinking no more than 16 ounces at a time (due to sugar content).
> ★ Avoid if you suffer from a sugar related health condition.
> ★ If planning to do a watermelon only cleanse, limit to 3 days maximum.
> ★ If doing a 3-day watermelon cleanse, it may be easier to juice a larger amount at a time (about half watermelon or more depending on size). That being said, I suggest juicing no more than what you plan to drink by the end of that day. Pour the extra in airtight glass containers and store in the fridge.
> ★ Even though you're drinking lots of juice, don't forget to drink plenty of purified, filtered water. This will help to dilute and flush.

Kidney Cleanser Juice #3

- ★ 1 cucumber
- ★ 1 apple (seeded)
- ★ 2 C packed parsley

Optional Additions

- ★ ½ inch piece ginger root
- ★ ½ lemon

Kidney Cleanser Juice #4

- ★ 2 apples (seeded)
- ★ 2 C packed parsley

Optional Addition

- ★ ½ inch piece ginger root

- ½ lemon

Kidney Cleanser Juice #5

- 1 apples (seeded)
- 2 carrots (tops removed)
- 2 C packed parsley

Optional Additions

- ½ inch piece ginger root
- ½ lemon

Bladder & UTI Buster

- 3-4 apples (seeded)
- ½ C cranberries (fresh or frozen)

> **Juicing Notes:**
> - Drink in divided doses throughout the day (at least 16 ounces per day).
> - Be sure to drink lots of purified, filtered water.
> - Limit or avoid if you suffer from a sugar related health condition.

Liver Cleanser Juice #1

- 1 apple (seeded)
- 2 carrots (tops removed)
- 1 small beet (including tops)

Optional Additions

- ¼-½ inch piece ginger root
- 1 small garlic clove

Liver Cleanser Juice #2

- 1 apple (seeded)
- 2 carrots (tops removed)
- ½ small beet
- 2 C packed dandelion, collard, kale, and/or spinach

Optional Additions

- ¼-½ inch piece ginger root
- 1 small garlic clove

Liver Cleanser Juice #3

- ★ 1 cucumber
- ★ 2 celery stalks
- ★ 2 carrots (tops removed)
- ★ ½ beet

Liver Cleanser Juice #4

- ★ 1 apple (seeded)
- ★ 2 carrots (tops removed)
- ★ 1 C packed dandelion
- ★ ½ lemon

Citrus Gallbladder Squeeze Juice #1

- ★ 2 grapefruits, peeled (include as much of the white pith as possible)
- ★ 1 lemon
- ★ ½-1inch piece ginger root

Citrus Gallbladder Squeeze Juice #2

- ★ 1 grapefruit, peeled (include as much of the white pith as possible)
- ★ 1 apple (seeded)

Lymphatic Lifter Juice #1

- ★ 1 apple (seeded)
- ★ 1 pear
- ★ 2 C grapes (including the seeds & stems)
- ★ ½ lemon

Optional Addition

- ★ ¼-½ inch piece ginger root

Lymphatic Lifter Juice #2

- ★ 2 apples (seeded)
- ★ 2 carrots (tops removed)
- ★ 2 celery stalks
- ★ ½ beet

Blood Buster Juice #1

- ★ 1 beet (including tops)
- ★ 1 apple (seeded)
- ★ 2 carrots (tops removed)

- 3-4 celery stalks
- 1-inch piece ginger root
- 1 lemon

Blood Buster Juice #2
- 1 burdock root
- 4 celery stalks
- 1 cucumber
- 2 C packed cilantro (and/or parsley)

Optional Addition
- 1 bell pepper for sweetness (if needed)

Lung Rejuvenator Juice #1
- 1 cucumber
- 2 celery stalks
- 1 C packed watercress
- ½-1 lemon

Lung Rejuvenator Juice #2
- 1 jewel yam or sweet potato
- 1 C packed parsley
- ½ C packed watercress

Optional Addition
- 1-2 carrots (tops removed) for added sweetness (due to potency of watercress)

Skin Beautifier Juice #1
- 1 cucumber
- 2 celery stalks
- 3-4 radish
- 1 burdock root
- 2 C packed cilantro
- ½ lemon

Skin Beautifier Juice #2
- 1 cucumber
- 2 celery stalks
- 1 apple (seeded)
- ¼ pineapple (including skin & core)

Optional Addition

★ ¼-½ inch piece ginger root

> **Juicing Notes:** Thoroughly wash pineapple, and then cut top and bottom off before cutting in half and then in half again in order to quarter.

Skin Beautifier Juice #3

★ ½-1 papaya (skinned & seeded)
★ 1 pear

Optional Additions

★ 1 lime or lemon

> **The sky is the limit when it comes to juicing recipes.** The above is just a teaser of some of my all-time favorites when it comes to the routine cleansing of our major detoxifying organs and the body systems they belong to. Some great books entirely dedicated to the art of juicing are:
>
> ★ *Complete Book of Juicing: Your Delicious Guide to Youthful Vitality* by Michael T. Murray
>
> ★ *Total Juicing: Over 125 Healthful and Delicious Ways to Use fresh Fruit and Vegetable Juices and Pulp* by Elaine LaLanne and Richard Benyo
>
> ★ *Juicing For Life: A Guide to the Benefits of Fresh Fruit and Vegetable Juicing* by Cherie Calbom and Maureen Keane

SOUPER SCRUMPTIOUS SOUPS

Raw fruit and veggie soups are a great alternative to juices. They retain the pulp and can offer an abundance of dietary fiber; something we can all use a little more of. With just a cutting board, knife and blender at your fingertips, you can be on your way to a satisfying appetizer or meal that is souper easy, souper fun, and souper scrumptious!

Please Note: Use the measurements provided in each recipe as a guideline to get started. Please understand that when you are dealing with fresh, raw ingredients of different shapes and sizes – some with a higher content of water and some with lower – the herbs, spices and addition of fluid may need to be fine-tuned. Be sure to taste test along the way until the desired balance of flavors has been reached.

Quick Soup Tips:

Due to the amount and bulkiness of veggies in some recipes, it may take two separate blending cycles to make a soup – but these can easily be combined later. In these cases, I suggest having a one-gallon pitcher handy (like a Rubbermaid ice tea pitcher), and then you can just pour back and forth.

When given a range in a recipe (e.g., ¼-½ tsp sea salt, 1-2 TBS of a spice blend or 1-3 tsp of an individual herb), I suggest starting with the smaller amount first and then tasting it. This will give you room to individualize. Even if not given a range, if you feel a spice or herb may be too much for you, feel free to start with a smaller amount (e.g., 1-2 tsp when 1 TBS is called for), and then taste test before adding the 2nd or 3rd tsp. Stop when the taste is just where you like it and make a note for future reference.

> **Please Note:** This also goes for the amount of purified water added. Start with the smaller amount called for and add the rest (or more) slowly until the desired consistency has been reached. Personally, I like most of my soups on the thicker side; therefore, I tend to stay right within the range given. However, others may like a thinner soup and may find themselves wanting to add a bit more water (which, by the way, can be done to either the entire batch or each individual serving).
>
> Another reason to leave a soup a bit thicker from the start is so a couple of ounces of warm water can be added to individual serving when a warmer soup is desired. I feel it's better to add after, for individual tastes and preferences, then to have added something "to the point of no return" at the start.

For warm soup: You could either do as suggested in the box above, or let a covered bowl of soup sit at room temperature in a bath of warm water, stirring occasionally until ready to eat. You may also wish to add up to 8 oz of warm water during the blending step, out of the specific amount called for. Just be sure the preheated water you add doesn't go above 150-160°F. You never want to add boiling water, as this can be very damaging to all the living enzymes and whole food nutrients we are trying to preserve and protect.

> **Please Note:** Due to much blending being required during the soup making process, these soups will often be warm straight out of your high-speed blender (just don't allow them to become too hot). Warm, yet still raw soups are very comforting and satisfying in the wintertime.

I love using cucumbers in soups, as they are not just water rich, but nutrient rich as well. To get the most out of your cucumbers, I advise not peeling them. Cucumber skins are where you find most all the nutrients (like magnesium). The skins also contain extremely high levels of collagen boosting and bone-building silica. Without adequate silica, our bodies cannot properly use calcium. When our bodies are not utilizing calcium properly, it can cause calcium to be leached from our bones.

Any and all home-grown sprouts make tremendous toppings to soup creations. Sprouts have one of the highest concentrations of nutrition per calorie of any known food on the planet. They are a rich source of live vitamins, minerals, enzymes, dietary fiber, chlorophyll, antioxidants and bio-available protein. They also give that bit of texture and crunch that will make your spectacular soup even more spectacular!

SAVORY SOUP IDEAS

Creamy Cucumber Soup

Chop veggies into small chunks, place in <u>high-speed blender</u> along with all other ingredients, and then blend until smooth:

- ★ 2 medium cucumbers
- ★ 1-2 celery stalks
- ★ 1 large avocado (peeled & pitted)
- ★ 1 TBS dried oregano, dill weed or Spicy Infusion Blend
- ★ 1 tsp sea salt (or to taste)
- ★ ¼ tsp asafoetida (or to taste)
- ★ 2 TBS lemon juice
- ★ 2 TBS extra virgin olive oil
- ★ 8-12 oz purified, filtered water (or until desired consistency)

Optional Additions

- ★ 1-2 collard or lacinato kale leaves (stems removed) or one handful baby spinach
- ★ 1 TBS spirulina

Thai Cucumber Soup

Chop veggies into small chunks, place in <u>high-speed blender</u> along with all other ingredients, and then blend until smooth:

- ★ 2 medium cucumbers
- ★ 3-4 medium carrots (peeled & tops removed)
- ★ ¾ C cashews
- ★ ½ jalapeno pepper (or chili pepper of choice)
- ★ 1-inch piece ginger root (or 1 tsp lemongrass)
- ★ 1 TBS Curry Blend (or turmeric)
- ★ 1 tsp sea salt (or to taste)
- ★ ¼ tsp asafoetida (or to taste)
- ★ 1 dash cayenne (or to taste)
- ★ 1 whole lime, juiced
- ★ 1-2 TBS coconut aminos
- ★ 1-2 TBS raw honey or agave
- ★ 2 TBS coconut oil (liquefied)
- ★ 12-16 oz purified, filtered water (or until desired consistency)

Optional Additions & Topping Ideas

- ★ Finely chopped fresh Thai basil leaves (if Thai basil is unavailable, substitute with ½ regular basil and ½ mint leaves)

- Finely chopped fresh cilantro leaves
- Diced roma tomatoes

Carrot Curry Soup

Chop veggies into small chunks, place in <u>high-speed blender</u> along with all other ingredients, and then blend until smooth:

- 6 large carrots (peeled & tops removed)
- 2-3 celery stalks
- ¾ C pumpkin seeds
- 1 TBS Curry Blend
- ½ inch piece ginger root (or 2-3 drops ginger essential oil)
- 1 tsp sea salt (or to taste)
- ¼ tsp asafoetida (or to taste)
- 1 dash cayenne (or to taste)
- 1-2 TBS coconut vinegar
- 2 TBS coconut oil (liquefied)
- 12-16 oz purified, filtered water (or until desired consistency)

Optional Variations

- Substitute 1 TBS Spicy Infusion Blend for Curry Blend.
- Substitute ¾ C hemp seeds for pumpkin seeds.

Optional Topping Ideas

- Mung bean, fenugreek, sunflower, lentil or pea sprouts
- Shredded carrots

Carrot Ginger Soup

Chop veggies into small chunks, place in <u>high-speed blender</u> along with all other ingredients, and then blend until smooth:

- 6 large carrots (peeled & tops removed)
- 1 large avocado (peeled & pitted)
- 1 TBS dried dill weed
- ½ inch piece ginger root (or 2-3 drops ginger essential oil)
- 1 tsp sea salt (or to taste)
- ¼ tsp asafoetida (or to taste)
- 1 dash cayenne (or to taste)
- 2 TBS lemon juice
- 2 TBS extra virgin olive oil
- 12-16 oz purified, filtered water (or until desired consistency)

Optional Variations

- ★ Substitute 1 TBS dried cilantro or tarragon for dill weed.

Optional Topping Ideas

- ★ Mung bean, fenugreek, sunflower, lentil or pea sprouts
- ★ Shredded carrots
- ★ Diced avocado

> **Make once, eat twice!** Many of these soup recipes will make a lot, but there is a method to my madness. Being in the business of owning a café, you learn quickly that it basically takes the same amount of time to make more as it does to make less. You can always freeze any leftovers or simply make a half batch. I suggest reserving the addition of spices until the very end, according to taste, when making a half batch.

Cream of Bell Pepper

Chop veggies into small chunks, place in <u>high-speed blender</u> along with all other ingredients, and then blend until smooth:

- ★ 2 medium red bell peppers
- ★ 1-2 celery stalks
- ★ 1 medium cucumber
- ★ 1 C cashews (or Brazil nuts)
- ★ 2 TBS chickpea miso paste
- ★ 1-2 TBS Spicy Infusion Blend
- ★ ½ tsp sea salt (or to taste)
- ★ ¼ tsp asafoetida (or to taste)
- ★ 8-12 oz purified, filtered water (or until desired consistency)

Optional Topping Ideas

- ★ Blend together (or use individually) any of the following:
    - o Hemp seeds and/or pumpkin seeds
    - o Cayenne to taste
    - o Nutritional yeast flakes

Spicy Bell Pepper

Chop veggies into small chunks, place in <u>high-speed blender</u> along with all other ingredients, and then blend until smooth:

- ★ 2 medium red bell peppers
- ★ 1-2 celery stalks
- ★ 2 medium avocados (peeled & pitted)

- 1 medium cucumber
- 2 TBS chickpea miso paste
- 1 TBS Chili Blend
- 1 TBS dried cilantro and/or oregano
- ½ tsp sea salt (or to taste)
- ¼ tsp asafoetida (or to taste)
- 8-12 oz purified, filtered water (or until desired consistency)

Optional Topping Ideas

- Blend together (or use individually) any of the following:
    - Chopped avocado
    - Chopped sun-dried olives
    - Chopped jalapeños (or chili pepper of choice)
    - Cilantro and/or oregano
    - Nutritional yeast flakes

Creamy Tomato Basil

Chop veggies into small chunks, place in <u>high-speed blender</u> along with all other ingredients, and then blend until smooth:

- 8 medium roma tomatoes
- 1-2 celery stalks
- ½ orange (peeled & seeded)
- ¾ C hemp seeds
- ½ C sun-dried tomatoes (presoaked)
- 1-2 TBS dried basil
- ½ tsp sea salt (or to taste)
- ¼ tsp asafoetida (or to taste)
- 1 dash cayenne (or to taste)
- ¼ C hemp or chia seed oil
- 12-16 oz purified, filtered water (or until desired consistency)

Optional Variations

- Substitute 1-2 TBS dried rosemary or thyme for basil.
- Substitute 2 medium carrots for 2 roma tomatoes.
- Substitute ¾ C pumpkin or sunflower seeds for hemp seeds.

Creamy Corn Soup

First, blend the following ingredients in a <u>high-speed blender</u> until smooth, and then poor into a mixing bowl, leaving at least eight ounces in the blender for the next step:

- ★ Corn kernels from 3 fresh, organic (GMO free) cobs of corn. Carefully remove kernels lengthwise using a sharp knife. For easy containment of kernels, I suggest doing over a large plate or bowl cover.
- ★ ¼ C red onion, chopped
- ★ 1 C raw cashews
- ★ 2 TBS chickpea miso
- ★ ½ tsp sea salt (or to taste)
- ★ ½ tsp paprika
- ★ ¼ tsp asafoetida
- ★ 12-16 oz purified, filtered water (or until desired consistency)

Second, add the ingredients below to the eight ounces of mixture left in blender from first step above. For a nice chunky texture, give a few quick pulses only:

- ★ Corn kernels from 3 additional fresh, organic (GMO free) cobs of corn
- ★ ¼ C red onion, chopped

Third, poor the chunky corn mixture in with the smooth corn mixture and enjoy!

Optional Additions & Topping Ideas

- ★ 1-3 tsp of dried herb leaves of choice (such as basil, cilantro, dill, parsley and/or tarragon)

Bali-Flower Soup

Chop veggies into small chunks, place in <u>high-speed blender</u> along with all other ingredients, and then blend until smooth:

- ★ 2-3 C packed cauliflower florets (leaves & core removed); chopped into small enough pieces to pack measuring cup
- ★ 1 medium red bell pepper
- ★ 1 medium carrot (peeled & tops removed)
- ★ ¾ C cashews
- ★ 1-2 TBS Garam Masala Blend
- ★ 1 tsp sea salt (or to taste)
- ★ ¼ tsp asafoetida (or to taste)
- ★ ½ lime, juiced
- ★ 1-2 TBS raw honey or agave
- ★ 2 TBS coconut oil (liquefied)
- ★ 12-16 oz purified, filtered water (or until desired consistency)

Optional Topping Ideas

- ★ Blend together (or use individually) any of the following:
  - ○ Fenugreek, sunflower, lentil or pea sprouts
  - ○ Shredded carrots

- o Cayenne to taste

Creamy Cauliflower Soup

Chop veggies into small chunks, place in <u>high-speed blender</u> along with all other ingredients, and then blend until smooth:

- ★ 2-3 C packed cauliflower florets (leaves & core removed); chopped into small enough pieces to pack measuring cup
- ★ 1 C macadamia nuts
- ★ 1-2 tsp dried oregano
- ★ 1-2 tsp dried rosemary
- ★ 1-2 tsp dried thyme
- ★ 1 tsp sea salt (or to taste)
- ★ ¼ tsp asafoetida (or to taste)
- ★ 2 TBS lemon juice (or 1-2 TBS coconut vinegar)
- ★ 12-16 oz purified, filtered water (or until desired consistency)

Optional Topping Ideas

- ★ Blend together (or use individually) any of the following:
  - o Minced broccoli florets
  - o Shredded carrots
  - o Paprika and/or cayenne to taste
  - o Nutritional yeast flakes

Cream of Choice Soup

Creamy Base

Blend the following ingredients in <u>high-speed blender</u> until smooth and use as a base for a creatively creamy soup of your choosing:

- ★ 4-6 celery stalks
- ★ ¾ C cashews (or macadamia nuts)
- ★ ½ tsp sea salt (or to taste)
- ★ ¼ tsp asafoetida (or to taste)
- ★ 1 dash cayenne (or to taste)
- ★ 1-2 dashes green leaf stevia powder (or ¼-½ tsp whole leaf)
- ★ 2 TBS lemon juice
- ★ ¼ C hemp or chia seed oil
- ★ 12-24 oz purified, filtered water (or until desired consistency)

Optional Ideas for Cream of Choice Soup

- ★ For **Cream of Collard Soup**: add 4-5 collard greens (stems removed). Addition of other veggies, herbs, spices and superfoods as desired.

- For **Cream of Kale Soup**: add 4-5 curly or lacinato kale leaves (stems removed). Addition of other veggies, herbs, spices and superfoods as desired.
- For **Cream of Spinach Soup**: add 2-3 large handfuls of baby spinach. Addition of other veggies, herbs, spices and superfoods as desired.
- For **Cream of Broccoli Soup**: add 2-3 C packed broccoli florets (chopped into small enough pieces to pack measuring cup), reserving a bit to mince and garnish the top. Great additions are a roma tomato (or two) and a bit of basil, oregano or rosemary.
- For **Cream of Wild Mushroom Soup**: add ¼ C chaga or shiitake mushroom powder or ½-¾ C fresh or rehydrated (from dried) shiitakes. This soup is excellent with a bit of ginger, cilantro and coconut aminos, and then topped with finely sliced shiitakes and shredded carrots.

> **Recipe Notes & Quick Tips:** Feel free to add a bit of bell pepper, carrot or tomato to any leafy green soup if you desire a bit of sweetness, any blend of herbs and spices for variation, and then top with nutritional yeast flakes for a bit of delicious cheesiness!

Fiesta Chili

Smooth Portion

First, chop veggies into small chunks, place in <u>high-speed blender</u> along with all other ingredients, and then blend into a paste:

- 6 medium roma tomatoes
- 1-2 celery stalks
- 1 jalapeno pepper (or habanera pepper for more intense heat)
- 2 C sun-dried tomatoes (presoaked)
- 2 TBS chickpea miso paste
- 1 TBS Chili Blend
- ½ tsp sea salt (or to taste)
- 1 tsp asafoetida (or to taste)
- 1 whole lime, juiced
- 1 TBS raw honey or agave

Optional Additions

- 1-2 TBS chaga and/or shiitake mushroom powder

Chunky Portion

Second, chop the following veggies into medium-small chunks and set aside; place each of the following ingredients in <u>food processor</u> INDIVIDUALLY (and in the order I have listed). Pulse-chop each until finely chopped into tiny pieces or as described below. Once each ingredient is processed, transfer to a large mixing bowl in preparation for the next ingredient to be chopped:

1. 2 C walnuts – pulse-chopped into small pieces.
2. 2 medium carrots (peeled & tops removed) – pulse-chopped to look like orzo or rice.
3. 2 medium red bell peppers (add first) with 4 medium roma tomatoes – pulsed until chopped small, but not overly processed into a purée.
4. 1 C packed, fresh cilantro (leaves and tender stems only) – pulsed until finely chopped.

Third, combine all your chunky ingredients with your smooth chili paste and stir together until well combined.

Optional Serving Ideas

- In a food processor, pulse-chop any of the following to the size of orzo or rice: jicama, turnip, cauliflower or zucchini. Serve under your chili as a bed of rice.
- Top chili with a dollop of Sour Nut Crème (page 345).
- Sprinkle with a combo of nutritional yeast flakes, hemp seed and sea salt for the flavor of sprinkle cheese. Mmm! My favorite!
- Serve with your favorite chia crackers (bought or home-made).

Macho Gazpacho

Chunky Portion

First, chop the following veggies into small chunks. Layer in <u>food processor</u> and pulse-chop until well and evenly combined, but still chunky. You may also slice and dice by hand if you don't want to use a food processor:

- ½ red onion, diced small
- 4 medium roma tomatoes, diced small
- 1 medium cucumber, seeded & diced small (reserve seeds for next step)
- 2 medium bell peppers, diced small (red, orange and/or yellow)

Smooth Portion

Second, chop veggies into small chunks, place in <u>high-speed blender</u> along with all other ingredients, and then blend until smooth:

- 6 medium roma tomatoes
- 3-4 celery stalks
- Reserved seeds from cucumber
- 1 TBS dried basil
- 1 TBS dried cilantro
- 1 TBS dried parsley
- ½ tsp sea salt (or to taste)
- ¼ tsp cayenne (or to taste)
- ¼ tsp asafoetida (or 1 garlic clove)
- 1 whole lime, juiced

- ★ 2 TBS coconut vinegar
- ★ 1 TBS raw honey or agave
- ★ ½ C extra virgin olive oil
- ★ Up to 4 oz purified, filtered water

Third, combine all your chunky ingredients with your blended ingredients and stir until well combined.

Optional Additions & Topping Ideas

- ★ Diced avocado; always a huge hit!
- ★ Additional diced veggies (such as reserved bell pepper and cucumber).

Optional Gazpacho Variation ideas

- ★ Add diced mango and/or strawberries (great with a sprig or two of fresh mint).
- ★ Add diced apple and/or pear (also great with a sprig or two of fresh mint).

Beet Borscht in the Raw

Chop veggies into small chunks, place in <u>high-speed blender</u> along with all other ingredients, and then blend until smooth:

- ★ 2-3 medium beets (peeled & tops removed)
- ★ 2-3 medium carrots (peeled & tops removed)
- ★ 1-2 celery stalks
- ★ 1 TBS dried dill weed
- ★ ½ tsp sea salt (or to taste)
- ★ ½ tsp asafoetida (or to taste)
- ★ ¼ tsp cayenne (or to taste)
- ★ 1-2 TBS raw honey or agave
- ★ 2 TBS lemon juice
- ★ ¼ C extra virgin olive oil
- ★ 16-24 oz purified, filtered water (or until desired consistency)

Optional Topping Ideas

- ★ Blend together (or use individually) any of the following:
    - o Shredded cabbage
    - o Shredded carrots
    - o Hemp and/or pumpkin seeds
    - o Chopped pecans and/or walnuts

Red Beet Borscht

Chop veggies into small chunks, place in <u>high-speed blender</u> along with all other ingredients, and then blend until smooth:

- ★ 2 medium beets (peeled & tops removed)
- ★ 2 medium carrots (peeled & tops removed)
- ★ 2 small sweet potatoes (peeled)
- ★ ½ C sun-dried tomatoes (presoaked)
- ★ 4 bay leaves
- ★ ½ tsp sea salt (or to taste)
- ★ ½ tsp asafoetida (or to taste)
- ★ ¼ tsp cayenne (or to taste)
- ★ 1-2 TBS raw honey or agave
- ★ 1-2 TBS apple cider vinegar
- ★ ¼ C extra virgin olive oil
- ★ 16-24 oz purified, filtered water (or until desired consistency)

Optional Topping Ideas

- ★ Blend together (or use individually) any of the following:
  - ○ Shredded cabbage
  - ○ Shredded carrots
  - ○ Hemp and/or pumpkin seeds
  - ○ Chopped pecans and/or walnuts

Sweet Potato Soup

Chop veggies into small chunks, place in <u>high-speed blender</u> along with all other ingredients, and then blend until smooth:

- ★ 2 large sweet potatoes (peeled)
- ★ 1 whole orange (peeled & seeded)
- ★ ½-1-inch piece ginger root (or 4-6 drops ginger essential oil)
- ★ ½ tsp Apple Pie Blend
- ★ ¼ tsp sea salt (or to taste)
- ★ 1 dash cayenne (or to taste)
- ★ 2 TBS raw honey or agave
- ★ 2 TBS coconut oil (liquefied)
- ★ 16-24 oz purified, filtered water (or until desired consistency)

Optional Variations & Topping Ideas

- ★ Add up to one red bell pepper to the blend above (reserving enough to dice and use as garnish) and substitute Curry or Garam Masala Blend (to taste) for Apple Pie Blend. **Note:** You will most likely need to use the smaller amount of water when adding bell pepper to the blend.

Zucchini Noodle Soup

First, add the following to a stainless-steel pot:

- ★ 3-4 medium zucchinis, spiralized (lightly chopped a few times after spiral cutting)
- ★ 1 large avocado (peeled, pitted & diced small)

Optional Additions & Variation Ideas

- ★ Chiffonade cut leafy greens such as collards, endive, escarole, lacinato kale and/or spinach. **FYI:** Chiffonade means to ribbon cut or finely cut into strips.
- ★ Add finely sliced radishes and shiitake mushrooms (fresh or rehydrated).
- ★ Add shredded carrots, parsnips and/or Chinese (Napa) cabbage.
- ★ Add diced bell pepper and/or tomato.

Soup Base

Second, chop veggies into small chunks and place in <u>high-speed blender</u> along with all other ingredients. Blend until smooth and then pour over spiralized zucchini in the large, stainless-steel pot:

- ★ 1 large bunch of celery
- ★ 1 large avocado (peeled & pitted)
- ★ 2-4 TBS Poultry Blend or Italian Blend
- ★ 1 tsp sea salt (or to taste)
- ★ ¼ tsp asafoetida (or to taste)
- ★ 1 dash cayenne (or to taste)
- ★ ¼ C lemon juice
- ★ ¼ C extra virgin olive oil
- ★ 24-32 oz purified, filtered water (or unit desired consistency)

Optional Topping Ideas

- ★ 1-3 tsp spirulina
- ★ Nutritional yeast flakes to taste

Sea-Veggie Miso Soup

First, add the following veggies to a large stainless-steel pot:

- ★ 2 medium zucchinis, spiralized (lightly chopped a few times after spiral cutting)
- ★ 1 medium cucumber, ribbon sliced (lightly chopped a few times after spiral slicing)
- ★ 1-2 bok choy stalks, finely sliced (including greens)
- ★ 1 large avocado (peeled, pitted & diced small)
- ★ 2-3 TBS sea vegetable flakes of choice (dulse, nori, wakame and/or triple blend flakes)

Optional Additions & Variation Ideas

- ★ Finely sliced shiitake mushrooms (fresh or rehydrated)
- ★ Shredded carrots and/or Chinese (Napa) cabbage

- ★ Finely sliced celery
- ★ Minced broccoli florets
- ★ Diced bell pepper (red, orange and/or yellow)

Miso Base

Second, chop the following veggies and place in <u>high-speed blender</u> along with all other ingredients. Blend until smooth and then pour over veggies in the large, stainless-steel pot:

- ★ 3-4 celery stalks
- ★ 1-2 medium carrots
- ★ 1 large avocado (peeled & pitted)
- ★ ⅓ C chickpea miso
- ★ ½ tsp sea salt (or to taste)
- ★ ¼ tsp asafoetida (or to taste)
- ★ 1 dash cayenne (or to taste)
- ★ 16 oz purified, filtered water

Optional Additions & Variation Ideas

- ★ 1-2 TBS chaga and/or shiitake mushroom powder
- ★ 1 TBS dried cilantro and/or parsley
- ★ 1 TBS spirulina

Third, prepare ONE of the following to be poured into the pot of veggies and miso base above:

- ★ 16 oz warm water (up to 150-160°F)
- ★ 16 oz brewed, loose-leaf gynostemma
- ★ 16 oz brewed, loose-leaf green tea

Finally, stir together and enjoy while still warm!

Optional Topping Ideas

- ★ Mung bean, fenugreek, sunflower, lentil or pea sprouts
- ★ Black sesame seeds
- ★ Paprika to taste

> **Allergies:** In the event that you have a known sensitivity or allergy to any of the nuts used in the creamy soup recipes (such as cashews or macadamia nuts), you may substitute with equal parts hemp seeds or sunflower seeds. These two will offer a similar consistency without altering the flavor.

Sweet Fruit Infusion Soup Ideas

Pineapple Chiller

Soup Base

Chop fruits and veggies into small chunks, place in <u>high-speed blender</u> along with all other ingredients, and then blend until smooth:

- 4 C fresh pineapple (peeled)
- 1 medium cucumber
- 2 celery stalks
- ¼ tsp sea salt (or to taste)
- 1 dash cayenne (or to taste)
- ½ lime, juiced
- ¼ C coconut crème (or 2 TBS coconut flakes with 2 TBS liquefied coconut oil)
- Up to 8 oz purified, filtered water (or until desired consistency)

Amazing Additions & Variations

- For **Pineapple-Cilantro Chiller Soup**: add 1-2 C packed, fresh cilantro (leaves and tender stems only). For a bit of a spicy kick, add ½ jalapeno pepper or up to ½ tsp of cayenne.
- For **Pineapple-Kale Chiller Soup**: add 2-3 curly or lacinato kale leaves and up to ¼ tsp of Apple Pie Blend. If needed, add a pinch or two of green leaf stevia or a drizzle of raw agave.
- For **Pineapple-Basil Chiller Soup**: add up to ¼ C fresh Thai basil leaves. If Thai basil is unavailable, substitute with ½ regular basil and ½ mint leaves. For a bit of a zesty zing, add a tad of coconut vinegar and asafoetida.

> **Recipe Notes & Quick Tips:** The best coconut crème on the market is by Vivapura. When unavailable, it is super easy to achieve the same results with coconut oil and coconut flakes (especially when making soups and smoothies in your high-speed blender). All you have to do is use half coconut oil and half coconut flakes. For instance, if the recipe calls for ¼ C coconut crème, replace with 2 TBS liquefied coconut oil and 2 TBS coconut flakes. In a couple of recipes, I only mark coconut oil as a suitable replacement. This is because the fruits (mango and papaya) add enough creaminess and texture to make up for the lack of meatiness in the coconut oil.

Tahitian Sunrise Soup

Chop fruits and veggie into small chunks, place in <u>high-speed blender</u> along with all other ingredients, and then blend until smooth:

- ★ 2 C mango (fresh or defrosted)
- ★ 1 medium red bell pepper
- ★ 1 tsp Curry Blend
- ★ ¼ tsp sea salt (or to taste)
- ★ 1 dash cayenne (or to taste)
- ★ 1 pinch whole ground vanilla bean powder
- ★ 2 TBS coconut crème (or liquefied coconut oil)
- ★ 2 TBS lemon juice
- ★ Up to 8 oz purified, filtered water (or until desired consistency)

Papaya Blush Soup

Chop fruits into small chunks, place in <u>high-speed blender</u> along with all other ingredients, and then blend until smooth:

- ★ ½ fresh papaya (seeded)
- ★ ½ C packed strawberries (fresh or defrosted)
- ★ ½ inch piece ginger root (or 2-3 drops ginger essential oil)
- ★ ¼ tsp Apple Pie Blend (or cinnamon)
- ★ 1 dash sea salt (or to taste)
- ★ 1 pinch whole ground vanilla bean powder
- ★ 1-2 whole limes, juiced (or 1 whole lemon, juiced)
- ★ 2 TBS coconut crème (or liquefied coconut oil)
- ★ Up to 8 oz purified, filtered water (or until desired consistency)

Optional Additions & Variations

- ★ 2 TBS of goji berries
- ★ Substitute a few sprigs of fresh mint leaves for the ginger and Apple Pie Blend

Spiked Blueberries & Crème Soup

Chop fruits and veggie into small chunks and place in <u>high-speed blender</u> along with all other ingredients. Blend until smooth:

- ★ 2 C wild blueberries (fresh or frozen)
- ★ 2 pears (or apples)
- ★ 2 celery stalks
- ★ ½ tsp Pumpkin or Apple Pie Blend
- ★ 1 dash sea salt
- ★ 1 pinch whole ground vanilla bean powder
- ★ 1-2 TBS raw honey or agave
- ★ 1-2 TBS coconut vinegar (or apple cider vinegar)
- ★ ¼ C coconut crème (or 2 TBS coconut flakes with 2 TBS liquefied coconut oil)
- ★ Up to 8 oz purified, filtered water (or until desired consistency)

Optional Additions

- ★ 1 TBS spirulina
- ★ Cayenne to taste

Optional Variation

- ★ For **Spiked Peaches & Crème Soup**, substitute 2 C sliced peaches (fresh or defrosted) for blueberries.

SPLENDID SALADS, SLAWS & RAWGHETTI

We've all heard it: "I'm so tired of eating salads" or "vegetables are boring." But have you really stopped to seriously think of all the fruits and vegetables there are in the world, not to mention the different varieties of each that have their own unique taste and texture to offer? What about all the various and different combinations you can creatively concoct?

Now what about what you put on your salads or vegetables? Are you using just some random oil and vinegar; maybe just a little salt and pepper? If so, then I can see how salads or a simple bowl of vegetables can get boring real fast.

We often hear that "variety is the spice of life." I would like to elaborate on this saying by stating the following: "spice is the simplest of ways to add flavor and variety to the foods in our life." If you look up the definition of salad, it goes beyond just lettuce, tomato and cucumber. I love the definition that describes salad as: "a varied mixture." This definition may be a bit generalized, but I love that it forces creativity and imagination. To think, even with the same vegetables on hand, one can quickly create a "new" salad (or "new" veggie dish) just by changing up the blend of herbs and/or spices.

Our imagination is allowed to stretch even further when we challenge ourselves to create home-made dressings from the numerous raw, plant-based foods (such as fruits, vegetables, nuts and seeds) and quality raw food condiments (such as cold-pressed oils, wholesome vinegars and natural sweeteners) that we are fortunate enough to have at our disposal today. Also, let's not forget about all the superfoods that can be utilized. Pull these precious babies out of your refrigerator and cupboards and start making good use of them!

Quick Recipe Tips:

I would like to reiterate, that although I give specific measurements at times, and at other times a range, when it comes to the more pungent of herbs and spices (such as sea salt, cayenne, asafoetida, etc.), I suggest always starting small and adding as you go. Get into the habit of tasting what you're making until the balance of flavors is just where you like it. This also goes for the addition and balance of acids (e.g., lemon, lime, apple cider vinegar or coconut vinegar), oils (e.g., extra virgin olive oil, hemp seed oil or chia seed oil) and sweeteners (e.g., raw honey or agave).

Being able to balance flavors is the key to creating a satisfyingly seasoned and perfectly flavored dish. Having simple raw ingredients, such as sea salt and natural sweeteners, can really help cover strong and pungent tastes. They can also help round out weak ones. For instance, we all know that adding sweetness to the sour and bitter tastes of lemons in lemonade can really take the edge off, but did you know that adding salt can do the same? That's right; salt can bring down the bitterness of a grapefruit or a tomato that is a bit under ripe. Salt really brings out and balances all flavors, but especially sweet. Therefore, when you want to bring out the natural sweetness of the fruits and vegetables in a recipe, try adding a pinch of salt before adding additional sweetener. On the other hand, if a recipe is a bit too salty, you're going to want to add a bit of sweet to balance the saltiness. To balance out both salty and sweet, add a food or condiment that is sour. What if a recipe is a bit too spicy from adding too much cayenne or other chili pepper? Have no fear, just add a bit more fat (e.g., avocado, nuts, seeds or oil) to absorb and tone down the heat. Where there is a will, there is always a way!

> **Please Note:** Be sure to review "Must Have Condiments" (page 29) when transforming your kitchen into one that exudes healthy, energetic and youthful living.
>
> I share only the best of the best for adding sweet, salty and sour flavors to your recipes and dishes.
>
> For only the best of the best in raw, whole food fats and quality concentrated oils, make certain to review "Getting to Know Your True "FAT" Friends" (page 81). For the best of the best of all the rest, I highly recommend a careful review of Chapter 5 (page 118). I share not only all the superfoods that will complete your raw food kitchen makeover, but many superfruits and superherbs that can have you living a longevity lifestyle!

If time allows, many salad, slaw and rawghetti recipes will be better when allowed to marinate and chill for a short while before serving. This is especially true for recipes that call for cruciferous vegetables (such as broccoli, cauliflower and cabbage) and some of the tougher root vegetables. The extra time allows the flavors to set in and the vegetables to soften and tenderize. If planning to eat within 30-45 minutes, feel free to let your dish sit covered on your countertop at room temperature. Just before serving, be sure to gently toss again, checking to see whether the dish needs additional moisture (in the form of water, acid and/or oil) or additional flavor (in the form of herbs and spices). Serve, eat and enjoy!

Although it is not necessary, you may wish to prepare certain recipes several hours before serving or the night before. I find this to be especially true for broccoli, cabbage and root veggie slaws.

SUMPTUOUS SALADS

Step 1: Go-To Garden Salad

Before exploring the more specialized and ethnic salad creations, I would like to share how easy it can be to create your very own garden salad with any combination of the following ingredients. Use the amounts I give as a guideline and don't be afraid to add a little less or a little more. In addition, by alternating your leafy greens, veggie combinations, dressings and toppings, you can have a different salad just about any day of the week!

Choose Your Leafy Green Base

Chiffonade (or finely cut into ribbon strips) large leafy greens, then place in a large mixing bowl:

- ★ Choose from either 4 C packed, mixed baby greens (aka baby spring mix); 4 C packed baby spinach; or 4 C packed, chopped endive, escarole, green leaf, red leaf, romaine, Boston bibb or any other lettuce of choice. Feel free to mix and match whatever you have on hand (for instance, red with green leaf, endive with escarole, etc.).

Choose Your Veggie Combo

Chop veggies into small bite size pieces and then add to leafy greens in mixing bowl:

- ★ 2 C (or more) of assorted chopped veggies such as cucumber, celery, roma tomato and bell pepper (red, yellow and/or orange).

Optional Additions & Variations

- Add or substitute with shredded carrots and/or cabbage; spiralized and chopped zucchini and/or summer squash; groomed and chopped snap peas, snow peas or green beans; and/or finely chopped cauliflower, broccoli, broccoli rabe, asparagus, etc.

Step 2: Go-To Salad Dressing

You may choose from any variety of salad toppers or dressings, which I explicitly and enthusiastically detail in "Mouthwatering Stove Stoppers" (page 332). In a pinch, you can very simply add any of the following ingredients to your leafy greens and veggies of choice. Just add to mixing bowl and quickly toss together until well combined and coated.

Choose Your Acid & Oil and Herbs & Spices

- Add lemon juice, lime juice, coconut vinegar or apple cider vinegar to taste.
- Add extra virgin olive oil, hemp seed oil or chia seed oil to taste.
- Add fresh or dried herbs and spices, to taste (including asafoetida for onion/garlic flavor without the onion/garlic aftertaste and breath). You may also choose from one of the home-blended spice blends (e.g., Italian, Taco or Spicy Infusion Blend).
- Add sea salt, sea vegetable flakes and/or cayenne to taste.

Optional Additions, Variations & Topping Ideas

- Add home-grown sprouts of choice (such as alfalfa, broccoli, clover, fenugreek, sunflower, lentil, pea, adzuki bean, mung bean, etc.).
- Substitute diced avocado for oil, and then toss until blended and well combined.
- Add ¼ C hemp seeds and other seeds or nuts of choice when using hemp or chia seed oil.
- Add a few tablespoons of sauerkraut (like Beagle Bay brand).
- Add a couple tablespoons of sun-dried black olives when using olive oil.
- Add 2-3 tsp of spirulina, chlorella and/or other superfood green powder and then toss until well blended.
- Sprinkle generously with up to 2 TBS nutritional yeast flakes.

> Eating healthfully doesn't have to be a daunting or elaborate task. With the right raw food condiments and superfoods right at your fingertips, along with dried herbs and your favorite spice blends, there is absolutely no excuse for not making a colorful and vibrant salad! One that is as tasty as it is good for you – and in less than 15 minutes!

Prawma Sprinkle (my raw version of parmesan sprinkle cheese)

This little combo is super easy to put together and absolutely amazing as a salad or rawghetti sprinkle. Place all the following ingredients into an airtight, glass mason jar, shake to blend together, and then refrigerate until ready to use:

- ★ ¾ C hemp seeds
- ★ 2 TBS nutritional yeast flakes (Premier Research Labs)
- ★ 1 TBS dried parsley
- ★ ½ tsp sea salt

Optional Addition

- ★ ¼ tsp cayenne (or to taste)

> **Recipe Notes & Quick Tips:** If paying attention to proper food combining, for the ultimate in proper digestion and assimilation of whole food nutrients, I highly suggest only choosing one type of dense/oily protein per meal. For instance, if you plan to have avocado (which is a dense/oily protein from the fruit family), it would be best to not overwhelm your dish with concentrated oils and/or proteins of a different type (e.g., whole nuts or seeds, nut or seed oils or legumes). This also means you would not want to add a nut/seed-based pâté, cheeze, sauce or dressings to avocado dishes.
>
> An exception to food combining rules (at least in my book) is to combine a dense/oily protein with a small amount of concentrated oil that is within the same family. This may not fly with the super radical and natural hygiene raw foodists, but I have found it to be a realistic and reasonable compromise. One that not only works for the majority (for instance, those who may be new to raw foodism), but works for a great many seasoned, yet sensible, individuals who are dedicated to mindful eating as well. I have also found it to never hinder the progress of those working through minor to major health challenge.
>
> Therefore, when formulating a recipe for better digestion, I do my best to only combine whole nuts and seeds with concentrated nut and seed oils (not with avocados). For example, when using whole nuts and seeds in a recipe (including nut/seed pâtés), I will almost always opt for seed oils such as hemp seed or chia seed oil.
>
> What about avocado-based recipes? Personally, I prefer to not add any additional fat. However, when a very smooth and creamy texture is desired (like with raw soups), I will usually add extra virgin olive oil. My justification for pairing these two together is due to both being a fruit-based fat.
>
> Keep these little tips in mind, as they can be useful when making some of your favorite recipes from other sources as well. At the very least, make it a goal to keep dense/oily proteins down to one type per mealtime, which allows for proper digestion to take place (about 2-3 hours) before having another.
>
> (Please refer to **Appendix D** for my detailed charts on proper food combining and tips for better digestion.)

Tuscan Spinach Salad

Salad Base

Chop veggies into small, bite-sized pieces and place in a large mixing bowl with all other ingredients:

- ★ 1 large bunch mature spinach (leaves & tender stems only); chiffonade cut into thin ribbons
- ★ 2-3 roma tomatoes, diced
- ★ 1 medium zucchini, diced
- ★ ⅓ C sun-dried tomatoes, presoaked & sliced into thin strips
- ★ ⅓ C sun-dried black olives, pitted (left whole or chopped in half)

Optional Additions

- ★ Add 1 diced bell pepper (red, orange or yellow).
- ★ Add ½-1 bunch finely chopped broccoli rabe (or minced broccoli florets).

Dressing

Add the following ingredients to salad base in mixing bowl and toss together until well combined and coated:

- ★ 1-2 TBS extra virgin olive oil
- ★ 1-2 TBS lemon juice
- ★ Up to 1 TBS Italian or Mediterranean Blend
- ★ 1 dash asafoetida (or 1-2 minced garlic cloves)
- ★ Sea vegetable flakes, sea salt and/or cayenne to taste

If time allows, cover and chill before serving to allow flavors to set in and veggies to soften. Then gently toss again just before serving and enjoy!

Optional Additions & Topping Ideas

- ★ Add home-grown sprouts of choice (such as alfalfa, broccoli, clover, fenugreek, sunflower, lentil, pea, adzuki bean, mung bean, etc.).
- ★ Add up to one diced avocado and then toss until blended and well combined.
- ★ Add 2-3 tsp of spirulina.
- ★ Sprinkle generously with nutritional yeast flakes.

Miso Caesar Salad

Salad Base

Chop or slice veggies into small, bite-sized pieces and place in a large mixing bowl with all other ingredients:

- ★ 1 head romaine lettuce, finely chopped
- ★ 3-4 celery stalks, finely sliced
- ★ ⅓ C sun-dried black olives, pitted (left whole or chopped in half)

Additions & Toppings

- ★ Add wakame and/or nori flakes, to taste (as replacement for anchovies).
- ★ Add nutritional yeast flakes, to taste (as replacement for parmesan).

Dressing

Please see page 361 for Miso Caesar Dressing. Another fantastic dressing (which is one of my favorites) is Hemp Caesar (page 362). Be sure to read recipes in their entirety, as I share some variations and serving ideas.

> **Please Note:** The dressing recipe for Miso Caesar (page 361) is meant to serve 1-2 people. If preparing for a large salad (as shown above), I suggest doubling the dressing recipe to make sure you have enough to cover salad. You may forgo whisking the dressing in a glass measuring cup and blend in a high-speed blender. Whichever you decide, this dressing is super simple to make. Refrigerate any that is unused. It will keep for at least 3-5 days.

Greek Isles Salad

Salad Base

Chop veggies into small, bite-sized pieces and place in a large mixing bowl with all other ingredients:

- ★ 4 C packed, mixed baby greens or 1 head romaine lettuce, finely chopped
- ★ 2-3 roma tomatoes, diced
- ★ 1 medium cucumber, diced
- ★ ⅓ C sun-dried black olives, pitted (left whole or chopped in half)

Optional Additions & Toppings

- ★ Add ⅓ C red onion, diced.
- ★ Add 2-3 tsp of spirulina.
- ★ Sprinkle generously with nutritional yeast flakes.

Dressing

Two great dressings for this salad include "Betta than Feta" Cheeze (page 346) or Cucumber Tahini (page 364). Be sure to read recipe in its entirety, as I share some variations and serving ideas.

> **Recipe Notes & Quick Tips:** Depending on salad size and the amount of dressing you personally like, you may wish to double the Cucumber Tahini dressing recipe (page 364) and refrigerate any leftover to be used within 3-5 days. Add finely chopped fresh herbs of choice (such as parsley, basil, thyme, etc.), or choose one of the options listed under "Optional Variations & Serving Ideas" on page 364. Either may be added to salad base above or to dressing base prior to blending. Modify amounts according to taste.
>
> For "Betta than Feta" Cheeze (page 346), I suggest placing about ½ C (or more, depending on how much you plan to serve) in a glass measuring cup and adding 1-2 TBS at a time of purified, filtered water and lemon juice until a creamy-like dressing consistency is reached. Toss and coat salad ingredients, adding additional Mediterranean style herbs and spices according to desired taste.

Curried Cruciferous Salad

Salad Base

Chop veggies into small, bite-sized pieces and place in a large mixing bowl with all other ingredients:

- ★ 1 large bunch mature spinach (leaves & tender stems only); chiffonade cut into thin ribbons
- ★ 2 C packed cauliflower florets, minced
- ★ 2 roma tomatoes, diced
- ★ 1 bell pepper, diced (red, orange or yellow)

Optional Variation

- ★ Substitute 2 C broccoli florets for cauliflower.

Dressing

Add the following ingredients to salad base in mixing bowl and toss together until well combined and coated:

- ★ 2-3 TBS hemp seed oil
- ★ 2-3 TBS coconut vinegar
- ★ 1 TBS raw honey or agave (optional)
- ★ 2-3 tsp Curry or Garam Masala Blend
- ★ ½ tsp sea salt (or to taste)
- ★ 1 dash asafoetida (or to taste)
- ★ 1 pinch cayenne (or to taste)

If time allows, cover and chill before serving to allow flavors to set in and veggies to tenderize. Then gently toss again just before serving and enjoy!

Optional Additions & Topping Ideas

- ★ Add home-grown sprouts of choice (such as fenugreek, sunflower, lentil, pea, adzuki bean, mung bean, etc.).
- ★ Add ¼ C hemp seeds and/or pumpkin seeds.
- ★ Sprinkle generously with nutritional yeast flakes.

Asian Cabbage Salad

Salad Base

Chop, slice or shred veggies (as described below) into small, bite-sized pieces and place in a large mixing or serving bowl with all other ingredients:

- ★ 1 head Chinese (Napa) cabbage; chiffonade cut into thin ribbons
- ★ 2-3 bok choy stalks, finely sliced
- ★ 1 red bell pepper (thinly sliced or diced)
- ★ 1 medium zucchini (or cucumber). You may either finely chop by hand or spiral cut with Spirooli. Chop a few times before adding to bowl. I suggest using small shredder attachment for zucchini and slicer attachment for cucumbers.
- ★ 1 C snow peas
- ★ ½ C shredded carrots (peeled & tops removed)
- ★ 1-2 TBS sea vegetable flakes (such as dulse, kelp, nori, wakame, etc.)

Optional Addition

- ★ Add ½-1 bunch finely chopped broccoli rabe.

Dressing

In a small glass measuring cup, whisk the following ingredients together, then add to salad base in mixing bowl and toss together until well combined and coated:

- ★ 2 TBS chickpea miso paste
- ★ 2 TBS hemp seed oil
- ★ 2 TBS coconut vinegar
- ★ 2 TBS lemon juice
- ★ 1 TBS raw honey or agave (optional)
- ★ 1-2-inch piece ginger root, minced (or 1-2 drop ginger essential oil)
- ★ ½ tsp Asian Blend (optional)
- ★ 1 dash asafoetida (or to taste)
- ★ Sea salt and/or cayenne to taste

Optional Variations

- Use Asian Dipping Sauce (page 360) or Asian Dressing (page 360) in place of dressing above.

If time allows, cover and chill before serving to allow flavors to set in and veggies to tenderize. Then gently toss again just before serving and enjoy!

Optional Additions & Topping Ideas

- Add home-grown sprouts of choice (such as alfalfa, broccoli, clover, fenugreek, sunflower, lentil, pea, adzuki bean, mung bean, etc.).
- Add ¼ C hemp seeds and/or black sesame seeds.
- Add 2-3 tsp of spirulina.
- Sprinkle with a bit of bee pollen.

Sweet & Zesty Cabbage Salad

Salad Base

Chop or shred veggies (as described below) into small, bite-sized pieces and place in a large mixing or serving bowl with all other ingredients:

- 1 small head red cabbage; chiffonade cut into thin ribbons
- 1 small bunch endive, finely chopped
- 1 C shredded carrots (peeled & tops removed)
- ½ C currants
- ½ C walnuts, chopped
- ¼ C black sesame seeds

Optional Addition

- Add one yellow bell pepper (thinly sliced or diced).

Dressing

In a <u>high-speed blender</u>, blend the following ingredients together, and then add to salad base in mixing bowl and toss together until well combined and coated:

- 2 oranges (peeled & seeded)
- ¼ C raw sesame tahini
- 2 TBS chickpea miso paste
- 2 TBS black sesame seed, hemp seed or chia seed oil
- 2-3 tsp Garam Masala Blend
- 1 TBS raw honey or agave (optional)
- 1 dash asafoetida (or to taste)
- Sea salt and/or cayenne to taste

Optional Variation

- ★ Use Island Pineapple Chutney (page 350) in the place of dressing above.

If time allows, cover and chill before serving to allow flavors to set in and veggies to tenderize. Then gently toss again just before serving and enjoy!

Optional Additions & Topping Ideas

- ★ Add home-grown sprouts of choice (such as fenugreek, sunflower, lentil, pea, adzuki bean, mung bean, etc.).
- ★ Sprinkle with raw coconut flakes and/or bee pollen.

Mexican Spring Corn Salad

Salad Base

Chop veggies into small, bite-sized pieces and place in a large mixing bowl with all other ingredients:

- ★ Corn kernels from 4 fresh, organic (GMO free) cobs of corn. Carefully remove lengthwise using a sharp knife. For easy containment of corn kernels, do over a large plate or bowl cover.
- ★ ½ C packed, fresh cilantro (finely chopped leaves & tender stems only)
- ★ 2 roma tomatoes, diced
- ★ 1 red or orange bell pepper, diced (for color variation choose orange)
- ★ 1 jalapeno pepper (seeds removed & minced)
- ★ ¼ C sun-dried black olives, pitted (left whole or chopped in half)

Dressing

Add the following ingredients to salad base in mixing bowl and toss together until well combined and coated:

- ★ 1 whole lime, juiced
- ★ 1-2 TBS coconut vinegar
- ★ 1-2 TBS extra virgin olive oil
- ★ 1-2 tsp Chili or Taco Blend
- ★ ½ tsp sea salt (or to taste)
- ★ ¼ tsp asafoetida (or to taste)

If time allows, cover and chill before serving to allow flavors to settle in. Then gently toss again just before serving and enjoy!

Optional Additions, Variations & Topping Ideas

- ★ Add home-grown sprouts of choice (such as sunflower, lentil, pea, adzuki bean, etc.).

- ★ Add 1-2 diced avocados, and then toss until blended and well combined.
- ★ Substitute chia seed oil for extra virgin olive oil and ½ C sprouted quinoa (either home-sprouted or presprouted TruRoots brand) for avocado.
- ★ Serve over a bed of baby spinach and/or chopped romaine.
- ★ Serve in Boston bibb or romaine lettuce leaves.
- ★ Sprinkle with nutritional yeast flakes and/or spirulina.
- ★ Add additional paprika and/or cayenne to taste.

Fennel & Grapefruit Salad

Salad Base

Chop or slice veggies (as described below) into small, bite-sized pieces and place in a large mixing or serving bowl with all other ingredients:

- ★ Baby arugula (whole 5 oz container)
- ★ 1-2 fennel bulbs (fronds removed & thinly sliced)
- ★ ½ C packed, fresh parsley (finely chopped leaves & tender stems only)
- ★ ¼ C packed, fresh mint (finely chopped leaves & tender stems only)
- ★ 1 pink grapefruit (peeled, seeded & finely chopped)
- ★ 2 avocados (peeled, pitted & diced)
- ★ 2-3 TBS golden berries

Optional Variations

- ★ Substitute one head finely chopped endive, escarole or romaine lettuce for arugula.
- ★ Substitute 2-3 finely chopped blood oranges (peeled & seeded) for grapefruit.
- ★ Substitute 2-3 TBS goji berries for golden berries.

Dressing

Add the following ingredients to salad base in mixing bowl and toss together until well combined and coated:

- ★ 1-2 TBS coconut vinegar
- ★ 1-2 TBS raw honey or agave (optional)
- ★ 1 ½-1-inch piece ginger root, minced (optional)
- ★ ¼ tsp sea salt (or to taste)
- ★ 1 dash cayenne (or to taste)
- ★ 1 pinch asafoetida (or to taste)

If time allows, cover and chill before serving to allow flavors to set in and veggies to tenderize. Then gently toss again just before serving and enjoy!

Optional Additions & Topping Ideas

- ★ Add home-grown sprouts of choice (such as fenugreek, sunflower, etc.).

- ★ Add a few chopped Turkish figs and/or apricots.
- ★ Add 1-2 TBS Hunza golden raisins and/or currants.
- ★ Sprinkle with raw coconut flakes and/or bee pollen.

Sprouted Quinoa Salad

Salad Base

Chop veggies (as described below) into small, bite-sized pieces and place in a large mixing or serving bowl with all other ingredients:

- ★ 4 C packed, mixed baby greens
- ★ ¾ C packed, fresh parsley, oregano, and/or cilantro (finely chopped leaves & tender stems only)
- ★ 2 roma tomatoes, diced
- ★ 1 bell pepper, diced (red, orange or yellow)
- ★ 1 medium cucumber, diced
- ★ ¾ C sprouted quinoa (home-sprouted or presprouted TruRoots brand)

Dressing

In a small glass measuring cup, whisk the following ingredients together, then add to salad base in mixing bowl and toss together until well combined and coated:

- ★ 2 TBS coconut vinegar
- ★ 2 TBS hemp seed or chia seed oil
- ★ 1 TBS chickpea miso paste
- ★ 1-2 tsp Chili Blend
- ★ ½ tsp sea salt (or to taste)
- ★ 1 dash asafoetida (or to taste)

If time allows, cover and chill before serving to allow flavors to settle in. Then gently toss again just before serving and enjoy!

Optional Additions & Topping Ideas

- ★ Add home-grown sprouts of choice (such as sunflower, lentil, pea, adzuki bean, etc.).
- ★ Sprinkle generously with nutritional yeast flakes and/or spirulina.
- ★ Add additional paprika and/or cayenne to taste.

Massaged Kale & Avocado Salad

Please see and follow step-by-step instructions below BEFORE placing all ingredients in a large mixing or serving bowl:

- ★ 1 bunch curly kale (stems removed)
- ★ 2-3 roma tomatoes, diced
- ★ 2 avocados (peeled, pitted & diced)

- ¼ C lemon juice
- 1-2 TBS Italian or Mediterranean Blend
- 1 dash asafoetida (or to taste)
- Sea salt and/or cayenne to taste

Optional Variations

- Substitute single fresh or dried herbs of choice (such as rosemary, thyme, basil, cilantro, etc.) for spice blend.

Instructions:

1. Chiffonade cut kale and place in a large mixing bowl by itself.
2. Sprinkle finely chopped kale with sea salt and massage for 2-3 minutes with your hands until kale begins to soften and wilt.
3. Cut avocados in half, remove seed, and with a knife slice a tic-tac-toe like grid through the avocado. Using a spoon, scoop avocado out of the peel.
4. Add diced avocados and gently message through the kale with your hand. If you would rather not massage with your hand, just be sure to smash up avocados a bit with two forks and toss with the kale.
5. Add diced roma tomatoes, lemon juice, herbs and spices straight into mixing bowl and toss again until all the ingredients are well combined.

If time allows, cover and chill before serving to allow flavors to set in and veggies to tenderize. Then gently toss again just before serving and enjoy!

Topping Ideas

- Sprinkle with nutritional yeast flakes and/or spirulina.

Massaged Kale & Tropical Fruit Salad

Please see and follow step-by-step instructions below BEFORE placing all ingredients in a large mixing or serving bowl:

- 1 bunch lacinato kale (stems removed)
- 2 avocados (peeled, pitted & diced)
- 1-2 C fresh mango, diced (or papaya)
- 2 whole limes, juiced
- 1 dash asafoetida (or to taste)
- Sea salt and/or cayenne to taste

Optional Additions

- Add a few sprigs of finely chopped fresh mint, cilantro and/or Thai basil (leaves & tender stems only).

Instructions:

1. Chiffonade cut kale and place in a large mixing bowl by itself.
2. Sprinkle finely chopped kale with sea salt and massage for 2-3 minutes with your hands until kale begins to soften and wilt.
3. Cut avocados in half, remove seed, and with a knife slice a tic-tac-toe like grid through the avocado. Using a spoon, scoop avocado out of the peel.
4. Add diced avocados and gently message through the kale with your hand. If you would rather not massage with your hand, just be sure to smash up avocados a bit with two forks and toss with the kale.
5. Add diced mango (or papaya), lime juice, herbs and spices straight into mixing bowl and toss again until all the ingredients are well combined.

If time allows, cover and chill before serving to allow flavors to set in and veggies to tenderize. Then gently toss again just before serving and enjoy!

Topping Ideas

- ★ Sprinkle with raw coconut flakes, bee pollen and/or spirulina.

Spiraled Beet Salad

Salad Base

Using the small shredder blade of a Spirooli (spiral 3-in-1 slicer), spiral cut the following veggie(s) and then place in a large mixing or serving bowl:

- ★ 3-4 medium-large beets (peeled & tops removed)

Optional Additions

- ★ Add 1-2 spiral cut carrots (peeled & tops removed).
- ★ Add 1 spiral cut daikon radish (peeled & tops removed).

Dressing

In a small glass measuring cup, whisk the following ingredients together, then add just enough dressing to salad base in mixing bowl to thoroughly coat spiralized veggie(s) when tossing. Reserve any additional dressing for adding when ready to serve:

- ★ 2 TBS hemp seed oil
- ★ 2 TBS lemon juice
- ★ 1 TBS coconut vinegar
- ★ 1 TBS chickpea miso paste
- ★ 1 TBS raw honey or agave (optional)
- ★ ½-1-inch piece ginger root, minced (or 1-2 drop ginger essential oil)
- ★ ¼ tsp sea salt (or to taste)

- ★ 1 dash asafoetida (or to taste)
- ★ 1 pinch cayenne (or to taste)

Optional Variations

- ★ Use Asian Dipping Sauce (page 360) or Asian Dressing (page 360) in the place of dressing above.

If time allows, cover and chill before serving to allow flavors to set in and veggies to tenderize. Then gently toss again just before serving and enjoy!

Serving & Topping Ideas

- ★ Serve on a bed of mixed baby greens, baby spinach or chiffonade cut leafy greens of choice, along with a side of additional dressing for drizzling.
- ★ Sprinkle with hemp seeds and/or coconut flakes.

SPLENDIFEROUS SLAWS

Cabbage Slaw

Slaw Base

Remove outer leaves of cabbage (including tough part of core) and prep carrots as described. Finely shred veggies in a <u>food processor</u> (using the specified blades for doing so) and place in a large mixing or serving bowl with a cover. Follow the instructions below before adding dressing:

- ★ 1 small head green cabbage
- ★ ½ small head red cabbage
- ★ 4 carrots (peeled & tops removed)

Marinade/Dressing Choices

- ★ **Maconaise** (page 352): This is my favorite all-around dressing for a basic cabbage slaw.
- ★ **Pucker-Up Mustard** (page 353): This is wonderful for a mustardy twist. Delish as a Honey Mustard Slaw when you add raw honey or agave to taste.
- ★ **"A Thousand Islands" Dressing** (page 363): I love this one for the sweet and tangy flavor it has to offer. Just another twist to traditional slaw.

Instructions:

1. Once cabbage and carrots have been shredded, sprinkle with sea salt and massage for 2-3 minutes with your hands to help soften cabbage.

2. Pick a marinade or dressing for cabbage slaw from the list above. Add enough to completely coat cabbage and carrots as you are tossing.

   Please Note: If dressing is a bit too thick, you can either add 1-2 TBS of water at a time to the actual dressing, until a desired (more pourable) consistency is reached; or you can wait and add 1-2 ounces of water to the already dressed slaw. The goal is to add just enough moisture to see your slaw go from dry and tacky to moist and creamy. You may also wish to add part water and part lemon juice or vinegar of choice. This will volumize the flavor and help tenderize the cabbage more. You can also add a bit more oil and spice if desired.

3. The final step is to cover and allow your cabbage slaw to marinate for several hours or overnight in the refrigerator. This will allow the flavors to set in and the cabbage to further soften. If just marinating for a few hours, I suggest doing this at room temperature. Gently toss again just before serving, add more moisture if needed and enjoy!

Serving & Topping Ideas

- ★ Serve on a bed of mixed baby greens, baby spinach or chiffonade cut leafy greens of choice, along with a side of additional dressing for drizzling.
- ★ Sprinkle and toss with unhulled back sesame seeds, pumpkin seeds and/or hemp seeds.
- ★ Sprinkle with nutritional yeast and/or spirulina.

Asian Root Veggie Slaw

Slaw Base

Scrub, wash and peel the root veggies below. Finely shred veggies in a <u>food processor</u> (using the specified blade for doing so) and place in a large mixing or serving bowl with a cover. Follow the instructions below before adding dressing:

- ★ 1 celery root (peeled & top removed)
- ★ 3-4 carrots (peeled & tops removed)
- ★ 2-3 daikon radishes (peeled & tops removed)

Optional Variation

- ★ Toss a handful of groomed snap or snow peas, some finely chopped fresh Thai basil leaves and some cilantro into the bowl. You now have a Thai Infused Root Veggie Slaw.

Marinade/Dressing Choices

- ★ **Asian Dipping Sauce** (page 360): This is my favorite marinade for making Thai Slaw. Although the recipe calls for ginger, I sometimes like to substitute a few drops

of lime peel oil for the ginger, then add the herbs and peas I suggest above under "Optional Variations."
- ★ **Asian Dressing** (page 360): I make this dressing often for salads, cabbage slaws, root veggie slaws and broccoli slaw. It is one of my favorites. When adding to a large slaw, feel free to add a bit more Asian Blend. Don't go overboard though, as a little goes a long way. Start by adding ¼ tsp at a time if you desire more spice.
- ★ **Thai-Hini Dressings** (page 363): Another go-to dressing that I love for salads and slaws of all kinds. Feel free to add in extra cayenne or fresh chili peppers of choice to up the heat!

Instructions:

1. Once all the root veggies have been shredded, sprinkle with sea salt and massage for 2-3 minutes with your hands to help soften.
2. Pick a marinade or dressing for root veggie slaw from the list above. Add enough to completely coat root veggies as you are tossing.

    Please Note: If dressing is a bit too thick, you can either add 1-2 TBS of water at a time to the actual dressing, until a desired (more pourable) consistency is reached; or you can wait and add 1-2 ounces of water to the already dressed slaw. The goal is to add just enough moisture to see your slaw go from dry and tacky to moist and creamy. You may also wish to add part water and part lemon juice or vinegar of choice. This will volumize the flavor and help to tenderize the root veggies more. You can also add a bit more oil and spice if desired.

3. The final step is to cover and allow your root veggie slaw to marinate for several hours or overnight in the refrigerator. This will allow the flavors to set in and the root veggies to further soften. If just marinating for a few hours, I suggest doing so at room temperature. Gently toss again just before serving, add more moisture if needed and enjoy!

Serving & Topping Ideas

- ★ Serve on a bed of mixed baby greens, baby spinach or chiffonade cut leafy greens of choice, along with a side of additional dressing for drizzling.
- ★ Sprinkle and toss with unhulled back sesame seeds, hemp seeds and/or cashews.
- ★ Sprinkle with nutritional yeast and/or spirulina.

Broccoli Slaw

Slaw Base

Remove outer leaves of cabbage (including tough part of core), prep carrots and broccoli as described (please see full instructions below), and finely shred cabbage, carrots and broccoli stalk in a <u>food processor</u> (using the specified blades for doing so). Then place shredded veggies and minced broccoli florets in a large mixing or serving bowl with a cover:

- 1 bunch broccoli
- 4 carrots (peeled & tops removed)
- ½ small head red cabbage

Marinade/Dressing Choices

Please read recipes in their entirety for other ideas and inspiration. Also read my notes for each of these dressings under Cabbage Slaw (page 325) and Asian Root Veggie Slaw (page 326):

- Maconaise (page 352)
- Pucker-Up Mustard (page 353)
- Asian Dipping Sauce (page 360)
- Asian Dressing (page 360)
- Thai-Hini Dressings (page 363)
- "A Thousand Islands" Dressing (page 363)

Instructions:

1. Chop broccoli florets from the stalk (reserving stalk), and then finely chop florets until minced. Place minced broccoli florets into mixing bowl.
2. Next, cut 1-2 inches off the bottom of the reserved broccoli stalk (or stem) and then peel outer tough skin using a vegetable peeler.
3. Use the same blade that would be used for shredding carrots to shred your broccoli stalk. Add shredded broccoli stalk to minced broccoli florets in your mixing bowl.
4. Shred peeled carrots and red cabbage using appropriate blades and then add them to broccoli in mixing bowl.
5. Sprinkle shredded, minced and chopped veggies with sea salt and massage for 2-3 minutes with your hands to help soften.
6. Pick a marinade or dressing for broccoli slaw from the list above. Add enough to completely coat your veggies as you are tossing.

   Please Note: If dressing is a bit too thick, you can either add 1-2 TBS of water at a time to the actual dressing, until a desired (more pourable) consistency is reached; or you can wait and add 1-2 ounces of water to the already dressed slaw. The goal is to add just enough moisture to see your slaw go from dry and tacky to moist and creamy. You may also wish to add part water and part lemon juice or vinegar of choice. This will volumize the flavor and help tenderize veggies more. You can also add a bit more oil and spice if desired.

7. The final step is to cover and allow your broccoli slaw to marinate for several hours or overnight in the refrigerator. This will allow the flavors to set in and the veggies to further soften. If just marinating for a few hours, I suggest doing at room temperature. Gently toss again just before serving, add more moisture if needed and enjoy!

Serving & Topping Ideas

- ★ Serve on a bed of mixed baby greens, baby spinach or chiffonade cut leafy greens of choice, along with a side of additional dressing for drizzling.
- ★ Sprinkle and toss with unhulled back and tan sesame seeds and/or hemp seeds.
- ★ Sprinkle with nutritional yeast and/or spirulina.

RAWLICIOUS RAWGHETTI

My idea of rawghetti is any vegetable that can be created into noodle-like strands. The two best vegetables that take home the title for best rawghetti creators are zucchini and summer squash. They have a perfect texture (not too soft and not too hard) and a perfect mild to bland taste. Two other contenders are actually sea vegetables. Mineral rich kelp noodles and arame seaweed come prepackaged and ready to blow your old nutritionless pasta and rice noodles away. Arame is seaweed, but one that gets a thumbs up from sea vegetable newbies for its mild flavor; and kelp noodles have zero taste, zero fat and zero gluten! They are also extremely low in carbohydrates and calories.

Whether you choose zucchini, summer squash, kelp noodles or arame seaweed, all of the above will bring back the joy of twirling noodles around a fork. Each are also mild in taste, making these the perfect base for your raw sauce or dressing creation. I truly love how they allow for the wholesome flavors to soak in, stand out and really pop! On page 331 I share some favorite raw spin-offs of cooked classics, but in reality any sauce or dressing under "Mouthwatering Stove Stoppers" (page 332) can be utilized as a mouthwatering rawghetti topper. Explore your favorite flavors and enjoy the fun of the process.

Zucchini & Summer Squash Rawghetti

Follow the following step-by-step instructions for spiral cutting zucchini or summer squash when planning to make a rawghetti dish with either of these two vegetables:

1. For Zucchini & Summer Squash Rawghetti you will need a Spirooli (spiral 3-in-1 slicer).
2. Choose the smaller of the two shredder blades and follow the illustrated instructions on the box for spiralizing. You may choose to peel zucchini or summer squash or keep the skin intact (which is what I prefer). Just be sure to thoroughly wash the outer skin and chop the ends off before placing zucchini or summer squash in position for spiraling. Also, be careful when locking the blades in position, as they are sharper than they look.
3. For a personal serving, I usually like to use two medium zucchinis or two medium summer squashes. If you are making rawghetti for more than one person, or would like to prep for more than one meal ahead of time, plan to spiral cut two zucchini or summer squashes per serving.
4. Once you are done spiralizing, give the long strands a few course chops for easier twirling.

5. Pour your dressing of choice over your spiralized veggies, allowing them to marinate for at least 20-30 minutes (if time permits).
6. Remove the amount you plan to eat and store the remainder in the fridge for your next meal. Marinated spiralized veggies are great eaten alone or tossed onto a bed of mixed greens.
7. Feel free to add any combinations of chopped, diced and/or shredded veggies to the mix (such as bell peppers, carrots, tomatoes, etc.) to make this meal as colorful as it is complete!

Kelp Noodle Rawghetti

Follow the following step-by-step instructions when preparing kelp noodles for your rawghetti or Asian noodle dishes:

1. For Rawghetti made with Kelp Noodles you will need to look for a supplier that carries the Sea Tangle brand. I like the 1 lb bags, which is the perfect amount for preparing enough for 2-3 servings.
2. A real simple way of preparing these noodles is to rinse them thoroughly in a large fine mesh strainer. I love using a salad spinner for this task. I can soak them for a few minutes, while detangling them, and then rinse, drain and spin the excess water out quickly and easily.
3. Once rinsed, detangled and drained, I suggest giving the noodles a couple of course chops to shorten the strands a bit. This will make it easier to twirl around a fork.
4. Pour your dressing of choice over the kelp noodles and allow them to marinate for at least 20-30 minutes. Remove the amount you plan to eat and store the remainder in the fridge for your next meal.
5. Marinated kelp noodles are great on their own or tossed onto a bed of mixed greens.
6. Feel free to add any combinations of chopped, diced and/or shredded veggies to the mix (cabbage, carrots, radishes, etc.) to make this meal as colorful as it is complete!

Arame Seaweed Rawghetti

Follow the following step-by-step instructions when preparing arame seaweed for your rawghetti or Asian noodle dishes:

1. For Rawghetti made with Arame Seaweed you will need to look for arame in the seaweed section of your natural grocery store. I recommend the brand Emerald Cove. They offer an Organic Pacific Arame that is wonderful.
2. A simple way to prepare these noodles is to place the contents of the entire bag into a glass bowl.
3. Pour just enough room temperature to slightly warmer water over them in order to just cover them. Then allow soaking for 10-15 minutes.
4. When time is up, drain the water out using a fine mesh strainer, and then place the rehydrated arame back into the bowl.

5. Pour your dressing of choice over the arame and allow it to marinate for at least 20-30 minutes. Remove the amount you plan to eat and store the remainder in the fridge for your next meal. Marinated arame seaweed is great by itself or tossed onto a bed of mixed greens.
6. Feel free to add any combinations of chopped, diced and/or shredded veggies to the mix (bell pepper, celery, cucumber, etc.) to make this meal as colorful as it is complete!

Rawghetti Sauce & Dressing Options

My inspiration for creating the following sauces and dressings came from a longing for classic flavors. I wanted flavors reminiscent of my childhood. Believe it or not, I actually enjoy these raw renditions better than traditional cooked versions, but please don't tell my nana that! I suggest starting out with what I have listed below, and then feel free to experiment with all the others found under "Sexy Sauces & Dressings" on page 357.

- ★ Hemp Pesto Sauce (page 357)
- ★ Popeye's Pesto Sauce (page 357)
- ★ Alfrawdo Sauce (page 358)
- ★ Marawnara Sauce (page 358)
- ★ Asian Dressing (page 360)
- ★ Miso Caesar Dressing (page 361)
- ★ Hemp Caesar Dressing (page 362)
- ★ Thai-Hini Dressing (page 363)

Serving & Topping Ideas

- ★ Serve on a bed of mixed baby greens, baby spinach or chiffonade cut leafy greens of choice.
- ★ For even more Mediterranean infusion when using Hemp Pesto Sauce, Popeye's Pesto Sauce or Alfrawdo Sauce, top with some fresh, chopped roma tomatoes, a few presoaked and thinly sliced sun-dried tomatoes and several chopped, sun-dried black olives. Finish with a generous sprinkle of nutritional yeast flakes.
- ★ Rawghetti with Alfrawdo Sauce is divine with minced broccoli rabe (or even minced broccoli florets), presoaked and thinly sliced sun-dried tomatoes and chopped, sun-dried black olives.
- ★ Rawghetti with Marawnara Sauce, Miso Caesar Dressing or Hemp Caesar Dressing is beautiful when tossed with fresh, finely chopped herbs (such as Italian parsley, basil or rosemary) and chopped, sun-dried black olives.
- ★ If you have a dehydrator, I highly suggest making Italian-style nut/seed balls (page 345) out of the Italian Stallion Pâté (page 341). These make a rawsome alternative to traditional meatballs that will have your family and friends marveling!

★ When marinating with Asian Dressing or Thai-Hini Dressing, toss in some finely sliced bell peppers (red or yellow for color variation), shredded carrots, chopped asparagus and some finely sliced shiitakes (fresh or rehydrated from dried). Then sprinkle with black sesame and/or hemp seeds.

Mouthwatering Stove Stoppers

From pâtés and spreads to sauces and dressings, these creatively satisfying raw food fillers and toppers will have you convinced that raw food is not just for rabbits! The recipes you are about to explore are super easy to make and super scrum-delicious to eat. What's more, they can serve many purposes. Left thick, with the least amount of water, and you have a perfect pâté or dip; thinned out, by adding a bit more water, and now you have a divine dressing. The sky is the limit as to what you can create.

Remixing old favorites is not just for deejays!

Herbs and spices are the movers and the shakers that can really seal the deal in any recipe conception! With just the right blend, you can be totally transcended to a different part of the world any day of the week. Furthermore, you can quickly and easily revolutionize any combination of whole food ingredients into flavorful, raw vegetarian dishes. Dishes that will tantalize your taste buds while you satisfyingly reminisce about old cooked and comfort food favorites.

If you learn and take anything from the recipes I share, promise that you will not be afraid to experiment with the many herbs and spices of the world. Fresh or dried, herbs and spices can bring new life to the same foods, transform others completely, and take some to the next stratosphere!

Quick Recipe Tips:

I like to use chickpea miso paste for the touch of creaminess, natural sweetness, and saltiness it has to offer many savory recipes. I also love the idea of sneaking in fermented foods in any way I can. With digestion being one of the most complicated bodily processes, it is really a great idea to incorporate foods that can give the digestive system a leg-up. Through all the friendly bacteria fermented foods produce, we can significantly increase our ability to breakdown carbohydrates, proteins and fats much more efficiently, not to mention boost our absorption and assimilation capacity of essential vitamins and minerals.

Fermented foods have been used for centuries throughout Asia, Europe and the Middle East for not only providing a good amount of probiotics, but prebiotics as well.

> **Please Note:** Although I highly encourage the regular use of a high-quality, organic chickpea miso (South River Co. or Miso Master), if unavailable, you can always substitute with additional sea salt (for flavor balance) and oil (for creaminess and consistency). I've found the following to work best: 1 TBS chickpea miso paste = ¼ tsp sea salt and 1 TBS oil. Liquefied coconut oil is my 1st choice, but you may also use hemp seed oil, chia seed oil or a combo (such as coconut and hemp seed oil). Therefore, if a recipe calls for 2 TBS chickpea miso paste, replace with an additional ½ tsp sea salt and 2 TBS oil of choice. Add more if needed until desired taste and texture is reached.

Some of my recipes call for raw sesame tahini, which is ground sesame seeds made into a paste. Tahini is very popular in Greek, Middle Eastern, North African and Turkish cuisine. Raw sesame tahini is rich in whole food calcium and makes for a great spread or quick dressing straight out of the jar. It is heavenly with raw honey and/or just a squeeze of lemon. That being said, a high-quality raw sesame tahini can get a bit pricey when using ½ C (or more) at a time. If you love tahini as much as I do, I suggest having one bottle of high-quality sesame tahini for snacking, special occasions, and for making simple tahini specific dressings. For all other occasions, there is no reason why you cannot substitute with tan sesame seeds (pre-soaked preferred) and a bit of a complimentary oil as needed; especially when a recipe calls for using a high-speed blender and includes other nuts, seeds and/or oil in the mix.

> **Please Note:** In recipes that call for raw sesame tahini, feel free to substitute every ¼ with ⅓ C unhulled, tan sesame seeds. Why do I say unhulled rather than hulled? The hull is where all the calcium is, that's why. Just be sure to presoak sesame seeds in sea salted water at room temperature, drain, and then rinse thoroughly before using in a recipe. This will neutralize the protective anti-nutrients, thereby increasing digestibility of all the essential nutrients.
>
> So, if a recipe calls for ½ C raw sesame tahini, replace with ⅔ C unhulled, tan sesame seeds. In addition, for every ¼ C of raw sesame tahini that is called for, add up to 1 TBS of oil for better emulsification and consistency. Therefore, in a recipe that calls for ½ C raw sesame tahini, you may either add 1-2 TBS oil of choice, or increase the oil already called for by 1-2 TBS. During a six-month period where there was no raw sesame tahini to be found (due to supply and demand issues), this was my solution. It worked out beautifully and never altered any of my blended recipes.
>
> Although I encourage the use of omega-3 rich oils (such as hemp seed and chia seed oil) to help counterbalance the higher amounts of omega-6 naturally found in most foods, I sometimes make an exception when using sesame seeds in savory recipes. For a richer and more intense sesame flavor, that is sure to compliment the intention behind the use of sesame seeds, I suggest nothing less than the highest quality <u>black</u> sesame seed oil on the market. One that is organic, raw and truly cold-pressed (not toasted). The two brands I recommend are Alive Foods and Andreas Oils (which are the same two I recommend for chia seed oil). **FYI:** <u>Black</u> sesame seed oil is abundantly rich in antioxidants. Furthermore, <u>black</u> sesame seed oil is the most suitable for medicinal purposes out of all sesame seed/oil varieties.

When making any recipe (e.g., pâtés, dips or dressings) in a high-speed blender, use a thick silicone spatula (with strong, defined edges) to carefully push down contents that are accumulating along the sides of the pitcher. This will keep all your ingredients moving toward the center. Just be sure to keep a good grip on your spatula, and don't push it directly down the center towards the spinning blade. Do the same with recipes you plan to make in a food processor. Every so often take the cover off and push the contents down.

Always taste recipes for seasoning before serving. Depending on your goal – dip or spread versus sauce or dressing – you may need to add more liquid. This can easily be done by adding small amounts of water at a time. On the other hand, if planning to use a recipe as a dressing or marinade that will need to cover a large amount of veggies, you can always add additional lemon juice, lime juice or vinegar for a bit more zing, and/or more oil for some slippery coating action.

> **Please Note:** Many times, when a recipe is left to sit in the fridge, it will naturally congeal and thicken. This often happens with nuts and/or seeds that have not been presoaked. It will also happen with drier root veggies and cruciferous veggies (such as cabbage, cauliflower and broccoli). These ingredients lack fluid content and, as a result, will sponge up a lot of the liquid that was added during the recipe making and/or marinating process.
>
> **With the laws of nature come the laws of balance.**
>
> What do you do when a recipe thickens that was intended to be used as pourable dressing? Simply add small amounts of fluid until desired consistency is reached. Then check to make sure herbs and spices are to your liking and have not become diluted. I suggest adding only 1 TBS of water at a time. In most cases a recipe will only need 1-2 oz of additional fluid, which equates to 2-4 TBS.
>
> What do you do if this happens to a finished marinated cabbage slaw or veggie dish? Simply add more of the dressing being used as the marinade, and maybe a bit more water if needed. You can also choose to add extra lemon, lime, vinegar and/or oil. Don't forget to taste and add more seasoning if needed.
>
> Another great tip is to pull out the amount you plan to eat or serve that mealtime and let it sit on your countertop at room temperature for a while. Sometimes it's just a matter of the oils (saturated and monounsaturated) needing to warm up to room temperature in order to soften and reliquify.

While on the topic of water content, I would like to further explain why a range (rather than an exact measurement) is given when it comes to the addition of water. It basically comes down to this – the amount of water needed will vary, and by how much (or how little) can depend upon a number of things: the type of blender and food processor you currently possess (horsepower, speed, blade quality, etc.); whether or not you choose to presoak nuts and seeds; the size and juiciness (or lack thereof) of fruits and vegetables; the purpose and intended use the recipe is to serve (a thicker dip or spread versus a thinner sauce or dressing); and/or personal preference when it comes to consistency (do you like it thick, thin or somewhere in between?). Giving a range not only allows for the unforeseen, but for more options and preferences. Who can't appreciate the freedom to choose!

Many recipes will keep up to one week or longer when stored properly in a tightly closed container (preferably glass) in the refrigerator. Unless otherwise stated, I suggest planning out your meals. This way certain recipes can be appropriately paired and leftovers can be finished within one week. In fact, you will find that many recipes become more flavorful the longer they sit and marinate. I actually love leftovers for this reason. With the laws of nature in full effect, a new experience can be appreciated and enjoyed with each passing meal.

Protein Packed Pâtés

Brazilian Sunrise Pâté

Chop veggies into small chunks and then combine with all other ingredients in a food processor. Process until well combined. Be sure to add water a little at a time for a consistency that is wet and creamy, yet still thick, rich and spreadable:

- 2 C Brazil nuts (rinsed only)
- 2 celery stalks
- 1 red bell pepper
- 1 ½ TBS Curry Blend
- 1 ½ TBS dried basil
- 1 ½ TBS dried cilantro
- 1 tsp sea salt (or to taste)
- ¼ tsp asafoetida
- 1 dash cayenne (or to taste)
- 2 TBS coconut vinegar

Optional Serving Ideas

- Heavenly as a salad topper; as a spread for kale, lettuce or collard wraps; or as dips for veggies, flax and/or chia seed crackers.
- If you have a dehydrator, the following is fabulous: cut one (or more) bell peppers in half and stuff each half generously with nut pâté. Dehydrate at 115°F for 4-6 hours. Serve and enjoy! This is easily one of my favorite little dishes!

"Hold the Chicken" Salad Pâté

Chop celery into small chunks and then combine with all other ingredients in a food processor. Process until well combined. Be sure to add water a little at a time for a consistency that is wet and creamy, yet still thick, rich and spreadable:

- 1 ½ C Brazil nuts (rinsed only)
- ½ C sunflower seeds
- 2 celery stalks
- 2 TBS Poultry Blend
- 1 tsp sea salt (or to taste)
- ¼ tsp asafoetida
- ¼ tsp paprika
- ¼ tsp cumin
- 1 dash ground mustard seeds
- ¼ C lemon juice
- 2 TBS hemp seed or chia seed oil
- 3-4 oz purified, filtered water (more as needed)

Optional Variations

- ★ Substitute 1-2 TBS apple cider vinegar and a ½ juiced lemon for a ¼ C juiced lemon.
- ★ Substitute 1 tsp Curry blend for cumin and mustard seeds.
- ★ Substitute 1 ½ C pecans for Brazil nuts.
- ★ Substitute ½ C hemp or pumpkin seeds for sunflower seeds.

FYI: The 1 ½ C pecan and ½ C pumpkin seed combo is one of my favorite variations to this recipe. Brazil nuts (or pecans) with pumpkin seeds make a perfect tasting pâté for the holidays.

Transfer the above pâté into a mixing bowl, add the following veggies as described and then stir until well combined:

- ★ ¼ C shredded carrots
- ★ 1-2 finely sliced and diced celery stalks
- ★ 1-2 finely sliced and diced radishes (optional)

Optional Serving Ideas

- ★ Yummy as a salad topper; as a spread for kale, lettuce or collard wraps; or as dips for veggies flax and/or chia seed crackers.
- ★ Try tossed in a colorful blend of Boston bib, radicchio and arugula lettuce.
- ★ Serve in whole radicchio leaves as "stuffed radicchio cups."
- ★ For a sweet variation: add some shredded carrot, finely sliced celery and a sweet red apple (such as Jonalgold, McIntosh or Pink Lady) to your favorite chiffonade cut leafy greens (like kale) and then smother with a scoop or two of pâté.
- ★ If you have a dehydrator: divide this pâté into four portions on a sheeted tray; mold into oval shaped mounds that look like mini loafs. Dehydrate at 105-115°F until the outside has formed a brown crust. Remove from sheeted tray and place directly on mesh screen to dry and brown the underneath. Try the Brazil nut (or pecan) and pumpkin seed combo and you will really have something special to be thankful for on Thanksgiving! I call this my "Go-To Pâté for the Holidays."

"Hold the Egg" Salad Pâté

Blend the following ingredients together in a <u>high-speed blender</u> until smooth and creamy:

- ★ 1 C cashews
- ★ ½ C macadamia nuts
- ★ 1 tsp turmeric
- ★ 1 tsp ground mustard seeds
- ★ ½ tsp sea salt (or to taste)
- ★ ½ tsp paprika
- ★ ¼ tsp asafoetida
- ★ 1 TBS apple cider vinegar
- ★ ¼ C lemon juice

- ★ 4 oz purified, filtered water (more if desired)

Transfer the above pâté into a mixing bowl, add the following veggies as described and then stir until well combined:

- ★ ½ C finely chopped daikon radish or red radish (pulse-chop in a mini food processor to make this task quick and easy)
- ★ ½ diced red bell pepper and/or 1 diced roma tomato
- ★ 1-2 finely sliced and diced celery stalks

Optional Serving Ideas

- ★ Scrumptiously satisfying tossed in a baby spinach or spring mix salad along with a combo of your favorite salad veggies. Trust me. You will not need a drip of any other dressing, as this pâté covers it all!
- ★ Great as a spread in a kale, lettuce or collard wrap along with diced veggies of choice and a handful of baby spring mix. This is a Rawk Star Café favorite!
- ★ Awesome as the dip for an appetizer of chopped veggies. How about with flax or chia crackers? Even kids love this raw creation!

"Hold the Tuna" Salad Pâté

Chop veggies into small chunks and then combine with all other ingredients in a food processor. Process until well combined. Be sure to add water a little at a time for a consistency that is wet and creamy, yet still thick, rich and spreadable:

- ★ 2 C sunflower seeds
- ★ 2 celery stalks
- ★ 2 roma tomatoes
- ★ 2 TBS chickpea miso paste
- ★ 1 TBS kelp (flakes or power)
- ★ 1 TBS dulse flakes (or Triple Blend Flakes)
- ★ 1 TBS Spicy Infusion Blend
- ★ ½ tsp sea salt (or to taste)
- ★ ¼ tsp asafoetida
- ★ ¼ C lemon juice
- ★ 3-4 oz purified, filtered water (more only if desired)

Transfer the above pâté into a mixing bowl, add the following veggies as described and then stir until well combined:

- ★ 1-2 finely sliced and diced celery stalks

Optional Variations & Serving Ideas

- ★ Substitute 1 tsp only of Asian Blend and 1 dash of 100% wasabi powder (optional) for the 1 TBS of Spicy Infusion Blend. This is great served on Chinese (Napa) cabbage leaves and sprinkled with additional dulse or Triple Blend Flakes. Also great as a spread with the addition of finely sliced veggies in a nori wrap.
- ★ Substitute 2-3 tsp dried dill weed for Spicy Infusion Blend. This variation is delish when served on a bed of finely chopped lettuces and cucumber that has been ribbon sliced with a Spirooli. I suggest lightly chopping your ribbons before dispersing through your salad. Sprinkle with additional dill, dulse and/or Triple Blend Flakes for a colorful garnish.
- ★ All variations are amazing as salad toppers, as spreads for leafy green and nori wraps, or as dips for veggies, flax and/or chia seed crackers.

Re-Fined Bean Pâtés

First, add the following veggies (as described and in the order I have listed) to a <u>food processor</u>. Process until finely chopped/shredded and well combined:

- ★ ¼ head of red cabbage; chopped a few times and distributed evenly at the bottom of food processor
- ★ 2 C packed baby spinach; distributed evenly on top of red cabbage
- ★ 1 C sun-dried tomatoes (presoaked); distributed evenly on top of red cabbage

Second, place all the following ingredients on top of veggies already in food processor. Process until well combined. Be sure to add water a little at a time for a consistency that is wet and creamy, yet still thick, rich and spreadable:

- ★ 2 C sunflower seeds
- ★ 2 TBS chickpea miso paste
- ★ 1 TBS Chili Blend
- ★ ½ tsp coriander
- ★ ½ tsp sea salt (or to taste)
- ★ ½ tsp asafoetida
- ★ 3-4 oz purified, filtered water (more as needed)

Optional Serving Ideas

- ★ Delish as a salad topper; as a spread for kale, lettuce or collard wraps; or as dips for veggies, flax and/or chia seed crackers.

- Using a large collard, or 2 large overlapping lettuce leaves, create a veggie burrito or enchilada! Start by adding pâté first, and then top with your choice of jicama, turnip or cauliflower rice (page 348). For a burrito style wrap, sprinkle with nutritional yeast flakes and add a dollop or two of Sour Nut Crème (page 345). For more of an enchilada style, layer with Enchilada Sauce instead (page 359). Now you're ready to garnish with any or all of the following, and then tuck one end as you tightly roll up: diced roma tomatoes, diced bell pepper (red, orange or yellow), chopped black olives, minced jalapenos, shredded carrots, baby spinach leaves and/or sprouted legumes. No doubt, this will become a family fun fiesta night tradition!
- If you have a dehydrator you can go one step further by placing your burritos or enchiladas in the dehydrator for a few hours at 115°F. This really helps to bring out all the savory Mexican flavors.

Raw Rancho Taco Pâtés

Add the following ingredients to <u>food processor</u>. Process until well combined. Be sure to add water a little at a time for a consistency that is wet and creamy, yet still thick, rich and spreadable:

- 2 C walnuts
- 2 roma tomatoes
- 2 TBS chickpea miso paste
- 1 TBS Taco Blend
- ½ tsp coriander
- ½ tsp sea salt (or to taste)
- ¼ tsp asafoetida
- 3-4 oz purified, filtered water (more if desired)

Optional Serving Ideas

- Fiesta fabulous as a salad topper; as a spread for kale, lettuce or collard wraps; or as dips for veggies, flax and/or chia seed crackers.
- Make tacos by using romaine, cabbage or smaller sized collard leaves as the shells. Start by adding pâté first, and then top with diced roma tomatoes, diced bell peppers (red, orange or yellow), chopped black olives and minced jalapenos. As an alternative or addition to individual diced veggies, top with fresh Tomato Salsa (page 348). Sprinkle the top with nutritional yeast flakes, a dollop of Sour Nut Crème (page 345) or Macho Nacho Cheeze (page 346), and you have another fiesta-filled night!
- Prior to serving, you can place a bowl of this pâté in the dehydrator for a couple of hours in order to warm and lightly brown it up. It will help amplify the flavors a bit as well.

Italian Stallion Pâtés

Chop celery into small chunks and then combine with all other ingredients in a <u>food processor</u>. Process until well combined. Be sure to add water a little at a time for a consistency that is wet and creamy, yet still thick, rich and spreadable:

- ★ 1 ½ C walnuts
- ★ ½ C pumpkin seeds
- ★ 2 celery stalks
- ★ 1-2 TBS Italian Blend
- ★ 1 tsp dried fennel seed
- ★ 1 tsp sea salt (or to taste)
- ★ ¼ tsp asafoetida
- ★ ¼ tsp cayenne (or to taste)
- ★ ¼ tsp cumin
- ★ 2 TBS hemp seed or chia seed oil
- ★ 3-4 oz purified, filtered water (more as needed)

Optional Variations

- ★ Substitute sunflower seeds for pumpkin seeds or use all walnuts.

Optional Serving Ideas

- ★ Great as a salad topper; as a spread for kale, lettuce or collard wraps; or as dips for veggies, flax and/or chia seed crackers.
- ★ If you have a dehydrator, this pâté makes for a fabulous raw version to traditional Italian-style meatballs (see box on page 345 for instructions). Your Italian-style nut/seed balls will be a hit served with kelp or zucchini noodles marinated in Marawnara (page 358) or Alfrawdo Sauce (page 358). Now that's amore!
- ★ Another idea is to form pâté into patties prior to dehydrating. Now you have Italian-style mini burgers! If you would like them to be more of a traditional size, just use a 3-4 oz squeeze handle disher instead (see box on page 345).

Greek Gyraw Pâtés

Chop apple and bell pepper into small chunks and then combine with all other ingredients in a <u>food processor</u>. Process until well combined. Be sure to add water a little at a time for a consistency that is wet and creamy, yet still thick, rich and spreadable:

- ★ 1 ½ C pecans
- ★ ½ C pumpkin seeds
- ★ 1 small red apple (Braeburn, Fuji, Gala, Pink Lady, etc.)
- ★ ½ red bell pepper
- ★ 2 TBS chickpea miso paste
- ★ 1 TBS Mediterranean Blend
- ★ 1 TBS Poultry Blend

- ★ ½ tsp sea salt (or to taste)
- ★ ¼ tsp asafoetida
- ★ ¼ tsp cayenne (or to taste)
- ★ ¼ tsp cumin
- ★ 3-4 oz purified, filtered water (more as needed)

Optional Variations

- ★ Substitute walnuts for pumpkin seeds or use all pecans.
- ★ Add up to 1 tsp dried fennel seed.

Optional Serving Ideas

- ★ Scrumptious as a salad topper; as a spread for kale, lettuce or collard wraps; or as dips for veggies, flax and/or chia seed crackers.
- ★ This pâté is satisfyingly yummy served as is, yet it also makes the perfect base for creating a tasty raw version to the traditional gyro burger when you have a dehydrator (see box on page 345 for instructions).
- ★ Try this pâté, either as is or as a dehydrated burger, served up in a romaine lettuce leaf, drizzled with a simple Cucumber Tahini Dressing (page 364), and alongside a generous serving of Hemp Tabouli Salad (page 352) and cucumber slices. This combo is also spectacular all wrapped up in a collard leaf.

Marvelous Mediterranean Falafel Pâtés

Chop celery into small chunks and then combine with all other ingredients in a <u>food processor</u>. Process until well combined. Be sure to add water a little at a time for a consistency that is wet and creamy, yet still thick, rich and spreadable:

- ★ 1 ½ C walnuts
- ★ ½ C sunflower seeds
- ★ 2 celery stalks
- ★ 2 TBS chickpea miso paste
- ★ 1-2 TBS Mediterranean Blend
- ★ 1-2 tsp dried thyme
- ★ ½ tsp sea salt (or to taste)
- ★ ½ tsp paprika
- ★ ¼ tsp asafoetida
- ★ 3-4 oz purified, filtered water (more as needed)

Optional Variations

- ★ Substitute pumpkin seeds for sunflower seeds or use all walnuts.

Optional Serving Ideas

- ★ Heavenly as a salad topper; as a spread for kale, lettuce or collard wraps; or as dips for veggies, flax and/or chia seed crackers.
- ★ Delicious served as is! However, if you have a dehydrator, this pâté makes the perfect base for creating a delectable raw version to traditional falafel balls (see box on page 345 for instructions).
- ★ Whether serving as is or as dehydrated falafel balls, this pâté is delish when drizzled with a simple Cucumber Tahini Dressing (page 364) and served alongside a generous serving of Hemp Tabouli Salad (page 352) and cucumber slices. This exact combo is also delightful all wrapped up in a collard leaf.

Rawkin' Burgers (dehydrator needed)

First, chop veggies into small chunks. Place in <u>high-speed blender</u> along with all other ingredients, blend until smooth and then set aside for the next step:

Smooth Burger Mixture

- ★ 2-3 carrots (peeled & tops removed)
- ★ 1-2 celery stalks
- ★ ¼ C shiitake mushroom powder
- ★ 1-2 tsp dried parsley
- ★ 1-2 tsp dried sage
- ★ 1-2 tsp dried summer savory
- ★ 1-2 tsp dried thyme
- ★ 1 tsp sea salt (or to taste)
- ★ 1 tsp cumin
- ★ ½ tsp coriander
- ★ ¼ tsp asafoetida
- ★ 2 TBS coconut oil (liquefied)
- ★ 4-6 oz purified, filtered water

Second, place the following ingredients in a <u>food processor</u>. Process until all nuts and seeds are well broken down and then slowly add the above mixture, while continuing to process nuts and seeds. This step is done when above and below ingredients are well combined and have formed a thick pâté consistency:

Burger Base

- ★ 1 C walnuts
- ★ ½ C pumpkin seeds
- ★ ½ C sunflower seeds
- ★ 2 TBS chia seeds

- Purified, filtered water as needed for consistency. Only add water if mixture is not moving enough to be evenly distributed. To help keep the mixture moving, take cover off and push down and redistribute contents with a spatula. Mixture should be moist, yet still thick enough to scoop and dish without losing its form.

Optional Variations

- Substitute pecans for walnuts (or use ½ C walnuts and ½ C pecans).
- Substitute hemp seeds for pumpkin or sunflower seeds.
- Add 4-6 presoaked sun-dried tomatoes or ¼ C Snazzy Ketchup (page 354) to the smooth burger mixture. When adding Snazzy Ketchup, you can subtract about 2 ounces of water to the blending process.

Finally, follow the instructions for Traditional Style Burger Patties (see box on page 345).

CREATIVE PÂTÉ TRANSFORMATIONS & DEHYDRATING TIPS:

For Nut/Seed Balls and Mini Burger Patties: Using a 2-ounce stainless-steel squeeze handle disher (or scooper), scoop up pâté and dish onto dehydrator trays with sheets. Dehydrate at 105-115°F for about 4-6 hours, making sure to not over dehydrate. About halfway through, remove from the sheets and form them into balls (by gently rolling in your hands) or patties (by gently pressing down on them and reshaping as needed). Then place them directly onto mesh screened trays for the remainder of time. Look for nut/seed balls to be dry and slightly crisp on the outside, yet still soft on the inside. Now you know they are ready to be enjoyed. Refrigerate any remainder, as they are deliciously flavorful the next day!

For Traditional Style Burger Patties: Follow all the same steps as above, except use a 3-4-ounce squeeze handle disher instead. Dish onto dehydrator trays with sheets, and then press down and shape into patties. When half the time has passed, take a mesh screened tray (without a sheet), lay it upside down over the tray with the burgers on it, hold the sides firmly (but without squeezing too tight) and quickly flip over. Now just slowly peel the dehydrator sheet from the burgers and pop them back into the dehydrator for the remainder of the time. These patties are bigger, so they will need a bit of extra time. Just be sure to check on them hourly.

Please Note: Whenever planning to dehydrate or expose a recipe to heat, I suggest adding a little coconut oil (at least 1 tsp) or using coconut oil in the place of the concentrated oil called for (e.g., hemp or chia seed oil). Even though the temperature may be considered rather low, coconut oil still contains the highest amount of stable fat of all oils. You may also choose to replace just 1 TBS of called for oil with 1 TBS of coconut oil. For instance, if 2 TBS of hemp seed oil is called for, use 1 TBS of hemp seed oil with 1 TBS coconut oil.

Just by adding a small amount of coconut oil (even 1 tsp) to all recipes that will be warmed or dehydrated, you can increase the stabilizing potential and integrity of all monounsaturated and polyunsaturated fats. As a result, the benefits these fats have to offer our health are not lost or degraded.

NUT CRÈMES & CHEEZES

Sour Nut Crème

Place the following ingredients in high-speed blender and blend until smooth and creamy:

- ★ 2 C macadamia nuts
- ★ ½ tsp sea salt (or to taste)
- ★ ¼ C lemon juice
- ★ 6-8 oz purified, filtered water (more as needed for thinner consistency)

Optional Serving Ideas

- ★ This recipe is extremely versatile! Serve as an appetizer to dip chopped veggies, flax and/or chia crackers in; as a topper for raw vegetarian chili, tacos and burritos; or as a base for any herb dressing you desire.

Mozzarawlla Cheeze

Place the following ingredients in high-speed blender and blend until smooth and creamy:

- ★ 2 C macadamia nuts
- ★ 2-3 tsp Italian Blend
- ★ ½ tsp sea salt (or to taste)
- ★ 1 dash asafoetida (or to taste)
- ★ ¼ C lemon juice
- ★ 6-8 oz purified, filtered water (more as needed for thinner consistency)

Optional Serving Ideas

- ★ The recipe is exactly the same as Sour Nut Crème except we are adding a touch of herbs and spices. This recipe is "delizioso" on Italian-style raw vegetarian pizza! In a small bowl, toss a small amount of Mozzarawlla with whatever veggies you plan to top on your pizza before actually layering it on your crust (page 438) already layered with Marawnara (page 358). This way you get creamy, crunchy and savory goodness in every bite!

"Betta than Feta" Cheeze

Place the following ingredients in high-speed blender and blend until smooth and creamy:

- ★ 2 C Brazil nuts
- ★ 2-3 tsp Mediterranean Blend, dried thyme or dill weed
- ★ ½ tsp sea salt (or to taste)
- ★ 1 dash asafoetida (or to taste)
- ★ ¼ C lemon juice
- ★ 6-8 oz purified, filtered water (more as needed for thinner consistency)

Optional Serving Ideas

- ★ Another great option as a dip, salad dressing or pizza cheeze. This cheeze is perfect for a Greek themed pizza! Just top crust (page 438) and Marawnara (page 358) with thinly sliced cucumber, chiffonade cut spinach and sun-dried olives.

Macho Nacho Cheeze

Chop veggies into small chunks, place in high-speed blender along with all other ingredients and then blend until smooth and creamy:

- ★ 1 red bell pepper
- ★ 2 C macadamia (or Brazil nuts)
- ★ 1 tsp Taco Blend
- ★ ½ tsp sea salt (or to taste)
- ★ 1 dash asafoetida (or to taste)
- ★ ¼ C lemon juice
- ★ 3-4 oz purified, filtered water (more as needed for thinner consistency)

Optional Serving Ideas

- ★ Whether it is for an intimate gathering or blowout party, Macho Nacho Cheeze is sure to be a conversation starter amongst guests! Keep it thick for a dip or thin it out for a drizzly dressing. What's more, you have another cheeze for pizza; except this time, it's for a Mexican tostada pizza night!

Crème Cheeze

Place the following ingredients in <u>high-speed blender</u> and blend until smooth and creamy:

- ★ 2 C macadamia nuts
- ★ ½ tsp sea salt (or to taste)
- ★ ½ tsp whole ground vanilla bean powder (optional)
- ★ ¼ C raw honey or agave
- ★ ¼ C lemon juice
- ★ 4-6 oz purified, filtered water (more as needed for thinner consistency)

Optional Serving Ideas

- ★ When thick, this lightly sweetened crème cheeze is the perfect dip for fruits. It is also a great variation for fruit and nut parfaits (page 266) and makes a fabulous crème cheeze frosting for cakes and brownies as well.
- ★ Thinned out, this concoction is a divine pourable dressing for those hot summer nights when you find yourself craving a huge bowl of bitter greens contrasted with tropical fruits or berries. Then go ahead and top with your favorite superfoods such as spirulina, goji berries, golden berries, coconut flakes, cacao beans and/or bee pollen. Mmm! Luscious, superfood heaven in a bowl!

DELECTABLE DIPS, SIDE DISHES & CONDIMENTS

Guacamole

Combine the following ingredients in a mixing bowl (as described), following the instructions below:

- ★ 4 avocados (peeled & pitted)

- 1 whole lime, juiced
- ¼ C packed, fresh cilantro (finely chopped leaves & tender stems only)
- ½-1 red serrano chili pepper (seeds removed & minced)
- ½ tsp sea salt (or to taste)
- ¼ tsp asafoetida

Instructions:

1. Cut avocados in half, remove seed and with a knife slice a tic-tac-toe like grid through the avocado. Use a spoon to scoop out avocado from the peel and into the mixing bowl.
2. Add the rest of the ingredients and, using a fork, roughly mash the avocado – but don't overdo it, as guacamole should be a little chunky. I suggest adding only ½ of the chili pepper to start, adding the other half if you desire a higher level of heat. If you prefer no chili pepper, or to sprinkle with cayenne instead, it will still be delicious.
3. Prior to serving, add 2 chopped roma tomatoes and stir through. Now your simple guacamole is ready to be served with chopped and sliced veggies, chia cracker or whatever your little heart hungers for!

Fresh & Spicy Tomato Salsa

Combine the following ingredients in a mixing bowl (as described) and serve:

- 8 diced roma tomatoes
- 1 diced red, orange or yellow bell pepper (for color variation choose orange or yellow)
- 1 whole lime, juiced
- 1 C packed, fresh cilantro (finely chopped leaves & tender stems only)
- 1 small-medium jalapeno pepper (seeds removed & minced)
- ½ tsp sea salt (or to taste)
- ¼ tsp asafoetida (or to taste)

Optional Variations

- For more traditional salsa, substitute diced red onion (to taste) for asafoetida.
- For **Fresh Tomato & Pineapple Salsa**, substitute 1 C packed, diced pineapple for 4 roma tomatoes.
- For **Sweet & Spicy Mango Salsa**, substitute 1 diced cucumber and about 2 C packed, diced mangos for all 8 roma tomatoes.

Veggie-Style Rice

Choose ONE of the following veggies, chop into small chunks, place in food processor and then pulse-chop until it resembles the size of orzo or rice:

- Jicama (peeled)

- ★ Turnip (peeled)
- ★ Cauliflower (leaves & core removed)

Optional Serving Ideas

- ★ Jicama, turnip and cauliflower rice are all great low starch alternative that will make food combining easy on the brain as well as the digestive system. It is simple and quick to prepare and really pairs nicely with many Asian, Indian and Mexican dishes. For instance, you can serve veggie-style rice with a bowl of raw vegetarian chili or curry marinated veggies, layer in a burrito or enchilada wrap, or toss into a bowl of miso soup or to an Asian spice infused seaweed salad.

Mashed Turner Tots

Chop veggies into small chunks, place in <u>high-speed blender</u> along with all other ingredients, and then blend until smooth:

- ★ 2 C packed turnips (peeled); chopped into small enough pieces in order to pack measuring cup
- ★ 1 C macadamia nuts
- ★ 1-2 tsp dried parsley
- ★ 1-2 tsp rosemary
- ★ ½ tsp sea salt (or to taste)
- ★ 1 dash asafoetida
- ★ 1 pinch cayenne (or to taste)
- ★ 2 TBS coconut crème (or liquefied coconut oil)
- ★ 2 oz purified, filtered water

Optional Variations & Serving Ideas

- ★ A marvelous alternative to traditional mashed potatoes! Not to mention much less starchy and much more nutritious.
- ★ Substitute 2 C packed cauliflower florets (chopped small) for turnips.
- ★ Mashed Turner Tots make a great and grounding little side dish to pair with Pecan Mushroom Gravy (page 349), Cranberry-Goji Holiday Relish (page 350) and Go-To Pâté for the Holidays (described under "Hold the Chicken" Salad Pâté on page 336).
- ★ This recipe is also great dehydrated a bit. Place a glass bowl filled with Mashed Turner Tots in the dehydrator. Leave for a couple of hours at 105-115°F, stirring at least once per hour. A holiday feast you won't need a nap to recover from!

Pecan Mushroom Gravy

Place the following ingredients in <u>high-speed blender</u> and blend until smooth:

- ★ ⅔ C pecans
- ★ ⅓ C shiitake mushroom powder
- ★ 2-3 tsp dried sage

- ★ 2-3 tsp dried thyme
- ★ ½ tsp sea salt (or to taste)
- ★ ¼ tsp asafoetida
- ★ 2 TBS hemp seed or chia seed oil
- ★ 8 oz purified, filtered water

Optional Variations & Serving Ideas

- ★ Substitute 1-2 TBS of Poultry Blend for sage and thyme.
- ★ Replace sea salt with 1 TBS coconut aminos (or to taste).
- ★ Great as a gravy to compliment holiday creations and delish as a dressing for arame, zucchini or kelp noodles.

Cranberry-Goji Holiday Relish

Chop fruits into small chunks and then place in <u>food processor</u>. Pulse-chop until contents resembles relish and transfer to a glass storage container:

- ★ 2 C fresh cranberries
- ★ 1 pear
- ★ 1 orange (peeled & seeded)

Then, toss in the following and refrigerate unit ready to serve:

- ★ ⅓ C goji berries
- ★ ⅓ C golden raisins (or currants)

Optional Serving Ideas

- ★ Not just for holidays! Add 3-4 TBS hemp seeds and/or a sprinkle of bee pollen and you have an energy boosting breakfast.
- ★ Add this condiment to a bed of mixed baby greens, along with ¼ C of nuts, and you have a new tangy twist on a salad fit for lunch.

Island Pineapple Chutney

Combine the following ingredients in a large mixing bowl (as described), following the instructions below:

- ★ 1 fresh pineapple (peeled & cored)
- ★ 1-2-inch piece ginger root, minced
- ★ 1 TBS Curry Blend
- ★ 2 TBS coconut vinegar
- ★ ¼ tsp cayenne (or to taste)
- ★ ½ C coconut flakes
- ★ ½ C currants

Instructions:

1. Slice pineapple lengthwise and then into medium-large chunks. Evenly distribute chunks in food processor, and then process until finely chopped, yet not pureed into a sauce. May also finely chop pineapple by hand, using a sharp knife.
2. Place finely chopped pineapple in a large mixing bowl, then add minced ginger root (minced either by hand or with a garlic press) followed by the rest of the ingredients listed above.
3. Toss together until well combined and then cover and let sit for at least 30 minutes to allow flavors to infuse. This can be done either on a countertop at room temperature or in the fridge. If not planning to eat within an hour, then I suggest placing it in the fridge.

Optional Additions & Serving Ideas

- ★ Add finely chopped mango to above blend and/or macadamia nut pieces.
- ★ Makes a palate pleasing side dish or salad topper.
- ★ Quite flavorful at room temperature or slightly warmed in dehydrator.

Genie Zucchini Hummus

Chop veggies into small chunks, place in <u>high-speed blender</u> along with all other ingredients, and then blend until smooth:

- ★ 2 medium zucchini (peeled)
- ★ ⅔ C unhulled, tan sesame seeds
- ★ ½ C raw sesame tahini
- ★ 2 TBS chickpea miso paste
- ★ 1 tsp paprika
- ★ 1 tsp cumin
- ★ ½ tsp sea salt (or to taste)
- ★ ¼ tsp asafoetida
- ★ 1 dash cayenne (or to taste)
- ★ ½ C lemon juice
- ★ 1-2 TBS black sesame seed oil

Optional Variations & Serving Ideas

- ★ Replace lemon juice with a combo of 1 lemon and 2 limes, juiced.
- ★ Add to above 1 TBS Mediterranean Blend, dried parsley or thyme.
- ★ If replacing raw sesame tahini with unhulled, tan sesame seeds entirely, I suggest doing as follows: increase amount of unhulled, tan sesame seeds (presoaked) to 1 ¼ C in total and increase black sesame seed oil to 2-4 TBS in total. If black sesame oil is unavailable, may replace with extra virgin olive oil.

★ This is great as a dip, as a spread in collard or lettuce leaf wraps, tossed in a salad, or as the base for a Mediterranean themed pizza topped with chiffonade cut leafy greens, chopped sundried tomatoes, cucumber, bell pepper and sun-dried olives.

Hemp Tabouli Salad

First, chiffonade cut the following ingredients by hand or use a <u>food processor</u> to make this task easier. I suggest not packing the food processor. Divide into a few small to medium sized batches, transferring each batch into a large mixing bowl as you go. Be sure to evenly distribute herbs (including some spearmint sprigs to each batch) and pulse-chop until a fine consistency is reached:

- ★ 2 bunches fresh parsley (leaves & tender stems only)
- ★ 1 bunch fresh cilantro (leaves & tender stems only)
- ★ 10-12 spearmint sprigs (stems removed)

Second, prepare the following veggies as described and then transfer each into the large mixing bowl along with your herbs:

- ★ 2 cucumbers (seeded & diced)
- ★ 5-6 roma tomatoes (seeded & diced)

Third, add the following ingredients into the large mixing bowl of herbs and veggies and toss together until ingredients are evenly distributed and well combined:

- ★ 1 tsp sea salt (or to taste)
- ★ ½ tsp asafoetida (or to taste)
- ★ ½ C lemon juice
- ★ ½ C hemp seed oil

Last, add the following and toss again until well combined. Best when allowed to set for a few hours or overnight before serving, as the flavors really get a chance to set in:

- ★ 1 ½ C hemp seeds

Optional Variations & Serving Ideas

- ★ Replace lemon juice with a combo of 1 lemon and 2 limes, juiced.
- ★ Use all fresh parsley (3 bunches) instead of cilantro.
- ★ Substitute home-sprouted quinoa or presprouted TruRoots brand for hemp seeds
- ★ This is refreshing and flavorful as a side dish, a dip for flax or chia crackers or a filler for collard and lettuce leaf wraps (especially with Marvelous Mediterranean Falafel Pâté, page 342).

Maconaise

Place the following ingredients in <u>high-speed blender</u> and blend until smooth and creamy:

- ★ 1 C macadamia nuts
- ★ 1 C cashews
- ★ 1 TBS chickpea miso paste
- ★ ½ tsp sea salt (or to taste)
- ★ ¼ tsp asafoetida
- ★ 1 dash ground mustard seeds
- ★ 1 TBS raw honey or agave
- ★ 2 TBS apple cider vinegar
- ★ 2 TBS lemon juice
- ★ 6-8 oz purified, filtered water (more as needed for thinner consistency)

Optional Serving Ideas

- ★ This makes one dang good spread, if I must say-so myself! I love spreading this on chia crackers or lettuce leaves and then stacking with strips of apple smoked dulse, sliced roma tomatoes and thinly sliced cucumber.
- ★ When thinned out with water this makes the perfect marinade/dressing for cabbage or veggie slaws. To help soften cabbage and veggies for slaws, I suggest sprinkling them with sea salt. You may also wish to splash these with more apple cider vinegar and/or lemon juice, which will only add to the end flavor once everything is mixed together.
- ★ Try tossing cabbage and veggie slaws with a bed of salad greens, and then add enough extra dressing to moisten and coat. It is quite satisfying and enjoyable as a main meal.

Pucker-Up Mustard

Follow the instructions below and then combine the following ingredients in a high-speed blender until smooth:

- ★ ½ C mustard seeds
- ★ ½ tsp turmeric
- ★ ½ tsp sea salt (or to taste)
- ★ 2 TBS raw honey or agave
- ★ ½ C apple cider vinegar
- ★ 4 oz purified, filtered water

Instructions:

1. If using preground mustard seeds, just combine all the above ingredients in blender and blend until smooth. If you plan to use whole mustard seeds, then presoak mustard seeds overnight at room temperature and add a bit of sea salt to the water. You may use all brown mustard seeds (which are a bit spicier), all yellow mustard seeds, or half of each (¼ C brown and ¼ C yellow). It is totally up to you.
2. The next day: rinse and drain your mustard seeds, add them to blender with all other ingredients, and then blend until smooth.

3. When mustard is freshly made, it can be quite bitter; but have no fear, the longer it sits the less bitter it becomes. I suggest making mustard two or three days ahead of when you plan to use it. This will allow enough time for all the flavors to settle in. Store your mustard in a glass mason jar in the fridge for up to 2-3 months.
4. For more honey mustard flavor: add up to ¼ C more raw honey or agave. I suggest doing this after the flavors have had a chance to mellow. You may also wish to divide and store in two different mason jars so that you can have one that is more traditional and one that is sweet.

Optional Serving Ideas

- ★ This is a spectacular condiment that will serve more than just one purpose. Use it as a spread in wraps or thin it out for a mustardy dressing on salads. Thinned out and you have another amazing marinade for veggie and cabbage slaws.
- ★ If you're into making dehydrated nut/seed loafs and burgers, you can add a touch of this mustard to your recipe and/or spread it on once ready to eat.

Snazzy Ketchup

Chop veggies into small chunks, place in <u>high-speed blender</u> along with all other ingredients, and then blend until smooth:

- ★ 2 roma tomatoes
- ★ 1 C sun-dried tomatoes (presoaked)
- ★ ¼ tsp sea salt (or to taste)
- ★ 1 dash cayenne (or to taste)
- ★ 1 pinch asafoetida
- ★ 2 TBS raw honey or agave
- ★ 2 TBS apple cider vinegar
- ★ 2 TBS extra virgin olive oil
- ★ 4-8 oz purified, filtered water (more as needed for thinner consistency)

Optional Serving Ideas

- ★ If you have a dehydrator, this is a great little condiment to serve with jicama or sweet potato friez (page 453). It is also a tangy little spread for raw dehydrated burgers and wraps!
- ★ Also makes a great nut free marinade for veggies which can then be popped in the dehydrator for a few hours to soften and warm. I love doing this with chopped broccoli and cauliflower florets (which have a tendency to be a bit on the dry side when eaten as is). Also delish with thinly shredded cabbage.

Zany BBQ Sauce

Chop veggies into small chunks, place in <u>high-speed blender</u> along with all other ingredients, and then blend until smooth:

- ★ 2 roma tomatoes
- ★ 1 C sun-dried tomatoes (presoaked)
- ★ 2 TBS mesquite powder
- ★ ¼ tsp sea salt (or to taste)
- ★ 1 dash cayenne (or to taste)
- ★ 1 dash ground cloves
- ★ 1 pinch asafoetida
- ★ 2 TBS raw honey or agave
- ★ 2 TBS apple cider vinegar
- ★ 2 TBS extra virgin olive oil
- ★ 4-8 oz purified, filtered water (more as needed for thinner consistency)

Optional Serving Ideas

- ★ If you have a dehydrator, this is another awesome little condiment to serve with jicama or sweet potato friez (page 453). It also makes a tangy little spread for raw dehydrated burgers and wraps!
- ★ For warm and soft BBQ flavored veggies, marinate and pop in the dehydrator for a few hours. Do the same for a flavorful side of wilted kale or spinach.

Sicilian Tapenade

Chop bell pepper into small chunks, combine with all other ingredients in a <u>food processor</u> and then process into a paste:

- ★ 1 red bell pepper
- ★ 1 C sun-dried tomatoes (presoaked)
- ★ ½ C raw sun-dried black olives (pitted)
- ★ 2 TBS Italian Blend
- ★ ¼ tsp sea salt (or to taste)
- ★ ¼ tsp cayenne (or to taste)
- ★ ¼ tsp asafoetida (or to taste)
- ★ 2 TBS lemon juice
- ★ 2 TBS extra virgin olive oil

Optional Serving Ideas

- ★ This makes a savory and scrumptious spread. I absolutely love it wrapped up in a lettuce leaf with sliced avocado.
- ★ It also makes a divine spread for zucchini slices. Top with a pitted sun-dried olive and now you have an amazing appetizer.

Curry Spread

Place the following ingredients in a <u>high-speed blender</u> and blend until well combined and a buttery paste forms:

- ★ 1 C pumpkin seeds
- ★ 1 TBS Curry Blend
- ★ ½ C coconut oil (liquefied)
- ★ ¼ tsp sea salt (or to taste)
- ★ 1 pinch asafoetida

Optional Additions & Serving Ideas

- ★ This spread is food therapy for intestinal parasites and can be consumed to help in the process of gently expelling intestinal worms. For the purpose of parasite cleansing, I would include 2-4 garlic cloves to the above recipe. You may also wish to include a ½-1-inch piece of ginger root.
- ★ Use as a veggie dip for carrots, cauliflower, bell pepper slices and/or broccoli florets; spread on sliced apples for a sweet and savory snack; or use as a spread in nori, collard or lettuce leaf wraps.

Cilantro Pesto: for Heavy Metal Cleansing

Place the following ingredients in <u>high-speed blender</u>, blend into a paste, and then follow instructions below:

- ★ ½ C Brazil nuts
- ★ ¼ C hemp seeds
- ★ ¼ C pumpkin seeds
- ★ 2 C packed, fresh cilantro (or 2 bunches)
- ★ 4 garlic cloves
- ★ 1 TBS kelp (powder or flakes)
- ★ ¼-½ tsp sea salt
- ★ ¼ C lemon juice
- ★ 1 C hemp seed oil

Instructions:

1. Once all ingredients are well combined and have formed a paste, use a spatula to scoop every bit out into a couple of pint-sized, wide mouth mason jars. Plan to store one of your jars in the freezer, as this pesto freezes well.
2. The process of heavy metal detoxification can be slow (anywhere from 3-6 months or longer). However, when utilizing all the right tools, at the appropriate times, the cleansing and detoxification process can go much smoother and much safer. The recipe above is a powerful tissue cleanser, making it a great addition to your self-detoxification program.

Please Note: Before a safe and effective chelation protocol can be put into practice, I strongly advise having all amalgam fillings properly removed (please review "Chelation & Heavy Metal Detoxification: Wellness Tips and Tools to Live By" on page 111). Once all the proper steps have been followed, I highly suggest heavy metal cleansing (more intensively) at least once a year as maintenance. When I do this cleanse, I spend one month doing the Medicardium, Glytamins and Xeneplex suppositories nightly. During that time, I also increase my chlorella intake to 1 TBS three times per day and take 1 TBS of the cilantro pesto three times per day at least 30 minutes after taking my chlorella. I also increase my sea vegetable intake at mealtime and take extra capsules of Modifilan, XenoStat and/or Medi-Clay-FX throughout the day.

SEXY SAUCES & DRESSINGS

Hemp Pesto Sauce

Place the following ingredients in <u>high-speed blender</u> and blend until smooth and creamy:

- ★ ½ C hemp seeds
- ★ ¼ C dried basil
- ★ 2 TBS dried cilantro
- ★ ¼ tsp sea salt (or to taste)
- ★ 1 dash asafoetida
- ★ 2 TBS lemon juice
- ★ ½ C hemp seed oil
- ★ 4-6 oz purified, filtered water (more as needed for thinner consistency)

Optional Serving Ideas

- ★ Savory and satisfying as a dip for chopped veggies, flax and/or chia crackers.
- ★ Add a bit more water (up to ½ C more) and you have the perfect sauce for arame seaweed, spiralized zucchini or kelp noodles.
- ★ Spectacular smothered over shredded and chopped veggies before topping on salad or dehydrated pizza crusts.

Popeye's Pesto Sauce

Place the following ingredients in <u>high-speed blender</u> and blend until smooth and creamy:

- ★ ½ C walnuts
- ★ 3 large handfuls baby spinach
- ★ 1 TBS spirulina
- ★ ¼ tsp sea salt (or to taste)
- ★ 1 dash asafoetida
- ★ 2 TBS lemon juice
- ★ ½ C hemp seed or chia seed oil
- ★ 4-6 oz purified, filtered water (more as needed for thinner consistency)

Optional Variations & Serving Ideas

- ★ Pesto does not always have to made with basil, so step out of the box and add any herb or combo of herbs you wish (such as a 3:1 ratio of rosemary to parsley, 3:1 ratio of oregano to parsley or 3:1 ratio of sage to parsley). For example, try adding 1 TBS dried rosemary and 1 tsp dried parsley to the recipe above.
- ★ For a totally different spin to this pesto sauce, replace spirulina and spinach with any herb combo listed above, but in a larger quantity than in the example just given. For instance, use 3 heaping TBS dried rosemary and 1 heaping TBS dried parsley.
- ★ Replace walnuts with pecans, hemp or pumpkin seeds for even more variation and to learn what combos you like best. **FYI:** Pecans go really well with the sage and parsley combo. You may use as little as 1 TBS of dried sage to 1 tsp of dried parsley for a lighter flavor or go a bit bolder and use as much as 3 heaping TBS of dried sage to 1 heaping TBS of dried parsley.

Alfrawdo Sauce

Place the following ingredients in <u>high-speed blender</u> and blend until smooth and creamy:

- ★ 2 C macadamia nuts
- ★ 3 TBS dried tarragon
- ★ 1 TBS dried thyme
- ★ ½ tsp sea salt (or to taste)
- ★ ¼ tsp asafoetida
- ★ ¼ C lemon juice
- ★ ½ C hemp seed or chia seed oil
- ★ 8-10 oz purified, filtered water (more as needed for thinner consistency)

Optional Serving Ideas

- ★ Creamy and heavenly rich as a dip for chopped veggies, flax and/or chia crackers.
- ★ Add a bit more water (up to ½ C more) and you have the perfect sauce for arame seaweed, spiralized zucchini or kelp noodles.
- ★ Even try smothered over shredded and chopped veggies before topping on salad or dehydrated pizza crusts.

Marawnara Sauce

Chop veggies into small chunks (in the order I have listed), layer the following ingredients in a <u>food processor</u>, and then process until well combined and semi-smooth:

- ★ 2 C sun-dried tomatoes (presoaked)
- ★ 7-8 roma tomatoes
- ★ 1-2 celery stalks
- ★ 1 whole orange (peeled & seeded)
- ★ 2 TBS Italian Blend

- ½ tsp sea salt (or to taste)
- ¼ tsp cayenne (or to taste)
- 1 dash asafoetida
- 1-2 TBS apple cider vinegar
- 2 TBS extra virgin olive oil

Optional Variations & Serving Ideas

- Substitute 1 red bell pepper for 2 roma tomatoes.
- Add to zucchini or kelp noodles, served either alone or with dehydrated nut/seed balls and you will never long for nutritionless pasta again! Now just give it a touch of cheesy flare by sprinkling with nutritional yeast flakes or Prawma Sprinkle (page 312) and this dish is complete!
- This sauce is perfect for Italian-style pizza. Generously layer on top of dehydrated pizza crusts (page 438) and then add your favorite veggies with Mozzarawlla Cheeze (page 346).
- For a different themed pizza, substitute Mediterranean Blend for Italian Blend and use "Betta than Feta" Cheeze (page 346). How about substituting 1 TBS Mexican or Taco Blend (more or less to taste) for Italian Blend, using Macho Nacho Cheeze (page 346)? It is a simple as that!

Enchilada Sauce

Chop veggies into small chunks, place in <u>high-speed blender</u> along with all other ingredients, and then blend until smooth:

- 2 roma tomatoes
- 1 C sun-dried tomatoes (presoaked)
- 2 TBS chickpea miso paste
- 2 TBS Chili Blend
- 1 tsp dried oregano
- ½ tsp coriander
- ½ tsp sea salt (or to taste)
- ¼ tsp asafoetida (or to taste)
- 1 dash cinnamon or Apple Pie Blend (optional)
- 2 TBS extra virgin olive oil
- 6-8 oz purified, filtered water (more as needed for thinner consistency). Add water slowly and just enough to keep it blending smoothly. Enchilada sauce should be thick enough to coat a spoon, yet thin enough to pour.

Optional Variations & Serving Ideas

- Feel free to add a bit of sweetness if desired. You may wish to add 1-2 TBS raw agave, a few pinches of green leaf stevia, or whatever other natural sweetener you prefer.

- ★ This sauce was inspired by the idea of creating a spicy sauce for raw vegetarian enchiladas, but has proved to be a great addition to so much more. For instance, it's delicious drizzled on Mexican-style pizza topped with Re-fined Bean Pâté (page 339) instead of sauce.
- ★ I love anything spicy, so I tend to add a lot more cayenne or add a habanera pepper to the batch. Feel free to add as much heat as you can handle.
- ★ Two sauces in one! Take a small amount from the batch made above (about ½ C) and add 1-2 TBS raw cacao powder to turn this into a mole-like sauce. I suggest adding a touch of sweetener (of choice and to taste) with the addition of raw cacao. This will balance out the bitterness.

Asian Dipping Sauce

Place the following ingredients in a glass measuring cup and whisk with a fork (or small whisk) until well combined and smooth:

- ★ ¼ C coconut vinegar
- ★ ¼ C coconut aminos
- ★ 1-2-inch piece ginger root, minced (or 1 drop ginger essential oil)
- ★ 1 pinch asafoetida (optional)
- ★ 1 TBS raw honey or agave

Optional Variations & Serving Ideas

- ★ Add sea vegetable flakes and cayenne to taste for a bit of color and spicy zip!
- ★ As is, this sauce makes the perfect little dip for raw vegetarian nori rolls. Add ¼ C of hemp seed oil, a squeeze or two of lemon and/or lime, and you now have an incredible tangy dressing for salads. This variation also makes a fabulous marinade for cabbage, cruciferous and root veggies slaws.
- ★ In a food processor: shred carrots, celery root and daikon radish. Blend together in a large mixing bowl and then pour this entire dressing (more as needed) over the shredded veggies for Asian Root Veggie Slaw (page 326). Toss in a handful of fresh and groomed snap or snow peas, some finely chopped fresh Thai basil leaves (and/or cilantro), and now you have a Thai Infused Root Veggie Slaw.

Asian Dressing

Place the following ingredients in <u>high-speed blender</u> and blend until smooth:

- ★ ½ C hemp seeds
- ★ ½ C shiitake mushroom powder
- ★ 1 tsp Asian Blend
- ★ ½ tsp sea salt
- ★ ¼ C coconut vinegar
- ★ ¼ C hemp seed oil
- ★ 6 oz purified, filtered water

Optional Serving Ideas

- ★ Delish as a basic salad dressing or as a marinade for a cabbage slaw made with shredded Chinese (Napa) cabbage, shredded carrots and minced broccoli. Top with sea veggie flakes and black sesame seeds for a beautiful presentation that will have people talking.
- ★ This dressing is also amazing for making a quick and simple arame seaweed salad. Just soak arame for 10-15 minutes in enough room temperature-warm water to cover. Rinse, drain and chop a few times before tossing with Asian Dressing, shredded carrots, and a generous sprinkle of hemp seeds. Mmm! A mineral rich meal or satisfying snack good for any day of the week!

Miso Caesar Dressing

Place the following ingredients in a glass measuring cup and whisk with a fork (or small whisk) until well combined and smooth:

- ★ ¼ C raw sesame tahini
- ★ 1 TBS chickpea miso paste
- ★ ¼ tsp sea salt (or to taste)
- ★ 1 dash asafoetida (or to taste)
- ★ 1 pinch ground mustard seeds (or to taste)
- ★ ¼ C lemon juice
- ★ 1-2 oz purified, filtered water (more as needed for thinner consistency)

Dressing Additions

When smooth, creamy and thin enough to pour add the following and give it a few more whisks. You may also reserve adding it to the dressing and just sprinkle on top of dressed salad greens:

- ★ Wakame and/or nori flakes, to taste (as replacement for anchovies)
- ★ Nutritional yeast flakes or Prawma Sprinkle, to taste (as replacement for parmesan)

Optional Variations & Serving Ideas

Please Note: Feel free to adjust spices to your liking. I have added more and less and have liked them all; therefore, I basically gave the average of all the various amounts I have tried.

- ★ Try substituting 2 TBS coconut vinegar and 2 TBS lemon juice for the ¼ C of lemon juice.
- ★ Double or triple recipe in a high-speed blender if you desire leftovers or would like enough for 4-6+ servings.
- ★ Serve over chopped romaine lettuce, finely sliced celery and sun-dried olives (optional). Whatever you do, don't forget to add the sea veggie flakes and Prawma Sprinkle (page 312).

- ★ For croutons, crumble some flax or chia crackers on top. I suggest the SeaVeg Chia Chips by Oh So Pure! They are oh so delicious!
- ★ This dressing is also great when used to marinate fresh baby spinach or chiffonade cut mature spinach leaves. Let it marinate for a while for a great wilted spinach side dish.

Hemp Caesar Dressing

Place the following ingredients in <u>high-speed blender</u> and blend until smooth:

- ★ ½ C hemp seeds
- ★ 1 TBS nutritional yeast
- ★ 1 TBS wakame and/or nori flakes
- ★ ½ tsp sea salt (or to taste)
- ★ ¼ tsp ground mustard seeds (or to taste)
- ★ 1 dash asafoetida (or to taste)
- ★ 1 pinch green leaf stevia powder (or ¼ tsp whole leaf)
- ★ ¼ C lemon juice
- ★ ¼ C hemp seed oil
- ★ 4 oz purified, filtered water

Ranch Dressing

Chop veggies into small chunks, place in <u>high-speed blender</u> along with all other ingredients, and then blend until smooth:

- ★ 1-2 celery stalks
- ★ 1 C macadamia nuts
- ★ ½ C cashews
- ★ 1 TBS dried dill weed
- ★ 1 TBS dried parsley
- ★ 1 TBS dried thyme
- ★ ½ tsp sea salt (or to taste)
- ★ ¼ tsp asafoetida
- ★ 2 TBS apple cider vinegar
- ★ ¼ C lemon juice
- ★ ½ C hemp seed or chia seed oil
- ★ 4-6 oz purified, filtered water (more as needed for thinner consistency)

Optional Variations & Serving Ideas

- ★ Substitute 2-3 tsp dried oregano or cilantro for thyme.
- ★ Add paprika and/or cayenne to taste.
- ★ Serve as a dip with chopped veggies, flax and/or chia crackers, or thin it out a bit and use as a salad dressing.

- ★ When made thinner, another great option with this recipe is to use it as a marinade for a minced broccoli salad! In a food processor: pulse-chop broccoli, cauliflower and carrots (separately) until minced; sprinkle veggies with extra sea salt and/or splash with extra apple cider vinegar or lemon juice (in order to help tenderize); transfer to a bowl and add diced red bell peppers and celery; stir in a generous amount of ranch dressing and allow to marinate until ready to serve. This is great as a side served in cabbage leaves or tossed in a chopped leafy green salad. When broccoli rabe is available, use in place of broccoli.
- ★ This raw version of ranch dressing will have you convinced that you don't need Hidden Valley to make everything taste better!

Thai-Hini Dressing

Chop veggies into small chunks, place in <u>high-speed blender</u> along with all other ingredients, and then blend until smooth:

- ★ 4 roma tomatoes
- ★ 1 C cashews
- ★ ½ C raw sesame tahini
- ★ 1 TBS Garam Masala Blend
- ★ ½ tsp sea salt (or to taste)
- ★ ¼ tsp cayenne (or to taste)
- ★ 1 dash asafoetida
- ★ 1 TBS raw honey or agave
- ★ 1-2 TBS coconut vinegar
- ★ 2 limes, juiced
- ★ ¼ C black sesame seed, hemp seed or chia seed oil
- ★ Purified, filtered water until desired consistency is reached (about 2 oz at a time)

Optional Variations & Serving Ideas

- ★ Substitute hemp or sunflower seeds for cashews.
- ★ Replace raw sesame tahini with ⅔ C tan sesame seeds.
- ★ This dressing serves many purposes. Serve thick for a dip, or thin it out and drizzle over a basic leafy green salad made with chiffonade cut lettuce, lacinato kale or collard leaves.
- ★ It is also great for Thai inspired veggie or salad dishes made with spiralized zucchini, shredded red cabbage and carrots, and minced broccoli and/or cauliflower florets.

"A Thousand Islands" Dressing

Chop veggies into small chunks, place in <u>high-speed blender</u> along with all other ingredients, and then blend until smooth:

- ★ 2 roma tomatoes

- ★ 1 red bell pepper
- ★ 1 C pumpkin seeds
- ★ ½ C raw sesame tahini
- ★ 1-2 TBS dried parsley
- ★ 1 TBS dried dill weed
- ★ ½ tsp sea salt (or to taste)
- ★ ¼ tsp paprika
- ★ ¼ tsp asafoetida
- ★ 1 dash ground mustard seeds
- ★ 1-2 TBS apple cider vinegar
- ★ ¼ C lemon juice
- ★ ¼ C black sesame seed, hemp seed or chia seed oil
- ★ Purified, filtered water until desired consistency is reached (about 2 oz at a time)

Optional Variations & Serving Ideas

- ★ Substitute hemp or sunflower seeds for pumpkin seeds.
- ★ Replace raw sesame tahini with ⅔ C tan sesame seeds.
- ★ Another dressing that serves many purposes. Leave it thick and it's a delectable dip. Thin it out and it's a delish dressing. Pour over shredded or chiffonade cut veggies and you have another marinade for slaws and salads.
- ★ Toss in a chopped salad with romaine leaves, cucumbers, bell peppers (red, orange and/or yellow) and tomatoes. Then garnish with additional dill weed and paprika.

Cucumber Tahini Dressing

Chop veggies into small chunks, place in <u>high-speed blender</u> along with all other ingredients, and then blend until smooth:

- ★ 1 cucumber
- ★ ¼ C raw sesame tahini
- ★ ¼ tsp sea salt
- ★ 1 dash paprika
- ★ 1 pinch asafoetida
- ★ ¼ C lemon juice
- ★ Purified, filtered water as needed for thinner consistency (about 1-2 oz at a time)

Optional Variations & Serving Ideas

- ★ Add to above 2-3 tsp Mediterranean Blend, 1-2 tsp dried thyme and/or dill weed.
- ★ Refreshing as a dressing for a simple cucumber salad, Greek salad (page 316) or as a drizzle and plate scaper for Mediterranean themed dishes.
- ★ Double recipe if you desire leftovers or would like enough for 4-6+ servings.

Very Berry Vinaigrette Dressing

Place the following ingredients in high-speed blender and blend until smooth:

- ★ 1 C packed raspberries, strawberries or mixed berries (fresh or defrosted)
- ★ 2 TBS goji berries
- ★ 2 tsp dried basil
- ★ 1 tsp sea salt (or to taste)
- ★ ½ tsp dried oregano
- ★ ¼ tsp dried thyme
- ★ 1 dash asafoetida (or to taste)
- ★ 1-2 TBS raw honey or agave
- ★ ¼ C coconut vinegar
- ★ ½ C hemp seed or chia seed oil
- ★ 2 oz purified, filtered water (more as needed for thinner consistency)

Optional Variations & Serving Ideas

- ★ Delicious drizzled and tossed with a bowl of chopped Boston bibb, radicchio and/or arugula and accompanied by chopped cucumber and finely sliced celery.
- ★ Add walnut pieces and strawberry slices for a spectacular summer salad.
- ★ Add nuts/seeds of choice (such as almonds, pecans, pumpkin seeds and/or hemp seeds) with some chopped apple and/or pear for a fabulous fall salad.
- ★ Top with additional goji berries, coconut flakes, cacao nibs, bee pollen and/or spirulina for a superfood salad fit for superheroes!

Citrus Gold Vinaigrette Dressing

Place the following ingredients in high-speed blender and blend until smooth:

- ★ 2 oranges or 1 pink grapefruit (peeled & seeded)
- ★ 2 TBS golden berries
- ★ 2 tsp dried basil
- ★ 1 tsp sea salt (or to taste)
- ★ ½ tsp dried oregano
- ★ ¼ tsp dried thyme
- ★ 1 dash asafoetida (or to taste)
- ★ 1-2 TBS raw honey or agave
- ★ ¼ C coconut vinegar
- ★ ½ C hemp seed or chia seed oil
- ★ 2 oz purified, filtered water (more as needed for thinner consistency)

Optional Variations & Serving Ideas

- ★ Fabulous drizzles and tossed with a bowl of your favorite leafy greens (such as arugula, endive, escarole, romaine, etc.), complimented with some chopped cucumber and finely sliced celery.

- ★ Add some chopped apple and/or pear for a fall and winter delight good enough for breakfast, lunch or dinner.
- ★ Add Brazil nuts (or other nuts/seeds of choice) for protein and crunch appeal.
- ★ Top with additional golden berries, coconut flakes, cacao nibs, bee pollen and/or spirulina for another superfood salad fit for superheroes!

DECADENT DESSERTS & SWEET TREATS

If you find yourself gravitating towards the recipes under this chapter, then it may be safe to assume that dessert, chocolates and everything sweet is your #1 weakness. They certainly are mine. Have no fear though, as from this day forward you will no longer feel the need to punish yourself by taking your sweets away! Besides, deprivation will almost always lead to setbacks, binges, emotional let-downs and a return of excess weight.

For those with a fondness and craving for something sweet, I say this: know your weakness, embrace it, and then ask yourself what it is that makes you crave it. Then choose a healthy raw vegetarian alternative – that tastes good – to replace it. Just by switching the ingredients that make up your favorite desserts and treats, you can be on your way to a healthier, glowing, energized and slimmer you! It truly does work. How, you ask? Because you're actually not giving up all the taste and flavors you are craving and lusting over, just all the processed, refined and toxic-laden chemical ingredients that went into making it.

Processed and refined ingredients will eventually destroy one's health. They also can cause major mood swings and are the main culprits for weight gain. They actually cause fat cells to multiply as they blow up with foreign toxic substances. Who wants that!

If I thought for even one minute that a piece of chocolate or dessert could never touch my lips again, I know for a fact that I would have failed miserably at becoming a raw vegetarian. Instead, here I am almost 10 years later writing about how I made it happen. Yup, I was one of the guilty ones. I was notorious for binging on worthless, sugar-laden, nutrient-devoid junk food and was always at my worst just days before entering into a mini-cleanse; something I did to ramp up my athletic performance a few times per year. I behaved like a true addict being sent off to rehab. My body would feel so awful, and my brain so fuzzy, that I would vow to never do it again. At least until the next mini-cleanse, of course.

It wasn't until I tasted my first bite of a raw chocolate brownie that I realized how delicious raw chocolate and raw desserts really were. This is when I knew I could commit. I was inspired to become a full-on raw vegetarian. I literally thought that I had gone to heaven! Raw desserts truly do taste better! One of my friends expressed it best when he sat back after his first few bites of a raw brownie, with a dumbfounded look on his face, and asked "this is legal?" **FYI:** Many of the people in my life are not raw foodists, or health nuts for that matter, by any means. So, making simple switches like these can really work with family and friends.

Quick Dessert & Sweet Treat Tips:

For a lot of my dessert recipes, I prefer to use nuts and seeds that are ready to enjoy and don't have to be soaked (or at least not for long periods of time). However, with the exception of hemp seeds and chia seeds, I do recommend giving nuts and seeds that you don't plan to soak at least a quick rinse, especially tree nuts. This will help to remove any surface debris. You may even spritz them with a little 3% food grade hydrogen peroxide (H_2O_2) and then rinse again.

> **Please Note:** In general, most all nuts and seeds can be used interchangeably. Just be sure to plan ahead if you choose to use nuts and/or seeds which should ideally be soaked for optimal health benefits.
>
> To review "The Science Behind the Soak," "General Soaking Schedule for Nuts & Seeds" and other great tips, please refer to page 26.

It is not necessary to soak raw cashews or hazelnuts. However, if time allows, I do recommend soaking for certain dessert recipes (e.g., cheeze cake, crème cake and ice cream recipes). Presoaking can really improve the texture and creaminess. It will also make blending a bit easier (especially with creations that use very little liquid such as cake and frosting recipes). So, if time allows, consider soaking cashews for 1-2 hrs and hazelnuts overnight in room temperature water. In addition, due do these nuts not posing the same degree of enzyme inhibitor issues as many other nuts (such as almonds, pecans and walnuts), it is totally acceptable to utilize their soak water for any amount of water called for in the recipe.

> **Please Note:** When blending ingredients in a high-speed blender, especially those going into making raw cakes and pies, I suggest starting out at a low speed. Once all the dry/solid ingredients break down, and start coming together with all the wet/liquid ingredients, you can start increasing the speed to a higher level. Increasing the speed at the right time will make the entire dessert making experience "a piece of cake." Pun intended!

For molding raw cakes and pies, I suggest investing in silicone cake pans of various shapes and sizes. I prefer cake pans over pie dishes, as their straight up and down shape makes cutting much neater. I prefer silicone due to their non-stick surface. It makes removing a snap. Silicone cake molds also come in deeper sizes that can hold a lot more, which comes in handy when making layered cakes. Because nothing sticks to it, you also won't risk your masterpiece falling apart prematurely.

> **Please Note:** Most of the following recipes will require a 9 ½ inch round or 9-inch square pan; therefore, I suggest investing in a couple of round silicone pans that measure 9 ½ inches in diameter and at least 2 ¼ inches tall. I also suggest having at least one 9-inch square pan (for brownies, bars and squares).
>
> Although all my cake recipes call for round silicone cake pans or molds, you may also use the deeper round (or square) 9-inch Springform pans, which also make for easy molding and serving. I suggest the Springform pans put out by Norpro. The base is actually made from a tempered glass, noted to be scratch resistant. Tempered glass is a much better material to be cutting on than the many questionable metals and non-stick materials. For instance, many of the Springform pans on the market are made of aluminum and have a nonstick coated surface. This may be acceptable for some, but I do not recommend it; especially at the base where a knife can scratch the material and increase the chances of ingesting aluminum or nonstick coating particles. Not good!

Keep the following in mind when you get to food processor recipes that call for nuts and dried fruits (such as bars, brownies, cakes, cookies, etc.): the need for a bit of water will depend on a few different factors. For instance, certain recipes call for dried fruits that are stickier and, as a result, will not need any water – while others may need 1-4 TBS of water added. Other factors that will determine the need for water include the fat content of nuts and whether or not the nuts have been soaked. For instance, nuts with a higher fat content add more moisture (such as Brazil nuts, macadamia, pecans and walnuts) and, as a result, may not need the addition of water.

> **Please Note:** The mixture should not need water if you can pinch it and it sticks together between your fingers (it may even start to form a ball right in the food processor). If the mixture completely crumbles apart when you squish it (too dry and floury), then you may need to add a bit of water (1 TBS at a time). The mixture should be moistened enough to hold a shape, yet not so wet that it is gooey. For cake and bar recipes that are going to be placed in a pan, rather than shaped in your hand, it is okay if they do not completely ball together. On the other hand, if you are trying to shape cookies or balls, you will have to test a small amount first.
>
> If a mixture ever comes out too wet, you may add some ground chia seeds to absorb the excess moisture. You may also add some extra dry ingredients such as coconut flakes. Be sure to always add a small amount at a time until desire texture is reached. Remember, for every problem there is a solution.
>
> Another trick I tend to use when a mixture is too wet is to simply place the mixture in the fridge for a short period. This allows the oils and sticky/tacky fruit pectin to harden up a bit, which in turn makes the mixture much easier to work with when molding and shaping by hand. Another trick is to use coconut oil. Coconut oil serves several culinary purposes in raw food recipes. It adds moisture when liquefied to help in the blending process and when cold it solidifies to assist in the molding and holding together process. Let's also not forget all the nutritional purposes it serves in increasing the potential of omega-3 and the absorption of fat-soluble vitamins and minerals.

You will find that I utilize sun-dried cane juice crystals quite often in dessert recipes. This is done purposely. For culinary purposes, using sun-dried cane juice crystals (versus raw honey or agave) helps to cut down on the amount of liquid, which in turn helps in the molding process and the texture of the end product. It also adds a real, natural sweetness that is not only well balanced in glucose and fructose, but highly mineralized. The cane juice crystals I speak of are from sugar cane that is grown in extremely mineralized volcanic soil in a pristine region of Ecuador. This particular region of Ecuador is also known for being one of the most pristine areas on the planet. Quality is of the essence! Learn more about this unique sweetener (including all the others I recommend) by reviewing "Sweet Flavor for Your Creations, Being Sweet Savvy with Nature's Best" on page 34.

> **Please Note:** If trying to cut down on sugar, or if you suffer from a sugar related condition, you can simply substitute sun-dried cane juice crystals for equal amounts of xylitol. Getting the flavor right with stevia (whole leaf, powder or liquid) can be very tricky when it comes to certain dessert recipes; therefore, I highly advise the use of xylitol instead. It makes for a great low glycemic option. Look for a xylitol product that is derived from organic hardwood trees and not corn. Smart Sweet Xylitol is the brand I recommend.
>
> To obtain the benefits that both sun-dried cane juice crystals and xylitol have to offer, you may use half-and-half of each. You may even use a larger portion of one and a smaller portion of the other. For instance, in a recipe that calls for ¾ C sun-dried cane juice crystals, you can use ½ C sun-dried cane juice crystals and ¼ C xylitol. **FYI:** If you decide to use xylitol in a recipe that does not require a blender or food processor (like any one of the raw chocolate recipes that start on page 430), please note that xylitol will not melt and break down as well as sun-dried cane juice crystals. It will not affect the flavor or texture, but you will notice flecks of white throughout your chocolate. To do a better job at breaking down the xylitol, I suggest using an electric milk frother. This little gadget works great for breaking up clumps of caked up powders.

The consistency and texture when making homemade raw desserts can be a bit tricky in the beginning and may take a little trial and error. Therefore, just remember to always have fun and be forgiving of yourself. With a little patience and creativity, what started out as a mistake may just lead to a deliciously decadent masterpiece!

RAW CAKES, FROSTINGS, ICINGS & PIES

Basic Cheeze Cake

Crust

Pulse-chop the following dry ingredients in a <u>food processor</u> until medium ground:

- ★ 1 ½ C macadamia nuts
- ★ ½ C coconut flakes
- ★ ¼ tsp whole ground vanilla bean powder
- ★ 1 dash sea salt

Optional Variations

- ★ Substitute 1 ½ C pecans or walnuts for macadamia nuts.

Then, add the following to the above ingredients in <u>food processor</u> and process until mixture begins to stick together when pressed between your fingers:

- ★ 1 C packed, dried mulberries (presoaked for 5-10 minutes & then drained)

> Crust Instructions: Place a deep, 9 ½ inch round silicone cake mold on a plate for stability. Transfer crust mixture into silicone cake mold, and then spread and press in evenly using a spatula and your hands. Place plate with cake mold in the refrigerator (or freezer) for a short time while you prepare filling.

Cheeze Cake Filling

Blend the following ingredients in a <u>high-speed blender</u> until smooth and creamy. Stop and scrape down sides as needed:

- ★ 2 C cashews
- ★ 1 C raw sun-dried cane juice crystals
- ★ ½ tsp whole ground vanilla bean powder
- ★ ½ tsp sea salt
- ★ ¾ C lemon juice
- ★ 4-6 oz purified, filtered water

Then, add the following very slowly (which you may do while blender is still running), increase speed and blend until thick, smooth and creamy:

- ★ Additional 1 C cashews
- ★ ¾ C coconut oil (liquefied)

> Filling Instructions: Take plate with cake mold out of fridge (or freezer) and pour in your cheeze cake filling over the crust. Jiggle the plate to help easily distribute filling, and then use the back end of a spoon or a spatula to help smooth and evenly distribute the top.
>
> Molding Instructions: Place plate and cake mold back into the freezer to firm up overnight. If you have a lightweight plate or large bowl cover (larger than cake pan), I suggest placing it over the top of the cake while forming in the freezer. This will help prevent the light frost that tends to form along the edges.
>
> Serving & Storing Instructions: Remove from mold while cake is still frozen (which is easily done using your hands); place on a cutting board and cut into 8-10 slices; transfer slices onto a plate and thaw in fridge until ready to serve. When ready to serve, choose one (or more) of your favorite toppings (page 372-374) and pour over the top of individual slices. Store leftover slices in an airtight, glass container for up to one week in the fridge or up to three months (or longer) in freezer.
>
> Optional Decorating Ideas: If you would like a topping to be molded as a top layer on your cheeze cake, then choose whichever topping you wish and pour and smooth over the top of the cheeze cake. Then let set in freezer as instructed above. You may also decorate the flavored top layer with a sprinkle of cacao nibs, coconut flakes, goji berries and/or mulberries for color contrast and texture just prior to freezing.

Chocolate Topping

Place the following ingredients in a glass measuring cup, whisk with a fork (or small whisk) until well combined and smooth and then drizzle over individual slices:

- ★ ½ C raw cacao powder
- ★ 1 dash whole ground vanilla bean powder
- ★ 1 pinch sea salt
- ★ ½ C raw agave
- ★ 2 TBS coconut oil (liquefied)

Optional Additions for Variation

- ★ Top cheeze cake with additional superfoods (such as cacao nibs, coconut flakes, goji berries, mulberries, etc.).
- ★ Substitute 1-2 TBS chia seed oil, hemp seed oil, black sesame seed oil or extra virgin olive oil for coconut oil.

La-Caramel Topping

Place the following ingredients in a glass measuring cup, whisk with a fork (or small whisk) until well combined and smooth and then drizzle over individual slices:

- ★ ½ C lucuma powder
- ★ 1 dash whole ground vanilla bean powder

- ★ 1 pinch sea salt
- ★ ½ C raw agave
- ★ 2 TBS coconut oil (liquefied)

Optional Serving Idea

FYI: This topping is amazing by itself, but even more amazing when drizzled along with the chocolate topping above!

Strawberry Topping

Blend together the following ingredients in a <u>high-speed blender</u> until smooth, and then pour over individual slices for a fabulous presentation:

- ★ 1 C packed strawberries (fresh or defrosted)
- ★ 2 TBS raw agave (or to taste)
- ★ 1 TBS chia seeds

Optional Additions for Variation

- ★ Add sliced fresh strawberries all around the top outer edge of cheeze cake (which can be done before or after slicing).
- ★ If you would like a pulpy topping, add about ½ C more strawberries to smooth mixture above and gently pulse them through. Just a few quick pulses will be enough. Taste and add additional sweetener if needed.

Raspberry Topping

Blend together the following ingredients in a <u>high-speed blender</u> until smooth, and then pour over individual slices for a fabulous presentation:

- ★ 1 C packed raspberries (fresh or defrosted)
- ★ 2-3 TBS raw agave (or to taste)
- ★ 1 TBS chia seeds

Optional Additions for Variation

- ★ Add whole raspberries all around the top outer edge of cheeze cake (which can be done before or after slicing).
- ★ If you would like a pulpy topping, add about ½ C more raspberries to smooth mixture above and gently pulse them through. Just a few quick pulses will be enough. Taste and add additional sweetener if needed.

Blueberry Topping

Blend together the following ingredients in a <u>high-speed blender</u> until smooth, and then pour over individual slices for a fabulous presentation:

- 1 C packed blueberries (fresh or defrosted)
- 2-3 TBS raw agave (or to taste)
- 1 TBS chia seeds

Optional Additions for Variation

- Add sliced fresh strawberries all around the top outer edge of cheeze cake (which can be done before or after slicing). The color variation is beautiful.
- If you would like a pulpier topping, add about ⅓ C more blueberries to smooth mixture above and gently pulse them through. Just a few quick pulses will be enough. Taste and add additional sweetener if needed.

Cherry Topping

Blend together the following ingredients in a <u>high-speed blender</u> until smooth, and then pour over individual slices for a fabulous presentation:

- 1 C packed, frozen cherries (defrosted)
- 2 TBS raw agave (or to taste)
- 1 TBS chia seeds

Optional Additions for Variation

- If you would like a pulpier topping, add about ½ C more cherries to smooth mixture above and gently pulse them through. Just a few quick pulses will be enough. Taste and add additional sweetener if needed.

> **Recipe Notes & Quick Tips:** Store leftover topping(s) in an airtight glass jar in the fridge. Chocolate & La-Caramel Topping will keep for up to two weeks in the fridge and all fruit-based toppings will keep for up to one week in fridge. All may be stored in freezer for up to three months or longer.
>
> Place glass jar in a bowl filled with warm water to help thin out before serving again (especially Chocolate & La-Caramel Topping).

Karen's Chocolate Crème Cake

Crust

Pulse-chop the following dry ingredients in a <u>food processor</u> until medium ground:

- 1 ½ C walnuts
- ½ C coconut flakes
- ½ C cacao beans or nibs
- ¼ tsp whole ground vanilla bean powder
- 1 dash sea salt

Optional Variations

- ★ Substitute 1 ½ C Brazil nuts or pecans for walnuts.

Then, add the following to the above ingredients in <u>food processor</u> and pulse through until well incorporated. Be sure to not over process into a paste:

- ★ ¼ C raw agave

> Crust Instructions: Place a deep, 9 ½ inch round silicone cake mold on a plate for stability. Transfer crust mixture into silicone cake mold, and then spread and press in evenly using a spatula and your hands. Place plate with cake mold in the refrigerator (or freezer) for a short time while you prepare filling.

Crème Cake Filling

Please Note: Make chocolate base layer first. Then move on to top layer while base layer is firming up.

Chocolate Base Layer

Blend the following ingredients in a <u>high-speed blender</u> until smooth and creamy. Stop to scrape down sides as needed:

- ★ 1 C cashews
- ★ ¾ C raw sun-dried cane juice crystals
- ★ ¾ C raw cacao powder
- ★ ½ tsp whole ground vanilla bean powder
- ★ ¼ tsp sea salt
- ★ 8-12 oz purified, filtered water

Then, add the following very slowly (which you may do while blender is still running), increase speed and blend until thick, smooth and creamy. Stop to scrape down sides as needed:

- ★ Additional 1 C cashews
- ★ ¾ C coconut oil (liquefied)

Optional Variation

- ★ Replace ¼ C of coconut oil with melted cacao butter: ½ C of coconut oil + ¼ C melted cacao butter.

> Base Layer Filling Instructions: Take plate with cake mold out of fridge (or freezer) and pour the chocolate base layer over the crust. Jiggle the plate to help easily distribute filling. Use the back end of a spoon or a spatula to smooth and evenly distribute the top if needed. Place in freezer for at least one hour (or until firm) before pouring on the vanilla top layer (below).

Vanilla Top Layer

Blend the following ingredients in a <u>high-speed blender</u> until smooth and creamy. Stop to scrape down sides as needed:

- ★ 1 C cashews
- ★ ¼ C raw sun-dried cane juice crystals
- ★ ½ tsp whole ground vanilla bean powder
- ★ 1 dash sea salt
- ★ ¼ C coconut oil (liquefied)
- ★ 6-8 oz purified, filtered water

Optional <u>Top Layer</u> Additions & Variations

- ★ For **Chocolate Chai Crème Cake:** add 1 TBS of loose-leaf chai tea prior to blending.
- ★ For **Chocolate Goji-Orange Crème Cake:** add 1-2 TBS goji berries and about 2-3 drops of sweet orange essential oil (or to taste) prior to blending.
- ★ For **Chocolate Matcha Crème Cake:** add 1 TBS of matcha green tea powder prior to blending.
- ★ For **Chocolate Mocha Crème Cake:** add 1 TBS of shilajit (for coffee-like flavor) prior to blending.
- ★ For **Chocolate Mint Crème Cake:** add ¼ tsp spirulina and about 2-3 drops of peppermint essential oil (or to taste) prior to blending.

> Top Layer Instructions: Take plate with cake mold out of freezer and pour vanilla top layer evenly over chocolate layer. Gently jiggle the plate to help easily distribute, and then use the back end of a spoon or a spatula to help smooth and evenly distribute the top.
>
> Decorating Ideas: Sprinkle top layer with cacao nibs or crushed cacao beans. You may also add coconut flakes, goji berries or whatever you wish before placing back into the freezer to mold.
>
> Molding Instructions: If you have a lightweight plate or large bowl cover (larger than cake pan), place over the top of the cake while firming up in the freezer. Allow to set overnight.
>
> Serving & Storing Instructions: Remove from mold while cake is still frozen (which is easily done using your hands); place on a cutting board and cut into 8-10 slices; transfer slices onto a plate and thaw in fridge until ready to serve. Store leftover slices in an airtight, glass container for up to two weeks in the fridge or 3-6 months (or longer) in the freezer.

Chocolate Hazelnut Dream Cake

Crust

Pulse-chop the following dry ingredients in a <u>food processor</u> until medium ground:

- ★ 1 ½ C hazelnuts
- ★ ½ C coconut flakes
- ★ ½ C cacao beans or nibs
- ★ ¼ tsp whole ground vanilla bean powder
- ★ 1 dash sea salt

Then, add the following to the above ingredients in <u>food processor</u> and pulse through until well incorporated. Be sure to not over process into a paste:

- ★ ¼ C raw agave

> Crust Instructions: Place a deep, 9 ½ inch round silicone cake mold on a plate for stability. Transfer crust mixture into silicone cake mold, and then spread and press in evenly using a spatula and your hands. Place plate with cake mold in the refrigerator (or freezer) for a short time while you prepare filling.

Hazelnut Filling

Blend the following ingredients in a <u>high-speed blender</u> until smooth and creamy. Stop to scrape down sides as needed:

- ★ 2 C hazelnuts
- ★ 1 C raw sun-dried cane juice crystals
- ★ ¾ C raw cacao powder
- ★ 1 tsp whole ground vanilla bean powder

- ½ tsp Pumpkin Pie Blend
- ¼ tsp sea salt
- 12-14 oz purified, filtered water

Then, add the following very slowly (which you may do while blender is still running), increase speed and blend until thick, smooth and creamy. Stop to scrape down sides as needed:

- 1 C cashews
- ¾ C coconut oil (liquefied)

Optional Variation

- Replace ¼ C of coconut oil with melted cacao butter: ½ C of coconut oil + ¼ C melted cacao butter.

> Filling Instructions: Take plate with cake mold out of fridge (or freezer) and pour in the hazelnut filling. Jiggle the plate to help easily distribute filling. Use the back end of a spoon or a spatula to smooth and evenly distribute the top if needed.
>
> Decorating Ideas: Sprinkle top layer with cacao nibs, crushed cacao beans and/or coconut flakes before placing back in the freezer to mold. You may also circle the outer top edge with dried mulberries, fresh raspberries or sliced fresh strawberries if desired.
>
> Molding Instructions: If you have a lightweight plate or large bowl cover (larger than cake pan), place over the top of the cake while firming up in the freezer. Allow to set overnight.
>
> Serving & Storing Instructions: Remove from mold while cake is still frozen (which is easily done using your hands); place on a cutting board and cut into 8-10 slices; transfer slices onto a plate and thaw in fridge until ready to serve. Store leftover slices in an airtight, glass container for up to two weeks in the fridge or 3-6 months (or longer) in the freezer.

Tiramisu Crème Cake

Crust

Pulse-chop the following dry ingredients in a <u>food processor</u> until medium ground:

- 1 ½ C pecans
- ½ C coconut flakes
- ½ C cacao beans or nibs
- ¼ tsp whole ground vanilla bean powder
- 1 dash sea salt

Then, add the following to the above ingredients in <u>food processor</u> and pulse through until well incorporated. Be sure to not over process into a paste:

* ¼ C raw agave

> Crust Instructions: Place a deep, 9-inch square silicone cake mold on a plate for stability. Transfer crust mixture into silicone cake mold, then spread and press in evenly using a spatula and your hands. Place plate with cake mold in the refrigerator (or freezer) for a short time while you prepare filling.

Tiramisu Filling

Blend the following ingredients in a <u>high-speed blender</u> until smooth and creamy. Stop to scrape down sides as needed:

* 1 C almonds
* ½ C raw sun-dried cane juice crystals
* ¼ C lucuma powder
* 2 TBS raw cacao powder
* 2 TBS shilajit (for coffee-like flavor)
* 1 tsp whole ground vanilla bean powder
* ½ tsp cinnamon
* ¼ tsp sea salt
* 10-12 oz purified, filtered water

Then, add the following very slowly (which you may do while blender is still running), increase speed and blend until thick, smooth and creamy. Stop to scrape down sides as needed:

* 1 C cashews
* ¾ C coconut oil (liquefied)

Optional Variation

* Replace ¼ C of coconut oil with melted cacao butter: ½ C of coconut oil + ¼ C melted cacao butter.

> Filling Instructions: Take plate with cake mold out of fridge (or freezer) and pour in the tiramisu filling. Jiggle the plate to help easily distribute filling. Use the back end of a spoon or a spatula to smooth and evenly distribute the top if needed.

Tiramisu Topping

In a small bowl, combine the ingredients below. Then, sprinkle evenly over the entire top of the cake (can be done prior to placing in the freezer or right before serving):

* 1 TBS raw cacao powder
* 1 TBS cinnamon
* 1 TBS lucuma powder

- ★ 1 TBS shilajit

Optional Additions

- ★ In addition to the above, you may sprinkle top layer with cacao nibs or decorate edges with whole cacao beans.

> Molding Instructions: Once topping has been added, place back in the freezer to set overnight. If you have a lightweight plate or large bowl cover (larger than cake pan), place over the top of the cake while firming up in the freezer.
>
> Serving & Storing Instructions: Remove from mold while cake is still frozen (which is easily done using your hands); place on a cutting board and cut into desired number of squares; transfer pieces onto a plate and thaw in fridge until ready to serve. Store leftover pieces in an airtight, glass container for up to two weeks in the fridge or 3-6 months (or longer) in freezer.

Vanilla Cake Envy

Pulse-chop the following dry ingredients in a <u>food processor</u> until medium-well ground:

- ★ 3 C almonds
- ★ 1 C coconut flakes
- ★ ¼ C sun-dried cane juice crystals
- ★ 1 tsp whole ground vanilla bean powder
- ★ ½ tsp Pumpkin Pie Blend (optional or to taste)
- ★ ¼ tsp sea salt

Then, add the following to the above ingredients in <u>food processor</u> and process until mixture begins to stick together when pressed between your fingers:

- ★ 1 C packed Hunza golden raisins (presoaked for 5-10 minutes & then drained)

Optional Variations

- ★ Substitute 1 C packed Turkish apricots, currants or other dried fruit of choice for Hunza golden raisins.

Last, add the following to the above ingredients in <u>food processor</u> and process again until well incorporated. Mixture should be moistened just enough to hold together when pinched between fingers and may even start to form a ball in food processor:

- ★ ¼ C coconut oil (liquefied)
- ★ Purified, filtered water as needed. Only add water if necessary (1 TBS at a time). Mixture should be moist and sticky enough to hold together when squished in your hand.

> Molding Instructions: Place a round or square silicone cake mold (smaller than 9 inches for thicker cake) on a plate for stability. Transfer cake mixture into silicone mold, and then spread and press in evenly using a spatula and your hands. If you have a lightweight plate or large bowl cover (larger than cake pan), place over the top of the cake while firming up in the freezer. Let sit in freezer for several hours or overnight. **Quick Tip:** For a cupcake or muffin rendition, use silicone muffin pans.
>
> Decorating Ideas: Remove from mold while cake is still frozen (which is easily done using your hands); place on a plate or cutting board; apply a frosting or icing of choice (pages 383-386); decorate frosting with whatever you choose (fresh fruit, dried fruit, nuts, cacao nibs, coconut flakes, etc.). You may also choose to leave plain.
>
> Serving & Storing Instructions: Allow cake to thaw in fridge until ready to serve. Cut into desired number of slices or squares, and then store leftover pieces in an airtight, glass container for up to two weeks in the fridge or 3-6 months (or longer) in the freezer.

Chocolate Cake Envy

Pulse-chop the following dry ingredients in a <u>food processor</u> until well ground:

- ★ 3 C Brazil nuts
- ★ 1 C coconut flakes
- ★ ¾ C raw cacao powder
- ★ ¼ C lucuma powder
- ★ ¼ C sun-dried cane juice crystals
- ★ ½ tsp whole ground vanilla bean powder
- ★ ¼ tsp Pumpkin Pie Blend (optional or to taste)
- ★ ¼ tsp sea salt

Optional Variations

- ★ Substitute 3 C almonds for Brazil nuts.
- ★ Substitute 3 C walnuts and/or pecans (e.g., 2 C walnuts and 1 C pecans) for Brazil nuts.

Then, add the following to the above ingredients in <u>food processor</u> and process until mixture begins to stick together when pressed between your fingers:

- ★ 2 C packed Hunza golden raisins (presoaked for 5-10 minutes & then drained)

Optional Variations

- ★ Substitute 2 C packed Turkish apricots, currants or other dried fruit of choice for Hunza golden raisins.

Last, add the following to the above ingredients in <u>food processor</u> and process again until well incorporated. Mixture should be moistened just enough to hold together when pinched between fingers and may even start to form a ball in food processor:

- ★ ¼ C coconut oil (liquefied)
- ★ Purified, filtered water as needed. Only add water if necessary (1 TBS at a time). Mixture should be moist and sticky enough to hold together when squished in your hand.

Molding Instructions: Place a 9 ½ inch round or a 9-inch square silicone cake mold on a plate for stability. Transfer cake mixture into silicone mold, and then spread and press in evenly using a spatula and your hands. If you have a lightweight plate or large bowl cover (larger than cake pan), place over the top of the cake while firming up in the freezer. Let sit in freezer for several hours or overnight. **Quick Tip:** For a cupcake or muffin rendition, use silicone muffin pans.

Decorating Ideas: Remove from mold while cake is still frozen (which is easily done using your hands); place on a plate or cutting board; apply a frosting or icing of choice (starting on page 383); decorate frosting with whatever you choose (fresh fruit, dried fruit, nuts, cacao nibs, coconut flakes, etc.). You may also choose to leave plain.

Serving & Storing Instructions: Allow cake to thaw in fridge until ready to serve. Cut into desired number of slices or squares, and then store leftover pieces in an airtight, glass container for up to two weeks in the fridge or 3-6 months (or longer) in the freezer.

Carrot Cake Envy

First, process the following in a <u>food processor</u> until finely chopped or, if you prefer, use the shredding disc instead. Process enough to obtain 2 C, packed. Remove from processor and set aside to add along with dried fruit later:

- ★ Carrots (peeled & tops removed)

Second, pulse-chop the following ingredients in a <u>food processor</u> until medium-well ground:

- ★ 3 C walnuts
- ★ 1 C coconut flakes
- ★ ¼ C white chia seeds
- ★ ¼ C sun-dried cane juice crystals
- ★ 1 tsp Pumpkin Pie Blend
- ★ ½ tsp whole ground vanilla bean powder
- ★ ¼ tsp sea salt

Optional Variation

- ★ Replace up to half the amount of walnuts (about 1-1 ½ C) with pecans.

Third, add the following to the above ingredients in <u>food processor</u> and process until mixture begins to stick together when pressed between your fingers:

- ★ 2 C packed carrots (already chopped fine or shredded)
- ★ 1 C packed Hunza golden raisins (presoaked for 5-10 minutes & then drained)

Optional Variations

- ★ Substitute 1 C packed Turkish apricots or currants for Hunza golden raisins.

Last, add the following to the above ingredients in <u>food processor</u> and process again until well incorporated. Mixture should be moistened just enough to hold together when pinched between fingers and may even start to form a ball in food processor:

- ★ ¼ C coconut oil (liquefied)
- ★ Purified, filtered water as needed. Only add water if necessary (1 TBS at a time). Mixture should be moist and sticky enough to hold together when squished in your hand.

Molding Instructions: Place a 9 ½ inch round or a 9-inch square silicone cake mold on a plate for stability. Transfer cake mixture into silicone mold, and then spread and press in evenly using a spatula and your hands. If you have a lightweight plate or large bowl cover (larger than cake pan), place over the top of the cake while firming up in the freezer. Let sit in freezer for several hours or overnight. **Quick Tip:** For a cupcake or muffin rendition, use silicone muffin pans.

Decorating Ideas: Remove from mold while cake is still frozen (which is easily done using your hands); place on a plate or cutting board; apply Spiced Walnut Crème Frosting (page 384); decorate with walnuts and shreds of carrot.

Serving & Storing Instructions: Allow cake to thaw in fridge until ready to serve. Cut into desired number of slices or squares, and then store leftover pieces in an airtight, glass container for up to two weeks in the fridge or 3-6 months in the freezer.

Vanilla Crème Frosting

Blend the following ingredients in a <u>high-speed blender</u> until smooth and creamy. Stop to scrape down sides as needed:

- ★ 2 C cashews
- ★ ½ tsp whole ground vanilla bean powder
- ★ 1 dash sea salt
- ★ ¼ C raw honey or agave
- ★ ¼ C coconut oil (liquefied)
- ★ 4-6 oz purified, filtered water (as needed)

Optional Additions for Variation

- ★ Add 2-3 drops (or to taste) of one of the following therapeutic quality essential oils: sweet orange, lemon, lime peel, ginger or peppermint.

> **Recipe Notes & Quick Tips:** Chill for at least one hour to thicken, and then spread as desired onto cakes, brownies, bars, etc. Great as a cookie dip too! Store frosting in an airtight container in the fridge for up to two weeks.

Crème Cheeze Frosting

Blend the following ingredients in a high-speed blender until smooth and creamy. Stop to scrape down sides as needed:

- ★ 2 C macadamia nuts
- ★ ½ tsp sea salt (or to taste)
- ★ ¼ C raw honey or agave
- ★ ¼ C lemon juice
- ★ 4-6 oz purified, filtered water (as needed)

> **Recipe Notes & Quick Tips:** Chill for at least one hour to thicken, and then spread as desired onto cakes, brownies, bars, etc. Great as a cookie dip too! Store frosting in an airtight container in the fridge for up to two weeks.

Spiced Walnut Crème Frosting

Blend the following ingredients in a high-speed blender until smooth and creamy. Stop to scrape down sides as needed:

- ★ 2 C walnuts
- ★ ½ tsp Pumpkin Pie Blend (or to taste)
- ★ 1 dash sea salt
- ★ ¼ C raw honey or agave
- ★ ¼ C coconut oil
- ★ 4-6 oz purified, filtered water (as needed)

> **Recipe Notes & Quick Tips:** Chill for at least one hour to thicken, and then spread as desired onto cakes, brownies, bars, etc. Great as a cookie dip too! Store frosting in an airtight container in the fridge for up to two weeks.

Vanilla Icing

Blend the following ingredients in a high-speed blender until smooth and creamy (be sure to start at a slow speed and increase slowly). Stop and scrape down sides as needed:

- ★ ½ C coconut crème
- ★ ¼ C raw agave

- ★ ¼ tsp whole ground vanilla bean
- ★ 1 pinch sea salt
- ★ 4-6 oz purified, filtered water (as needed)

> **Recipe Notes & Quick Tips:** Use immediately once made, and then store leftover in an airtight glass jar in the fridge for up to two weeks. Once refrigerated, icing will become hard and need to be thawed or warmed. I suggest placing glass jar in a bowl filled with hot tap water and stir contents on occasion. When oils warm up the frosting will become soft and spreadable again.

Chocolate Icing

Blend the following ingredients in a <u>high-speed blender</u> until all ingredients are completely broken down and smooth. Be sure to start at a slow speed and increase slowly. Stop and scrape down sides as needed:

- ★ 1 C packed dates, pitted (presoaked for at least one hour & then drained)
- ★ ¼ C raw cacao powder
- ★ ¼ tsp whole ground vanilla bean
- ★ 1 pinch sea salt
- ★ ¼ C coconut oil (liquefied)
- ★ 6-8 oz purified, filtered water (as needed)

> **Recipe Notes & Quick Tips:** Use immediately once made, and then store leftover in an airtight glass jar in the fridge for up to two weeks. Once refrigerated, icing will become hard and need to be thawed or warmed. I suggest placing glass jar in a bowl filled with hot tap water and stir contents on occasion. When oils warm up the frosting will become soft and spreadable again.

Go-To Raw Icings

Please Note: The following raw icing recipes are my absolute favorites. They are super easy and take almost no time to whip up. No blender or food processor required! All you need is a 16 oz glass measuring cup or small mixing bowl, a fork for whisking, your ingredients and a little wrist action!

Ecstasy Icing

This chocolate icing is pure ecstasy and so much better for you than Betty Crocker or Duncan Hines!

- ★ ¾ C raw honey (high-quality local or Premier Research Labs Canadian Gold)
- ★ ¼ C coconut oil (liquefied)
- ★ ¼ C raw cacao powder

- ½ tsp whole ground vanilla bean powder
- 1 dash sea salt

Emerald Icing

Don't let the addition of spirulina scare you off. The flavor of this icing concoction is scrumptiously irresistible and the color is enchanting!

- ¾ C raw honey (high-quality local or Premier Research Labs Canadian Gold)
- ¼ C coconut oil
- 2 TBS spirulina
- 2 TBS baobab powder
- ½ tsp whole ground vanilla bean powder
- 1 dash sea salt

Blonde Icing

Yum! The subtle flavors of lucuma and mesquite make this icing lusciously mouth-watering.

- ¾ C raw honey (High-quality local or Premier Research Labs Canadian Gold)
- ¼ C coconut oil (liquefied)
- 2 TBS lucuma powder
- 2 TBS mesquite powder
- ½ tsp whole ground vanilla bean power
- 1 dash sea salt

> **Recipe Notes & Quick Tips:** Use immediately once made, and then store leftover in an airtight glass jar in the fridge for up to two weeks. Once refrigerated, icing will become hard and need to be thawed or warmed. I suggest placing glass jar in a bowl filled with hot tap water and stir contents on occasion. When oils warm up the frosting will become soft and spreadable again. You may substitute ⅔ C raw agave for honey if desired.

Pecan Pie

Crust

Pulse-chop the following dry ingredients in a <u>food processor</u> until medium ground:

- 1 ½ C almonds
- ½ C coconut flakes
- ¼ tsp whole ground vanilla bean powder
- 1 dash sea salt

Optional Variation

- Replace ½ C of almonds with ½ C of pecans.

Then, add the following to the above ingredients in <u>food processor</u> and process until mixture begins to stick together when pressed between your fingers:

- ★ ½ C packed dates, pitted (presoaked for 5-10 minutes & then drained)

> Crust Instructions: Place a deep, 9 ½ inch round silicone cake mold on a plate for stability. Transfer crust mixture into silicone cake mold, and then spread and press in evenly using a spatula and your hands. Place plate with cake mold into the refrigerator (or freezer) for a short time while you prepare filling.

Date Filling

Process the following in a <u>food processor</u> until all ingredients are well broken down into what looks like a thick, but smooth paste. Stop and scrape down sides as needed:

- ★ 3 C packed dates, pitted (presoaked for at least one hour & then drained)
- ★ 2 TBS lucuma powder
- ★ 1 tsp Pumpkin Pie Blend
- ★ ½ tsp whole ground vanilla bean
- ★ ¼ tsp sea salt
- ★ Purified, filtered water as needed. Add water a little at a time just to keep it moving enough to break down into a smooth paste

Add the following next and then process again until well incorporated:

- ★ 2 TBS coconut oil (liquefied)

Filling Instructions: Take plate with cake mold out of fridge (or freezer); transfer date filling to the crust; spread and press in evenly using the back end of a spoon or a spatula.

Decorating Instructions: Use ½-1 C of pecans to decorate the top. You may circle around the edges and go inward towards the center with whole pecans (absolutely beautiful) or, to save time, you can coarsely chop pecans and generously sprinkle over the entire top (still very beautiful). Once pecans have been applied (whole or pieces), gently press them down into the date paste mixture to stick.

Molding Instructions: If you have a lightweight plate or large bowl cover (larger than cake pan), place over the top of the pie while firming up in the freezer. Let set for several hours or overnight in freezer.

Serving & Storing Instructions: Remove from mold while pie is still frozen (which is easily done using your hands); place on a cutting board and cut into 8-10 slices; transfer slices onto a plate and thaw in fridge until ready to serve. Store leftover slices in an airtight, glass container for up to two weeks in the fridge or 3-6 months (or longer) in the freezer.

Lemon Chia Pie

Crust

Pulse-chop the following dry ingredients in a <u>food processor</u> until medium ground:

- ★ 1 ½ C macadamia nuts
- ★ ½ C coconut flakes
- ★ ¼ tsp whole ground vanilla bean powder
- ★ 1 dash sea salt

Then, add the following to the above ingredients in <u>food processor</u> and process until mixture begins to stick together when pressed between your fingers:

- ★ ½ C packed golden berries (presoaked for 5-10 minutes & then drained)

Optional Variations

- ★ Substitute ½ C packed Hunza golden raisins or currants for golden berries. May also choose Turkish apricots or figs (chopped).

> Crust Instructions: Place a 9 ½ inch round silicone cake mold (for pie) or a 9-inch square silicone cake mold (for squares) on a plate for stability. Transfer crust mixture into silicone mold, and then spread and press in evenly using a spatula and your hands. Place plate with cake mold into the refrigerator (or freezer) for a short time while you prepare filling.

Lemon Chia Filling

Blend the following in a <u>high-speed blender</u> until well emulsified, thick and creamy. Stop to scrape down sides as needed:

- ★ 3 whole lemons (peeled)
- ★ ½ C white chia seeds
- ★ ¼ C coconut flakes
- ★ 6 drops lemon essential oil
- ★ ¼ tsp whole ground vanilla bean powder
- ★ 1 dash turmeric
- ★ 1 pinch sea salt
- ★ ½ C raw agave
- ★ ¼ C coconut oil (liquefied)
- ★ 4 oz purified, filtered water

> Filling Instructions: Take plate with cake mold out of fridge (or freezer) and pour lemon chia filling over crust immediately. Jiggle the plate to help easily distribute filling, and then use the back end of a spoon or a spatula to help smooth and evenly distribute the top if needed.

Crunch Topping

Coarsely pulse-chop the below in a <u>food processor</u> and sprinkle evenly over the top of the lemon chia filling. Then gently press the topping down using the back end of a spoon or a spatula so topping sticks firmly to the filling:

- ★ ⅔ C macadamia nuts
- ★ 2 TBS coconut flake

> Molding Instructions: If you have a lightweight plate or large bowl cover (larger than cake pan), place over the top while molding in the freezer. Let set for several hours or overnight in freezer.
>
> Serving & Storing Instructions: Remove from mold while pie is still frozen (which is easily done using your hands); place on a cutting board and cut into 8-10 slices (for pie) or 9-12 squares; transfer pieces onto a plate and thaw in fridge until ready to serve. Store leftover slices in an airtight, glass container for up to one week in the fridge or up to three months (or longer) in the freezer.

Sweet Potato Pie

Crust

Pulse-chop the following dry ingredients in a <u>food processor</u> until medium ground:

- ★ 2 C Brazil nuts
- ★ ½ C coconut flakes
- ★ ¼ tsp Pumpkin Pie Blend
- ★ 1 dash sea salt

Then, add the following to the above ingredients in <u>food processor</u> and pulse through until well incorporated. Be sure to not over process into a paste:

- ★ ¼ C raw agave

> Crust Instructions: Place a deep, 9 ½ inch round silicone cake mold on a plate for stability. Transfer crust mixture into silicone cake mold, and then spread and press in evenly using a spatula and your hands. Place plate with cake mold into the refrigerator (or freezer) for a short time while you prepare filling.

Sweet Potato Filling

Blend the following ingredients in a <u>high-speed blender</u> until smooth:

- ★ 1 large sweet potato (peeled)
- ★ 1 whole orange (peeled & seeded)
- ★ ¼ C raw agave
- ★ 4 oz purified, filtered water

Then, add the following to the above mixture and blend again until thick and smooth. Stop to scrape down sides as needed:

- ★ ½ C packed Turkish apricots (presoaked for 5-10 minutes & then drained)
- ★ ½ C packed currants (presoaked for 5-10 minutes & then drained)
- ★ ¼ tsp Pumpkin Pie Blend
- ★ 1 dash sea salt

- ¼ C coconut oil (liquefied)

> Filling Instructions: Take plate with cake mold out of fridge (or freezer) and pour in sweet potato filling. Jiggle the plate to help easily distribute filling. Use the back end of a spoon or a spatula to smooth and evenly distribute the top if needed.
>
> Decorating Ideas: Sprinkle top layer with coconut flake. You may also decorate the top outer edge with chopped Brazil nuts, whole pecans, chopped Turkish apricots and/or currants if desired.
>
> Molding Instructions: If you have a lightweight plate or large bowl cover (larger than cake pan), place over the top of the pie while firming up in the freezer. Let set for several hours or overnight in freezer.
>
> Serving & Storing Instructions: Remove from mold while pie is still frozen (which is easily done using your hands); place on a cutting board and cut into 8-10 slices; transfer slices onto a plate and thaw in fridge until ready to serve. Store leftover slices in an airtight, glass container for up to one week in the fridge or three months (or longer) in the freezer.

Amazing Apple Pie

Crust

Pulse-chop the following dry ingredients in a <u>food processor</u> until medium ground:

- 2 C walnuts
- ½ C coconut flakes
- ¼ tsp whole ground vanilla bean powder
- 1 dash sea salt

Then, add the following to the above ingredients in <u>food processor</u> and process until mixture begins to stick together when pressed between your fingers:

- ½ C packed Hunza golden raisins (presoaked for 5-10 minutes & then drained)

Optional Variations

- Substitute ½ C packed Turkish apricots, figs, currants or other dried fruit of choice for Hunza golden raisins.

> Crust Instructions: Transfer crust mixture into a 9-inch Springform pan, then spread and press in evenly using a spatula and your hands. Refrigerator while you prepare filling.

Apple Filling

Process the following in a <u>food processor</u> until smooth and then transfer to large mixing bowl. Stop and scrape down sides as needed:

- ★ 2 sweet red apples (chopped)
- ★ 1 C Hunza golden raisins (not soaked)
- ★ ¼ C white chia seeds
- ★ 1 TBS mesquite powder
- ★ 1 TBS lucuma powder
- ★ 1 tsp Apple Pie Blend
- ★ 1 dash sea salt
- ★ 2 TBS lemon juice

Optional Variation

- ★ Substitute 1 C currants (not soaked) for Hunza golden raisins.

Then, add the following to mixing bowl until all apple pieces are blended in and evenly coated. Transfer to Springform pan, and then spread mixture evenly over crust:

- ★ 2 additional sweet red apples sliced thin and then chopped into small pieces. To make this task easier, coarsely pulse-chop into small-medium chunks in <u>food-processor</u>.

Crunch Topping

Coarsely pulse-chop the following in a <u>food processor</u> and sprinkle evenly over the top of apple filling. Then gently press the topping down using the back end of a spoon or a spatula so topping sticks firmly to the filling:

- ★ ⅔ C almonds
- ★ 2 TBS coconut flakes
- ★ 1 dash Apple Pie Blend

> Molding & Storing Instructions: If you have a lightweight plate or large bowl cover (larger than cake pan), place over the top of the pie while firming up. Let sit in freezer for a few hours, and then transfer to refrigerator until ready to serve. Store any remaining slices in an airtight, glass container for up to one week in the fridge or three months (or longer) in the freezer.
>
> Optional Serving Ideas: If you desire warm apple pie, slice pie while partially frozen and still firm, place slices onto dessert dishes and then place dessert dishes into the dehydrator (set at 105-115°F). Remove when pie slices are warm and starting to brown. If desired, drizzle with La-Caramel Topping (page 372) and/or serve with ice cream of choice (page 417).

BRAWNIES, RAWKIES, BARS & BITES

If you haven't guessed, "brawnies" are my raw version of traditional brownies and "rawkies" are my raw version of traditional cookies. I'm also excited to share a few other traditional favorites that I have had the pleasure of creatively remixing into raw delights, as well as a few new and cutting-edge creations!

Quick Recipe Tips:

Although it is not necessary, I highly suggest pregrinding certain seeds before adding them into the food processor to be incorporated with all the other ingredients. A food processor does many things; however, it will not completely flour down smaller seeds such as chia and sesame seeds. If you've never tried the actual recipe with the seeds both ways (i.e., thrown in whole versus preground), it probably wouldn't really matter, as both will taste delicious. Having tried them both ways myself though, I can say that when you pregrind the smaller seeds, the flavor is richer, has more depth and the texture is richer and more uniform. Furthermore, having a richer and more uniform texture influences how well it molds and holds up to a fork or spoon. It is certainly well worth the extra minute it takes to pregrind.

> **Please Note:** A coffee grinder will do just fine for small amounts (like a few ounces), but for larger amounts, I advise using a blender. A Blendtec blender will grind all nuts and seeds into powder, but if you own or are looking into a Vitamix, you will need to purchase the dry container separately for milling seeds. That said, I actually have a better recommendation that I feel will come in handy for more than just one use: the Nutribullet! The Nutribullet comes with a milling blade that will make pregrinding your chia seeds and sesame seeds a fast and easy task. It makes chopping nuts really easy as well. You can even powder down spice seeds and whole leaf herbs with the milling blade. What's more, the Nutribullet is actually a high-powered blender that is perfect for making smaller portions of dips, dressings, smoothies and elixir drinks. So instead of buying a coffee grinder, or separate dry container for your Vitamix, I highly recommend investing in a Nutribullet. With all the pieces you get, you may find yourself using it more than you think. Oh, and how could I forget how super easy it is to clean as well!

Why do some recipes call for white chia, others black and yet others are indiscriminant? Let me first start out by stating that both white and black chia seeds have the same exact nutrients and provide the human body with the same health benefits. Nutritionally they are almost identical. So nutritionally, they can be used interchangeably. According to expert researchers who have studied the quality and health benefits of both types, the main culprits behind the higher ratings for white chia are the manufacturers of white chia themselves. Commercial competition confuses consumers yet again!

Be that as it may, many prefer to use white chia over black; especially in white and light-colored recipes. It's more of a culinary preference than having anything to do with health. Aesthetically speaking, the ability of white to blend in is more appealing to the eye than seeing flecks of black (at least in certain recipes). For instance, if white chia is available, I prefer it to black in chia pudding recipes. On the other hand, I prefer to use black over white in deep, dark chocolaty recipes. It really just comes down to personal preference upon presentation. When I'm making these same treats for just myself, or for an informal gathering, I never let the color of the chia seeds stop me.

Chia seeds are a wonderful recipe addition when you want to thicken or bind ingredients together but do not wish to alter the flavor. Because chia seeds are virtually tasteless, they are extremely versatile, making them an easy add-in for a nutritional up-grade. Whether eaten whole or ground, chia seeds are the highest plant-based source of omega-3 known to man – even higher than flax seeds if you recall. This fact alone should place chia on everyone's most wanted list!

> **Please Note:** I highly recommend grinding your own whole chia seeds versus buying into the convenience factor of milled chia seeds. It takes literally less than a minute to grind your own. Besides, it's really only necessary for a smoother texture and mouth feel; not for any gain in nutrition. You can always store any unused ground chia in an airtight, glass container in your fridge, which can easily be used in smoothies or other recipes within the week. Due to their unique chemical composition and high content of antioxidants, whole chia seeds are extremely shelf stable and will keep for long periods when stored in a cool, dark and dry place. Milled chia seeds may seem like a good idea, but any time a larger surface area is exposed to the elements (fatty acids in this case), susceptibility to oxidation increases. Please refer back to page 122 for more on the benefits of chia seeds.

Black sesame seeds are amazing and synergistically enhanced when combined with raw cacao. From a culinary standpoint, I find black sesame gives raw chocolate treats that fresh-baked taste, which is why they are featured in my Fudge Brawnie recipe. I also use them to make my raw rendition of Oreos. Oreo Rawkie Bars are a personal favorite of mine. They are not overly sweet and the black sesame gives these bars a unique and interestingly rich and smoky flavor. The extreme nutritional value of each individual ingredient, coupled with the synergism of all the ingredients together, will have every cell in your body singing "hallelujah!"

> **Please Note:** Black sesame seeds are super rich in calcium and magnesium and are also a great source of copper, manganese, copper, iron, phosphorus, vitamin B1, zinc and selenium. In addition to being super high in nutrients, sesame seeds contain two unique substances: sesamin and sesamolin. Both of which belong to a group of beneficial fibers called lignans and have been shown to have cholesterol-lowering effects in humans. Sesamin has also been found to protect the liver from oxidative damage.

Fudge Brawnies (raw brownies)

First, pregrind the following in a high-speed blender (I suggest the use of a Blendtec, Nutribullet with milling blade or Vitamix dry container for this task). Then transfer ground seeds to a food processor in order to thoroughly combine and evenly distribute all the rest of the ingredients:

- ★ ¾ C black sesame seeds

Second, add the following to the above ingredients in food processor and process again until well combined and blended in (mixture should look like chocolaty flour):

- ★ 2 C walnuts
- ★ ¾ C raw cacao powder
- ★ ½ C coconut flakes
- ★ ½ C sun-dried cane juice crystals
- ★ 1 TBS mesquite powder
- ★ 1 TBS lucuma powder
- ★ ½ tsp whole ground vanilla bean powder
- ★ ¼ tsp Pumpkin Pie Blend
- ★ ¼ tsp sea salt

Optional Variations

- ★ Substitute 2 C Brazil nuts or pecans for walnuts.

Third, add the following to the above ingredients in <u>food processor</u> and process until mixture begins to stick together when pressed between your fingers. Stop and scrape down sides as needed:

- ★ 1 ½ C packed Hunza golden raisins (presoaked for 5-10 minutes & then drained)

Optional Variations

- ★ Substitute 1 ½ C packed Turkish apricots, currants and/or other dried fruit of choice for Hunza golden raisins.

Last, add the following to the above ingredients in <u>food processor</u> and process again until well incorporated. Mixture should be moistened just enough to hold together when squished between fingers:

- ★ ¼ C coconut oil (liquefied)
- ★ Purified, filtered water as needed. Only add water if necessary (1 TBS at a time). Mixture can be semi-moist for molding in a cake pan, but should be a bit stickier for molding into balls.

> Molding Instructions: Place a 9-inch square silicone cake mold on a plate for stability. Transfer brownie mixture into silicone mold, and then spread and press in evenly using a spatula and your hands. Cover and let sit for at least one hour or overnight in freezer. This can be done either before or after decorating, depending on what you choose (see below).
>
> Decorating Ideas: Decorate the top with whole or chopped walnuts (or pecans), cacao nibs, coconut flakes, mulberries and/or goji berries <u>before</u> placing in freezer. Frost the top with your favorite frosting or icing <u>after</u> removing from freezer (pages 383-386). Also delish with La-Caramel Topping (page 372).
>
> If you decide to frost: remove brownies from mold while cold and firm from freezer (which is easily done using your hands); place onto a plate or cutting board; apply a frosting or icing of choice (pages 383-386); then either leave plain or decorate frosting with whatever you choose (fresh fruit, dried fruit, nuts, cacao nibs, coconut flakes, etc.).
>
> Serving & Storing Instructions: Allow brownies to thaw in fridge until ready to serve, and then cut into desired number of squares. Scrumptious when served with raw ice cream (page 417). Store any leftover pieces in an airtight, glass container for up to two weeks in the fridge or 3-6 months (or longer) in the freezer.
>
> Molding & Serving Variations: Instead of molding in a cake pan, form into **Brawnie Bites**! Using a 1 oz stainless-steel squeeze handle disher (or scooper): scoop up mixture, pack and level each half sphere and then dish onto a plate until there is no mixture left. You may either serve plain or top with 1-2 cacao beans or one whole nut (such as a walnut or pecan).
>
> You may also go one step further and make **Fudge Brawnie Truffles**! Take each 1 oz brawnie bite and gently roll in the palm of your hand to form a ball. If you desire, you can then roll each truffle in a small bowl of one (or more) of the following superfoods: cacao nibs, cacao powder, lucuma powder, mesquite powder, coconut flakes and/or hemp seeds.
>
> **Quick Tip:** If mixture is ever not cooperating when you want to shape and mold by hand, try placing bowl of mixture in the freezer for a few minutes before handling.

Oreo <u>Rawkie</u> Bars (my raw version of Oreo-like <u>cookie</u> bars)

Pregrind the following TWO ingredients (which can be done together) in a <u>high-speed blender</u> (I suggest using a Blendtec, Nutribullet with milling blade or Vitamix dry container for this task). Then transfer ground seeds to a <u>food processor</u> in order to thoroughly combine and evenly distribute all the rest of the ingredients:

- ★ 2 C black sesame seeds
- ★ ¾ C black chia seeds

Then, add the following to the above ingredients in <u>food processor</u> and process again until well combined and blended in (mixture should look like chocolaty flour):

- ★ 1 C sun-dried cane juice crystals

- ¾ C raw cacao powder
- ½ tsp whole ground vanilla bean powder
- ¼ tsp sea salt

Last, add the following to the above ingredients in <u>food processor</u> and process again until very well incorporated (stopping to scrape down sides as needed):

- ¼ C coconut oil (liquefied)

> Molding Instructions: Place a 9-inch square silicone cake mold on a plate for stability. Transfer mixture into silicone mold, and then spread and press in evenly using the back end of a spoon or a spatula. Cover and let sit for a few hours or overnight in freezer.
>
> Decorating & Serving Ideas: Remove from mold while still frozen (which is easily done using your hands); place on a plate or cutting board; cut into desired number of bars or squares; frost with Vanilla Crème Frosting (page 383) or Vanilla Icing (page 384). Sprinkle frosting with cacao nibs if desired. Also fabulous when served with raw ice cream (page 417).
>
> Storing Instructions: Store remaining pieces in an airtight, glass container for up to two weeks in fridge or 3-6 months (or longer) in freezer.

Key Lime Bars

Blend the following in a <u>high-speed blender</u> until well emulsified, thick and creamy. Stop to scrape down sides as needed:

- 1 C cashews
- 1 C raw macadamia nuts
- ½ C sun-dried cane juice crystals
- ¼ tsp whole ground vanilla bean powder
- 1 dash sea salt
- ½ C lime juice
- ½ C coconut oil (liquefied)
- 2-4 oz purified, filtered water

> Molding Instructions: Place a 9-inch square silicone cake mold on a plate for stability. Transfer key lime mixture into silicone mold. Jiggle the plate to help easily distribute, and then use the back end of a spoon or a spatula to help smooth and evenly distribute the top. If desired, you may sprinkle with coconut flakes and/or macadamia nut pieces. Cover and let set for several hour or overnight in freezer.
>
> Serving & Storing Instructions: Remove from mold while still frozen (which is easily done using your hands); place on a plate or cutting board; cut into desired number of bars or squares. Store leftovers in an airtight, glass container for up to two weeks in fridge or 3-6 months (or longer) in freezer.

Amazonian Energy Bars

Process the following ingredients in a <u>food processor</u> until well combined:

- ★ 1 C jungle peanuts
- ★ 1 C pumpkin seeds
- ★ ½ C coconut flakes
- ★ ¼ C chia seeds
- ★ ¼ C hemp protein powder
- ★ ¼ C sun-dried cane juice crystals
- ★ 1 TBS spirulina
- ★ 1 TBS maca
- ★ 1 TBS mesquite
- ★ ¼ tsp whole ground vanilla bean powder
- ★ 1 dash sea salt

Optional Additions & Variations

- ★ Add 1 TBS of vine-ripened banana powder.
- ★ Substitute ¼ C Sunwarrior Classic Protein (natural) for hemp protein.

Then, add the following to the above ingredients in <u>food processor</u> and process until mixture begins to stick together when pressed between your fingers. Stop and scrape down sides as needed:

- ★ 1 ½ C packed Hunza golden raisins (presoaked for 5-10 minutes & then drained)

Optional Variations

- ★ Substitute 1 ½ C packed Turkish apricots, currants and/or other dried fruit of choice for Hunza golden raisins.

Last, add the following to the above ingredients in <u>food processor</u> and process again until well incorporated. Mixture should be moistened just enough to hold together when squished between fingers and may even start to form a ball in food processor:

- ¼ C coconut oil (liquefied)

> Molding Instructions: Place a 9-inch square silicone cake mold on a plate for stability. Transfer mixture into silicone mold, and then spread and press in evenly using a spatula and your hands. Cover and let sit for at least one hour or overnight in freezer.
>
> Serving & Storing Instructions: Remove from mold while cold and firm (which is easily done using your hands); place on a plate or cutting board; cut into desired number of bars or squares. Store leftovers in an airtight, glass container for up to two weeks in fridge or 3-6 months (or longer) in freezer.

Hemp Fudge Power Bites

Process the following ingredients in a <u>food processor</u> until well combined:

- 2 C coconut flakes
- 1 C hemp seeds
- ½ C raw cacao powder
- ¼ C hemp protein powder
- 2 TBS maca powder
- 1 TBS mesquite powder
- ½ tsp whole ground vanilla bean powder
- ¼ tsp Pumpkin Pie Blend
- ¼ tsp sea salt

Then, add the following to the above ingredients in <u>food processor</u> and process again until well incorporated. Stop and scrape down sides as needed:

- 1 C goji berries
- ¼ C raw agave
- ½ C coconut oil (liquefied)

> Molding Instructions: Place a 9-inch square silicone cake mold on a plate for stability. Transfer mixture into silicone mold, and then spread and press in evenly using a spatula and your hands. Cover and let sit for at least one hour or overnight in freezer.
>
> Serving & Storing Instructions: Remove from mold while cold and firm (which is easily done using your hands); place on a plate or cutting board; cut into 16 bite-sized pieces. Store leftovers in an airtight, glass container for up to two weeks in the fridge or 3-6 months in freezer.

Chocolate Chip <u>Raw</u>kie Dough Balls (real, raw <u>cook</u>ie dough)

Pulse-chop the following ingredients in a <u>food processor</u> until medium ground:

- 1 C macadamia nuts
- 1 C hemp seeds

- ½ C coconut flakes
- ½ C cacao beans (or nibs)
- ½ tsp whole ground vanilla bean powder
- ¼ tsp sea salt

Then, add the following to the above ingredients in <u>food processor</u> and process until mixture begins to stick together when pressed between your fingers. Stop and scrape down sides as needed:

- 1 C packed Hunza golden raisins (presoaked for 5-10 minutes & drained)

Last, add the following to the above ingredients in <u>food processor</u> and process again until well incorporated. Mixture should be moistened just enough to hold together when squished between fingers and may even start to form a ball in food processor:

- 2 TBS coconut oil (liquefied)

> **Molding & Storing Instructions:** Using a 1 oz stainless-steel squeeze handle disher (aka scooper), scoop up mixture and pack and level each half sphere. Then dish onto a plate until there is no mixture left. Take each 1 oz half sphere and gently roll in the palm of your hand to form a ball. Store balls in an airtight, glass container for up to two weeks in the fridge or 3-6 months in freezer. **Quick Tip:** If mixture is ever not cooperating, try placing it in the freezer for a few minutes before handling.

Maca-Roons

Pulse-chop the following ingredients in a <u>food processor</u> until medium ground:

- 1 C coconut flakes
- ½ C cashews
- ½ C macadamia nuts
- 2 TBS maca powder
- 1 TBS mesquite powder
- ¼ tsp whole ground vanilla bean
- 1 dash sea salt

Then, add the following to the above ingredients in <u>food processor</u> and process again until well incorporated. Stop and scrape down sides as needed. Mixture should be moistened just enough to hold together when squished between fingers:

- 2 TBS raw agave
- 2 TBS coconut oil (liquefied)

> Molding & Storing Instructions: Using a 1 oz (or slightly larger) stainless-steel squeeze handle disher, scoop up mixture and pack and level each half sphere. Then dish onto a plate until there is no mixture left. Store remainder in an airtight, glass container for up to two weeks in the fridge or 3-6 months in freezer. **Quick Tip:** If mixture is ever not cooperating, try placing it in the freezer for a few minutes before handling.

Mulberry Maca-Roons

Pulse-chop the following ingredients in a <u>food processor</u> until medium ground:

- ★ 1 C coconut flakes
- ★ 1 C dried mulberries
- ★ ½ C cashews
- ★ ½ C macadamia nuts
- ★ 2 TBS maca powder
- ★ ¼ tsp whole ground vanilla bean
- ★ 1 dash sea salt

Then, add the following to the above ingredients in <u>food processor</u> and process again until well incorporated. Stop and scrape down sides as needed. Mixture should be moistened just enough to hold together when squished between fingers:

- ★ 2 TBS raw agave
- ★ 2 TBS coconut oil (liquefied)

> Molding & Storing Instructions: Using a 1 oz (or slightly larger) stainless-steel squeeze handle disher, scoop up mixture and pack and level each half sphere. Then dish onto a plate until there is no mixture left. Store remainder in an airtight, glass container for up to two weeks in the fridge or 3-6 months in freezer. **Quick Tip:** If mixture is ever not cooperating, try placing it in the freezer for a few minutes before handling.

Christmas Goji-Roons

Pulse-chop the following ingredients in a <u>food processor</u> until medium ground:

- ★ 1 C coconut flakes
- ★ 1 C goji berries
- ★ ½ C cashews
- ★ ½ C macadamia nuts
- ★ 1 tsp spirulina
- ★ ¼ tsp whole ground vanilla bean
- ★ 1 dash sea salt

Then, add the following to the above ingredients in <u>food processor</u> and process again until well incorporated. Stop and scrape down sides as needed. Mixture should be moistened just enough to hold together when squished between fingers and may even start to form a ball in food processor:

- ★ 2 TBS raw agave
- ★ 2 TBS coconut oil (liquefied)

> Molding & Storing Instructions: Using a 1 oz (or slightly larger) stainless-steel squeeze handle disher, scoop up mixture and pack and level each half sphere. Then dish onto a plate until there is no mixture left. Store remainder in an airtight, glass container for up to two weeks in the fridge or 3-6 months in freezer. **Quick Tip:** If mixture is ever not cooperating, try placing it in the freezer for a few minutes before handling.

Jungle Peanut Balls

Pulse-chop the following ingredients in a <u>food processor</u> until medium ground:

- ★ 2 C jungle peanuts
- ★ 2 TBS maca powder
- ★ 2 TBS mesquite powder
- ★ ¼ tsp whole ground vanilla bean
- ★ 1 dash sea salt

Then, add the following to the above ingredients in <u>food processor</u> and process again until well incorporated. Stop and scrape down sides as needed. Mixture should be moistened just enough to hold together when squished between fingers and may even start to form a ball in food processor:

- ★ ¼ C raw honey or agave
- ★ ¼ C coconut oil (liquefied)

> Molding Instructions: Using a 1 oz stainless-steel squeeze handle disher, scoop up mixture and pack and level each half sphere. Then dish onto a plate until there is no mixture left. Take each 1 oz half sphere and gently roll in the palm of your hand to form a ball. **Quick Tip:** If mixture is ever not cooperating, try placing it in the freezer for a few minutes before handling.
>
> Decorating Ideas: Roll each ball in a small bowl of cacao nibs. Add in some coconut flakes and/or bee pollen for variety.
>
> Storing Instructions: Store balls in an airtight, glass container for up to two weeks in the fridge or 3-6 months in freezer.

Goji Christmas Balls

Pulse-chop the following ingredients in a <u>food processor</u> until medium ground:

- ★ 2 C pistachio nuts

- ★ 1 C coconut flakes
- ★ 2 TBS sun-dried cane juice crystals
- ★ ½ tsp whole ground vanilla bean powder
- ★ ¼ tsp sea salt

Then, add the following to the above ingredients in <u>food processor</u> and process until mixture begins to stick together when pressed between your fingers. Stop and scrape down sides as needed:

- ★ 1 ½ C goji berries

Last, add the following to the above ingredients in <u>food processor</u> and process again until well incorporated. Mixture should be moistened just enough to hold together when squished between fingers and may even start to form a ball in food processor:

- ★ ¼ C coconut oil (liquefied)
- ★ Purified, filtered water as needed. Only add water if necessary (1 TBS at a time). Should be moist and sticky enough to roll into balls.

> Molding & Storing Instructions: Using a 1 oz stainless-steel squeeze handle disher, scoop up mixture and pack and level each half sphere. Then dish onto a plate until there is no mixture left. Take each 1 oz half sphere and gently roll in the palm of your hand to form a ball. Store balls in an airtight, glass container for up to two weeks in the fridge or 3-6 months in freezer. **Quick Tip:** If mixture is ever not cooperating, try placing it in the freezer for a few minutes before handling.

Chocolate Hazelnut Snowballs

Pulse-chop the following ingredients in a <u>food processor</u> until medium ground:

- ★ 2 C Hazelnuts
- ★ 1 C coconut flakes
- ★ ½ C raw cacao powder
- ★ ½ tsp whole ground vanilla bean powder
- ★ ¼ tsp Pumpkin Pie Blend
- ★ ¼ tsp sea salt

Then, add the following to the above ingredients in <u>food processor</u> and process until mixture begins to stick together when pressed between your fingers. Stop and scrape down sides as needed:

- ★ 1 C packed, dried mulberries (presoaked for 5-10 minutes & then drained)
- ★ ¼ C raw agave

Last, add the following to the above ingredients in <u>food processor</u> and process again until well incorporated. Mixture should be moistened just enough to hold together when squished between fingers and may even start to form a ball in food processor:

- ¼ C coconut oil (liquefied)
- Purified, filtered water as needed. Only add water if necessary (1 TBS at a time). Should be moist and sticky enough to roll into balls.

> Molding Instructions: Using a 1 oz stainless-steel squeeze handle disher, scoop up mixture and pack and level each half sphere. Then dish onto a plate until there is no mixture left. Take each 1 oz half sphere and gently roll in the palm of your hand to form a ball. **Quick Tip:** If mixture is ever not cooperating, try placing it in the freezer for a few minutes before handling.
>
> Decorating Ideas: Roll each ball in a small bowl of coconut flakes and/or cacao nibs.
>
> Storing Instructions: Store balls in an airtight, glass container for up to two weeks in the fridge or 3-6 months in freezer.

Halvah

Pregrind the following TWO ingredients (which can be done together) in a <u>high-speed blender</u> (I suggest using a Blendtec, Nutribullet with milling blade or Vitamix dry container for this task). Then transfer ground seeds to a <u>food processor</u> in order to thoroughly combine and evenly distribute all the rest of the ingredients:

- 1 C unhulled, tan sesame seeds
- 1 C white chia seeds

Then, add the following to the above ingredients in <u>food processor</u> and process again until well combined and blended in (mixture should look like flour):

- 1 C coconut flakes
- ¼ C mesquite powder
- 1 tsp whole ground vanilla bean powder
- ¼ tsp sea salt

Optional Addition for Variation

- Add up to ½ C of cacao nibs for **Chocolate Chip Halvah.**

Last, add the following to the above ingredients in <u>food processor</u> and process again until well incorporated. Stop and scrape down sides as needed (mixture should be nice and sticky and look like dough):

- 1 C raw sesame tahini
- 1 C raw honey

> Molding Instructions: Place a 9-inch square silicone cake mold on a plate for stability. Transfer mixture into silicone mold, and then spread and press in evenly using a spatula and your hands. Cover and let set for a few hours or overnight in freezer.
>
> Serving & Storing Instructions: Remove from mold while still frozen (which is easily done using your hands); place on a plate or cutting board; cut into desired number of bars or squares. Store leftovers in an airtight, glass container for up to two weeks in fridge or 3-6 months (or longer) in freezer.

Rawklava (my raw version of the Greek favorite: baklava)

Pregrind the following TWO ingredients (which can be done together) in a <u>high-speed blender</u> (I suggest using a Blendtec, Nutribullet with milling blade or Vitamix dry container for this task). Then transfer ground seeds to a <u>food processor</u> in order to thoroughly combine and evenly distribute all the rest of the ingredients:

- ★ 1 ½ C unhulled, tan sesame seeds
- ★ 2 TBS white chia seeds

Then, add the following to the above ingredients in <u>food processor</u> and process again until well combined and blended in (mixture should look like flour):

- ★ 1 ½ C coconut flakes
- ★ 1 C walnuts
- ★ ½ tsp whole ground vanilla bean powder
- ★ ¼ tsp cinnamon
- ★ 1 dash sea salt

Last, add the following to the above ingredients in <u>food processor</u> and process again until well incorporated. Mixture should be moistened just enough to hold together when squished between fingers and may even start to form a ball in food processor:

- ★ ½ C raw honey
- ★ ¼ C coconut oil (liquefied)

> Molding Instructions: Place a 9-inch square silicone cake mold (or smaller for thicker pieces) on a plate for stability. Transfer mixture into silicone mold, and then spread and press in evenly using a spatula and your hands. Cover and let set for at least 2-3 hours or overnight in freezer.
>
> Decorating & Serving Ideas: Remove from mold while still cold and firm from freezer (which is easily done using your hands); place on a plate or cutting board; cut into desired number of bars or squares and place in fridge to thaw until ready to serve. When ready to serve, top individual pieces with a light layer of raw honey. Then generously sprinkle with chopped walnut pieces. For a different variation, substitute pecans for walnuts (or use half-and-half of each).
>
> Storing Instructions: Store leftover base pieces (undecorated) in an airtight, glass container for up to two weeks in fridge or 3-6 months (or longer) in freezer. Decorate prior to serving.

Afternoon Delight Scones (nut free)

First, pregrind the following in a high-speed blender (I suggest the use of a Blendtec, Nutribullet with milling blade or Vitamix dry container for this task). Then transfer ground seeds to a food processor in order to thoroughly combine and evenly distribute all the rest of the ingredients:

- ★ ½ C white chia seeds

Second, add the following dry ingredients to the above ingredients in food processor and process until very well ground into flour:

- ★ 4 C coconut flakes
- ★ ½ C sun-dried cane juice crystals
- ★ 1 tsp whole ground vanilla bean powder
- ★ ½ tsp Pumpkin Pie Blend
- ★ ¼ tsp sea salt

Third, add the following to the above ingredients in food processor and process until mixture begins to stick together when pressed between your fingers. Stop and scrape down sides as needed:

- ★ 2 C packed, Hunza golden raisins (presoaked for 5-10 minutes & then drained)

Optional Variations

- ★ Substitute 2 C packed Turkish apricots, figs, currants and/or other dried fruit of choice for Hunza golden raisins.

Last, add the following to the above ingredients in food processor and process again until well incorporated. Mixture should be moistened just enough to hold together when squished between fingers and may even start to form a ball in food processor:

- ★ ½ C coconut oil (liquefied)

> Molding Instructions: Place a 9-inch square silicone cake mold on a plate for stability. Transfer mixture into silicone mold, and then spread and press in evenly using a spatula and your hands. Cover and let set for a couple of hours or overnight in freezer.
>
> Decorating & Serving Ideas: Remove from mold while cold and firm (easily done using your hands); place on a plate or cutting board; cut into four squares and cut each square into triangles. Store in fridge until ready to serve or place them in the dehydrator (at 105-115°F) until warm and starting to brown. When ready to serve: drizzle individual pieces with Chocolate and La-Caramel Topping (page 372), top with Vanilla Icing or Chocolate Icing (pages 384-385) or serve with your favorite raw jam (pages 268-269).
>
> Storing Instructions: Store any remaining pieces (undecorated) in an airtight, glass container for up to two weeks in fridge or 3-6 months (or longer) in freezer. Decorate prior to serving.

Super Seed Power Balls

First, pulse-chop the following ingredients in a <u>food processor</u> until medium ground:

- ★ 1 C pumpkin seeds
- ★ 1 C sunflower seeds
- ★ 1 C coconut flakes
- ★ ¼ C sun-dried cane juice crystals
- ★ 2 TBS mesquite powder
- ★ ½ tsp whole ground vanilla bean powder
- ★ ¼ tsp Apple Pie Blend
- ★ 1 dash sea salt

Second, add the following ingredients to the above already in <u>food processor</u> and pulse through until well incorporated:

- ★ ½ C hemp seeds
- ★ ½ C chia seeds

Third, add the following to the above ingredients in <u>food processor</u> and process until mixture begins to stick together when pressed between your fingers. Stop and scrape down sides as needed:

- ★ 1 C packed Hunza golden raisins (presoaked for 5-10 minutes & then drained)
- ★ ½ C packed goji berries

Optional Variations

- ★ Substitute 1 C packed Turkish apricots, figs, currants and/or other dried fruit of choice for Hunza golden raisins.

Last, add the following to the above ingredients in <u>food processor</u> and process again until well incorporated. Mixture should be moistened just enough to hold together when squished between fingers and may even start to form a ball in food processor:

- ¼ C coconut oil (liquefied)
- Purified, filtered water as needed. Only add water if necessary (1 TBS at a time). Should be moist and sticky enough to roll into balls.

> Molding Instructions: Using a 1 oz stainless-steel squeeze handle disher, scoop up mixture and pack and level each half sphere. Then dish onto a plate until there is no mixture left. Take each 1 oz half sphere and gently roll in the palm of your hand to form a ball. **Quick Tip:** If mixture is ever not cooperating, try placing it in the freezer for a few minutes before handling.
>
> Decorating Ideas: If you desire, you can then roll each power ball in a small bowl of one (or more) of the following superfoods: cacao nibs, cacao powder, lucuma powder, maca powder, coconut flakes and/or hemp seeds.
>
> Storing Instructions: Store balls in an airtight, glass container for up to two weeks in the fridge or 3-6 months in freezer.

Chocolate Fudge Truffles

Process the following ingredients in a <u>food processor</u> until very well ground into what looks like a chocolate flour:

- 1 ½ C cashews
- ½ C raw cacao powder
- ¼ tsp whole ground vanilla bean powder
- 1 dash sea salt

Optional Additions for Variation

- Add 1 tsp mesquite powder, ½ tsp cinnamon and 1 dash cayenne (or to taste) for **Chocolate Mayan Fudge Truffles.**

Then, add the following to the above ingredients in <u>food processor</u> and process until mixture begins to stick together when pressed between your fingers. Stop and scrape down sides as needed:

- 1 C packed Hunza golden raisins (presoaked for 5-10 minutes & then drained)
- Substitute 1 C packed Turkish apricots, currants and/or other dried fruit of choice for Hunza golden raisins.

> Molding Instructions: Using a 1 oz stainless-steel squeeze handle disher, scoop up mixture and pack and level each half sphere. Then dish onto a plate until there is no mixture left. Take each 1 oz half sphere and gently roll in the palm of your hand to form a ball. **Quick Tip:** If mixture is ever not cooperating, try placing it in the freezer for a few minutes before handling.
>
> Decorating Ideas: If you desire, you can then roll each truffle in a small bowl of one (or more) of the following superfoods: cacao nibs, cacao powder, lucuma powder, maca powder, coconut flakes and/or hemp seeds.
>
> Storing Instructions: Store balls in an airtight, glass container for up to two weeks in the fridge or 3-6 months in freezer.

Go-To Rawkies (raw cookies)

Pulse-chop the following ingredients in a food processor until coarsely ground into small chunky pieces. Be sure to not over process into flour:

- ★ 2 C nuts and seeds of choice
- ★ ½ tsp whole ground vanilla bean powder (or to taste)
- ★ ¼-½ tsp Pumpkin or Apple Pie Blend (optional)
- ★ ¼ tsp sea salt (or to taste)

Then, add the following to the above ingredients in food processor and process until mixture begins to stick together when pressed between your fingers. Mixture should be moist and sticky enough to roll into balls:

- ★ 2 C packed, dried fruit of choice (presoaked for 5-10 minutes & then drained)
- ★ 1-2 TBS sweetener of choice (as needed)

> **Quick Tip:** Use sun-dried cane juice crystals, xylitol and/or green leaf stevia powder when there is enough stickiness. Use raw honey or raw agave when more stickiness is needed (e.g., when using mulberries and/or goji berries, which tend to be a bit drier).

Rawkie Combo Favorites

- ★ Almonds & either Turkish apricots, Turkish figs or Hunza golden raisins.
- ★ Brazil nuts & either currants, Turkish figs or Hunza golden raisins.
- ★ Macadamia nuts & either Turkish apricots, jackfruit, mulberries or Hunza golden raisins.
- ★ Pecans & either Turkish apricots, currants, dates or Hunza golden raisins.
- ★ Walnuts & either currants, dates, Turkish figs or Hunza golden raisins.

Optional Variations

- ★ Replace ½ C nuts with cashews or coconut flakes.

- ★ Replace ½ C nuts with pumpkin seed or hemp seeds.
- ★ Replace ½ C Hunza golden raisins with goji berries or golden berries (add additional sweetener as needed due to mild sweetness of goji berries and tartness of golden berries).

Molding, Serving & Storing Instructions:

1. Using a 1 oz stainless-steel squeeze handle disher (aka scooper), scoop up mixture and pack and level each half sphere. Then dish onto a plate until there is no mixture left. If you desire larger sized rawkies, then feel free to double the scoop.
2. Roll each half sphere (or two for one larger sizes rawkie), and then press into evenly shaped round rawkies.
3. If desired, press the top of each rawkie into cacao nibs, coconut flakes, hemp seeds or sesame seeds.
4. Store rawkies in an airtight, glass container for up to two weeks in the fridge or 3-6 months in freezer.

Quick Recipe Tips & Variation Ideas

- ★ If mixture is ever not cooperating, place it in the freezer for a few minutes before handling.
- ★ Utilizing silicone standard muffin pans makes for perfectly round shaped rawkies.
- ★ For a cupcake or muffin rendition, use silicone mini muffin pans and frost with a frosting or icing of choice from pages 383-386.
- ★ For raw balls, follow steps 1 and 2 above, and then roll each ball in a small bowl of one (or more) of the following superfoods: cacao nibs, cacao powder, lucuma powder, maca powder, mesquite powder, coconut flakes, bee pollen and/or hemp seeds.

Pure Indulgent Puddings & More!

Bliss Kiss Pudding

Process the following ingredients in a <u>food processor</u> until very well broken down and smooth:

- ★ 2 avocados (peeled & pitted)
- ★ ½ C raw agave

Then, add the following to the above ingredients in <u>food processor</u> and process until well incorporated. Stop to scrape down sides as needed:

- ★ ½ C raw cacao powder
- ★ 2 TBS mesquite powder
- ★ 2 TBS lucuma powder
- ★ ¼ tsp whole ground vanilla bean powder

- ★ 1 dash Pumpkin Pie Blend
- ★ 1 dash sea salt

Last, add the following to the above ingredients in <u>food processor</u> and process again until smooth and creamy:

- ★ 4-6 oz purified, filtered water
- ★ 2 TBS coconut oil (liquefied)

Optional Additions for Variation & Serving Ideas

- ★ Add a dash (or two) of cayenne for some heat and an extra little kick.
- ★ Add 2-3 drops (or to taste) of one of the following therapeutic quality essential oils for a completely different flavor experience: sweet orange, lavender, lemon, lime peel, ginger or peppermint.
- ★ For more of a chocolate mousse like texture, substitute 2 TBS melted cacao butter for coconut oil and don't go over the 4 oz of water (aim for the lesser amount).
- ★ For a parfait presentation, layer in a clear glass of choice with any of the following superfoods: coconut flakes, cacao nibs, bee pollen, goji berries and/or mulberries. You may also choose to layer with coconut flakes and fresh fruit (blackberries, raspberries, sliced strawberries, sliced kiwi, etc.).
- ★ Pour into popsicle molds and freeze for a fantastic frozen summer treat!
- ★ Bliss Kiss Pudding will keep for 2-3 days in an airtight, glass container the fridge. If it even lasts that long!

Vanilla Lime Pudding

Process the following ingredients in a <u>food processor</u> until very well broken down and smooth. Stop to scrape down sides as needed:

- ★ 2 avocados (peeled & pitted)
- ★ 2 whole lime, juiced
- ★ ½ tsp whole ground vanilla bean powder
- ★ 1 dash sea salt
- ★ ¼ C raw honey or agave (or to taste)

Then, add the following to the above ingredients in <u>food processor</u> and process until well incorporated:

- ★ 2 TBS coconut oil (liquefied)

Optional Serving Ideas

- ★ For a parfait presentation, layer in a clear glass of choice with any of the following superfoods: coconut flakes, cacao nibs, goji berries and/or golden berries. You may also choose to layer with coconut flakes and fresh fruit (blackberries, raspberries, sliced strawberries, sliced kiwi, etc.).

- Vanilla Lime Pudding will keep for 2-3 day in an airtight, glass container in the fridge.

Maca Mineral Pudding

Process the following ingredients in a <u>food processor</u> until very well broken down and smooth. Stop to scrape down sides as needed:

- 2 avocados (peeled & pitted)
- 1 whole lime, juiced
- 2 TBS maca powder
- 2 tsp spirulina
- ½ tsp whole ground vanilla bean powder
- 1 dash sea salt
- ¼ C raw honey or agave (or to taste)

Then, add the following to the above ingredients in <u>food processor</u> and process until well incorporated:

- 2 TBS coconut oil (liquefied)

Optional Serving Ideas

- For a parfait presentation, layer in a clear glass of choice with any of the following superfoods: coconut flakes, cacao nibs, goji berries and/or Hunza golden raisins. You may also choose to layer with coconut flakes and fresh fruit (blackberries, raspberries, sliced strawberries, sliced kiwi, etc.).
- Maca Pudding will keep for 2-3 day in an airtight, glass container in the fridge.

Matcha Pudding

Process the following ingredients in a <u>food processor</u> until very well broken down and smooth. Stop to scrape down sides as needed:

- 2 avocados (peeled & pitted)
- 1 whole lemon, juiced
- 1 TBS matcha powder
- ½ tsp whole ground vanilla bean powder
- 1 dash sea salt
- ¼ C raw honey or agave (or to taste)

Then, add the following to the above ingredients in <u>food processor</u> and process until well incorporated:

- 2 TBS coconut oil (liquefied)

Optional Serving Ideas

- ★ For a parfait presentation, layer in a clear glass of choice with any of the following superfoods: coconut flakes, cacao nibs, goji berries and/or mulberries. You may also choose to layer with coconut flakes and fresh fruit (blackberries, raspberries, sliced strawberries, sliced kiwi, etc.).
- ★ Matcha Pudding will keep for 2-3 day in an airtight, glass container in the fridge.

Chia "Tapioca" Pudding

Place the following in either a large glass storage bowl (one with a cover) or a wide mouth mason jar (quart size) and then set aside:

- ★ ⅓ C white chia seeds

Optional Additions

- ★ Add ¼ C of one of the following dried fruits: Hunza golden raisins, goji berries, mulberries or currants. This may be done either prior to pouring in hemp seed mixture (see below) or right after.

Then, blend the following ingredients in a <u>high-speed blender</u> until smooth and creamy. Stop to scrape down sides as needed, and then follow instructions below:

- ★ ¾ C hemp seeds
- ★ ¼ C sun-dried cane juice crystals
- ★ 2 TBS baobab powder
- ★ 2 tsp whole ground vanilla bean powder
- ★ 1 tsp Pumpkin Pie Blend
- ★ 1 dash sea salt
- ★ 2 TBS coconut oil (liquefied)
- ★ 16 oz purified, filtered water

Optional Variations

- ★ Substitute 2 TBS lucuma or vine-ripened banana powder for baobab.

Instructions:

1. Pour blended hemp seed mixture over chia seeds in bowl or jar. If you have not done so already, add in your dried fruit of choice (optional).
2. **If using a bowl:** gently stir or whisk until mixture starts to become gelatinous (couple of minutes), then cover and let sit until ready to serve. **If using a mason jar:** cover and gently swirl and shake until chia seeds are well dispersed from top to bottom.

3. Place covered bowl or jar in the refrigerator and let sit for a couple hours. Although it is ready within 20-30 minutes, giving it 1-2 hours will allow flavors to settle in nicely and the mixture to thicken to its full potential.
4. Stir, swirl and/or shake again to evenly distribute ingredients right before serving. Any remaining chia pudding will keep for up to one week in the fridge.
5. Feel free to sprinkle with additional Pumpkin Pie Blend (if desired) and/or top with whatever superfoods you wish (such as coconut flakes, cacao beans, bee pollen, etc.).

> **Recipe Notes & Quick Tips:** Chia "Tapioca" Pudding makes for phenomenal morning porridge! I actually call it my "raw power porridge." Many times, I will prep a batch the night before an anticipated day of high physical active and being on the go; a day when time and/or space to make my usual monstrous salad or smoothie is not feasible. I just store my filled mason jar in a cooler, along with some ice packs, and eat throughout the day with a sprinkle of goji berries and/or bee pollen. Even during a long day of intense fitness and physical activity, this alone can keep me fueled!

O-Mega Yougurt (my raw & dairy free version of yogurt)

Blend the following ingredients in a high-speed blender until smooth and creamy. Stop to scrape down sides as needed:

- ★ 1 C hemp seeds
- ★ ¼ C sun-dried cane juice crystals
- ★ 3 TBS chia seeds
- ★ ¼ tsp whole ground vanilla bean powder
- ★ 1 dash sea salt
- ★ ¼ C lemon juice
- ★ 2 TBS coconut oil
- ★ 6-8 oz purified, filtered water

Then, add ONE of the following fruits (fresh or defrosted). Blend again until well broken down and smooth:

- ★ 1 C blueberries
- ★ 1 C strawberries
- ★ 1 C mixed berries
- ★ 1 C mango
- ★ 1 C peaches

Optional Serving Ideas

- ★ For a parfait presentation, layer in a clear glass of choice with any of the following superfoods: coconut flakes, cacao nibs, bee pollen, goji berries and/or golden berries. You may also choose to layer with fresh fruit (blackberries, raspberries, sliced strawberries, sliced kiwi, etc.) and/or your favorite nuts and seeds.
- ★ Another great option is to serve with Fruit N' Nut Crumbles (page 415). Super simple to make with a multitude of uses!
- ★ O-Mega Yougurt will keep for 2-3 day in an airtight, glass container in the fridge.

Fruit N' Nut Crumbles

Choose equal amount of nuts and dried fruits (1:1 ratio) and in any combination you choose, then pulse-chop together in a <u>food-processor</u> to create a well combined course-ground sprinkle. Be sure to not over process into flour. **Quick Tip:** Coarsely pulse-chop nuts <u>first</u> (just enough to create chunky pieces), then add dried fruit and process slightly again (just enough to mix well).

Take it to the next level with a touch of whole ground vanilla bean powder (¼ tsp or to taste) and add Apple or Pumpkin Pie Blend (¼ tsp or to taste) for some warmth and spicy sweetness. You may even add up to 1 TBS of mesquite, lucuma or sun-ripened banana powder for a different flavor twist that is subtly delightful. **Quick Tip:** Add and pulse through any of these dry ingredients <u>before</u> adding dried fruit. This will make certain that flavors get evenly distributed and don't stick to the fruit.

Example #1

- ★ 1 C almonds
- ★ ¾ C Hunza golden raisins
- ★ ¼ C goji berries
- ★ 1 dash sea salt (or to taste)

Example #2

- ★ 1 C Brazil nuts
- ★ ¾ C Hunza golden raisins
- ★ ¼ C golden berries
- ★ 1 dash sea salt (or to taste)

Example #3

- ★ 1 C cashews
- ★ ½ C goji berries
- ★ ½ C mulberries
- ★ 1 dash sea salt (or to taste)

Example #4

- ★ 1 C macadamia nuts
- ★ 1 C mulberries
- ★ 1 dash sea salt (or to taste)

Uses & Serving Ideas

- ★ Use as a topping over a bowl of fresh sliced fruit for a simple and satisfying home-made cobbler (apple, berry, peach, pear, pineapple, etc.).
- ★ Delicious as a crumble over O-Mega Yougurt (page 414) and any combination of fresh fruit.
- ★ Crumble over or into your favorite ice cream (page 417) or use as a topping for ice cream sundaes.
- ★ Roll into balls or press into rawkies (aka raw cookies) for a fast and easy sweet treat that can be enjoyed at any time of the day.
- ★ Store leftover in an airtight, glass container for up to two weeks in the fridge.

Spirulina Pear-Mango Pudding

Blend the following ingredients in a <u>high-speed blender</u> until smooth:

- ★ 2 pears (chopped)
- ★ 3 TBS hemp seeds
- ★ 2 TBS Tocotriene Ultra (Premier Research Labs)
- ★ 1 TBS spirulina
- ★ ½ tsp whole ground vanilla bean powder
- ★ ¼ tsp Pumpkin Pie Blend
- ★ 1 dash green leaf stevia (whole leaf)
- ★ 1 TBS coconut oil (liquefied)
- ★ 4 oz purified, filtered water

Add the following frozen fruit, and then blend again until well broken down and smooth:

- ★ 1 C frozen mango

Optional Additions & Variations

- ★ Add 1 TBS of baobab or vine-ripened banana powder.
- ★ Stir in some bee pollen after blending.
- ★ Substitute 2 apples for pears and Apple Pie Blend for Pumpkin Pie Blend and you have **Apple-Mango Pudding.**

Souped-Up Applesauce

Blend the following ingredients in a <u>high-speed blender</u> until smooth:

- ★ 2 sweet red apples (chopped)
- ★ 2 TBS goji berries
- ★ 1 TBS chia seeds
- ★ ½ tsp Apple Pie Blend
- ★ ¼ tsp green leaf stevia (whole leaf)
- ★ 1 TBS coconut oil (liquefied)
- ★ 4 oz purified water

Optional Variations

- ★ Substitute 1 pear for 1 of the apples and you have **Apple-Pear Sauce.**
- ★ Substitute 2 TBS golden berries for goji berries or use half-and-half of each.

Luscious Raw Ice Creams

I scream, you scream, we all scream for ice cream!

Indulge yourself in ice cream that is 100% guilt free! Like all the recipes in this book, the following ice cream recipes are 100% free of eggs, dairy, refined sugars and trans-fats. Guess what else? No gluten, corn or soy! Did you know that many commercial ice creams contain modified corn starch as a thickening agent? Genetically modified corn and soy are in just about everything. So, for the sake of your health and well-being, I suggest "going against the grain!"

Transcend to heaven!

These luscious raw ice cream recipes are the real deal. What's more, they make a special treat for just about any occasion at any time of the day. They are delicious all by themselves, great for creating sundaes, and make a fabulous addition to any slice of raw pie, piece of raw cake and, of course, brownies! You can even use raw ice creams as a base for making cool mylk-shakes and frappes. You will notice that the base of many raw ice cream recipes almost always involves nuts, seeds, coconut or a combination. Hands down, my #1 nut of choice is raw cashews. Cashews are considered by many in the raw food realm to be the "dairy" nut. They offer a subtle sweetness that is perfect for making raw ice cream and other creamy sweet treats. Macadamia nuts and hemp seeds are my two alternate choices. I will also sometimes choose to use a portion of cashews along with macadamia nuts or hemp seeds.

Quick Recipe Tips:

An ice cream maker can be great for making sure your homemade ice cream freezes uniformly but is not necessary for any of the recipes I share below. Stirring (or whisking) your homemade ice cream can offer the same results, as it redistributes the heavier solid ingredients that have slightly separated from the liquid. Just by stirring or whisking once or twice during the freezing process (every 1-2 hours), will discourage an icy top layer. What also helps, dramatically, is the use of ingredients that act as natural emulsifiers. This is why I use baobab, lucuma and maca in almost all my ice cream recipes. What's more, each one of these ingredients is insanely nutrient rich. This way you can have your ice cream and feel amazing about eating it too!

If you decide to presoak raw cashews (which can step-up the creaminess), then I suggest soaking the amount of cashews called for in the amount of water called for in the recipe (i.e., soak raw cashew for 1-2 hrs in 12 oz of purified, filtered water). Then utilize the cashews, along with all the soak water, in the blending process (i.e., pour soaked cashews and soak water into blender with all other ice cream ingredients). Feel free to add the recipe's sea salt to cashews while they are soaking. Otherwise, add along with all other ingredients just prior to blending.

> **Please Note:** Although it is not necessary to soak raw cashews or macadamias for optimal health and nutritional benefits, soaking these two varieties will hydrate them and, as a result, improve upon the texture and creaminess of the recipe. That being said, fats add to the texture and creaminess of a recipe as well, and presoaking nuts and seeds draw out some of the fat. Using the soak water of cashew and macadamia nuts are the only two exceptions to the "nut soaking" rule. These two particular nuts do not pose the same degree of enzyme inhibitor issues as many other nuts (such as almonds, pecans and walnuts); therefore, it is totally acceptable to utilize their soak water. Just be sure to not over-soak. I suggest 1-2 hrs maximum for nuts such as these.
>
> To review "The Science Behind the Soak," "General Soaking Schedule for Nuts & Seeds" and other great tips, please refer to page 26.

If you suffer from a sugar related condition (such as cancer, Candida or diabetes), please know that you do not have to deny yourself something that is sweet to the taste. Although I enjoy using sun-dried cane juice crystals the most, you can always replace with equal amounts of xylitol. Xylitol will not alter the flavor whatsoever. In fact, it actually duplicates the sweetness and taste of real sugar. To learn more about these unique and natural sweeteners (including all the others I recommend), please review "Sweet Flavor for Your Creations, Being Sweet Savvy with Nature's Best" on page 34.

Dreamy Vanilla Bean #1

Blend the following ingredients in a high-speed blender until well broken down and very smooth. Stop to scrape down sides as needed. Then follow molding and serving instructions in the box on page 424:

- ★ 1 ½ C cashews
- ★ ¼ C sun-dried cane juice crystals
- ★ 2 tsp whole ground vanilla bean powder
- ★ 1 dash sea salt
- ★ 12 oz purified, filtered water

Add the following next, and then blend until thick, smooth and creamy. Stop to scrape down sides as needed:

- ⅓ C baobab powder
- ¼ C coconut oil (liquefied)

Dreamy Vanilla Bean #2

Blend the following ingredients in a <u>high-speed blender</u> until well broken down and very smooth. Stop to scrape down sides as needed. Then follow molding and serving instructions in the box on page 424:

- 1 C cashews
- ½ C baobab
- ¼ C sun-dried cane juice crystals
- 2 tsp whole ground vanilla bean powder
- 1 dash sea salt
- 12 oz purified, filtered water

Add the following next, and then blend until thick, smooth and creamy. Stop to scrape down sides as needed:

- ¼ C coconut oil (liquefied)

Optional Additions & Variations for Dreamy Vanilla Bean

- Add 1 TBS matcha green tea powder prior to blending for **Matcha Green Tea Ice cream**.
- Add 2-3 TBS cacao nibs (stirred in prior to freezing) for **Cacao Chip Ice cream**.
- Add ¼ tsp spirulina and 2-3 drops (or to taste) of peppermint essential oil prior to blending for **Mint Ice cream**. For **Mint Chip Ice cream**, stir in 2-3 TBS of cacao nibs prior to freezing.
- Add mulberries and crushed macadamia nuts (stirred in prior to freezing or as a topper) for **Mulberry-Macadamia Crunch**.
- Add coconut flakes and goji berries (stirred in prior to freezing or as a topper) for **Coconut-Goji**.

Jacked Up Jackfruit

Blend the following ingredients in a <u>high-speed blender</u> until well broken down and very smooth. Stop to scrape down sides as needed. Then follow molding and serving instructions in the box on page 424:

- 1 C cashews
- ½ C packed jackfruit
- ¼ C sun-dried cane juice crystals
- 2 TBS baobab powder

- ½ tsp whole ground vanilla bean powder
- 1 dash sea salt
- 12 oz purified, filtered water

Add the following next, and then blend until thick, smooth and creamy. Stop to scrape down sides as needed:

- ¼ C coconut oil (liquefied)

Succulent Strawberry

Blend the following ingredients in a <u>high-speed blender</u> until well broken down and very smooth. Stop to scrape down sides as needed. Then follow molding and serving instructions in the box on page 424:

- 1 C cashews
- 1 C frozen strawberries
- ¼ C sun-dried cane juice crystals
- 2 TBS baobab powder
- ½ tsp whole ground vanilla bean powder
- 1 dash sea salt
- 12 oz purified, filtered water

Add the following next, and then blend until thick, smooth and creamy. Stop to scrape down sides as needed:

- ¼ C coconut oil (liquefied)

Optional Addition for Variation

- Add ¼ C goji berries (stirred in prior to freezing) for **Goji-Strawberry.**

Black Forest Cherry

Blend the following ingredients in a <u>high-speed blender</u> until well broken down and very smooth. Stop to scrape down sides as needed. Then follow molding and serving instructions in the box on page 424:

- 1 C cashews
- 1 C frozen pitted cherries
- ¼ C raw cacao powder
- ¼ C sun-dried cane juice crystals
- ½ tsp whole ground vanilla bean powder
- 1 dash sea salt
- 12 oz purified, filtered water

Add the following next, and then blend until thick, smooth and creamy. Stop to scrape down sides as needed:

- ¼ C coconut oil (liquefied)

Optional Addition for Variation

- Add 2-3 TBS cacao nibs (stirred in prior to freezing) for **Black Cherry Chip.**

Chocolate Exotica

Blend the following ingredients in a high-speed blender until well broken down and very smooth. Stop to scrape down sides as needed. Then follow molding and serving instructions in the box on page 424:

- 1 ½ C cashews
- ¼ C sun-dried cane juice crystals
- ½ tsp whole ground vanilla bean powder
- 1 dash sea salt
- 12 oz purified, filtered water

Add the following next, and then blend until thick, smooth and creamy. Stop to scrape down sides as needed:

- ⅓ C raw cacao powder
- ¼ C lucuma powder
- ¼ C coconut oil (liquefied)

Optional Additions & Variations for Chocolate Exotica

- Add 2-3 TBS cacao nibs (stirred in prior to freezing) for **Chocolate Cacao Chip.**
- Add 1-2 dashes of cayenne and cinnamon (or to taste) for **Chocolate Mayan Fire.**
- Add 2-3 drops (or to taste) of peppermint essential oil prior to blending for **Mint Chocolate.** For **Mint Chocolate Chip**, stir in 2-3 TBS of cacao nibs prior to freezing.
- Add crushed macadamia nuts (stirred in prior to freezing or as a topper) for **Chocolate-Macadamia Crunch.**
- Add goji berries (stirred in prior to freezing or as a topper) for **Chocolate-Goji.**

Luscious La-Caramel

Blend the following ingredients in a high-speed blender until well broken down and very smooth. Stop to scrape down sides as needed. Then follow molding and serving instructions in the box on page 424:

- 1 C cashews
- ½ C lucuma powder
- ¼ C sun-dried cane juice crystals
- ½ tsp whole ground vanilla bean powder
- 1 dash sea salt
- 12 oz purified, filtered water

Add the following next, and then blend until thick, smooth and creamy. Stop to scrape down sides as needed:

- ★ ¼ C coconut oil (liquefied)

Optional Additions for Variation

- ★ Add crushed pecans (stirred in prior to freezing or as a topper) for a **Pecan Caramel** flavor experience.
- ★ Add crushed walnuts (stirred in prior to freezing or as a topper) for a **Maple Walnut** flavor experience.

Chocolate La-Caramel

Blend the following ingredients in a <u>high-speed blender</u> until well broken down and very smooth. Stop to scrape down sides as needed. Then follow molding and serving instructions in the box on page 424:

- ★ 1 C cashews
- ★ ⅓ C lucuma powder
- ★ ¼ C raw cacao powder
- ★ ¼ C sun-dried cane juice crystals
- ★ ½ tsp whole ground vanilla bean powder
- ★ 1 dash sea salt
- ★ 12 oz purified, filtered water

Add the following next, and then blend until thick, smooth and creamy. Stop to scrape down sides as needed:

- ★ ¼ C coconut oil (liquefied)

Optional Additions for Variation

- ★ Add crushed pecans (either stirred in prior to freezing or as a topper) for **Chocolate Pecan Crunch.**
- ★ Add crushed walnuts (either stirred in prior to freezing or as a topper) for **Chocolate Walnut Crunch.**

Majestic Mocha

Blend the following ingredients in a <u>high-speed blender</u> until well broken down and very smooth. Stop to scrape down sides as needed. Then follow molding and serving instructions in the box on page 424:

- ★ 1 C cashews
- ★ ⅓ C lucuma powder
- ★ ¼ C raw cacao powder
- ★ ¼ C sun-dried cane juice crystals

- ★ 1 TBS shilajit (for a subtle coffee-like flavor) or 2 TBS shilajit (for a more intense coffee-like flavor)
- ★ ½ tsp whole ground vanilla bean powder
- ★ 1 dash sea salt
- ★ 12 oz purified, filtered water

Add the following next, and then blend until thick, smooth and creamy. Stop to scrape down sides as needed:

- ★ ¼ C coconut oil (liquefied)

Optional Addition for Variation

- ★ Add 2-3 TBS cacao nibs (stirred in prior to freezing) for **Mocha Chip.**

Maca Madness

Blend the following ingredients in a <u>high-speed blender</u> until well broken down and very smooth. Stop to scrape down sides as needed. Then follow molding and serving instructions in the box on page 424:

- ★ 1 C cashews
- ★ ⅓ C maca powder
- ★ ¼ C lucuma powder
- ★ ¼ C sun-dried cane juice crystals
- ★ ½ tsp whole ground vanilla bean powder
- ★ 1 dash sea salt
- ★ 12 oz purified, filtered water

Add the following next, and then blend until thick, smooth and creamy. Stop to scrape down sides as needed:

- ★ ¼ C coconut oil (liquefied)

Optional Addition

- ★ Add 1 TBS mesquite powder for a subtle smoky/sweet flavor.

Chocolate Malt

Blend the following ingredients in a <u>high-speed blender</u> until well broken down and very smooth. Stop to scrape down sides as needed. Then follow molding and serving instructions in the box on page 424:

- ★ 1 C cashews
- ★ ⅓ C maca powder
- ★ ¼ C raw cacao powder
- ★ ¼ C sun-dried cane juice crystals

- ★ ½ tsp whole ground vanilla bean powder
- ★ 1 dash sea salt
- ★ 12 oz purified, filtered water

Add the following next, and then blend until thick, smooth and creamy. Stop to scrape down sides as needed:

- ★ ¼ C coconut oil (liquefied)

Optional Addition

- ★ Add 1 TBS mesquite powder for a subtle smoky/sweet flavor.

> **ICE CREAM MOLDING INSTRUCTIONS:**
>
> Once your ice cream is completely blended to a smooth and creamy consistency, transfer to a freezable container with an airtight cover. You may also wish to utilize a few smaller sized freezable containers (instead of one) that you can pull out and thaw individually. If time allows, stir or whisk at least once or twice within the first two hours of freezing.
>
> **If using an ice cream maker:** once ice cream is completely blended to a smooth and creamy consistency, pour ice cream into ice cream maker, and then follow manufacturer's directions.
>
> Serving Instructions: Allow ice cream to thaw for either a few hours in fridge or for at least 30 minutes at room temperature before serving. This will allow it to soften a bit and make it easier to scoop and serve if you don't have an ice cream scooper. Store any remaining ice cream in the freezer where it will keep for up to 3-6 months or longer.
>
> Optional Serving Ideas: You can choose not to freeze any of these ice cream recipes, as they all will make amazingly creamy and decadent raw puddings or mousses instead. No matter how you choose to enjoy, you will find all are deliciously satisfying. If you are looking for a succulent sundae experience, feel free to top with chopped nuts, seeds, dried superfruits, fresh sliced fruits and/or any of the toppings found under Basic Cheeze Cake, starting on page 372. For a chocolate chip rendition (using something other than cacao nibs), try stirring in broken pieces of homemade raw chocolate (page 430) prior to freezing. How about smothering with chocolate shavings prior to serving? Mm!

RAW CHOCOLATE PLEASURES

Cacao as a catalyst: the deliverer of medicines

When we eat raw cacao with certain foods, spices and herbs we increase our body's ability to absorb and assimilate the essential nutrients in that substance. In other words, by utilizing the power of raw cacao as a medicinal delivery system, we can intensify the nutritional benefits and healing potential of a specific food and herb without having to eat more of it.

Raw cacao is one of the highest sources of antioxidants in nature (more than red wine or even green tea). It also is one of the highest food sources of the mineral magnesium, needed for more than 300 biochemical reactions in the body. Cacao also contains anandamide (the brain bliss chemical), PEA (the love chemical), MAO inhibitors (known to curb one's appetite) and theobromine (known to increases mental clarity and focus while being gentle on the nervous system). To learn more about this wonderful food and its utterly great chemical complexity, I highly suggest referring back to my section on "Cacao" (page 127).

Quick Recipe Tips:

Depending on what you plan to make (which may depend on what you have on hand), you may choose to use raw cacao paste or raw cacao powder together with raw cacao butter. In most instances, either can be used interchangeably. Raw cacao paste is brown in color and differs from raw cacao butter, which is white. Raw cacao paste is the closest to whole cacao beans. It is the product of stone-grinding down raw cacao beans at low temperatures until a smooth and buttery consistency is reached and is then sold in bars, chunks or pieces for culinary purposes. On the other hand, raw cacao butter is the low-temperature extracted oil made from pure cacao beans. The leftover solids are low-temperature dried into what we know as raw cacao powder.

Raw cacao butter is white (hence, white chocolate) and is great to use when you desire a firmer texture than you would get from something like coconut oil, for example. This is due to cacao butter having a higher melting point than coconut oil. Raw cacao butter is also a great choice when you do not wish to alter the color of your creation, nor want to overwhelm it with a deep chocolaty flavor.

Both cacao paste and cacao butter need to be liquefied before adding to your recipe. This can be accomplished one of three ways: 1) Utilize a double boiler over a stove top burner at extremely low heat. Although this method may be the quickest, it is not one I prefer. The risk of cooking the cacao paste or butter and damaging its prized properties is great. 2) Place the amount you need in a glass bowl or measuring cup and let it melt down in your dehydrator. This method takes longer but doesn't require as much watching. 3) Set a glass bowl or measuring cup in a bath of warm to hot water (not boiling) and stir occasionally until it is completely melted down. This method is my most preferred, but may require changing out the water once or twice in order to completely melt the contents in the measuring cup.

> **Please Note:** If planning to use the double boiler method, I suggest using a glass double boiler instead of metal. Glass is not only a good heat conductor that will distribute heat evenly, it will also not leach impurities into the food. I also suggest bringing the water to just below a boil, and then turning the element completely down or off. If you choose to work directly over the heat source, I advise the use of a cooking thermometer to make sure the temperature of your cacao paste/butter never exceeds 115°F.
>
> As stated above, my method of choice is to utilize a simple glass measuring cup in a bath of preprepared warm to hot water. It is similar to the double boiler method, but without the use of a double boiler or stove. Everything can be done in a bowl right on your kitchen countertop instead. The cacao paste or butter can be left alone to melt while you're prepping and getting your add-ins together.

Caution: Whatever you do, be careful not to splash water in the chocolate. The tiniest bit of water will change the texture and cause it to become unpourable. It will still be edible, but will not be easy to work with, nor will the molded outcome be the same. Therefore, if planning to add presoaked nuts and/or seeds which have not been dehydrated, be sure to thoroughly pat them dry before adding them to your chocolates and bark candies.

Fabulous Fudges

Chocolate Ecstasy Fudge

Blend the following in a <u>high-speed blender</u> until well emulsified, thick and creamy. Stop and scrape down sides as needed. Then pour into mold(s) immediately. See step-by-step instructions and helpful recipe tips in the box on page 429:

- ★ 1 C cashews
- ★ ⅓ C cacao beans (or nibs)
- ★ ⅓ C raw cacao powder
- ★ 1 tsp whole ground vanilla bean powder
- ★ ¼ tsp sea salt
- ★ ⅔ C raw agave
- ★ 1 C cacao butter (liquefied)

Chocolate Malt Fudge

Blend the following in a <u>high-speed blender</u> until well emulsified, thick and creamy. Stop and scrape down sides as needed. Then pour into mold(s) immediately. See step-by-step instructions and helpful recipe tips in the box on page 429:

- ★ 1 C cashews
- ★ ⅓ C cacao beans (or nibs)
- ★ ⅓ C maca powder
- ★ 1 tsp whole ground vanilla bean powder

- ¼ tsp sea salt
- ⅔ C raw agave
- 1 C cacao butter (liquefied)

Chocolate Peanut Butter Fudge

Blend the following in a <u>high-speed blender</u> until well emulsified, thick and creamy. Stop and scrape down sides as needed. Then pour into mold(s) immediately. See step-by-step instructions and helpful recipe tips in the box on page 429:

- ½ C jungle peanuts
- ½ C cashews
- ⅓ C cacao beans (or nibs)
- 3 TBS maca powder
- 2 TBS mesquite powder
- 1 tsp whole ground vanilla bean powder
- ¼ tsp sea salt
- ⅓ C raw agave
- 1 C cacao butter (liquefied)

Mocha Fudge

Blend the following in a <u>high-speed blender</u> until well emulsified, thick and creamy. Stop and scrape down sides as needed. Then pour into mold(s) immediately. See step-by-step instructions and helpful recipe tips in the box on page 429:

- 1 C cashews
- 2 TBS raw cacao powder
- 1 TBS shilajit (for coffee-like flavor)
- 1 TBS lucuma powder
- ¼ tsp whole ground vanilla bean powder
- 1 dash sea salt
- ½ C raw agave
- 1 C cacao butter (liquefied)

Vanilla White Chocolate Fudge

Blend the following in a <u>high-speed blender</u> until well emulsified, thick and creamy. Stop and scrape down sides as needed. Then pour into mold(s) immediately. See step-by-step instructions and helpful recipe tips in the box on page 429:

- 1 C cashews
- 1 tsp whole ground vanilla bean powder
- 1 dash sea salt
- ½ C raw agave
- 1 C cacao butter (liquefied)

La-Caramel White Chocolate Fudge

Blend the following in a <u>high-speed blender</u> until well emulsified, thick and creamy. Stop and scrape down sides as needed. Then pour into mold(s) immediately. See step-by-step instructions and helpful recipe tips in the box on page 429:

- ★ 1 C cashews
- ★ ¼ C lucuma powder
- ★ ¼ tsp whole ground vanilla bean powder
- ★ 1 dash sea salt
- ★ ½ C raw agave
- ★ 1 C cacao butter (liquefied)

Goji-Orange White Chocolate Fudge

Blend the following in a <u>high-speed blender</u> until well emulsified, thick and creamy. Stop and scrape down sides as needed. Then pour into mold(s) immediately. See step-by-step instructions and helpful recipe tips in the box on page 429:

- ★ 1 C cashews
- ★ ½ C goji berries
- ★ ½ C raw agave
- ★ 2-3 drops sweet orange essential oil (or to taste)
- ★ 1 C cacao butter (liquefied)

Matcha Green Tea White Chocolate Fudge

Blend the following in a <u>high-speed blender</u> until well emulsified, thick and creamy. Stop and scrape down sides as needed. Then pour into mold(s) immediately. See step-by-step instructions and helpful recipe tips in the box on page 429:

- ★ 1 C cashews
- ★ 2 TBS matcha green tea powder
- ★ ¼ tsp whole ground vanilla bean powder
- ★ 1 dash sea salt
- ★ ½ C raw agave
- ★ 1 C cacao butter (liquefied)

Maple Walnut White Chocolate Fudge

Blend the following in a <u>high-speed blender</u> until well emulsified, thick and creamy. Stop and scrape down sides as needed. Then pour into mold(s) immediately. See step-by-step instructions and helpful recipe tips in the box on page 429:

- ★ ½ C pecans
- ★ ½ C cashews
- ★ 3 TBS lucuma powder
- ★ 1 TBS mesquite

- ★ ¼ tsp whole ground vanilla bean powder
- ★ 1 dash sea salt
- ★ ½ C raw agave
- ★ 1 C cacao butter (liquefied)

La-Caramel Pecan White Chocolate Fudge

Blend the following in a <u>high-speed blender</u> until well emulsified, thick and creamy. Stop and scrape down sides as needed. Then pour into mold(s) immediately. See step-by-step instructions and helpful recipe tips in the box on page 429:

- ★ ½ C pecans
- ★ ½ C cashews
- ★ 3 TBS lucuma powder
- ★ 1 TBS mesquite
- ★ ¼ tsp whole ground vanilla bean powder
- ★ 1 dash sea salt
- ★ ½ C raw agave
- ★ 1 C cacao butter (liquefied)

CACAO BUTTER MELTING INSTRUCTIONS FOR FUDGE MAKING:

1. To achieve 1 C of melted cacao butter: place approximately 1 ¾-2 C of cacao butter solids (chopped into small chunks and/or shaved into small pieces) in either a 32 oz glass measuring cup or an appropriate sized heat-resistant glass bowl. The reason for using approximately 2 C is due to the solids typically melting down to about half of their original volume.

2. Set a larger, heat-resistant glass bowl or stainless-steel pot on the countertop, and fill with water which is below boiling point. **Please Note:** Always use a type of glass that can tolerate heat (e.g., Pyrex). Otherwise you risk the glass shattering.

3. Place the heat-resistant glass cup or bowl which is holding the cacao butter into the preprepared bath of warm to hot water. Be careful not to splash water into chocolate.

4. Cover, stirring occasionally until cacao butter is completely melted. Change out water if needed in order to completely melt and liquefy contents.

5. Once completely melted, pour 1 C of liquefied cacao butter into blender with all other ingredients and follow recipe instructions.

6. Any unused cacao butter can be placed in silicone ice cube molds to solidify and then popped out and stored in an airtight, glass container until needed again.

> Molding Instructions: Place a 9-inch square silicone cake mold on a plate for stability. Transfer white chocolate fudge mixture into silicone mold, and then jiggle the plate to help easily and evenly distribute. Cover and let set in freezer until solid (which only takes 20-30 minutes tops). **Quick Tip:** May also use silicone ice cube or chocolate molds of various shapes and sizes in place of the silicone cake mold.
>
> Optional Additions for Variation: Prior to molding, sprinkle with chopped nuts, seeds, cacao nibs, coconut flakes and/or dried superfruits for added flavors and textures. Add broken pieces of homemade raw chocolate (page 430) to any white chocolate fudge recipe for a chocolate chip variation.
>
> Serving & Storing Instructions: Remove from mold while still frozen (which is easily done using your hands); place on a plate or cutting board; cut into desired number of fudge squares. Store leftovers in an airtight, glass container for up to two weeks in fridge or 3-6 months (or longer) in freezer.

HOMEMADE CHOCOLATES & BARKS

Below I give three raw chocolate recipes: one for beginners, one that is a bit more advanced, and one that is somewhere in-between. I suggest starting out with the beginner's recipe and then, as you become more comfortable with making your own chocolates, you can always graduate to the moderate and advanced techniques. It's not that they are more difficult, but they do require a bit more time and patience. Although I use chocolate base #3 most often, when I need a quick chocolate fix, chocolate base #1 is my go-to!

All three recipes are simple chocolate bases that can be flavored however you desire. Feel free to explore all your options when it comes to adding your favorite nuts, seeds, superfoods, superfruits, superherbs, spices and/or essential oils.

Raw Chocolates (using cacao powder & coconut oil)

Level of Difficulty: Easy

Chocolate Base #1

- ★ 1 C coconut oil (liquefied)
- ★ 1 C raw cacao powder
- ★ ½ C sun-dried cane juice crystals
- ★ ¼ C lucuma powder
- ★ ½ tsp whole ground vanilla bean powder
- ★ 1-2 dashes Pumpkin Pie Blend

Instructions:

1. Liquefy coconut oil by placing the coconut oil in a bowl or basin of warm-hot water.

2. Pour 1 C of coconut oil into a 16 oz measuring cup or an appropriately sized, heat-resistant glass bowl, then place this into a larger bowl or pan filled with warm water.
3. Add the rest of the ingredients to the coconut oil and whisk them together until well combined and smooth. Do this step while your glass cup or bowl of coconut oil is still in a bath of warm-hot water. The goal is to keep your chocolate base liquefied until ready to pour into molds.
4. Pour into silicone candy molds, ice cube molds or even some mini paper candy cups. **Please Note:** If using silicone molds, be sure to stabilize on a plate or cookie sheet.
5. Place molds in freezer to allow chocolate to set for 20-30 minutes (or less).
6. Remove from molds (which easily pop out when using silicone) and store in an airtight, glass container for up to two weeks in fridge or 3-6 months (or longer) in freezer.

Raw Chocolates (using cacao powder & cacao butter)

Level of Difficulty: Moderate

Chocolate Base #2

- ★ 1 C raw cacao butter (melted)
- ★ 1 C raw cacao powder
- ★ ½ C sun-dried cane juice crystals
- ★ 2 TBS lucuma powder
- ★ ½ tsp whole ground vanilla bean powder
- ★ 1-2 dashes Pumpkin Pie Blend
- ★ 1 pinch sea salt

Instructions:

1. Melt cacao butter and whisk in all the other ingredients according to the instructions found in the box on page 434.
2. **For Homemade Raw Chocolates:** pour into silicone candy molds, ice cube molds or even some mini paper candy cups. **For Chocolate Bark Candy:** pour into a 9-inch square silicone cake mold along with nuts, seeds, coconut flakes and/or dried fruits of choice. **Please Note:** If using silicone molds, be sure to stabilize on a plate or cookie sheet.
3. Place molds in freezer to allow chocolate to set for 20-30 minutes (or less).
4. Remove from molds (which easily pop out when using silicone) and store in an airtight, glass container for up to two weeks in fridge or 3-6 months (or longer) in freezer. **Note:** If making bark candy, break into small and/or large pieces right out of the freezer.

Raw Chocolates (using cacao paste & coconut oil)

Level of Difficulty: Advanced

Chocolate Base #3

- ★ 1 C raw cacao paste (melted)
- ★ ½ C sun-dried cane juice crystals
- ★ ¼ C coconut oil (liquefied)
- ★ 2 TBS lucuma powder
- ★ ½ tsp whole ground vanilla bean powder
- ★ 1-2 dashes Pumpkin Pie Blend
- ★ 1 pinch sea salt

Instructions:

1. Melt cacao paste and whisk in all the other ingredients according to the instructions found in the box on page 434.
2. For **Homemade Raw Chocolates:** pour into silicone candy molds, ice cube molds or even some mini paper candy cups. For **Chocolate Bark Candy:** pour into a 9-inch square silicone cake mold along with nuts, seeds, coconut flakes and/or dried fruits of choice. **Please Note:** If using silicone molds, be sure to stabilize on a plate or cookie sheet.
3. Place molds in freezer to allow chocolate to set for 20-30 minutes (or less).
4. Remove from molds (which easily pop out when using silicone) and store in an air-tight, glass container for up to two weeks in fridge or 3-6 months (or longer) in freezer. **Note:** If making bark candy, break into small and/or large pieces right out of the freezer.

Superfood Additions & Flavor Variation Ideas

Choose a flavor variation below and add to one of the above chocolate bases. Then whisk until well incorporated and smooth. Feel free to add additional sweetener and/or coconut oil as needed until desired taste and texture is reached:

- ★ For **Chia Crunch:** add up to ¼ C chia seeds (whisk directly into mixture or add to the bottom of mold before pouring in chocolate base).
- ★ For **Ginger & Spice:** add 1-2 tsp turmeric extract powder (95% curcumin) or 4-6 opened capsules (contents only) of Premier Research Labs Turmeric, along with 2-3 drops ginger essential oil (more to taste, adding 1 drop at a time).
- ★ For **Maca Malt:** add 2-3 TBS maca powder and 1 TBS mesquite powder (optional).
- ★ For **Mint Kiss:** add 1-2 TBS Sunwarrior Ormus Greens and 2-3 drops of peppermint essential oil (more to taste, adding 1 drop at a time).
- ★ For **Mocha Yogi:** add 2 tsp shilajit powder and 1 tsp ashwagandha powder.
- ★ For **Mylk Chocolate Muscle:** add 2-3 TBS of Surthrival Colostrum and 2-3 droppers full of Surthrival Pine Pollen.
- ★ For **Neuromancer:** add 2 tsp mucuna pruriens powder and 1 tsp shilajit powder.
- ★ For **Banana Orange:** add 1-2 TBS vine-ripened banana powder and 2-3 drops of orange essential oil (more to taste, adding 1 drop at a time).

- For **Shangri-La:** add 1-2 TBS spirulina and/or chlorella, along with 4-6 opened capsules (contents only) of Premier Research Labs Ginseng-FX or Dragon Herbs Siberian Ginseng.
- For **Shroom Immune:** add desired dosage of medicinal mushrooms of choice (such as a few droppers full and/or opened capsules [contents only] of Host Defense MyCommunity, Host Defense CordyChi, Dragon Herbs Siberian Chaga, etc.).
- For **Spicy Mayan:** add up to ¼ tsp cayenne powder (or to taste) and 1-2 TBS mesquite powder.

Optional Uses & Additions for Variation

- For **Ice Cream Bonbons:** pour a liquefied raw chocolate base of choice over one-ounce scoops of your favorite ice cream flavor (page 417). Try doing the same with any rawkie, maca-roon or raw ball recipe by dipping them in the liquefied raw chocolate base. Then let them harden up for about 15 minutes in the freezer. **Quick Tip:** Use a toothpick or skewer for dipping, then place on a nonstick silicone surface or natural parchment paper for molding.
- For **Nut Clusters:** cluster together about 1 TBS worth of nuts. Pour just enough chocolate over the nut cluster so that once it solidifies it holds the nuts together. Place in freezer to let harden up and then store in an airtight container in fridge. **Quick Tip:** Use a nonstick silicone surface or a natural parchment paper lined cookie sheet for molding.
- For flavor and texture variations, feel free to add one or more of the following ingredients to mold(s) either before or after pouring: desired amount of whole or coarsely ground nuts and/or seeds of choice, dried fruit pieces of choice, cacao beans (or nibs), coconut flakes, bee pollen, etc. **FYI:** These are best added to Chocolate Bark Candy.

CACAO PASTE & BUTTER MELTING INSTRUCTIONS FOR CHOCOLATES:

1. To achieve 1 C of melted cacao paste or butter: place approximately 1 ¾-2 C of cacao paste solids or butter solids (chopped into small chunks and/or shaved into small pieces) in either a 32 oz glass measuring cup or an appropriate sized heat-resistant glass bowl. The reason for using approximately 2 C is due to the solids typically melting down to about half of their original volume.

2. Set a larger, heat-resistant glass bowl or stainless-steel pot on the countertop, and fill with water which is below boiling point. **Please Note:** Always use a type of glass that can tolerate heat (e.g., Pyrex). Otherwise you risk the glass shattering.

3. Place the heat-resistant glass cup or bowl which is holding the cacao paste or butter into the preprepared bath of warm to hot water. Be sure not to splash water into chocolate.

4. Cover, stirring occasionally until completely melted. Change out water if needed in order to completely melt and liquefy contents.

5. Once completely melted into a smooth liquid, add all other chocolate base ingredients along with any superfood and flavor additions desired. Then stir or whisk until smooth. Do this step while your glass cup or bowl of cacao paste/butter is still in a bath of warm-hot water. The goal is to keep your chocolate base liquefied until ready to pour into molds.

Please Note: If following Chocolate Base #3 and cacao paste becomes too thick due to the addition of certain powders, feel free to add a bit more coconut oil. Taste and determine the need for additional sweetener.

Recipe Notes & Quick Tips: I love to experiment with different oils and oil combinations. Each raw, cold-pressed oil brings its own unique healing and health benefits to the mix. For this reason, when making raw chocolates with cacao paste (base #3), try replacing all (or a portion of) the coconut oil with extra virgin olive oil, black sesame seed oil, hemp seed oil or chia seed oil.

Sun-dried cane juice crystals can be substituted or mixed with Xylitol. You may also choose to work with raw honey or agave.

Based on personal wants and needs, feel free to formulate your very own medicinal raw chocolate masterpieces. Just start adding teaspoons or tablespoons (depending on desired dosage) of any superfood powder or combination of superfood powders you want (green powders, protein powders, Chinese herbs, Ayurvedic herbs, etc.). You may also add the suggested dosage of your favorite superfood extracts or tinctures (such as medicinal mushrooms, pine pollen, etc.). You can then add any additional sweetener and/or coconut oil (if needed) to your desired taste and texture.

CHAPTER 8
DEHYDRATED PIZZA CRUSTS, CRAKS & CHIPS

Why own a food dehydrator? Dehydrating is a wonderful way to warm, dry and preserve your foods without destroying all the living and vital nutrients within. With a dehydrator, you can make your very own crunchy "craks" (aka crackers) and "chipz" (aka chips). You can make your own gluten-free pizza crusts and breads. You can preserve fresh herbs, fruits and vegetables (and flavor them if you wish). You can even warm, marinate and soften foods for those days when you long for something reminiscent of a cooked favorite.

You can also form and then dehydrate any nut or seed pâté in order to make savory balls or burger patties. What about all the sweet treat recipes such as raw balls, maca-roons and rawkies? You can dehydrate any number of these for a raw cookie with a different texture. Dehydrate for less time and you have a warm and chewy inside and slightly crisp outside. Dehydrate longer and you have a crisp cookie throughout. The ideas are limitless!

What to buy: a 5-tray model or 9-tray model? I highly suggest a 9-tray model over a 5-tray. The following are my top picks out of all the dehydrators on the market: Excalibur 3900 Deluxe Non-Timer Series 9 Tray Food Dehydrator (or 3926T 9 Tray w/ 26 Hour Timer) and Sedona Digitally Controlled Food Dehydrator (SD-9000) by Tribest. With the amount of time you must wait for your masterpiece(s) to be ready to eat, you're going to want the extra space to make as much as you can at once. For instance, it can take overnight or longer for kale chipz to be ready and then less than 5 minutes to have the whole batch completely devoured. Plus, almost 90% of the people whom I have had the opportunity to work with have come back and stated that they wish they would have purchased the 9-tray model instead of the 5-tray.

Quick Recipe Tips:

The main focus of this chapter is to give a basic crust idea and a small variety of cracker and chip ideas. The crust recipe I offer makes the perfect base for layering all your savory pizza ingredients. Furthermore, it's simply seasoned and just enough to complement any ethnic-themed pizza night. Same goes for the crak and chip recipes. All it takes is a simple switch-up of just one or more ingredients (herbs, spices, nuts, seeds, etc.) for a twist of taste that is new and exciting!

You no longer have any more excuses! Start satisfying your craving for something crunchy without reaching for a box or bag of processed ingredients and chemical additives. Just remember, when eating dehydrated foods (or any dried food for that matter) you need to replace the fluid that the dehydrated food is going to absorb from your body. Be sure to drink plenty of fluids and eat a good amount of water rich fruits and vegetables when consuming dried foods of any kind.

What to use: chia or flax? I like using chia over flax seeds in the majority of my dehydrating recipes, but feel free to use either one. From a culinary point of view, both are gelatinous seeds that will bind all your ingredients, making them interchangeable. You may even wish to use half-and-half.

> **Please Note:** If you are looking to get more plant-based omega-3 in your diet, from a seed that is, look no further than chia or flax. However, you may want to consider the following when deciding which to use for raw food dehydrator recipes: 1) One of the big disadvantages of flax seeds is that they tend to spoil quickly. You must keep flax seeds in your fridge or freezer and even then, you must use them up in a short period of time before they oxidize and have the opportunity to go rancid. 2) You must grind flax seeds before consuming. If you don't grind flax seeds, your body will not be able to digest them and utilize the omega-3 fatty acids they contain. Furthermore, flax seeds oxidize so fast, their nutritional value starts declining as soon as they are ground. If you are going to consume flax, I highly suggest grinding the seeds yourself and in amounts small enough to be consumed within 2-3 days.
>
> With what I know about essential fatty acids, flax seeds do not stack up to be the best choice for obtaining much needed omega-3; especially once they have been exposed to oxygen and heat during the dehydration process. Yes, even low temperature heat.
>
> On the other hand, chia seeds can be digested either ground or whole, making it easy to take full advantage of their omega-3 fatty acids and other vital nutrients. Additionally, chia seeds do not need to be refrigerated and will keep for up to two years in your cupboards due to their super high levels of antioxidants (even more than blueberries). Compared to flax, chia seeds are richer in omega-3 fatty acids, which are then protected from spoilage due to their much higher levels of antioxidant. Chia seeds are also high in protein, dietary fiber and a host of much needed minerals, including calcium, magnesium, potassium, etc.
>
> To understand in greater detail why chia and hemp are a better choice than flax when it comes to seed sources of omega-3, please review "Essential Facts About Essential Fatty Acids" (page 70), "Getting to Know Your True 'FAT' Friends" (page 81), and "The Best of the Best" (page 118).

Flavors are always enhanced when dehydrating, so when adding the spicier of herbs and spices (onion, garlic, asafoetida, sea salt, cayenne, etc.), you may need a lot less than you think. Use the measurements that I give as a guideline (which I feel add a mild to medium amount of flavor that works for the majority); but if you find you like your craks or chipz more or less spicy, take note of the amounts used the first time, then add more or less the next time you make them. For instance, I love a lot of herby flavor and hot-heat type spices, so I tend to add a heaping amount of almost all the measurements given when making for just myself. Heck, I'll even add a bit of habanera powder for an extra kick!

Can savory and sweet foods be dehydrated together? Some are okay to dehydrate together and some should never be dehydrated together. For instance, I would never dehydrate garlic and onion foods at the same time as sweet foods. The flavors will combine. Although it really depends on the foods, herbs and spices chosen, I suggest always dehydrating sweet and savory foods separately. This way, you haven't spent hours preparing and then drying a variety of foods only to have them all taste the same!

> **Quick Flip Trick!** When it comes to flipping your partially dehydrate foods, there is a trick that most dehydrating fanatics do so well that they can do it with their eyes closed. As the time approaches to flip crusts, craks or chipz: take a clean, mesh screened tray (i.e., without a sheet); lay it topside down evenly and directly over the tray of craks or chipz; hold the sides firmly, without squeezing too tightly, and then quickly flip them over. Now, slowly peel the dehydrator sheet from the craks or chipz and pop the new tray back into the dehydrator for the remainder of the time it takes to completely dry. No need to be intimidated or afraid of losing your food to the floor. Just keep a good grip, do a quick flip and you're done!

Do you have produce that needs to be eaten before it goes bad? Do you not know what to do with all your fruit and vegetable juice pulp? No worries! Blend up whatever you have with some water and maybe some complementary fruits, vegetables, herbs and/or spice. Then for every 16-24 oz of mixture, you are going to use 1 C chia seeds to transform your concoction into crackers! All it takes is combining and thoroughly mixing your wet and dry ingredients in a bowl, allowing the mixture to set for about 30 minutes, and then spreading it onto sheeted dehydrator trays to dehydrate until dry and crisp. This is the easiest way to use up produce before it turns.

> **General Guideline for Making Craks & Chipz:** Use 1 C of chia seeds for every 16 oz of a liquid base that has a watery to nectar-like consistency (i.e. water rich fruits and vegetables that blend easily without the addition of much water). Add up to 8 oz of water (as needed) to the 16 oz liquid base for every 1 C of dry or solid ingredients you plan to add (nuts, seeds, powders, fruit pulp, fibrous vegetables, etc.). If your 16 oz liquid base is a bit on the thicker side (i.e., honey-like or spoon-thick consistency), then you will also want to add up to 8 oz of water (as needed) before adding the 1 C of chia seeds.

What about leftover raw soups or smoothies? I cannot tell you how many times I've used leftover soup to make crackers. I have even made double batches of soup just to have a side that is complimentary, yet offers a contrasting crunch. Again, just add 1 C of chia to every 16-24 oz of a liquid base and, voila, you have a new cracker recipe! I've even done this with leftover pâtés, dressings and dessert flops. Throw it in the blender with just enough water to bring the mixture up between 16 and 24 oz, doctor it up with herbs and spices as needed, and then add chia seeds and dehydrate until dry. Nothing ever has to go to waste again!

> **Please Note:** With the exception of Brazil nuts, hazelnuts, macadamia nuts, pine nuts, pistachio nuts and chia, flax and hemp seeds, all nuts and seeds should be presoaked, rinsed and drained for optimal absorption and assimilation of nutrients.
>
> To review "The Science Behind the Soak," "General Soaking Schedule for Nuts & Seeds" and other great tips, please refer to page 26.

Go-To Pizza Crust

First, process the following dry ingredients in a <u>food processor</u> until ground into flour:

- ★ 2 C Brazil nuts
- ★ 1 TBS dried oregano
- ★ 1 tsp sea salt

Optional Variations

- ★ Substitute 2 C of almonds, walnuts or sunflower seeds for Brazil nuts.

Second, add the following and process again until broken down and well incorporated:

- ★ 2 roma tomatoes
- ★ 2 TBS coconut oil (liquefied)

Optional Variation

- ★ Substitute 1 red bell pepper for roma tomatoes.

Third, pregrind the following in a <u>high-speed blender</u> (I suggest the use of a Blendtec, Nutribullet with milling blade or Vitamix dry container for this task). Then transfer ground seeds to the above ingredient in <u>food processor</u> and process again to thoroughly combine and evenly distribute:

- ★ 1 C chia seeds

Last, add the following to all the above ingredients in <u>food processor</u> (which can be done while processor is still running), but add slowly and only as needed. Then follow the step-by-step instructions in the box on page 439:

- ★ 16 oz (or more as needed) purified, filtered water. Add only a few ounces at a time until a dough-like consistency is reached.

INSTRUCTIONS FOR PIZZA CRUST:

1. Using a dry ½ C measuring cup as a serving size guide: scoop and level mixture and then dish contents into the center of each quadrant of a sheeted dehydrator tray. There should be four personal pizza crusts per tray – one per quadrant.

2. Shape doughy mixture to approximately 6 inch, ¼ inch thick rounds (continuously wet hands to help easily spread and shape – it really works). You should be able to get about 6-8 crusts out of the batch. The actual number will depend on how thick or thin you like your crust. If you don't have enough mixture to make one more crust, evenly distribute the remainder over the number of crusts you do have.

3. Dehydrate for several hours or overnight at 105-115°F.

4. Follow the "Quick Flip Trick" on page 437 in order to carefully (yet easily) transfer each crust from sheeted tray(s) to clean, mesh screened dehydrator tray(s). This will allow the underneath to thoroughly dry and start to brown and crisp.

5. Dehydrate for a few additional hours or until desired texture. Crusts should be fairly dry throughout (with a slightly soft and chewy inside, not wet and doughy). Don't worry if crusts become too dry and harden, they will naturally soften up with the addition of your toppings and when stored in the refrigerator.

6. Store in an airtight container in refrigerator with something like a natural parchment paper separating each crust. These will keep for up to one week. Crusts are best when served warm and fresh out of the dehydrator; therefore, feel free to pop leftovers back in for a short time before serving.

Recipe Notes & Quick Tips: If you desire one large pizza, this recipe allows for two large crusts. All you have to do is divide the mixture in half, mold one large crust per sheeted tray (round or square), and then follow the rest of the instructions (#s 3-6) in the box above. **Note:** Score desired number of slices while still soft and a bit doughy (8-10 triangles or 6-9 squares). I suggest doing this before the "Quick Flip Trick" (#4). Be sure to use a spatula or butter knife to score (i.e., nothing sharp that can damage your teflex or silicone sheets).

Whether personal size or large, this pizza crust is a great base for making Italian-style, Greek-style or Mexican-style pizzas. Please refer back to the sections of the book headed "Nut Crèmes & Cheezes" (page 345) and "Delectable Dips, Side Dishes & Condiments" (page 347), where I share some great serving ideas for each pizza style.

Once your pizza crust is topped with all your favorites, place back into the dehydrator for about 20-30 minutes (or so) to warm and soften veggies and allow marinating.

SAVORY CRAKS & CHIPZ

"Seeds of Change" Craks

Place the following whole seeds in a large mixing bowl and follow step-by-step instructions on page 441:

- ★ 1 ½ C chia seeds
- ★ ½ C pumpkin seeds
- ★ ½ C sunflower seeds
- ★ ¼ C black sesame seeds
- ★ ¼ C unhulled, tan sesame seeds
- ★ 2 TBS Spicy Infusion Blend
- ★ 2 tsp sea salt
- ★ ½ tsp asafoetida
- ★ 2 TBS coconut oil (liquefied)
- ★ 32-40 oz purified, filtered water (starting with 32 oz and adding more as needed)

Optional Variations

- ★ Substitute 2 TBS Italian Blend or Mediterranean Blend for Spicy Infusion Blend.

Cabbage N' Carrot Craks

Chop the following veggies into small chunks and place in a <u>food processor</u>. Process and pulse until finely chopped and shredded down and then transfer to a large mixing bowl:

- ★ 1 small head of red cabbage (cored)
- ★ 2-3 carrots (peeled & tops removed)

Then, add the following ingredients to the above veggies in large mixing bowl and follow the step-by-step instructions on page 441:

- ★ 1 ½ C chia seeds
- ★ 1 C pumpkin seeds
- ★ ½ C coconut flakes
- ★ 2 TBS Garam Masala Blend
- ★ 2 tsp sea salt
- ★ ½ tsp asafoetida
- ★ 2 TBS coconut oil (liquefied)
- ★ 32-40 oz purified, filtered water (starting with 32 oz and adding more as needed)

Optional Variations

- ★ Substitute ½ C unhulled, tan or black sesame seeds for coconut flakes.
- ★ Substitute 2 TBS Curry Blend or Spicy Infusion Blend for Garam Masala Blend.

INSTRUCTIONS FOR CRAKS:

1. Mix all the craks ingredients thoroughly by hand until well combined and entire mixture starts to become gelatinous. **Note:** Use 32 oz of water to start, reserving the rest.

2. Let mixture sit in the bowl at room temperature for 20-30 minutes. This will allow the chia seeds to absorb more of the liquid and the entire mixture to thicken.

3. Stir mixture one more time to make sure there are no lumpy clumps of chia seeds. Add reserved water if mixture is too thick to spread (2 oz at a time, as needed). Then spread evenly onto sheeted dehydrator tray(s). Personally, I like to use approximately 2 C per sheeted tray. **FYI:** You may use a spatula or your hands to evenly spread out mixture. If mixture is too doughy and tacky, cup some water in your hands and apply to mixture for more gliding action. Using wet hands really helps with easy and even spreading. Also, I suggest keeping mixture at least a half inch away from the edge of the tray.

4. Score to desired size and shape (such as bite-sized squares or triangles) and dehydrate at 105-115°F for 8-10+ hrs. Use a spatula or butter knife to score (not the sharp end of a regular knife, which can damage your teflex or silicone sheets).

5. Flip craks carefully (using "Quick Flip Trick" on page 437) onto a mesh screened tray without a sheet, and then peel dehydrator sheet from underside of craks. This will allow for more air circulation and faster drying.

6. Dehydrate for another 8-10 hrs or until completely dry and desired crispness is reached.

7. Store in an airtight container in a cool and dry place. Feel free to pop craks back in the dehydrator if they have lost some of their crunch.

Cheezy Craks

Pregrind the following in a <u>high-speed blender</u> (I suggest the use of a Blendtec, Nutribullet with milling blade or Vitamix dry container for this task). Then transfer ground chia seeds to a large mixing bowl:

- ★ 1 C white chia seeds

Then, blend the following ingredients in a <u>high-speed blender</u> until smooth and creamy, add entire mixture to bowl of chia seeds and follow the step-by-step instructions on page 445:

- ★ 1 C Brazil nuts
- ★ 2 TBS chickpea miso paste
- ★ 2 TBS nutritional yeast flakes
- ★ 1 red bell pepper (chopped)
- ★ ½ tsp sea salt
- ★ ½ tsp paprika
- ★ ¼ tsp asafoetida
- ★ 2 TBS coconut oil (liquefied)

- 16-24 oz purified, filtered water (using 16 oz to start, reserving 8 oz to be added as needed)

Optional Variations & Additions

- Substitute 1 C almonds for Brazil nuts.
- Add a dash or two of cayenne for a bit of spicy heat.

Mediterranean Pita Chipz

Pregrind the following in a <u>high-speed blender</u> (I suggest the use of a Blendtec, Nutribullet with milling blade or Vitamix dry container for this task). Then transfer ground chia seeds to a large mixing bowl:

- 1 C white chia seeds

Then, blend the following ingredients in a <u>high-speed blender</u> until smooth and creamy, add entire mixture to bowl of chia seeds and follow the step-by-step instructions on page 445:

- ½ C sunflower seeds
- ½ C unhulled, tan sesame seeds
- 2 TBS chickpea miso paste
- 1-2 TBS dried parsley
- 1-2 tsp dried thyme (optional)
- ½ tsp sea salt
- ½ tsp paprika
- ¼ tsp asafoetida
- 2 TBS coconut oil (liquefied)
- 16-24 oz purified, filtered water (using 16 oz to start, reserving 8 oz to be added as needed)

Optional Variations & Additions

- Increase sunflower or sesame seeds to 1 C and remove the ½ C of the other seeds.
- Add a dash or two of cayenne for a bit of spicy heat.

Chili-Lime Tortilla Chipz

Pregrind the following in a <u>high-speed blender</u> (I suggest the use of a Blendtec, Nutribullet with milling blade or Vitamix dry container for this task). Then transfer ground chia seeds to a large mixing bowl:

- 1 C white chia seeds

Then, blend the following ingredients in a <u>high-speed blender</u> until smooth and creamy, add entire mixture to bowl of chia seeds and follow the step-by-step instructions on page 445:

- 1 C sunflower seeds

- ★ 1 TBS dried cilantro
- ★ 1 tsp Chili Blend
- ★ 1 tsp sea salt
- ★ ¼ tsp asafoetida
- ★ 1 lime, juiced
- ★ 1 TBS raw agave
- ★ 2 TBS coconut oil (liquefied)
- ★ 16-24 oz purified, filtered water (using 16 oz to start, reserving 8 oz to be added as needed)

Optional Variations

- ★ Substitute 1 C unhulled, tan sesame seeds for sunflower seeds or use half-and-half of each.

Rosemary Craks

Place the following in a large mixing bowl:

- ★ 1 C chia seeds

Then, blend the following ingredients in a <u>high-speed blender</u> until smooth and creamy, add entire mixture to bowl of chia seeds and follow the step-by-step instructions on page 445:

- ★ 1 C almonds
- ★ 2 TBS chickpea miso paste
- ★ 2 roma tomatoes (chopped)
- ★ 1 TBS dried rosemary
- ★ 1 tsp dried thyme
- ★ ½ tsp sea salt
- ★ ½ tsp paprika
- ★ ¼ tsp asafoetida
- ★ 2 TBS coconut oil (liquefied)
- ★ 16-24 oz purified, filtered water (using 16 oz to start, reserving 8 oz to be added as needed)

Optional Variations & Additions

- ★ Substitute 1 C Brazil nuts or sunflower seeds for almonds.
- ★ Add 1-2 tsp of dried basil.
- ★ Add a dash or two of cayenne for a bit of spicy heat.

Bell Pepper Quinoa Chipz

Place the following in a large mixing bowl:

- ★ 1 C chia seeds

Then, blend the following ingredients in a <u>high-speed blender</u>, add entire mixture to bowl of chia seeds and follow the step-by-step instructions on page 445:

- ★ 1 C sprouted quinoa (either home-sprouted or presprouted TruRoots brand)
- ★ 2 TBS chickpea miso paste
- ★ 2 red bell peppers (chopped)
- ★ 1 TBS Curry Blend
- ★ 1 TBS dried cilantro
- ★ ½ tsp sea salt
- ★ ½ tsp paprika
- ★ ¼ tsp asafoetida
- ★ 2 TBS coconut oil (liquefied)
- ★ 16-24 oz purified, filtered water (using 16 oz to start, reserving 8 oz to be added as needed)

Optional Variations & Additions

- ★ Replace Curry Blend and cilantro for any of the following: 2 TBS Mediterranean Blend, 2 TBS Italian Blend or 1 TBS each of dried basil and cilantro, dried oregano and thyme or dried cilantro and parsley.
- ★ Add a dash or two of cayenne for a bit of spicy heat.

INSTRUCTIONS FOR CRAKS & CHIPZ:

1. Add blended mixture to chia seeds in large mixing bowl and thoroughly stir the two together until chia seeds are evenly distributed. **Note:** Blended mixture should include only 16 oz of water to start with, out of the 16-24 oz called for in recipe.

2. Add extra water, as needed (about 2-6 oz). I prefer to keep the mixture very thick and then add extra water as I spread the mixture out with my hands (see #4). However, if you desire thinner craks or chipz, feel free to add a few extra ounces to the mixture prior to blending.

3. Let mixture sit in the bowl at room temperature for 20-30 minutes. This will allow the chia seeds to absorb more of the liquid and the entire mixture to thicken.

4. Stir mixture one more time to make sure there are no lumpy clumps of chia seeds. Add additional water if mixture is too thick to spread (2 oz at a time, as needed). Then spread evenly onto sheeted dehydrator tray(s). Personally, I like to use approximately 2 C per sheeted tray. **FYI:** You may use a spatula or your hands to evenly spread out mixture. If mixture is too doughy and tacky, cup some water in your hands and apply to mixture for more gliding action. Using wet hands really helps with easy and even spreading. Also, I suggest keeping mixture at least a half inch away from the edge of the tray.

5. Score to desired size and shape (such as bite-sized squares or triangles) and dehydrate at 105-115°F for 8-10+ hrs. Use a spatula or butter knife to score (not the sharp end of a regular knife, which can damage your teflex or silicone sheets).

6. Flip craks or chipz carefully (using "Quick Flip Trick" on page 437) onto a mesh screened tray without a sheet, and then peel dehydrator sheet from underside of craks or chipz. This will allow for more air circulation and faster drying.

7. Dehydrate for another 8-10 hrs or until completely dry and desired crispness is reached.

8. Store in an airtight container in a cool and dry place. Feel free to pop craks or chipz back in the dehydrator if they have lost some of their crunch.

Cheezy Kale Chipz #1

Wash and spin dry the following (easily done in a salad spinner). Remove leaves from tough stem and tear into small to medium sized pieces before placing in a large mixing bowl:

- ★ 2 bunches curly kale

Then, blend the following ingredients in a high-speed blender until thick, smooth and creamy, add entire mixture to the bowl of kale and follow the step-by-step instructions on page 448:

- ★ 1 C Brazil nuts
- ★ 2 TBS chickpea miso paste

- ★ 2 TBS chia seeds
- ★ 1 red bell pepper (chopped)
- ★ ½ tsp sea salt
- ★ ¼ tsp paprika
- ★ 1 dash asafoetida
- ★ 2 TBS lemon juice
- ★ 1 TBS coconut oil (liquefied)
- ★ 8 oz purified, filtered water

Optional Additions for Variation

- ★ Add a pinch or two of cayenne for a bit of spicy heat.
- ★ Sprinkle coated kale chipz with nutritional yeast flakes just prior to dehydrating.

> How to De-Stem Kale: Hold the end of the kale stem and slide your hand down the stock. You should be able to easily remove the whole kale leaf in one quick swipe.

Cheezy Kale Chipz #2

Wash and spin dry the following (easily done in a salad spinner). Remove leaves from tough stem and tear into small to medium sized pieces before placing in a large mixing bowl:

- ★ 2 bunches curly kale

Then, blend the following ingredients in a <u>high-speed blender</u> until thick, smooth and creamy, add entire mixture to the bowl of kale and follow the step-by-step instructions on page 448:

- ★ 1 C hemp seeds
- ★ ¼ C nutritional yeast flakes
- ★ 2 TBS chia seeds
- ★ 1 tsp sea salt
- ★ ¼ tsp paprika
- ★ 1 dash asafoetida
- ★ 2 TBS lemon juice
- ★ 1 TBS coconut oil (liquefied)
- ★ 8-12 oz purified, filtered water (as needed)

Optional Variations & Additions

- ★ Substitute 1 C almonds, Brazil nuts or cashews for hemp seeds.
- ★ Add a pinch or two of cayenne for a bit of spicy heat.

Italian-Style Kale Chipz

Wash and spin dry the following (easily done in a salad spinner). Remove leaves from tough stem and tear into small to medium sized pieces before placing in a large mixing bowl:

- ★ 2 bunches curly kale

Then, blend the following ingredients in a <u>high-speed blender</u> until thick, smooth and creamy, add entire mixture to the bowl of kale and follow the step-by-step instructions on page 448:

- ★ 1 C almonds
- ★ 2 roma tomatoes
- ★ 2 TBS chia seeds
- ★ 2 TBS Italian Blend
- ★ 1 tsp sea salt
- ★ ¼ tsp asafoetida
- ★ 1 pinch cayenne
- ★ 2 TBS lemon juice
- ★ 1 TBS coconut oil (liquefied)
- ★ 8 oz purified, filtered water

Optional Addition for Variation

- ★ Sprinkle coated kale chipz with nutritional yeast flakes just prior to dehydrating.

Thai-Style Kale Chipz

Wash and spin dry the following (easily done in a salad spinner). Remove leaves from tough stem and tear into small to medium sized pieces before placing in a large mixing bowl:

- ★ 2 bunches curly kale

Then, blend the following ingredients in a <u>high-speed blender</u> until thick, smooth and creamy, add entire mixture to the bowl of kale and follow the step-by-step instructions on page 448:

- ★ 1 C cashews
- ★ 2 TBS chia seeds
- ★ 2 tsp dried basil
- ★ 2 tsp dried cilantro
- ★ 2 tsp dried parsley
- ★ 1 tsp Garam Masala Blend
- ★ 1 tsp sea salt
- ★ ¼ tsp asafoetida
- ★ 1 pinch cayenne
- ★ 1 TBS raw agave
- ★ 1 lime, juiced

- ★ 1 TBS coconut oil (liquefied)
- ★ 8-12 oz purified, filtered water (as needed)

INSTRUCTIONS FOR KALE CHIPZ:

1. Using your hands, massage blended mixture into kale and thoroughly coat each piece. Be sure to get inside all the little curls of kale.

2. Place onto sheeted dehydrator trays and don't worry about being too particular. It is not necessary to space each piece or flatten them. Having them clumped up is fine.

3. Dehydrate at 105°F overnight (or until coating is dry), then slide kale onto clean, mesh screened trays and dehydrate for another four hours (or until completely crisp). Total dehydrating time is approximately 12-14 hours.

4. Store in a cool and dry spot and consume before the humidity in the air decreases their crunchiness. This shouldn't be too hard to accomplish!

Recipe Notes & Quick Tips: Just about any dressing or sauce recipe under "Sexy Sauces & Dressings" (page 357) can be utilized as a kale chip flavor. The options are limitless! You can even coat your kale with Macho Nacho Cheeze (page 346) or any other cheeze recipe under "Nut Crèmes & Cheezes" (page 345). Just add your favorite herbs to a cheeze base and a tad more sea salt, to taste. How about marinating your kale in any one of the salsa variations (page 348) or Marawnara Sauce (page 358)? What about Zany BBQ Sauce (page 354) or "A Thousand Islands" Dressing (page 363)? Let's not forget about the various pesto sauces (page 357) or Caesar Dressings (page 362)!

Whatever you choose, you will want your kale chip coating to be pourable, yet thick enough to actually coat the kale. If a sauce or dressing is a bit too runny, blend it up with 1-2 TBS of chia seeds, and then allow it to sit for a short while until it thickens. This leads me to mention how any nut or seed pâté under "Protein Packed Pâtés" (page 336) will work as a kale chip coating as well. Only this time you will want to blend the pâté with a few ounces of water. Be sure to add any additional herbs and spices as needed (e.g., sea salt) and maybe some nutritional yeast flakes. You may even choose to just sprinkle any additional dried herbs, spices and/or nutritional yeast flakes right over the top of your freshly coated kale chips just prior to dehydrating. **Note:** Sprinkling over the top may be best if you are concerned about over spicing.

Review all the recipes in "Mouthwatering Stove Stoppers" (page 332) for all the endless flavoring possibilities you have at your fingertips for kale chipz!

SWEET CRAKS & CHIPZ

Chocolate Chia Craks

Place the following in a large mixing bowl:

- ★ 1 C chia seeds

Then, blend the following ingredients in a high-speed blender, add entire mixture to bowl of chia seeds and follow the step-by-step instructions on page 451:

- ★ 1 sweet red apple (chopped)
- ★ ⅔ C hemp seeds
- ★ ⅓ C raw cacao powder
- ★ ¼ tsp whole ground vanilla bean powder
- ★ 1 dash sea salt
- ★ 2 TBS raw agave
- ★ 2 TBS coconut oil (liquefied)
- ★ 16-20 oz purified, filtered water (as needed)

Optional Variations & Additions

- ★ Substitute 1 orange (peeled & seeded) for the apple.
- ★ Add a pinch or two of cinnamon and/or cayenne.

Last, add the following frozen fruit, then blend again until well broken down and smooth:

- ★ 1 C strawberries

Spiced Green Apple Chipz

Place the following in a large mixing bowl:

- ★ 1 C chia seeds

Then, blend the following ingredients in a high-speed blender, add entire mixture to bowl of chia seeds and follow the step-by-step instructions on page 451:

- ★ 1 granny smith apple (chopped)
- ★ 4 C packed baby spinach
- ★ ¾ C hemp seeds
- ★ ¼ tsp Apple Pie Blend
- ★ 1 dash sea salt
- ★ 2 TBS raw agave
- ★ 2 TBS coconut oil (liquefied)
- ★ 16-20 oz purified, filtered water (as needed)

Optional Variations & Additions

- ★ Substitute 1 pear or orange (peeled & seeded) for the apple.
- ★ Add a pinch or two of cinnamon and/or cayenne.

Sweet N' Berry Craks

Place the following in a large mixing bowl:

- ★ 1 C chia seeds

Then, blend the following ingredients in a <u>high-speed blender</u>, add entire mixture to bowl of chia seeds and follow the step-by-step instructions on page 451:

- ★ 1 C hemp seeds
- ★ 2 TBS mesquite powder
- ★ ¼ tsp Pumpkin Pie Blend
- ★ 1 dash sea salt
- ★ 2 TBS raw agave
- ★ 2 TBS coconut oil (liquefied)
- ★ 16-20 oz purified, filtered water (as needed)

Optional Variations & Additions

- ★ Substitute 1 C almonds or Brazil nuts for hemp seeds.
- ★ Add ¼-½ C of mulberries and/or goji berries.

Last, add the following frozen fruit, then blend again until well broken down and smooth:

- ★ 1 C mixed berries

INSTRUCTIONS FOR CRAKS & CHIPZ:

1. Add blended mixture to chia seeds in large mixing bowl and thoroughly stir the two together until chia seeds are evenly distributed. **Note:** Blended mixture should include only 16 oz of water to start with, out of the 16-20 oz called for in recipe.

2. Add extra water, as needed (about 2-6 oz). I prefer to keep the mixture very thick and then add extra water as I spread the mixture out with my hands (see #4). However, if you desire thinner craks or chipz, feel free to add a few extra ounces to the mixture prior to blending.

3. Let mixture sit in the bowl at room temperature for 20-30 minutes. This will allow the chia seeds to absorb more of the liquid and the entire mixture to thicken.

4. Stir mixture one more time to make sure there are no lumpy clumps of chia seeds. Add additional water if mixture is too thick to spread (2 oz at a time, as needed). Then spread evenly onto sheeted dehydrator tray(s). Personally, I like to use approximately 2 C per sheeted tray. **FYI:** You may use a spatula or your hands to evenly spread out mixture. If mixture is too doughy and tacky, cup some water in your hands and apply to mixture for more gliding action. Using wet hands really helps with easy and even spreading. Also, I suggest keeping mixture at least a half inch away from the edge of the tray.

5. Score to desired size and shape (such as bite-sized squares or triangles) and dehydrate at 105-115°F for 8-10+ hrs. Use a spatula or butter knife to score (not the sharp end of a regular knife, which can damage your teflex or silicone sheets).

6. Flip craks or chipz carefully (using "Quick Flip Trick" on page 437) onto a mesh screened tray without a sheet, and then peel dehydrator sheet from underside of craks or chipz. This will allow for more air circulation and faster drying.

7. Dehydrate for another 8-10 hrs or until completely dry and desired crispness is reached.

8. Store in an airtight container in a cool and dry place. Feel free to pop craks or chipz back in the dehydrator if they have lost some of their crunch.

Chocolate Kale Chipz

Wash and spin dry the following (easily done in a salad spinner). Remove leaves from tough stem and tear into small to medium sized pieces before placing in a large mixing bowl:

- ★ 2 bunches curly kale

Then, blend the following ingredients in a <u>high-speed blender</u> until thick, smooth and creamy, add entire mixture to the bowl of kale and follow the step-by-step instructions on page 453:

- ★ ¾ C cashews
- ★ ½ C raw cacao powder

- ¼ tsp whole ground vanilla bean powder
- 1 dash sea salt
- ½ C raw honey or agave
- 2 TBS coconut oil (liquefied)
- 4-6 oz purified, filtered water (as needed)

Optional Variations & Additions

- Substitute ¾ C hemp seeds for cashews.
- Add a dash or two of Pumpkin Pie Blend and/or cayenne.
- Add 1-3 tsp of spirulina.
- Sprinkle coated kale chipz with coconut flakes just prior to dehydrating.

Sesame Honey Kale Chipz

Wash and spin dry the following (easily done in a salad spinner). Remove leaves from tough stem and tear into small to medium sized pieces before placing in a large mixing bowl:

- 2 bunches curly kale

Then, place the following ingredients in a glass measuring cup, whisk with a fork (or small whisk) until well combined and smooth, add entire mixture to bowl of kale and follow the step-by-step instructions on page 453:

- ⅔ C raw sesame tahini
- ¼ tsp whole ground vanilla bean powder
- ¼ tsp sea salt
- 1 dash Pumpkin Pie Blend (optional)
- 1 pinch cayenne (optional)
- ⅓ C raw honey or agave
- 2-3 TBS lemon juice
- Purified, filtered water (as needed). Only add water if necessary (1 TBS at a time). Mixture should be thick, but still pourable.

INSTRUCTIONS FOR KALE CHIPZ:

1. Using your hands, massage blended mixture into kale and thoroughly coat each piece. Be sure to get inside all the little curls of kale.
2. Place onto sheeted dehydrator trays and don't worry about being too particular. It is not necessary to space each piece or flatten them. Having them clumped up is fine.
3. Dehydrate at 105°F overnight (or until coating is dry), then slide kale onto clean, mesh trays and dehydrate for another four hours (or until completely crisp). Total dehydrating time is approximately 12-14 hours.
4. Store in a cool and dry spot and consume before the humidity in the air decreases their crunchiness. This shouldn't be too hard to accomplish!

SAVORY SNACKIN' SIDES (DEHYDRATOR NEEDED)

Who needs cooked foods when you can create raw delectable versions of your baked, fried and steamed favorites! Yes, dehydrating may challenge pre-planning abilities and test patience, but as the saying goes – "anything worth having is worth waiting for" – and our health is certainly something worth having. If we ultimately want better health and to decrease our chances of developing allergies and disease, we need to learn to live by the following proverb: "good things come to those who wait." Ditch all the processed and refined flour, sugar and vegetable oil that make up our deep-fried and fast-food society and reap the rewards of successful aging, quality of life and longevity. The following recipes are super easy and make fantastic snacks, sides or raw tapas-like dishes! You will just have to tame the hungry beast within while you wait!

Rawkin' Friez

Gather the following ingredients, and then follow the step-by-step instructions on page 454:

- ★ 2-3 medium jicama roots (peeled)
- ★ ¼ C coconut oil (liquefied)
- ★ 1 tsp sea salt
- ★ ½ tsp turmeric
- ★ ¼ tsp asafoetida
- ★ ¼ tsp paprika
- ★ 1 dash cayenne (or to taste)

> **INSTRUCTIONS FOR FRIEZ:**
>
> 1. Thoroughly scrub jicama roots, peel outer skin with a vegetable peeler and then cut in half lengthwise. Now, take each half (flat side down) and make lengthwise slices that are spaced about a half inch apart. When you are done cutting and slicing, each jicama stick should resemble a french fry.
> 2. Liquefy the coconut oil and pour approximately ¼ C into an appropriately sized glass bowl. Place glass bowl into a larger bowl filled with warm water to ensure that the coconut oil stays liquefied if jicama is cold from being in the fridge.
> 3. Whisk all your herbs and spices into the liquefied coconut oil, then toss and massage jicama strips in the coconut oil mixture.
> 4. Place coated jicama strips onto mesh screened dehydrator trays (no sheet necessary); dehydrate at 105°F for approximately 2-3 hrs or until they have that crispy french fry look on the outside; then enjoy!

Optional Variations & Serving Ideas for Rawkin' Friez

- ★ Substitute sweet potatoes for jicama and add a couple of extra hours of dehydrating time.
- ★ These are a fabulous snack by themselves and make an awesome side when served with veggie burger patties and wrap creations. For burgers, burrito, enchilada and other veggie wrap ideas, please refer back to "Protein Packed Pâtés" (page 336).
- ★ Serve with a dipping side or your favorite condiment(s) found under "Delectable Dips, Side Dishes & Condiments" (page 347).

Optional Spice Variations for Rawkin' Friez

Gather the following ingredients, and then follow the step-by-step instructions listed on page 454 (above):

Rawkin' Spicy Friez

- ★ 2-3 medium jicama roots (peeled)
- ★ ¼ C coconut oil (liquefied)
- ★ 1 tsp sea salt
- ★ 1 tsp Chili Blend
- ★ ¼ tsp asafoetida

Rawkin' Masala Friez

- ★ 2-3 medium jicama roots (peeled)
- ★ ¼ C coconut oil (liquefied)
- ★ 1 tsp sea salt

- ★ 1 tsp Garam Masala Blend
- ★ ¼ tsp asafoetida
- ★ 1 dash cayenne (or to taste)

Italian Batter of Choice

Blend the following ingredients in a <u>high-speed blender</u> until thick, smooth and creamy, then pour into a large mixing bowl and follow the step-by-step instructions for each (pages 455-458):

- ★ 1 C almonds
- ★ 2 roma tomatoes
- ★ 2 TBS chia seeds
- ★ 2 TBS Italian Blend
- ★ 1 tsp sea salt
- ★ ¼ tsp asafoetida
- ★ 1 pinch cayenne
- ★ 2 TBS lemon juice
- ★ 1 TBS coconut oil (liquefied)
- ★ 8 oz purified, filtered water

Optional Addition for Variation

- ★ Sprinkle coated veggies with nutritional yeast flakes just prior to dehydrating.

> **Recipe Notes & Quick Tips:** The amount of batter above will fully coat one medium-large head of cauliflower, broccoli bunch or eggplant. Therefore, when working with less bulky vegetables (e.g., a bunch of asparagus or broccolini), you will have enough batter left over to play with some others (e.g., red onion, string beans, summer squash or zucchini). Once you have tried and tested all your options, I suggest preparing two or more batches of batter in the future. This way, you will have plenty of batter to go around and be able to work with more than just one vegetable at once. Make once, eat twice! Now that's being what I call kitchen savvy! What's more, your dehydration time will not go to waste. Trust me when I say, nothing will last long. They are all too scrumptiously delicious!

Italian Battered Asparagus Sticks:

These are a delicious alternative to asparagus fries. Totally healthy, totally full of nutrition and totally easy to make!

1. Chop tougher ends off of asparagus stalks (one or more bunches). Then gently wash each one in preparation for coating with batter.
2. Dip each asparagus stalk into the bowl of batter and thoroughly coat each one. Then place each coated asparagus stalk onto sheeted dehydrator trays.

3. Sprinkle with nutritional yeast flakes for a cheezy flavor, if desired.
4. Dehydrate at 105°F for approximately 2-3 hrs. Transfer to clean, mesh screened dehydrator trays (without a sheet) and dehydrate 1-2 hrs longer, or until coating on underside is brown and completely dry to the touch.
5. Enjoy while slightly softened and warm!

Italian Battered Broccolini:

These are a fabulous alternative to any fried or baked variation. Totally healthy, totally full of nutrition and totally easy to make!

1. Chop one inch off bottom of broccolini (one or more bunches). Then gently wash each broccolini spear in preparation for coating with batter.
2. Dip each broccolini spear into the bowl of batter and thoroughly massage and coat each one. Then place coated broccolini spears onto sheeted dehydrator trays.
3. Sprinkle with nutritional yeast flakes for a cheezy flavor, if desired.
4. Dehydrate at 105°F for approximately 2-3 hrs. Transfer to clean, mesh screened dehydrator trays (without a sheet) and dehydrate 1-2 hrs longer, or until coating on underside is brown and completely dry to the touch.
5. Enjoy while slightly softened and warm!

Italian Battered Broccoli & Cauliflower:

These are a scrumptious alternative to fried broccoli and cauliflower bites. Totally healthy, totally full of nutrition and totally easy to make!

1. Core cauliflower head and/or chop off the tougher part of each broccoli stalk. Now, chop florets into small-medium bite size pieces. Gently wash and spin dry the florets in preparation for coating with batter. **Note:** I like using a salad spinner for this task.
2. Dip each floret into the bowl of batter, thoroughly massage and coat each one, and then place coated florets onto sheeted dehydrator trays.
3. Sprinkle with nutritional yeast flakes for a cheezy flavor, if desired.
4. Dehydrate at 105°F for approximately 6-8 hrs or overnight. Transfer to clean, mesh screened dehydrator trays (without a sheet) and dehydrate for approximately 2-3 hrs longer for cauliflower and 3-4 hrs longer for broccoli – or until coating on underside is brown and completely dry to the touch. Be sure to not overdry florets.
5. Enjoy while warm and a bit soft and moist on the inside!

> **Recipe Notes & Quick Tips**: Unlike "Dehydrated Pizza Crusts, Craks & Chips" where the goal is to thoroughly dry your foods all the way through, the idea in Savory Snackin' Sides is to dry the batter coating on the outside, while retaining moistness on the inside. During the initial stages of dehydrating, the battered veggies are releasing moisture (sweating) and softening as a result. Therefore, as soon as the batter coating is thoroughly dry to the touch, these flavor popping finger foods are ready to be relished. It is at this stage where your raw and nutrient rich veggies are the most reminiscent of fried and baked favorites. Fully dehydrated, they tend to become too airy. Use the provided dehydrating temperatures and times as a guideline, but experiment and taste test along the way to learn at what stage you like your battered veggies best.

Italian Battered Eggplant:

This is an amazing alternative to eggplant parmesan. Totally healthy, totally full of nutrition and totally easy to make!

1. Wash the outer skin of a medium sized eggplant, thinly slice into approximately ¼ inch slices, and then place into a large mixing bowl.
2. Cover slices of eggplant with purified, filtered water, and then add juices of one lemon and one tsp of sea salt. Gently massage each slice and allow them to soak for at least one hour.
3. Drain water and rinse thoroughly in preparation for coating with batter.
4. Dip each eggplant slice into the batter, thoroughly massage and coat each one, and then place coated eggplant slices onto sheeted dehydrator trays.
5. Add a thinly sliced tomato to the top and sprinkle with nutritional yeast flakes.
6. Dehydrate at 105-115°F for approximately 6-8 hrs or overnight. Carefully flip eggplant slices onto clean, <u>sheeted</u> dehydrator trays this time (to prevent sticking) and then carefully peel dehydrator sheet from underside of eggplant slices.
7. Lower temperature to 105°F and dehydrate for approximately 3-4 hrs longer or until coating on underside is brown and completely dry to the touch. If time allows, you may wish to transfer eggplant slices onto clean, mesh screened dehydrator trays (without a sheet) about 1-2 hours in to the process. Do not overdry eggplant.
8. Enjoy while warm and still a bit moist and soft on the inside!

Italian Battered Red Onion Rings:

These are a fantastic alternative to deep fried versions and are super crunchy and full of flavor. Eat as a snack or crumble on your salads as croutons. Totally healthy, totally full of nutrition and totally easy to make!

1. Peel off outer layer of red onion(s), slice into approximately ¼ inch thick rings, and then place rings into a large mixing bowl.

2. Just cover rings with purified, filtered water, add the juices of one lemon and one tsp sea salt, and then gently massage onion rings and allow them to soak for at least one hour.
3. Drain water and rinse thoroughly in preparation for coating with batter.
4. Dip each onion ring into the bowl of batter, thoroughly massage and coat each one, and then place coated rings onto sheeted dehydrator trays.
5. Dehydrate at 105-115°F overnight (8-12+ hrs). Transfer to clean, mesh screened dehydrator trays (without a sheet) and then dehydrate until underside is completely dry and onion rings are completely crisp (usually takes one more overnight stay in the dehydrator). Total dehydrating time for "crispy onion ringz" is approximately 24-36 hrs in total.
6. Store in an airtight container in a cool and dry place and feel free to pop back into the dehydrator if they have lost some of their crunch.
7. Enjoy while they last!

Italian Batterer String Beans:

These are a scrumptious alternative to deep fried string beans. Totally healthy, totally full of nutrition and totally easy to make!

1. Thoroughly wash and pat dry string beans and remove the tip with the stem.
2. Dip each green bean into the bowl of batter, thoroughly coat each one, and then place onto a sheeted dehydrator tray.
3. Dehydrate at 105°F for approximately 2-3 hrs. Transfer to clean, mesh screened dehydrator trays (without a sheet) and dehydrate 1-2 hrs longer or until coating on underside is brown and completely dry to the touch.
4. Enjoy while still slightly soft and warm!

Italian Battered Summer Squash & Zucchini Sticks:

These are a delicious alternative to any fried variation. Totally healthy, totally full of nutrition and totally easy to make!

1. Thoroughly wash the outer skin of small-medium sized zucchinis and/or summer squashes.
2. Cut off the ends, cut in half widthwise, then cut each half in half again, lengthwise.
3. Take each quarter (flat side down) and make lengthwise slices that are spaced about a half inch apart. When you are done cutting and slicing, each stick should resemble french fries and measure 3-4 inches long and about a ½ inch wide.
4. Dip each zucchini and summer squash stick into the bowl of batter, thoroughly coat each one, and then place onto a sheeted dehydrator tray.
5. Dehydrate at 105°F for approximately 4-6 hrs. Transfer to clean, mesh screened dehydrator trays (without a sheet) and dehydrate 2-3 hrs longer or until coating on underside is brown and completely dry to the touch. Be sure not to overdry.
6. Enjoy while slightly soft and warm!

Optional Variations & Serving Ideas for Battered Veggies

- ★ Substitute one of the cheezy batters (page 459) for Italian batter. I love alternating between these three batters, and especially love the cheezy options when working with asparagus, broccoli, broccolini, cauliflower and string beans.
- ★ Serve any of the above with a side of Marawnara Sauce (page 358) for dipping. This is an especially fabulous option for battered broccoli and cauliflower bites and, of course, battered eggplant slices. You may also wish to serve your eggplant slices with a side of Mozzarawlla Cheeze (page 346) and sprinkle with additional nutritional yeast flakes for the complete flavor experience of a true Raw Eggplant Parmesan that is rawkin!

Other Savory Veggie Batter Favorites!

Cheezy Batter Choice #1

Blend the following ingredients in a <u>high-speed blender</u> until thick, smooth and creamy and pour into a large mixing bowl. Then follow the step-by-step instructions for each of the Italian Battered Veggies of Choice (pages 455-458).

- ★ 1 C Brazil nuts
- ★ 2 TBS chickpea miso paste
- ★ 2 TBS chia seeds
- ★ 1 red bell pepper (chopped)
- ★ ½ tsp sea salt
- ★ ¼ tsp paprika
- ★ 1 dash asafoetida
- ★ 2 TBS lemon juice
- ★ 1 TBS coconut oil (liquefied)
- ★ 8 oz purified, filtered water

Optional Additions for Variation

- ★ Sprinkle coated veggies with nutritional yeast flakes just prior to dehydrating for a more authentic cheezy flavor. You can also add 2 TBS of nutritional yeast flakes to the mixture above just prior to blending.
- ★ Add a pinch or two of cayenne for a bit of spicy heat. Can be added to the mixture above prior to blending or lightly sprinkled over the top prior to dehydrating.

Cheezy Batter Choice #2

Blend the following ingredients in a <u>high-speed blender</u> until thick, smooth and creamy and pour into a large mixing bowl. Then follow the step-by-step instructions for each of the Italian Battered Veggies of Choice (pages 455-458):

- ★ 1 C macadamia nuts

- ¼ C nutritional yeast flakes
- 2 TBS chia seeds
- 1 tsp sea salt
- ¼ tsp paprika
- 1 dash asafoetida
- 2 TBS lemon juice
- 1 TBS coconut oil (liquefied)
- 8-10 oz purified, filtered water (as needed)

Optional Variations & Additions

- Substitute 1 C almonds, Brazil nuts or cashew for macadamia nuts.
- Add herbs of choice to taste, if desired (dill weed, oregano, parsley, thyme, etc.).
- Add a pinch or two of cayenne for a bit of spicy heat. Can be added to the mixture above prior to blending or lightly sprinkled over the top prior to dehydrating.

Sweet Snackin' Sides (Dehydrator Needed)

Coconut-Fruit Crepes (nut free)

Blend any of the following combinations in a <u>high-speed blender</u> until thick and smooth, and then follow the step-by-step instructions on page 461:

Pear-Mango Crepes

- 1 medium pear (chopped)
- 1 C packed mango (fresh or defrosted)
- ¼ C coconut crème
- 2 TBS white chia seeds
- 1 TBS lucuma powder
- ½ tsp whole ground vanilla bean
- 4 oz purified, filtered water

Pear-Strawberry Crepes

- 1 medium pear (chopped)
- 1 C packed strawberries (fresh or defrosted)
- ¼ C coconut crème
- 2 TBS white chia seeds
- 1 TBS baobab powder
- ½ tsp whole ground vanilla bean
- 4 oz purified, filtered water

Tropical Mango Crepes

- 2 C packed mango (fresh or defrosted)
- ¼ C coconut crème
- 2 TBS white chia seeds
- 1 TBS lucuma powder
- ½ tsp whole ground vanilla bean
- 6 oz purified, filtered water

Optional Additions

- Add ¼-½ tsp of Pumpkin or Apple Pie Blend to any of the above.

INSTRUCTIONS FOR CREPES:

Once mixture is blended to a thick and smooth consistency, slowly pour a small amount (approximately ½ C) in the center of each quadrant of a sheeted dehydrator tray (4 crepes per tray). Gently and evenly spread in order to widen the circle to approximately 5-6 inches. I like using the back end of a spoon, but you may also use a spatula.

Dehydrate at 105-115°F overnight, carefully flip onto an unlined dehydrator tray to allow for more air circulation, and then peel dehydrator sheet from crepes.

Dehydrate for up to one additional hour (or until desired level of flexible dryness) and enjoy!

Please Note: Unlike craks and chipz, the texture of crepes should be soft and pliable. Due to the varying factors involved (temperature, precipitation, humidity, etc.), it is truly impossible to give an exact time to completion. Therefore, I suggest checking on crepes frequently once they have been flipped. The goal is to not overdry if you intend to roll or fold them. If they become a bit dry though, no worries! You can always mist them with some water or place them in the fridge until ready to eat. The moisture from refrigerating will soften crepes and bring back their pliable texture.

Store leftover crepes in an airtight container (separated by a piece of natural parchment paper). Crepes will keep in the fridge for 3-5 days.

Optional Variations & Serving Ideas for Crepes

- Place a light layer of thinly sliced fruit (or some whole berries) in the middle of the crepe; fold both ends toward the center; and then top with a Sweet Crème from any one of the recipes under "Raw Prana Parfaits" (page 266) or the Crème Cheeze recipe on page 347.
- Drizzle Chocolate and/or La-Caramel Topping (page 372) over the top of each crepe roll.
- In the place of fresh fruit, you may fill with a light layer of Raw Jam (pages 268-269).

- ★ Instead of making crepe rolls, what if you fold the crepe to form a half moon with filling inside? This is my favorite way to serve (and eat) crepes! Simple, stunning and scrumptious! I love filling one with fresh sliced strawberries and Sweet Crème, then folding into a half moon and drizzling with Chocolate and La-Caramel Topping. Mmm! How divine!
- ★ If you prefer larger (yet thinner) crepes, you can spread the entire mixture over the sheeted tray (making one big square). Carefully score into four smaller squares (before flipping over) and separate (by carefully tearing) once ready to fill and roll. Just make sure mixture is spread evenly to avoid large cracks forming while dehydrating, and keep mixture at least one inch away from the edge of the tray. **Please Note:** small cracks are normal, so don't worry about these. However, due to mixture being spread thinner, I do suggest keeping a closer eye. **Quick Tip:** If you like filling versus topping, the square shape and size versus the round is a bit easier to keep rolled.
- ★ Have fun experimenting with such versatile recipes and enjoy the rich flavors of real raw nutrition in the process. Creativity is king!

Candied Nuts & Seeds

Gather the following ingredients, and then follow the step-by-step instructions below.

- ★ 2 C nuts or seeds of choice
    - ○ Best choices for nuts are almonds, pecans and/or walnuts
    - ○ Best choices for seeds are pumpkin seeds or a pumpkin and sunflower seed combination.
- ★ ¼ C raw honey or agave
- ★ 1 tsp Apple or Pumpkin Pie Blend
- ★ ½ tsp whole ground vanilla bean powder
- ★ ¼ tsp sea salt

Optional Additions for Variation

- ★ Add 1 TBS of mesquite and/or 1 TBS of lucuma powder.
- ★ Add 1-2 TBS of raw cacao powder for a chocolaty variation.
- ★ Add a pinch or two of cayenne for a bit of spicy heat.
- ★ Squeeze a bit of fresh orange juice into the mixture.

Instructions for Candied Nuts & Seeds:

1. Place nuts or seeds of choice in a glass mixing bowl, add the rest of the above ingredients (including any additions, if desired), and then stir until thoroughly and evenly coated.

2. Spread coated nuts or seeds onto sheeted dehydrator trays, dehydrate at 105-115°F overnight, and then continue to dehydrate until completely dry. **Please Note:** Total dehydrating time can be anywhere from 12-24 hrs depending on whether you are using nuts or seeds (seeds take less time than nuts). Soaked raw almonds can take up to 48 hrs to thoroughly dry (especially on the inside). I suggest testing a few from the front, back and middle of the trays and rotating trays a few times within the day. It is also a good idea to dry almonds closer to the top of the dehydrator where foods tend to dry a bit quicker.
3. Once completely dry, store candied nuts and seeds in an airtight glass mason jar (4-6 months in fridge and 8-12 months in freezer).

CHAPTER 9
LONGEVITY ELIXIR DRINKS & TEAS

According to Merriam-Webster, an elixir is defined as "a substance held capable of prolonging life indefinitely." Elixir drinks and teas should not be seen as a replacement for medicine, professional counseling or spiritual guidance, but they certainly can provide additional support in one's journey toward healing, health and happiness.

Quick Recipe Tips:

I choose hemps seeds over all other nuts and seeds for my Longevity Elixirs due to their unique and astonishingly nutritional composition. They also bestow an amazing milk-like creaminess and are exceedingly convenient, to boot (no presoaking required)! That being said, raw cashews are another fun favorite for making creamy elixirs and specialty tea drinks.

> **Please Note:** When it comes to making superfood smoothies and warm elixir drinks, I like to add the contents of at least one capsule of MegaHydrate (by Phi Sciences) for extra assurance against oxidation. According to documented research, the antioxidant power of MegaHydrate can significantly improve intracellular absorption of vitamins, minerals, amino acids and the delicate omega-3 fatty acids our bodies so desperately need. This is also a genius way to effectively keep omega-3 fatty acids from oxidizing during the process of digestion, as well as keep more fragile nutrients from breaking down before reaching their purposeful destinations.
>
> Please refer to "Getting to Know Your 'FAT' Friends" (page 81) and "The Best of the Best" (page 118) to learn more about the restorative properties of hemp seeds and why they are my #1 choice, especially when it comes to choosing the best base for rejuvenating recipes.

When it comes to a sweetener used in my longevity elixir drinks, I prefer to use the highest quality of raw honey for all the powerful healing properties it can provide: anti-allergen, anti-inflammatory, anti-microbial, etc. What's more, a true, high-quality, raw honey can effectively revitalize one's energy and replenish certain important nutrients in the body, such as antioxidants, certain B vitamins, minerals and enzymes. Although not local, my absolute favorite honey is Canadian Gold by Premier Research Labs. It is not heated, refined, spun, whipped, stripped or treated in any way. This totally raw honey is out-of-this-world delicious, naturally thick, and has a texture that is delightfully creamy (without crystallization or granulation). Gathered from wildflowers in the remote and pristine wildlands of Northern Canada, there is no need for concern when it comes to toxic chemical or pesticide contamination.

> **Please Note:** If you are a strict vegan and not a honey advocate, please feel free to replace honey with a high-quality raw agave or sun-dried cane juice crystals. If you are avoiding sugar altogether or suffer from a sugar related condition, you may replace one of the above sweeteners with green leaf stevia and/or xylitol to taste. I also love a luo han guo fruit product by Dragon herbs called Sweetfruit Drops. I reserved mentioning it until now, because it is especially good when synergistically blended with tonic herbal elixirs and teas.
>
> Luo han guo (*Momordica grosvenori*) is about 300 times sweeter than refined cane sugar and has just five percent of the calories, to boot. Luo han guo glucoside (mogroside), the active immune supporting saponin in luo han guo, is a stable non-fermentable substance. It will sweeten any beverage it is added to, has no known side effects, and is safe for children and adults alike.
>
> Please refer to "Must Have Condiments" (page 29), to not only learn more about all but one (luo han guo) of the natural sweeteners mentioned above, but to learn more about the companies behind the brands I have come to respect and trust – and why.
>
> Use the measurements I give for sweeteners as a general guideline. Feel free to use less or more according to taste. For instance, with certain additions to a recipe (such as reishi), and how much you desire to use of these additions, you may need to add a little extra sweetener to balance the flavors.

When brewing up a loose-leaf tea intended as a base for elixir drinks, I recommend steeping a bit longer than traditionally recommended for tea that is to be drunk straight-up. Since I do not recommend brewing with high temperature water, the extra minutes go to good use without turning the tea bitter.

> **Are you a tea enthusiast?** If you are, then I suggest looking into the Pino Digital Kettle Pro. It is the perfect kettle for brewing all your favorite loose-leaf teas and for when you want to avoid the risk of bringing your water to a boil. Please read the box on page 478 for why you do not ever want to heat your water above 159-169°F.
>
> With the Pino Digital Kettle Pro, you can set the temperature with the digital controller and have the water heated to your desired temperature (+/- 3% of your desired target). **Quick Tip:** To keep the temperature of the water from rising above my end goal temperature of 159-169°F, I always keep my digital kettle set at 150°F.
>
> When it comes to the actual brewing process of your tea and tonic herbs, I highly suggest using a press made for coffee versus tea. The fine mesh screen makes it ideal for brewing up a wide variety of teas, from whole leaf to powder! I am a huge fan of the Brazil French Press coffee maker by Bodum.
>
> **What about the tea itself?** Organic or wild crafted loose-leaf tea is the best if you truly want therapeutic effects. With the exception of yerba mate and gynostemma, the two companies I always use for all of my certified organic loose-leaf teas are Mountain Rose Herbs and Starwest Botanicals. For more Yerba Mate information, please see page 197. For more details on Gynostemma, please view page 214.

Caution: When blending with warm to hot liquids, please be sure to secure the lid and keep a hand on it while blending. The steam from warm-hot liquids can cause the blender to erupt and blow the lid right off if not secured. Due to the design of the Nutribullet, blending with warm liquids should never be an issue as long as you snuggly screw the extractor blade on prior to placing the cup onto the power base. However, if you are going to use the Blendtec or Vitamix, please be sure to secure the lid and keep a hand on it while blending.

Mind Altering Mochaccino

Blend the following ingredients in a high-speed blender until smooth and creamy (Nutribullet is ideal for making personal elixir drinks):

- ★ 3 TBS hemp seeds
- ★ 2 TBS raw cacao powder
- ★ 1 TBS chia seeds
- ★ 1 TBS shilajit
- ★ 1-2 opened capsules (contents only) of MegaHydrate
- ★ 1-2 droppers full of Duanwood Reishi (Dragon Herbs) or reishi extract (Surthrival)
- ★ ½ tsp whole ground vanilla bean powder
- ★ ¼ tsp Pumpkin Pie Blend
- ★ 1 pinch sea salt
- ★ 2 TBS raw honey or agave
- ★ 1 TBS coconut oil (liquefied)
- ★ 10-12 oz of brewed loose-leaf tea (see instructions below)
    - o 1 TBS each of yerba mate, gynostemma & mucuna pruriens

- o 1 TBS each of yerba mate & mucuna pruriens
- o 1 TBS each of gynostemma & mucuna pruriens

Instructions:

1. Brew one of the above tea blends for about 8-10 minutes using water which is below boiling point (159-169°F). While tea is brewing, place all the other ingredients in the blender.
2. Once 8-10 minutes are up, strain your tea and pour liquid into blender.
3. Blend until smooth, pour and enjoy!

Vanilla Caramel Chaga Latte

Blend the following ingredients in a high-speed blender until smooth and creamy (Nutribullet is ideal for making personal elixir drinks):

- ★ 3 TBS hemp seeds
- ★ 2 TBS lucuma powder
- ★ 2 tsp shilajit and/or mesquite powder
- ★ 1-2 opened capsules (contents only) of MegaHydrate
- ★ 3-4 droppers full of chaga extract (Surthrival) or 3-4 opened capsules (contents only) of Siberian Chaga (Dragon Herbs)
- ★ ½ tsp whole ground vanilla bean powder
- ★ 1 pinch sea salt
- ★ 2 TBS raw honey or agave
- ★ 1 TBS coconut oil (liquefied)
- ★ 10-12 oz of brewed loose-leaf tea (see instructions below)
  - o 2 TBS yerba mate
  - o 1 TBS gynostemma
  - o 1 TBS each of yerba mate & gynostemma
  - o 2 TBS yerba mate & 1 TBS schizandra berries
  - o 1 TBS gynostemma & 1 TBS schizandra berries
  - o 1 TBS each of yerba mate, gynostemma & schizandra berries

Instructions:

1. Brew one of the above tea blends for about 8-10 minutes using water which is below boiling point (159-169°F). While tea is brewing, place all the other ingredients in the blender.
2. Once 8-10 minutes are up, strain your tea and pour liquid into blender.
3. Blend until smooth, pour and enjoy!

Spicy Mayan Infusion

Blend the following ingredients in a high-speed blender until smooth and creamy (Nutribullet is ideal for making personal elixir drinks):

- ¼ C hemp seeds
- 2 TBS raw cacao powder
- 2 tsp lucuma and/or maca powder
- 1 tsp mesquite powder
- 1-2 opened capsules (contents only) of MegaHydrate
- ½ tsp whole ground vanilla bean powder
- ¼ tsp cinnamon (or Pumpkin Pie Blend)
- 1-2 dashes cayenne (or to taste)
- 1 pinch sea salt
- 2 TBS raw honey or agave
- 1 TBS coconut oil (liquefied)
- 10-12 oz of brewed loose-leaf tea (see instructions below)
  - 2 TBS yerba mate
  - 1 TBS pu-erh
  - 1 TBS green rooibos
  - 1 TBS yerba mate & 1 TBS pu-erh
  - 1 TBS yerba mate & 1 TBS green rooibos

Instructions:

1. Brew one of the above tea blends for about 5-8 minutes using water which is below boiling point (159-169°F). While tea is brewing, place all the other ingredients in the blender.
2. Once 5-8 minutes are up, strain your tea and pour liquid into blender.
3. Blend until smooth, pour and enjoy!

Pu-erh tea from China's Yunnan Province undergoes a unique fermentation process where microbes act on the tea leaves, causing the leaves to darken and change the flavor profile. Over time this method increases the value of the pu-erh tea like a fine wine. Pu-erh tea is known to help lower blood cholesterol levels, enhance circulation, aid in proper digestion (especially the breakdown of fats), invigorate the spleen and remove toxins.

Rooibos is a South African tea and contains no caffeine. Rooibos is known for its anti-inflammatory and anti-allergen properties and may relieve fever, asthma, insomnia, colic in infants and skin disorders.

Hormone Balancing Macaccino

Blend the following ingredients in a <u>high-speed blender</u> until smooth and creamy (Nutribullet is ideal for making personal elixir drinks):

- ¼ C hemp seeds
- 2 TBS maca powder

- ★ 1 tsp shilajit powder
- ★ 1 tsp mesquite powder
- ★ 1-2 opened capsules (contents only) of MegaHydrate
- ★ ½ tsp whole ground vanilla bean powder
- ★ ¼ tsp Pumpkin Pie Blend
- ★ 1 pinch sea salt
- ★ 2 TBS raw honey or agave
- ★ 1 TBS coconut oil (liquefied)
- ★ 10-12 oz of brewed loose-leaf tea (see instructions below)
    - o 2 TBS yerba mate
    - o 1 TBS pu-erh
    - o 1 TBS yerba mate & 1 TBS pu-erh

Instructions:

1. Brew one of the above tea blends for about 5-8 minutes using water which is below boiling point (159-169°F). While tea is brewing, place all the other ingredients in the blender.
2. Once 5-8 minutes are up, strain your tea and pour liquid into blender.
3. Blend until smooth, pour and enjoy! Stir in 1-2 tsp of bee pollen if desired.

Matcha Tea Latte

Blend the following ingredients in a <u>high-speed blender</u> until smooth and creamy (Nutribullet is ideal for making personal elixir drinks):

- ★ ¼ C hemp seeds
- ★ 2 tsp matcha green tea powder
- ★ 1-2 opened capsules (contents only) of MegaHydrate
- ★ ½ tsp whole ground vanilla bean powder
- ★ 1 pinch sea salt
- ★ 2 TBS raw honey or agave
- ★ 1 TBS coconut oil (liquefied)
- ★ 10-12 oz of brewed loose-leaf tea (see instructions below)
    - o 2 TBS yerba mate & 1 TBS goji berries and/or schizandra berries
    - o 1 TBS each of green rooibos, goji berries and/or schizandra berries

Optional Additions

- ★ Add 1 tsp of Green Tea-ND (Premier Research Labs).
- ★ Add 1 dropper full of MyCommunity and/or CordyChi Extract (Host Defense).
- ★ Add 1 dropper full of chaga and/or reishi extract (Surthrival).
- ★ Add 2-3 opened capsules (contents only) of Siberian Chaga, Siberian Ginseng, Super Adaptogen and/or Will Power (Dragon Herbs).

Instructions:

1. Brew one of the above tea blends for about 5-8 minutes using water which is below boiling point (159-169°F). While tea is brewing, place all the other ingredients in the blender.
2. Once 5-8 minutes are up, strain your tea and pour liquid into blender.
3. Blend until smooth, pour and enjoy!

> **Matcha Better!** When you drink matcha you are ingesting the whole leaf and not just the brewed water. For this reason, the health benefits of matcha green tea powder far exceed regular green tea benefits.
>
> Matcha is loaded with antioxidants, including the catechin EGCg (epigallocatechin gallate). EGCg is the catechin with the most potent cancer-fighting properties. Researchers have found that the concentration of EGCg available from drinking matcha is up to 137 times greater than the amount of EGCg available from other green teas.
>
> Matcha is also rich in L-theanine, a rare and unique amino acid that actually promotes a state of relaxed alertness. Matcha green tea powder naturally contains up to 5 times more L-theanine than all other teas (including regular green tea). L-theanine is also well known for improving memory, concentration and focus.
>
> All in all, matcha has quite an impressive nutrient profile, including an immense amount of chlorophyll that can greatly help with the elimination of harmful toxins from the body.

Chocolate Hemp Nog

Blend the following ingredients in a high-speed blender until smooth and creamy (Nutribullet is ideal for making personal elixir drinks):

- ★ 3 TBS hemp seeds
- ★ 2 TBS raw cacao powder
- ★ 1 TBS chia seeds
- ★ 1 TBS lucuma
- ★ 1-2 opened capsules (contents only) of MegaHydrate
- ★ ½ tsp Apple Pie Blend
- ★ ¼ tsp whole ground vanilla bean powder
- ★ 1 pinch sea salt
- ★ 2 TBS raw honey or agave
- ★ 1 TBS coconut oil (liquefied)
- ★ 10-12 oz of brewed chai tea (see instructions below)

Instructions:

1. Brew 1 TBS of chai tea for about 5-8 minutes using water which is below boiling point (159-169°F). While tea is brewing, place all the other ingredients in the blender.
2. Once 5-8 minutes are up, strain your tea and pour liquid into blender.
3. Blend until smooth, pour and enjoy!

> Chai tea has a tremendous amount of beneficial properties. The black tea in chai is rich in antioxidants, and the spices it contains have been used for thousands of years to promote general health and well-being. According to numerous studies, the synergistic blend of spices in chai has been shown to have anti-inflammatory and chemo-preventative effects.

Chocolate Orange Hibiscus

Blend the following ingredients in a high-speed blender until smooth and creamy (Nutribullet is ideal for making personal elixir drinks):

- 1 whole orange (peeled & seeded)
- 3 TBS hemp seeds
- 2 TBS raw cacao powder
- 1 TBS chia seeds
- 1 TBS baobab powder
- 1-2 opened capsules (contents only) of MegaHydrate
- ½ tsp whole ground vanilla bean powder
- 1 dash sea salt
- 2 TBS raw honey or agave
- 1 TBS coconut oil (liquefied)
- 10-12 oz of brewed hibiscus flowers (see instructions below)

Optional Variation

- Substitute 1 TBS lucuma powder for baobab.

Instructions:

1. Brew 1 TBS of hibiscus for 5-10 minutes using below boiling point water (159-169°F). While tea is brewing, place all the other ingredients in the blender.
2. Once 5-10 minutes are up, strain your tea and pour liquid into blender.
3. Blend until smooth, pour and enjoy!

> A study published in the *Journal of Human Hypertension* has shown that drinking hibiscus tea can reduce high blood pressure in individuals with type 2 diabetes. Hibiscus flowers are also known for their ability to soothe the nervous system and relieve stomach and digestive issues.

Endocrine Elixir

Blend the following ingredients in a <u>high-speed blender</u> until smooth and creamy (Nutribullet is ideal for making personal elixir drinks):

- ★ 1 small jewel yam (peeled & chopped)
- ★ 1 TBS maca powder
- ★ 1 tsp ashwagandha powder
- ★ 1-2 opened capsules (contents only) of Ginseng-FX (Premier Research Labs)
- ★ 1-2 opened capsules (contents only) of MegaHydrate
- ★ ½ tsp Pumpkin Pie Blend
- ★ ¼ tsp whole ground vanilla bean powder
- ★ 1 dash sea salt
- ★ 2 TBS raw honey or agave
- ★ 1 TBS coconut oil (liquefied)
- ★ 10-12 oz of brewed chai tea (see instructions below)

Instructions:

1. Brew 1 TBS of chai for about 5-8 minutes using water which is below boiling point (159-169°F). While tea is brewing, place all the other ingredients in the blender.
2. Once 5-8 minutes are up, strain your tea and pour liquid into blender.
3. Blend until smooth, pour and enjoy! Stir in 1-2 tsp of bee pollen if desired.

Anti-inflammatory Elixir

Blend the following ingredients in a <u>high-speed blender</u> until smooth (Nutribullet is ideal for making personal elixir drinks):

- ★ 1 tsp turmeric extract powder (95% curcumin)
- ★ 1-2 opened capsules (contents only) of MegaHydrate
- ★ ½ tsp whole ground vanilla bean powder
- ★ 1 pinch sea salt
- ★ 1 pinch cayenne
- ★ 2 TBS raw honey or agave
- ★ 1 TBS coconut oil (liquefied)
- ★ 10-12 oz of brewed chai tea (see instructions below)

Instructions:

1. Brew 1 TBS of chai for about 5-8 minutes using water which is below boiling point (159-169°F). While tea is brewing, place all the other ingredients in the blender.
2. Once 5-8 minutes are up, strain your tea and pour liquid into blender.
3. Blend until smooth, pour and enjoy!

Longevity Iced Tea

Place the following ingredients in a wide mouth mason jar (quart size), then follow the step-by-step instructions below:

- ★ 1 TBS yerba mate
- ★ 1 TBS gynostemma
- ★ 1 TBS schizandra berries
- ★ 1 TBS beet powder
- ★ 1 tsp cayenne (more or less to taste)
- ★ 2 lemons, juiced
- ★ 24 oz purified, filtered water

Optional Additions

- ★ Add 1 TBS of organic detox tea (Starwest Botanicals) with above ingredients.
- ★ Add 2-3 droppers full of MyCommunity Extract (Host Defense) after straining.
- ★ Add 3 droppers full of Goji and Schizandra Drops (Dragon Herbs) after straining.
- ★ Add 3 droppers full of Sweetfruit Drops (Dragon Herbs) after straining.
- ★ Add 3 droppers full of Eucommia Drops (Dragon Herbs) after straining.

> **Recipe Notes & Quick Tips:** This tea is meant to be cold brewed, so I suggest making it the night before. Make up the number of batches you plan on drinking the following day and then allow to cold brew (steep) at room temperature on your countertop. However, if you prefer it cold, you may brew and store batches in the fridge.
>
> This is my remixed version of the Master Cleanse (lemonade diet). You may wish to drink this as a morning liver cleanser or throughout the day during a structured cleanse/detox. One or two batches should be plenty if you are only planning to drink it as a morning liver cleanser. Personally, I like to do 2 batches per day, one weekend a month as maintenance. Sometimes I will also juice on these 2 days, and sometimes I will drink only purified, filtered water and herbal teas.
>
> If planning for a mini-cleanse (3-5 days) or longer, I suggest making 3-4 batches which you can drink throughout the day. I also suggest including green juices and green powders (such as chlorella, spirulina, etc.), marine phytoplankton, herbal teas and plenty of purified, filtered water for flushing.
>
> Feel free to adjust the ingredients to your tolerance level. For instance, you may only be able to tolerate a pinch or two of cayenne, initially, and may even need to add a natural sweetener (such as raw honey and/or Sweetfruit Drops). Be patient, respect yourself, and live in the truth of the present moment.
>
> Remember this quote by Bonnie Mohn with all that you do: *"living life is not a race but indeed a journey."*
>
> **Please Note:** Always consult with a qualified holistic practitioner before embarking on any type of intensive cleansing, detoxification or fasting program, especially if you are currently on prescription medications.

Instructions:

1. Once all the ingredients have been placed into a sealed, 32 oz wide mouth mason jar, let it sit overnight in a cool, dark place.
2. The next morning, shake up your concoction, pour through a strainer and drink the entire thing followed by 8-16 oz of plain water. If you have more batches, spread them out throughout the day. If you are juicing or eating, be sure to drink this tea prior to your juice or eating food.
3. Although this counts as fluids for the day, don't forget to drink plenty of pure water and herbal teas to assist in flushing out the toxins. To find the ideal amount for your weight, multiply your weight by 0.66 and then convert to ounces. For example: 150 pounds x 0.66 = 99. Therefore, 99 oz of pure water (which includes herbal teas) should be drunk daily.

Morning Chlorella Detox Elixir

This elixir is potent and definitely has a bit of a bitter and unique taste that will take some time getting used to. Your taste buds may say no (at first), but every cell in your entire body will be saying yes, yes and yes! I actually do this 1-2 times per day. My day doesn't start until I drink my Morning Chlorella Detox Elixir. Chug-a-lug!

Place the following ingredients in a glass, drink it down, and then follow with 16-24 oz of additional pure water every morning:

- ★ 1 TBS OptiMSM
- ★ 1 TBS chlorella
- ★ 1 tsp camu camu powder
- ★ 1 tsp Max B-ND (Premier Research Labs)
- ★ 1 tsp Green Tea-ND (Premier Research Labs)
- ★ 1-2 droppers full of MyCommunity Extract (Host Defense)
- ★ Few drops to 1 dropper full of marine phytoplankton (Oceans Alive)
- ★ 8 oz purified, filtered water

Optional Addition

- ★ Add 1-2 opened capsules (contents only) of MegaHydrate.

> **Recipe Notes & Quick Tips:** During different stages of sleep throughout the night, our bodies are busy rejuvenating, revitalizing and rebuilding. They are concentrating on tasks such as replenishing energy to different organ systems, processing waste materials, and neutralizing and eliminating toxic chemicals. This is why it is so important that we drink plenty of pure water first thing in the morning. We need to hydrate our thirsty cells after a night of hard work and help our bodily systems flush out all the toxins and waste more effectively. I suggest at least 24-32 oz of pure water within the first 45 minutes of being awake and before eating.
>
> Chlorella is a powerful chelator of heavy metals and other toxins. Please use with caution if you still have amalgam (mercury) fillings. The goal is to remove toxins, not to continuously recirculate them. To understand more, I highly suggest reviewing "Chelation & Heavy Metal Detoxification: Wellness Tips and Tools to Live By" on page 111.

Digestive Elixir

Place the following ingredients in a glass and drink it down:

- ★ 1-2 oz of AloePro (Premier Research Labs)
- ★ 1 tsp Liver-ND (Premier Research Labs)
- ★ 1 tsp Gallbladder-ND (Premier Research Labs)
- ★ 1 tsp cayenne

- 6-8 oz purified, filtered water

> **Recipe Notes & Quick Tips:** In herbal medicine (aka herbalism), both aloe and cayenne have been used in the treatment of ulcers, as well as several other gastrointestinal disorders (such as gas, nausea, heartburn, indigestion and constipation).
>
> If you have not yet mastered cayenne pepper, start with a small amount (¼ tsp or less). Increase every few days and your body should soon become accustomed to its healing heat.
>
> Dr. Christopher, one of the leaders in American herbal medicine, recommends one teaspoon of cayenne pepper in a glass of water three times per day – and has cured many stomach ulcers.
>
> *"If you master only one herb in your life, master cayenne pepper. It is more powerful than any other."* – Dr. Richard Schulze, Medical Herbalist

Candida Kicker Elixir

Blend the following ingredients in a high-speed blender until smooth and creamy (Nutribullet is ideal for making personal elixir drinks):

- 3 TBS hemp seeds
- 1-2 TBS raw cacao powder (optional)
- 1 TBS chia seeds
- 1-2 opened capsules (contents only) of MegaHydrate
- 1-2 oz of AloePro (Premier Research Labs)
- 1-2 droppers full of MyCommunity Extract (Host Defense)
- 1-2 droppers full of CordyChi Extract (Host Defense)
- ½ tsp whole ground vanilla bean powder
- ¼ tsp Apple Pie Blend
- 1 pinch sea salt
- 1 TBS coconut oil (liquefied)
- Stevia, xylitol and/or Sweetfruit Drops (by Dragon Herbs) to taste
- 10-12 oz of brewed loose-leaf tea (see instructions below)
  - 2 TBS pau d'arco
  - 1 TBS pau d'arco & 1 TBS horsetail
  - 1 TBS pau d'arco & 1 TBS yerba mate

Instructions:

1. Brew one of the above tea blends for 30 minutes using water which is below boiling point (159-169°F). While tea is brewing, place all the other ingredients in the blender.
2. Once 30 minutes are up, strain your tea and pour liquid into blender.
3. Blend until smooth, pour and enjoy!

BREWING LOOSE-LEAF TEA IS EASY

In many respects the ritual of tea preparation is quite like the judgment of the tea itself: flexible, individual and unlimited. For your ultimate enjoyment, please experiment with the amount of tea leaves, water temperature (as long as it is not too hot to scald) and steeping time. Although there are no hard and fast rules, the following are some general suggestions that I feel can make a tremendous difference to the resulting brew.

TEA BREWING TIPS TO LIVE BY!

I suggest heating your water (for all teas and herbal tisanes) to no more than 159-169°F. It appears that when water is heated above 170°F it can provoke an increase in white blood cell activity called leukocytosis. According to David Wolfe, "the response by the human body is kind of an immune system response to an intruder or a foreign object."

Leukocytosis – a higher than normal white blood cell count – is typically triggered by a condition such as an allergic reaction, infection, inflammation, malignancy, tissue damage, stress (physical and emotional), etc. It is a reaction that is typically found only when the body is invaded by a dangerous pathogen or experiences some sort of physical and/or emotional trauma. So then, why would the temperature of drinking water be a concern? Please read on for a better understanding.

In the 1930s, at the Institute of Clinical Chemistry in Switzerland, Dr. Paul Kouchakoff conducted research which found the following: leukocytosis occurred anytime an individual consumed highly altered foods (such as processed and refined foods) – but would mysteriously not occur whenever whole, raw foods were consumed. However, if these same whole, raw (enzyme rich) foods were heated at too high a temperature, leukocytosis would then occur. The same phenomenon was observed with the consumption of water. Whenever water was heated beyond its critical temperature, the individual would experience leukocytosis.

In the research of Dr. Kouchakoff, the worst offenders of all (heated or not) were the following: foods which had been processed and refined (such as white flour, white rice and white sugar), and foods which had been homogenized (like milk), pasteurized (such as milk and juice) or preserved. Believe it or not, cooked and salt-cured meats brought on violent leukocytosis which was consistent with the ingestion of a poison.

If the above information is not concerning enough, what about the fact that drinking liquids which are too hot (such as hot coffee and tea) can severely irritate the esophagus, causing squamous cells to mutate or develop errors in their DNA – leading to esophagus cancer? According to a study published in March 2009 in the *British Medical Journal,* drinking liquids at a temperature of greater than 158°F was associated with an eight-fold increased risk of esophageal cancer compared to sipping warm or lukewarm liquids at less than 149°F.

In conclusion: In order to obtain all the benefits without the downsides, steep your health-giving teas and herbal tisanes in water that does not exceed 159-169°F. This will allow for a temperature which is high enough to extract the medicinal and healing properties of the tea, but low enough to prevent an unnecessary immune response. Furthermore, by the time the tea has completed brewing, the temperature of the steep water will have dropped down further and be at a temperature that cannot cause thermal injury to the lining of the throat.

Basic Black Tea Brewing Instruction (including pu-erh):
1. Measure the desired amount of tea leaves and place into a press or mesh tea strainer: 1 tsp of tea leaves for every 8 oz of water.
2. Bring purified, filtered water to a temperature that does not exceed 159-169°F and pour over tea leaves.
3. Steep tea leaves for 5-6 minutes.
4. Separate leaves from water by pressing or using an infusing device or strainer.

> **Tea Notes & Quick Tips:** If you like to add nut or seed mylk (or just like a stronger cup) add a bit more tea leaves.
>
> Steeping black tea longer than six minutes is typically not recommended.
>
> Adding a natural sweetener of choice is optional.
>
> For black iced tea, use 1 TBS (3 tsp) of black tea for every 8 oz of water and follow iced tea brewing instructions on page 481.

Basic Chai Tea Brewing Instruction:
1. Measure the desired amount of tea leaves and place into a press or mesh tea strainer.
    - For **Plain Chai:** use 1 tsp of tea leaves for every 8 oz of water.
    - For **Chai with nut/seed mylk:** use 1 ½ to 2 tsp of tea leaves for every 8 oz.
2. Bring purified, filtered water to a temperature that does not exceed 159-169°F and pour over tea leaves.
3. Steep tea leaves for 5-7 minutes.
4. Separate leaves from water by pressing or using an infusing device or strainer.
5. Add nut or seed mylk and sweetener of choice to taste, if desired.

> **Tea Notes & Quick Tips:** For chai iced tea, use 1 level to heaping TBS (3 level to rounded tsp) of chai for every 8 oz of water and follow iced tea brewing instructions on page 481.

Basic Oolong Tea Brewing Instruction:
1. Measure the desired amount of tea leaves and place into a press or mesh tea strainer: 2 tsp of oolong tea for every 8 oz of water.
2. Bring purified, filtered water to a temperature that does not exceed 159-169°F and pour over tea leaves.
3. Steep tea leaves for 4-6 minutes.
4. Save the leaves and re-steep. Each additional infusion will have its own unique individual character. Depending on personal taste, you may wish to add one minute for each additional brew (up to 2-3 total brews).

> **Tea Notes & Quick Tips:** Adding a natural sweetener of choice is optional.
>
> For oolong iced tea, use 1 heaping TBS (3 rounded tsp) of oolong for every 8 oz of water and follow iced tea brewing instructions on page 481.

Basic Green Tea Brewing Instruction:

1. Measure the desired amount of tea leaves and place into a press or mesh tea strainer: 2-3 tsp or 1 TBS of green tea for every 8 oz of water.
2. Bring purified, filtered water to a temperature that does not exceed 159-169°F and pour over tea leaves.
3. Allow tea leaves to steep 1-2 minutes for most Japanese greens and 2-3 minutes for most Chinese greens.
4. Save the leaves and re-steep. Each additional infusion will have its own unique individual character. Depending on personal taste, you may wish to add one minute for each additional brew (up to 3 total brews).

> **Tea Notes & Quick Tips:** Adding a natural sweetener of choice is optional.
>
> For green iced tea, use 2 TBS (6 tsp) of green tea for every 8 oz of water and follow iced tea brewing instructions on page 481.

Basic White Tea Brewing Instruction:

1. Measure the desired amount of tea leaves and place into a press or mesh tea strainer: 3-4 tsp or 1 heaping TBS of white tea for every 8 oz of water.
2. Bring purified, filtered water to a temperature that does not exceed 159-169°F and pour over tea leaves.
3. Steep for 4-6 minutes.
4. Save the leaves and re-steep. Each additional infusion will have its own unique individual character. Depending on personal taste, you may wish to add one minute for each additional brew (Silver Needles, 3-4 total brews. White Darjeeling or Peony, 2-3 total brews).

> **Tea Notes & Quick Tips:** Adding a natural sweetener of choice is optional.
>
> For white iced tea, use 2 heaping TBS (6 rounded tsp) of white tea for every 8 oz of water and follow iced tea brewing instructions on page 481.

Basic Tisane Brewing Instruction (rooibos & other herbal infusions):

1. Measure the desired amount of rooibos or herbs and place into a press or mesh tea strainer: 1 tsp (level or heaping depending on personal taste) for every 8 oz of water.
2. Bring purified, filtered water to a temperature that does not exceed 159-169°F and pour over tea leaves.

3. Allow rooibos to steep for 5-8 minutes and herbals for about the same or longer (up to 15 minutes or until the desired strength is reached).

> **Tea Notes & Quick Tips:** Adding a natural sweetener of choice is optional.
>
> For iced rooibos or herbals, use 1 level to heaping TBS (3 level to rounded tsp) for every 8 oz of water and follow iced tea brewing instructions on page 481.

Basic Yerba Mate Brewing Instructions:

1. Measure the desired amount of yerba mate and place into a press or mesh tea strainer: 1 TBS (level or heaping depending on personal taste) for every 8 oz of water.
2. Bring purified, filtered water to a temperature that does not exceed 159-169°F and pour over tea leaves.
3. Steep tea leaves for 4-6 minutes.
4. Save the leaves and re-steep. Each additional infusion will have its own unique individual character. Depending on personal taste, you may wish to add one minute for each additional brew (up to 2-3 total brews).

> **Tea Notes & Quick Tips:** Adding a natural sweetener of choice is optional.
>
> For yerba mate iced, use 2 level to heaping TBS (6 level to rounded tsp) for every 8 oz of water and follow iced tea brewing instructions on page 481.

Hot Brewing Method for Iced Tea

1. To make iced tea from a hot brew: double the amount of tea leaves recommended on the basic hot tea brewing instructions (please see Tea Notes & Quick Tips).
2. Follow the basic tea brewing instruction and be sure to not over steep tea leaves.
3. Place a natural sweetener of choice into a glass pitcher, if desired. Pour the hot tea over a strainer (if not already strained) into the glass pitcher and stir.
4. Place ice in cups and pour the hot tea over ice.
5. Let the tea chill for a few minutes before drinking.

> **Tea Notes & Quick Tips:** In general, the volume of ice added should equal the volume of water used to brew the tea.

Cold Brewing Method for Iced Tea, Simply Delicious!

1. To make cold brewed ice tea: double the amount of tea leaves recommended on the basic hot tea brewing instructions (please see Tea Notes & Quick Tips).
2. Place the tea leaves in a clean glass jug or pitcher and add the appropriate amount of purified, filtered water.
3. Let stand in the refrigerator overnight (or for at least six hours).

4. Remove tea leaves. If using a strainer, simply place strainer over a second clean glass jug or pitcher and pour.
5. Now just sip and enjoy!

How to Kick Caffeine from Your Cup Right at Home

Many commercial methods of extracting caffeine from tea (or any other beverage for that matter) can be rather harsh and affect the taste.

There is a Chinese method of infusing tea that has led to a simple way for anyone to remove most of the caffeine from their tea in less than one minute. It is called the Gongfu Decaffeination Method.

Because most of the caffeine found in tea leaves ends up on the outside of the leaf during the drying process, a simple "leaf washing" or "pre-brewing" is all that is needed to remove 80-90% of the caffeine from any black, oolong, green or white tea. Depending on the tea, this now leaves a minimal amount of caffeine (2-10 milligrams per cup), which is the same amount in most all decaffeinated beverages on the market. If you are looking for zero caffeine in your cup, then rooibos or an herbal tisane will be your best choice.

This technique allows decaf tea drinkers to experience the whole world of teas. Please read on.

Simple Decaffeination Method

1. Measure the correct amount of tea leaves (as usual) into your press.
2. Pour a small amount of hot water into your press (i.e., just enough to cover the measured tea leaves). So, don't fill up your press just yet.
3. Set your tea timer for 30-45 seconds.
4. Pour off this small amount of water when the 30-45 seconds is up. By doing this procedure, you allow the caffeine to dissolve. Then, pour the concentrated caffeine solution down the drain.
5. Now you may fill up your tea press with your hot water and brew as usual.

That's it! You've successfully decaffeinated your own fine quality loose tea right at home in less than one minute!

> **Tea Notes & Quick Tips:** You may notice a slight decrease in flavor or strength with certain teas after using this technique. If this is the case, simply add an extra teaspoon of tea to your press prior to the procedure.
>
> **Please Note:** Anything over one minute does not insure additional caffeine reduction.

Answers to Commonly Asked Tea Questions

How do I store my tea? All you need is a dark, dry and cool place. Tea does not like light or refrigeration (or anywhere there is moisture). Never put your tea in the freezer.

Does tea have caffeine? Yes, but the quantity varies depending on the type of tea, where it was picked, when it was picked, and its processing methods. Examples per 8 oz cup are as follows:

- ★ Black tea has approximately 50-60 milligrams
- ★ Oolong tea has approximately 25-30 milligrams
- ★ Green tea has approximately 10-20 milligrams
- ★ White tea has approximately 10-15 milligrams
- ★ Decaf tea has approximately 2-10 milligrams
- ★ Tisanes (rooibos & other herbals) have 0 milligrams

What is the caffeine content of tea versus coffee? Being so light in weight, tea leaves yield 180-200 liquid servings per lb, while coffee beans (being much heavier) yield 15-30 liquid servings per lb. As a result, a serving of tea contains a substantially smaller amount of caffeine compared to a serving of coffee.

Coffee, depending on the brewing method, contains 90-120 milligrams of caffeine per cup. For comparison, cola contains approximately 45 milligrams per 12 oz can.

A FINAL WORD

WILL YOU TAKE THE RED PILL OR THE BLUE PILL?

As you may have gathered, my biggest goal is not to restrict and become fanatical to the point of being a fascist raw foodist, vegan, vegetarian or whatever other new and different label someone may want to come along and create; especially when it comes to justifying what one eats, drinks and/or takes in as supplementation (and why). Rather, my biggest goal is to continuously learn and educate how one can properly nourish the body, mind and spirit with only the best possible fuel. It comes from a driving passion to continually research and gain the proper knowledge so that the right choice can be made at the right time. This is of pivotal importance when only the optimum in health and wellness will do. Who doesn't want restful, restorative and rejuvenative sleep, as well as a youthful vigor and everlasting energy?

Our Body, Our Temple

With every choice, there is a consequence; and I don't know about you, but I certainly don't want any choice to diminish my health, the quality of my life, or my longevity. If the food is not grown, picked or processed with integrity and high regard to the nutritional and health claims it holds for my health, I DON'T WANT IT! If the nutritional value is no longer present and doesn't hold the same benefit it did before being processed into a liquid, oil, powder, etc., I DON'T WANT IT! If a company, manufacturer or distributer cannot provide me with all the data I request regarding details on the start to finish process, quality assurance and control, lab reports, third party testing, etc., I DON'T WANT IT!

No matter how confusing, conflicting or intimidating the information, wouldn't you rather know the truth? We certainly have the right to know. Of course, there will <u>always</u> be variables to consider before making any choice in life; but when it comes to the overall health and wellness of myself and others, I take pride in knowing that I did my research and, therefore, did my best.

Understanding the biochemistry of the human body, and how nutrients and all the unique constituents of food are best assimilated and absorbed, is the ultimate key in helping each and every one of us make informed decisions – especially when it comes to choosing one food, product and/or supplement over another, even when called by the same name. Don't be fooled by sly marketing ploys; get to know the true quality behind the name of what you are buying. It may just make the difference between being a health damaging product versus a viable and healing one.

> *Humans are organic, highly complex and dynamic, so why should the food and fluid we fuel our bodies with be any different?*

How is it that under the scope of African, Native American, Indian Ayurvedic, traditional Chinese and Tibetan philosophies of medicine (to name but a few) practitioners treat their patients as complex beings, whose reality encompasses more than the mere physical? Now let us compare to our conventional model of Western medicine, and it appears that human beings are reduced down to machines made from flesh. Have we truly learned nothing from the undeniable successes of cultural traditions all over the globe? Could big business, greed, apathy and arrogance be to blame for bad medicine in America?

When nature provides a perfect food, why do we feel the need to mess with it? What good is there in consuming a substance that has been manipulated beyond its original intent? What good is there in taking a large amount of one nutrient if all the other components necessary for its proper breakdown and utilization are missing in action? This is why self-medicating with a bunch of isolated synthetic supplements, over-the-counter drugs and prescription medications doesn't work – especially if we are in for the long-haul. More times than not, they actually complicate matters by creating further imbalances and additional problems. This is also why a lifetime of processed, refined and cooked food does not work. There are so many essential vitamins, minerals and enzymes that are fragile and heat sensitive. When unnecessarily messed with, these necessary nutrients become damaged or cooked out, leaving us with an incomplete tool box.

I cannot tell you how many times I have heard "I eat a good diet, but I still don't feel good." Then I find out that the person eats most all of their foods cooked to death, they rely on taking a bunch of isolated supplementation in the hopes of filling in the blanks, they don't get enough variety, they eat more processed and refined foods than they were initially aware of, and don't put much importance on eating organic and GMO free. It may appear on the surface that people are eating better and making better choices; but if the essential building blocks, phytonutrients, enzymes, catalysts and cofactors (which are all necessary for proper brain and body function) are getting stripped away or destroyed, then guess what? None of it makes a bit of difference.

When we violate Mother Nature, we are assaulting ourselves!

Natural, whole food sources of any nutrient or chemical that are either naturally produced by the body or essentially required by the body should never be compared to and confused with artificially manufactured nutrients and chemical imposters. Whether they are over-the-counter or prescribed, bought legally at the grocery store or illegally on the streets, they are all counterfeit as far as I'm concerned! Any substance that has been isolated from nature, man-made in a lab to mimic the real thing, and/or manipulated or cut to create an abnormally intense response can be detrimental and dangerously life-threatening. Whenever you follow big business' siren call to use foreign, synthetic substances to step in and overthrow what your body was designed to handle and thrive on naturally, you are opening Pandora's Box. Every cell in our body contains receptor binding sites for what they need, and when those sites are continuously bombarded by synthetic isolates and foreign chemical substances –like a swarm of killer bees – the brain and body are starved of what they truly require to function properly: REAL FOOD WITH REAL NUTRITION. If this continues, chemical imbalances and nutrient deficiencies begin to develop and can set the stage for illness and disease.

Please Note: This is not to say that someone cannot have a negative reaction to a healthy, natural, whole food or – more specifically – any number of its many constituents. However, we should always consider the strong possibility of underlying issue(s) first. A negative reaction may have less to do with the actual food itself (especially if it is whole and natural) and more to do with a weakness or imbalance; most likely due to a lifetime of poor dietary choices (processed and refined foods), too much of one thing and/or too little of another, or toxins that have changed our natural chemistry and thrown off our equilibrium.

As I have said before, everybody's individual chemistry is unique and different. Therefore, how much of any one thing an individual can safely consume will totally depend on the level and combination of various nutrients, chemicals and enzymes they already have on board at that very moment. Remember the following saying: "one man's medicine is another man's poison." Another great aphorism to remember is: "the difference between medicine and poison is in the dosage."

ABOVE ALL, DO NO HARM

Attention! If you are reading between the lines, the information earlier in this book should raise some concerns and one very important question: "how is it that small groups of individuals get to decide and regulate what is right for all of us?" This question can be applied to so many aspects of our lives that directly influence our overall health and well-being and freedom of choice. For instance, I strongly believe that if we did not have so many environmental toxins poisoning the food we eat, the air we breathe and the water we bathe in, as a society we wouldn't be dealing with so many mysterious allergies and unexplainable sensitivities to a growing number of substances.

And what makes this scenario even worse? Our unhealthy society gets even worse with the artificial foods, vitamin and mineral isolates and synthetic medications we abuse our bodies with on a daily basis, without even batting an eye. Our bodies are so supersaturated with chemicals that we are rendering ourselves defenseless and vulnerable. We have become the creators of our own misery and internal wars; wars we have allowed to get so out of control that we've actually become afraid and completely lost sight of the need to do whatever it takes to reverse the tide.

Why do we fear taking responsibility when it comes to our health? Personally, I blame it on being so out of practice in our ability to logically reason, at least in what <u>really</u> matters. Marketers and greedy investors brainwash and condition us to the wrong set of priorities and practices. Furthermore, we don't ask enough of the right questions. Instead we give in, give up and tend to get annoyed with hard facts and details.

So, what inevitably happens? We get used to not trusting ourselves or standing on our own two feet; we behave like a herd of sheep and are led astray with our eyes closed and our ears shut. If we continue putting blind faith in liars, manipulators and profiteers, it's inevitable that we will find ourselves tangled in a nasty web of decay – many times with no clue how we got there. If you think these big bully and profit-greedy groups have little to do with how difficult it can be to be healthy, I challenge you to think again.

Please see **Appendices A & B** for more insight on how we are being blindsided by BIG business and BIG government on a daily basis.

> *"When small men begin to cast big shadows, it means that the sun is about to set." – Lyn Yutang*

TAKE THE 21-DAY CHALLENGE!

Whether your goal is to lose weight, improve upon your athletic performance, transition into an anti-aging lifestyle or fight disease with ease – raw foods, superfoods and superherbs are the answer! They are packed with all the vitamins, minerals, antioxidants and enzymes you will ever need. Furthermore, they can successfully satisfy your body's deficiencies so you can finally flush out the toxic waste stored in your fat cells and clogging up your tissues and joints.

"The greatest wealth is health." – Virgil

Do you wake up with aches, pains and stiffness? Detoxify your diet and your lifestyle and watch the simmering and smoldering fire of chronic inflammation finally die like a pit of hot embers doused by a bucket of water.

What about excess weight, chronic fatigue and hormonal imbalances? Again, if the fat cells are clogged and the receptor sites are blocked by foreign intruders and invaders, how can you expect your body to benefit from what it craves? Stop wasting your time and money on synthetic drugs and supplements (which may be adding to your toxic overload) and start decluttering your body.

Eating whole and health-giving food will equate to a whole and healthy body, mind and spirit!

The following is just an example of what your three weeks (or longer) of living it up on raw foods and live juices can look like. With the various recipes and options given throughout this book, you can make each meal time a unique experience and personalize it to your specific health and lifestyle goals.

WEEK ONE

Days 1-5

If you are new to raw and living foods, use this week as a transition period to become better oriented. Start your day with a superfood smoothie or any of the other all-day breakfast foods (page 245). There are plenty of nutritiously satisfying recipes to choose from that can easily be made for breakfast, brunch or lunch. To gratify your cravings for sweets, how about making a batch of Chia "Tapioca" Pudding (page 413) to snack on throughout the day? It's loaded with omega-3 for anti-inflammatory support and a protein powerhouse! To end the day, I suggest focusing on a protein packed pâté (page 336) wrapped in a collard or lettuce leaf from "Mouthwatering Stove Stoppers" (page 332) with either a raw soup from "Souper Scrumptious Soups" (page 293) or an amazing leafy green salad from "Splendid Salads, Slaws & Rawghetti" (page 309).

Be sure to drink plenty of water and tea throughout the day. You may even choose to start experimenting with any of the longevity elixir drinks under "Longevity Elixir Drinks & Teas" (page 464). I recommend utilizing this week to wean off sugar, coffee and other caffeinated beverages.

Days 1-5 or Days 6 & 7

If you are not new to raw and living foods, you may start here for cleansing and detoxing. Otherwise, start here on day 6 and 7, as it is time to start transitioning into more of a liquid diet. Start making at least 1-2 juices per day. If you plan on juicing in the morning, then it may be a good idea to end the day with a nice raw soup. If you plan on juicing at night, then start your day with a superfood smoothie with added plant-based protein. Remember, green-based juices with a bit of fruit for sweetness are an ideal way to start your day (unless you are restricting yourself from all sugar) and green-based vegetable juices are ideal any time of day. Use the juice recipes under "Jubilant Juices" (page 283) to get started. You may wish to juice with a focus on opening each of the primary detoxification pathways. This can be achieved by choosing one (or more) of the juice options listed per detoxification pathway and then spending at least 2-3 days working at each detoxification pathway in the order listed: colon, kidney and bladder, liver and gallbladder, lymphatic and blood and then lung and skin. You may also wish to make juicing simpler by choosing a go-to juice with add-ons of choice. Do whatever works best for you and your needs.

WEEK TWO

Days 8-14, 8-21 or 8-24

This is the week to go on a full-on juice fast. Drink only fresh fruit and vegetable juices, herbal teas and pure water throughout the day (no blended drinks or solids whatsoever). You may wish to strictly juice for a total of 3-5 days, then follow the suggestions for week three below; or you may wish to strictly juice for one, two or three weeks (7-21 days in total). How much you drink and what you drink will depend on your personal health challenges, activity level and lifestyle goals. Use the information provided throughout this book and under "Jubilant Juices" (page 283) as a guiding light and consult with a qualified practitioner if necessary.

During the juicing week(s) and beyond, I suggest incorporating Longevity Iced Tea (page 473), Morning Chlorella Detox Elixir (page 475) and Digestive Elixir (page 475). Any one or all of these recipes – and their individual ingredients – can offer great support throughout your juicing journey and thereafter. Feel free to add green powders (such as Organic Kamut Blend, Organic Barley Grass Juice, chlorella, spirulina, etc.) and marine phytoplankton to any juice, as desired.

Please Note: Remember to drink plenty of pure water and as much herbal tea as you wish. Staying away from caffeine is highly advised during this stage of cleansing and detoxing.

Week Three

Days 15-21, 22-28 or 25-31

Congratulations! You are over the hardest part and so close to the finish line. This is the week to slowly start introducing raw blended smoothies and soups, as well as some solid foods, back into your life. I suggest decreasing the number of juices and starting to bring back a simple superfood smoothie and/or raw soup for the first 1 or 2 days. On day 2 or 3 add a salad with maybe a ½ avocado if you wish. You can also increase your spectrum of teas (pu-erh, greens, whites, etc.) and start experimenting with more of the elixir drinks under "Longevity Elixir Drinks & Teas" (page 464). For those who had it in them to juice for two whole weeks, wait at least one full week before diving into all the desserts and dehydrated treats. For the warriors who went three solid weeks, wait at least 10-11 days in total. The key is to break your fast slowly to allow your metabolism to wake up.

Week Four & Beyond

Ahh! You did it! Now is the time to really evaluate how you feel physically, mentally, emotionally, socially and spiritually. Determine what the next step is and how you plan on maintaining your results. You may also be thinking of digging deeper in order to ultimately reach higher ground. Just remember to always respect your body and listen to what it is trying to tell you. Learn to honor your body's intelligence and trust in the signals you are receiving.

For instance, I know I am creative at work and athletically oriented at play; therefore, I am at my best when I nourish my brain and body by making superfood smoothies and raw cacao infused elixir drinks to power me through the day and improve my productivity. Then, when I'm ready to wind down and prepare myself for a night of deep and rejuvenative sleep, I calm my active mind by eating a gratifying leafy green salad for dinner and sipping on herbal concoctions prior to bed.

Get to know yourself through this journey. What are your passions? What drives and empowers you? Then nurture your body with organic whole foods, superfoods and superherbs that resonate with you the most. When it comes to amounts and combinations, remember, this will be very individualized. Use my suggestions as a guideline, and fine-tune according to your personal needs and desires.

> *"There are two mistakes one can make along the road to truth; not going all the way and not starting." – Buddha*

APPENDIX A

THE COMMINGLING OF BUSINESS & POLITICS

I recently found an informative graphic on www.cornucopia.org (Cornucopia Institute) showing which US government officials (past and present) have vested interests in the biotech and GMO giant Monsanto. No wonder we have yet to see the labeling of genetically modified foods! If this doesn't look to you like the pursuit of profit and power, then I don't know what does!

Monsanto strives to control the world's food supply by buying out all the seed companies and converting farmers to growing Roundup Ready crops. According to the article, "Farmers speak out: GMOs are a trap that Monsanto is using to take over agriculture," by Ethan A. Huff, posted August 19, 2011 on www.naturalnews.com, "As long as the US government continues to provide patent protection for GM crops, as well as allow monopoly control over the seed market by biotechnology companies, many American farmers will simply have to remain in the clutches of Monsanto to stay afloat."

Is the USDA a wholly-owned subsidiary of Monsanto?

Federal Government	Both	Monsanto
US Congressman (D)	Toby Moffett	Monsanto Consultant
US Senator (D)	Dennis DeConcini	Monsanto Legal Counsel
Dep Dir FDA, HFS (Bush Sr, Clinton)	Margaret Miller	Chemical Lab Supervisor
White House Senior Staff (Clinton)	Marcia Hale	Director, Int'l Government Affairs
Sec of Commerce (Clinton)	Mickey Kantor	Board Member
WH-Appt to CSA, Gore's SDR (Clinton)	Virginia Weldon	VP, Public Policy
White House Communications (Clinton)	Josh King	Director, Int'l Government Affairs
Gore's Chief Dom Policy Adv (Clinton)	David Beler	VP, Government & Public Affairs
WH-Appointed Consumer Adv (Clinton)	Carol Tucker-Foreman	Monsanto Lobbyist
Deputy Admin EPA (Clinton, Bush)	Linda Fisher	VP, Government & Public Affairs
USDA, EPA (Clinton, Bush, Obama)	Lidia Watrud	Manager, New Technologies
Dep Commissioner FDA (Obama)	Michael Taylor	VP, Public Policy
US Sen (D), Sec of State (Obama)	Hillary Clinton	Rose Law Firm, Monsanto Counsel
Dir, USDA NIFA (Obama)	Roger Beachy	Director, Monsanto Danforth Center
Ag Negotiator Trade Rep (Obama)	Islam Siddiqui	Monsanto Lobbyist

GEKE.US

www.cornucopia.org

APPENDIX B

For the People, or for Profit?

"Organic has undergone a transformation from a movement to a $20 billion a year industry in the United States," according to Philip H. Howard, an associate Professor in the Department of Community Sustainability at Michigan State University. Dr. Phil Howard is responsible for the creation and updating of the Organic Food Industry Structure Charts (2007-2013). The infographic below explores the latest changes in ownership and control of the U.S. organics industry.

To view this chart, as well as several other charts that focus on Dr. Phil Howard's investigative findings regarding the relationships between food, agriculture and public health, please go to his homepage: http://msu.edu/~howardp/index.html.

For a zoomable view of the chart below, visit Philip H. Howard's page on the Organic Processing Industry Structure (http://msu.edu/~howardp/organicindustry.html).

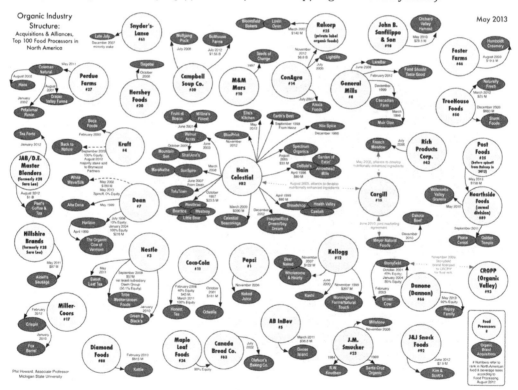

APPENDIX C

WHAT IS ESTROGEN DOMINANCE?

Dr. John R. Lee defines estrogen dominance as an overabundance of estrogen activity with insufficient progesterone to balance the effects of this activity in the body. Dr. John Lee is an authority on hormonal imbalances and estrogen dominance and the author of several best-selling books such as *Dr. John Lee's Hormone Balance Made Simple; What Your Doctor May Not Tell You about Menopause* and *What Your Doctor May Not Tell You about Premenopause*.

Estrogen dominance can cause a host of problems in both women and men. Page 494 lists some of the symptoms found to be related to estrogen dominance. If you can relate to more than just a few, there is a strong possibility that you may be estrogen dominant. According to Dr. Lee, many women between the ages of 40 and 50 suffer from this. You can have low estrogen (due to premenopause or menopause), but if you do not have enough progesterone to balance the effects of estrogen, then you can still suffer from symptoms of estrogen dominance.

Other Potential Causes of Estrogen Dominance

Estrogen dominance can be caused by more than the body's own production of hormones. For example, hormone replacement therapy (HRT), birth control pills, environmental estrogens (called xenoestrogens), plant estrogens (called phytoestrogens), stress, obesity, poor liver function, peri-menopause and glandular dysfunction are all potential causes of estrogen dominance.

Why Men Should Be Concerned About Estrogen Dominance?

Researchers, including Dr. John Lee, Dr. Jesse Hanley and Dr. Peter Eckhart, believe that the over-abundance of estrogenic compounds found in our environment are contributing to the growing number of health problems we see today. We are constantly assaulted by estrogens in our environment, from the food we eat to the air we breathe and the chemicals we use. A common misconception is that testosterone is the cause of an enlarged prostate and prostate cancer; but according to Dr. Lee, the primary offender appears to be overexposure to foreign environmental estrogens. The health of the prostate seems to be greatly influenced by the decline in testosterone (which we naturally see with increased age) in combination with the increase in estrogen levels due to chronic environmental and dietary exposure. Therefore, xenoestrogens and phytoestrogens may just be the prime culprits of an enlarged prostate and prostate cancer in men.

Progesterone Deficiency: A Problem for Both Sexes

Progesterone deficiency is the most common hormone imbalance among women of all ages. If you are progesterone deficient, it may be time to consult with your healthcare practitioner about getting off synthetic hormones (including birth control pills). It may also be time to change your diet. If you are consuming soy products, I highly suggest cutting them from your diet completely. I would also consider eliminating (or at least significantly decreasing) the amount of other phytoestrogens in your diet such as flax.

Progesterone is just as vital a hormone for men as it is for women. It is crucial to sustaining good hormone balance and health. Did you know that progesterone is essential in the synthesis of testosterone and other adrenal cortical hormones? Progesterone is the precursor to estrogen, testosterone and cortisol. Cortisol is a hormone produced by the adrenal glands that is responsible for keeping us alive. Cortisol helps the body respond to stress and illnesses. It is also responsible for maintaining our ability to process sugars, balancing our electrolytes, and keeping our blood pressure in check.

In my opinion, with the increase in environmental estrogens (xenoestrogens), there is no need to compound the issue by consuming foods rich in estrogenic compounds (e.g., soy and flax). Therefore, I absolutely recommend that everyone (especially men) look more toward hemp, chia, algae (such as marine phytoplankton, spirulina and chlorella) and bee pollen as a substitute for their protein, essential fatty acid and other vital nutrient needs.

Symptoms of Estrogen Dominance for Women

- Tender breasts
- Fibrocystic breasts
- Irregular periods
- Heavy bleeding
- Premenstrual syndrome (PMS)
- Infertility
- Early miscarriage
- Polycystic ovary syndrome (PCOS)
- Cervical dysplasia (abnormal pap smears)
- Fibroids
- Endometriosis
- Low libido
- Vaginal dryness
- Dry skin
- Night sweats
- Insomnia
- Fatigue
- Mood swings
- Irritability
- Foggy thinking
- Memory loss
- Weepiness
- Anxious depression
- Symptoms of hypothyroidism (low thyroid)
- Water retention/bloating
- Weight gain
- Cyclical migraine headaches
- Flushing of face
- Atherosclerosis
- Gallbladder issues

Symptoms of Estrogen Dominance for Men

- Prostate problems
- Man boobs
- Impotence
- Male patterned baldness
- Weight gain
- Low libido

Scientists have suggested that environmental estrogens (xenoestrogens) may reduce sperm count in men and cause breast cancer, fibroids and other reproductive diseases in women.

What Are Xenoestrogens?

Xeno- means foreign; therefore, xenoestrogens can simply be defined as foreign estrogens and hormone disruptors. Did you know that there are approximately 70,000 plus registered chemicals in use in the United States which have hormonal effects in addition to their toxic effects?

- ★ Many of these chemicals can be found in the items we use daily. For instance, household cleaning products, make-up, cosmetics and other body care products.
- ★ Xenoestrogens are also found in certain pesticides, plastics, fuels and drugs. All are synthetic and extremely difficult for the body to break down. These substances tend to increase the estrogen load in the body over time, are very difficult for the liver to detoxify and can place a tremendous amount of stress on several bodily systems.
- ★ Xenoestrogens can be found in much of our meat and dairy products in the form of the chemicals, antibiotics and growth hormones which are given to animals. When animal products are consumed, these estrogen-like hormones, hormone disruptors and growth hormones get passed on to us.

Sources of Xenoestrogens

- ★ Commercially raised meat (beef, chicken, pork, etc.)
- ★ Canned foods
- ★ Plastics, plastic food wraps and plastic drinking bottles
- ★ Styrofoam cups
- ★ Industrial wastes
- ★ Personal care products
- ★ Phytoestrogens (soybeans, soy-based products, flax seeds, etc.)
- ★ Car exhaust and indoor toxins
- ★ Cosmetics
- ★ Birth control pills and spermicides
- ★ Detergents
- ★ All artificial scents (air fresheners, perfumes, etc.)
- ★ Pesticides and herbicides
- ★ Paints, lacquers and solvents

What Are Phytoestrogens?

Phyto- means plant; therefore, the term phytoestrogens can be used to define naturally-occurring estrogenic compounds that are found in a variety of foods, herbs and spices. Their chemical structure resembles that of real estrogen. This makes it possible for phytoestrogens to mimic the action of estrogen produced in the body, with the potential of altering hormonal activity and balance. In comparison to real estrogen and xenoestrogens, these plant-derived estrogenic compounds are generally weak. However, in a body that is already experiencing too much estrogen (real or foreign) and possibly producing little to no progesterone, adding more estrogen can lead to more problems.

★ One of the strongest phytoestrogen containing substances is the class of isoflavones found in soy. Soy products include soybeans, soy milk, tofu, tempeh, textured vegetable protein, roasted soybeans, soy granules, miso and edamame. Another strong phytoestrogen is lignans found in flax seeds.

Getting to the Root of the Problem

Both women and men are often prescribed synthetic hormones, anti-depressants and a host of other drugs to relieve their symptoms of estrogen dominance without having addressed the underlying causes first. In addition, some of the latest research highlights the fact that some natural remedies, including progesterone cream, may not be working either. Why? Once again, because the root problem of estrogen dominance has not been addressed first.

Our hormones govern everything! Therefore, the root to our many problems could just be a blockage at the hormone receptor sites. In other words, our hormone receptor sites may be congested and being taken up by xenoestrogenic compounds that are known to mimic our natural hormones. Only once these receptor sites have been cleared and freed up can true hormonal balance be restored.

There are many options to consider when it comes to detoxifying the undesirable estrogenic compounds (xenoestrogens) from the body. Therefore, only once you have cleared your hormone receptor sites and know what you are truly dealing with would I consider an herbal formula or a more natural, topical progesterone cream for symptom relief. Otherwise, you could be just running in circles, wasting a lot of time and money.

> **Quick Tip:** Even if we are not regularly consume foods rich in estrogenic compounds (phytoestrogens) we are all still bombarded by estrogens and hormone disruptors in our environment (xenoestrogens) every day. For this reason alone, I suggest doing your best to consume foods – and/or take whole food supplements – that are high in very specific protective minerals, phytochemicals and compounds such as sea vegetables rich in iodine and cruciferous vegetable rich in DIM and I3C. These dual-action protectors not only keep hormone receptor sites clean and clear and ready to accept what they truly need, but can protect against hormone-dependent cancers.
>
> **How do they work?** A good analogy would be having the spark plugs in your car regularly cleaned for the proper functioning of your car's engine. This is just part of a good and regular maintenance plan if you desire to keep the engine in your car igniting properly. The only difference is that you are clean sweeping your hormone receptor sites for the harmony of your hormones instead.

The following is a list of ten excellent removers of <u>bad</u> estrogen I obtained while listening to an amazing lecture given by David Wolfe at the Longevity Now Conference in Costa Mesa, CA.

Bad Estrogen Removers

- ★ Agaricus bisporus (aka button mushrooms or white cap mushrooms)
- ★ Berries
- ★ Calcium D-Gluconate (C-D-G) – found in foods such as apples, oranges, broccoli, potatoes and Brussels sprouts
- ★ Citrus essential oils
- ★ Citrus peel
- ★ Cruciferous vegetables – such as broccoli, cauliflower, Brussels sprouts, kale and cabbage
- ★ Diindolylmethane (DIM) – found in cruciferous vegetables
- ★ Indole-3-carbinol (I3C) – found in cruciferous vegetables
- ★ Iodine – abundantly found in sea vegetables such as kelp, dulse and nori
- ★ Melatonin

Along with eating a diet rich in the above, there are two products I love to include as part of my own personal protocol against bad estrogens: XenoStat by Premier Research Labs and EstoGuard by Rejuvenation Science Labs. EstroGuard can be found at Longevity Warehouse.

In Closing

Estrogen and progesterone work synergistically with one another in order to achieve hormonal harmony in both women and men. I feel it is important, yet again, to point out the importance of balance. Why? Because it appears to not be the absolute deficiency of estrogen or progesterone that causes the majority of health problems, but rather the relative dominance of estrogen and relative deficiency of progesterone. According to Dr. John Lee, the key to optimum health is to keep the progesterone to estrogen ratio between 200 and 300 to 1.

Please Note: It is highly advisable to always consult with a qualified healthcare or holistic practitioner well-versed in the area of hormones. At the very least, I suggest seeing a holistic hormone specialist to get all your blood work done. Then actively participate in all the necessary steps toward hormone balance and management.

How to Reduce the Symptoms Associated with Estrogen Dominance

- ★ Avoid chemical sources of estrogen (xenoestrogens).
- ★ Avoid food sources of estrogen (phytoestrogens).
- ★ Cleanse the liver and colon. Do this as regular maintenance, as you would an oil change for your car.
- ★ Exercise daily (enough to work up a good sweat).
- ★ Reduce stress; at least any and all that are controllable (i.e., lifestyle choices).
- ★ Drink out of glass containers; not plastic water bottles or Styrofoam.
- ★ Store food in glass whenever possible. When not possible, store all food and liquid in BPA free plastic or food grade plastics with the following label and number: HDPE (#2), LDPE (#4) or PP (#5). Avoid all plastics with the following labels and numbers, as they have been found to leach toxic chemicals: PETE or PET (#1), PVC or V (#3), PS (#6) and polycarbonates (#7), which contain bisphenol A (BPA).
- ★ Avoid synthetic chemicals found in cosmetics, deodorants, shampoos, household cleaning supplies, car care chemicals, etc.
- ★ Use only natural detergents and soaps.
- ★ Don't use or subject yourself to chemical pesticides, herbicides or fungicides.
- ★ Purchase produce grown without the use of pesticides, herbicides, fungicides or synthetic fertilizer. Be sure to look for organic and GMO free. If organic, the produce sticker should always start with the number 9 and be 5 digits long.
- ★ If you eat meat, purchase only organic and grass fed meats raised without hormones.
- ★ Don't use condoms with spermicides.

APPENDIX D

FOOD COMBINING FOR OPTIMAL DIGESTION

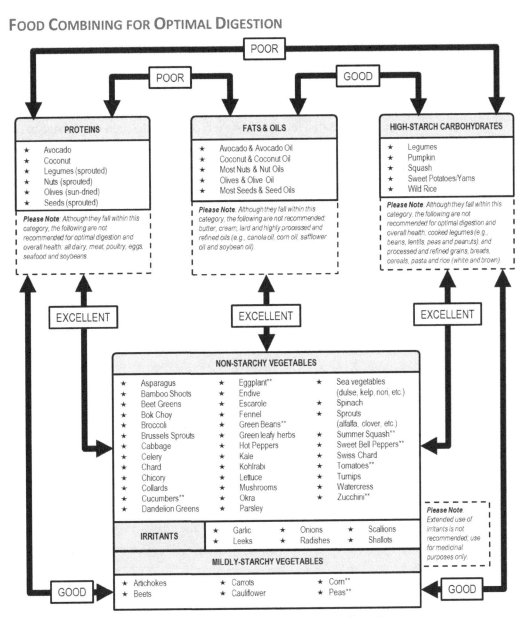

** Botanically classified as a fruit, but its biochemical composition places it in a non-fruit food combining category.

Quick Tips:

- ★ Non-Starchy vegetables combine well with all food groups, especially leafy greens and celery.
- ★ Ideally, protein and high starch carbohydrates should never be eaten together or within the same meal. These two groups of foods need totally different environments for digestion. Proteins require an acid environment and carbohydrates require an alkaline environment. When eaten together, neither starches nor proteins will be fully digested. The proteins will putrefy and the starch sugars will ferment.
- ★ It is best to choose either one concentrated protein or one concentrated fat per meal. Concentrated proteins are foods which contain a higher percentage of protein in their makeup. Concentrated fats are foods which contain a high percentage of fat or oil in their makeup. Both have longer transit (digestion) times and when eaten together will not fully digest.
- ★ Tomatoes only combine well with non-starchy vegetables, cucumbers, sweet peppers, avocados, olives, nuts and seeds – not with mild to high starch vegetables and other high carbohydrate foods (such as bread, pasta or rice).
- ★ With the exception of lemons and limes, it is best to eat acid foods away from concentrated proteins and high starch carbohydrates.

FRUITS

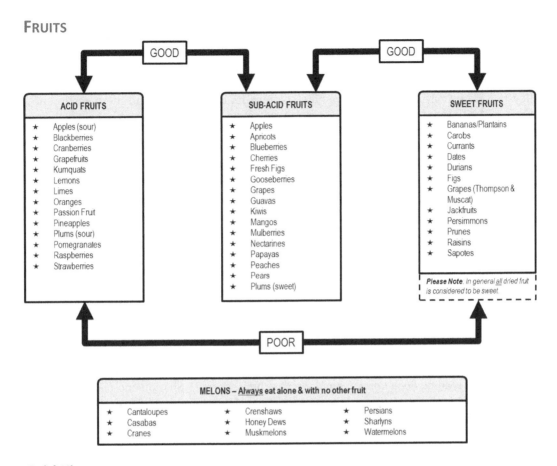

Quick Tips:

Depending on personal digestive fire and constitution, all fruits may be best eaten alone and on an empty stomach. Out of all the food categories, fruits digest the fastest (about 30-60 minutes). This is especially true for melons. Melons have the shortest transit time (about 20 minutes); therefore, when eaten with foods that digest slowly, such as proteins or fats, they will be held up in the stomach for hours and will literally begin to ferment. Unlike fermented (aka cultured) foods, where the sugars get eaten up by the bacteria cultures, fermenting sugars in the body are not properly assimilated and can halt the digestion of foods (like proteins), causing them to putrefy. For this reason, you should eat melons alone or with other melons, not with any other fruit or food category.

It is best to eat fruits early in the day (e.g., for breakfast), or at least several hours before or after consuming a meal that includes concentrated proteins, fats, mild to high starchy vegetables and/or other high carbohydrate foods (like grain-based foods). This rule is especially important to follow if eating cooked proteins, fats and/or high starch carbohydrates. It comes down to each food group (and individual food items within) requiring a different set of enzymes in order to properly digest. For example, fats require lipase, proteins require pepsin and starches require ptyalin and amylase. When two foods are eaten with different and opposite digestive needs, the precise adjustment of enzymes and gastric juices to digestive requirements becomes impossible. **Please Note:** There is a great difference between the digestion of a single food (no matter how complex its composition) and the digestion of a mixture of different foods. The body can easily adjust its juices to the digestive requirements of a single food, but not when two totally different foods are eaten with completely different digestive needs.

- ★ Fruits combine exceptionally well with raw, non-starchy vegetables; especially leafy greens, celery and cucumbers.
- ★ When combining fruits, sub-acid fruits combine well with either acid fruits or sweet fruits, but acid fruits combine poorly with sweet fruits.
- ★ While not ideal, small amounts of sub-acid or acid fruits may be eaten with nuts and seeds without digestive upset.

Please Note: The above are some great general guidelines to follow (especially during cleansing and detoxifying or when you are trying to correct a particular digestive problem), but not all of these food combining rules will apply to everyone. What is proper food combing for one, may not be proper food combing for another. I feel the best way to find out what works for your individual digestive system is to experiment with different food combinations at different times of the day. I also suggest keeping a food journal to learn what works best at different times in your life. If interested in learning more about proper food combining, I suggest reading *Food Combining Made Easy* by Herbert M. Shelton and *Food Combining & Digestion: 101 Ways to Improve Digestion* by Steve Meyerowitz and Rick Meyerowitz. Both of these books are a great resource for understanding the human digestion system.

APPENDIX E

ACID-ALKALINE FOODS FOR OPTIMAL HEALTH

Alkaline	Acid
Kindness, Gratitude, Love Meditation and Peace	**Anger, Fear, Jealousy, Overwork and Stress**
Extremely Alkaline Forming Foods pH 8.5 to 9.0	Extremely Acid Forming Foods pH 5.0 to 5.5
9.0 Lemons, Watermelon	5.0 Artificial Sweeteners
8.5 Agar-Agar, Asparagus, Cantaloupe, Cayenne (Capsicum), Dates (dried), Endive, Figs (dried), Fruit Juices (fresh), Kelp, Kiwi Fruit, Grapes (sweet), Limes, Mango, Melons, Papaya, Parsley, Passion Fruit, Pears (sweet), Pineapple, Raisins, Sea Vegetables, Seedless Grapes (sweet), Umeboshi Plum, Vegetable Juices (fresh), Watercress	5.5 Beef, Beer, Black Tea, Brown Sugar, Carbonated Soft Drinks and Fizzy Drinks, Chicken, Chocolate (processed), Cigarettes (tailor made), Coffee, Custard (commercial and made with refined sugar), Deer, Drugs (pharmaceutical and recreational), Flour (white and wheat), Goat, Jams and Jellies (commercial), Lamb, Liquor, Pasta (processed and refined), Pastries and Cakes (commercial and made from white or wheat flour), Pork, Semolina, Table Salt (refined and iodized), Turkey, Wheat Bread, White Rice, White Sugar, White vinegar (processed)
Moderate Alkaline pH 7.5 to 8.0	Moderate Acid pH 6.0 to 6.5
8.0 Apples (sweet), Apricots, Alfalfa Sprouts, Arrowroot (flour), Avocados, Bananas (ripe), Berries, Carrots, Celery, Currants, Dates (fresh), Figs (fresh), Garlic, Gooseberries, Grapes (less sweet), Grapefruit, Guava Fruit, Herbs (leafy green), Lettuce (leafy green), Nectarine, Peaches (sweet), Pears (less sweet), Peas (fresh, sweet), Persimmons, Pumpkin (sweet), Spinach, Vegetable Sea Salt	6.0 Breads (refined and made of corn, oats, rice or rye), Cereals (commercial and refined), Cigarette Tobacco (roll your own), Cream of Wheat (unrefined), Fish, Fruit Juices (commercial and sweetened), Maple Syrup (processed), Molasses (sulphured), Pickles (commercial), Shellfish, Wheat Germ, Whole Wheat Products, Wine, Yogurt (sweetened)
7.5 Apples (sour), Bamboo Shoots, Beans (fresh, green), Beets, Bell Peppers, Broccoli, Cabbage, Carob, Cauliflower, Daikon, Ginger (fresh), Grapes (sour), Kale, Kohlrabi, Lettuce (pale green), Oranges, Parsnips, Peaches (less	6.5 Bananas (unripe), Breads (unrefined and made of corn or rice), Buckwheat, Cheeses (sharp), Eggs (whole, hard cooked), Ketchup, Mayonnaise, Oats, Pasta (whole grain), Pastries and Cakes (whole grain and naturally sweetened with fruit, honey or maple syrup), Pea-

Alkaline	Acid
Kindness, Gratitude, Love Meditation and Peace	**Anger, Fear, Jealousy, Overwork and Stress**
sweet), Peas (less sweet), Potatoes (with skin), Pumpkin (less sweet), Raspberries, Sapote, Squash, Strawberries, Sweet Corn (fresh, organic), Tamari (organic), Turnips, Vinegar (apple cider)	nuts, Potatoes (without skins), Popcorn (with salt and butter), Rice (basmati), Rice (brown), Soy Sauce (commercial), Tapioca, Wheat Bread (sprouted, organic)
Slightly Alkaline to Neutral pH 7.0	Slightly Acid to Neutral pH 7.0
7.0 Almonds, Artichokes (Jerusalem), Brown Rice Syrup, Brussels Sprouts, Cherries, Coconut (fresh), Cucumbers, Eggplant, Honey (raw), Leeks, Miso, Mushrooms, Okra, Olives (ripe), Onions, Pickles (home-made), Radishes, Sea Salt, Spices, Taro, Tomatoes (sweet), Vinegar (sweet brown rice), Water Chestnuts, Amaranth, Artichokes (globe), Chestnuts (dry roasted), Egg Yolks (soft cooked), Essene Bread, Goat's Milk and Whey (raw), Horseradish, Mayonnaise (home-made), Millet, Olive Oil, Quinoa, Rhubarb, Sesame Seeds (whole), Soy Beans (dry, organic), Soy Cheese (organic), Soy Milk (organic), Sprouted Grains, Tempeh (organic), Tofu (organic), Tomatoes (less sweet), Yeast (nutritional flakes)	7.0 Agave Nectar, Barley, Barley Malt Syrup, Blueberries, Bran, Brazil Nuts, Butter (salted), Cashews, Cereals (unrefined and naturally sweetened with fruit, honey or maple syrup), Cheeses (mild and crumbly), Cornmeal, Crackers (unrefined and made of rice, rye or wheat) Cranberries, Dried Beans (mung, adzuki, pinto, kidney and garbanzo), Dried Coconut, Egg Whites, Goats Milk (homogenized), Honey (pasteurized), Lentils, Macadamia Nuts, Maple Syrup (unprocessed), Milk (homogenized and most other processed dairy products), Molasses (unsulphured, organic), Mustard Seed, Nutmeg, Olives (pickled), Pecans, Pistachios, Plums, Popcorn (plain, organic), Prunes, Rye (grain), Rye Bread (sprouted, organic), Seeds (pumpkin and sunflower), Spelt, Walnuts

Neutral – pH 7.0

Butter (fresh, unsalted), Cream (fresh and raw), Cow's Milk and Whey (raw), Oils (except olive), Whey, Yogurt (plain)

Please Note: There are several versions of acid and alkaline food charts and lists to be found in different books and on the internet. The above chart has been slightly modified from several different internet sources, and is intended only as a general guide to alkalizing and acidifying foods. Therefore, please do not feel as though you must adhere strictly to the alkaline side of the chart. There are many foods that fall on the acid side that are still considered healthful (e.g. certain fruits, nuts, seeds, etc.). Just be sure to make conscious choices, with a good percentage of the foods you eat being more alkaline. Remember, moderation in everything. Achieving a healthy balance is the true key to success!

Quick Tips:

The optimum ratio of alkaline forming foods to acid forming foods is approximately 3:1. Therefore, 75-80% of the diet should be alkaline forming food and 20-25% acid forming foods to maintain optimal health.

- ★ Generally, alkaline forming foods include: most fruits, leafy green vegetables, cruciferous vegetables, sea vegetables, sprouts, herbs and spices.
- ★ Always choose foods that are organic and free from genetically modified organisms (GMOs). Genetically modified foods include, but are not limited to: corn and soy.

Generally, acid forming foods include: artificial sweeteners, alcohol, coffee, soft drinks, meat, poultry, fish, pasteurized dairy, eggs, grains and legumes.

- ★ Raw, living, sprouted grains and legumes are an exception, as they are actually much more alkaline forming; therefore, more beneficial for internal health and balance.
- ★ Raw nuts and seeds that have been soaked and sprouted are also more alkaline forming.

Recreational, prescription and over-the-counter (OTC) drugs are very acidifying and can decrease the absorption of minerals and other nutrients. Their contribution to blood and body acidity can reduce the body's ability to repair damaged cells, detoxify chemicals and heavy metals, and may even encourage the growth of tumor cells.

If you are interested in monitoring your body's pH, you may wish to purchase and use pH test strips designed for checking the pH of saliva and urine in the privacy of your own home. Please keep in mind, everyone's normal (healthy) pH range is individual, so don't compare yourself to friends and family members. In addition, you may notice your pH rise and fall depending on the foods and beverages you are taking in, stress levels, sleeping habits, etc.

Also, I feel it is worth mentioning, that when your body is dumping stored up toxins during a period of cleansing, don't be surprised if your pH drops into the acid range (temporarily) until your body has successfully detoxified itself. Just be sure to continue flooding your body with alkaline foods full of oxygen and minerals, and as the saying goes, "this too shall pass."

With that said, an optimal saliva pH is between 6.8 and 7.2 +. An optimal urine pH is between 6.5 and 7.0+. Morning readings are generally lower, with the rest of the day proving to be higher.

Using pH test strips on a regular basis (and according to their individual instructions) can be a great tool in evaluating how well your body is mineralized and how your body is working to maintain the proper pH of your blood.

APPENDIX F

Ayurveda Made Easy

Ayurveda is an ancient system of holistic medicine in India that is becoming increasingly popular in our Western world. According to Ayurveda, an individual's state of health is not defined by yearly checkups and lab work. Instead, health is a continuous process that embraces ALL aspects of life: physical, mental, emotional, behavioral, spiritual, familial, social and universal. Achieving balance on all levels of being is the true measure of vital health and well-being.

The Three Doshas: Vata, Pitta, & Kapha

The doshas are dynamic energies that constantly change in response to our actions, thoughts, emotions, foods we eat, seasons, and any other sensory input that feeds our body, mind and spirit.

Through birth and prolonged specific behavior(s), one dosha may dominate. For some, a combination of two doshas is dominant (dual-dosha). Dual-dosha constitutions seem to be the most common. Some individuals (but not many), have all three doshas in relative balance (tri-dosha). Whether you have a dual-dosha constitution, or a tri-dosha constitution, it is a good idea to make note of which one or two predominate over the other(s).

Vata

Vata dominant individuals tend to be relatively thin and find it difficult to gain weight. Due to this, vata types tend to have very little energy reserves and can tire fairly easily. Vata types should make sure to get sufficient rest, not overdo things, and surround themselves with tranquility. Staying warm is important, as they tend to be always cold. It is also important for them to keep regular routines.

The vata dosha controls all movement in the body, including breathing, digestion and nerve impulses from the brain. When vata is out of balance, fear, anxiety and other nervous system disorders usually manifest. Other common signs of vata imbalance include: bodily disorders related to dryness, such as stiffness, dry skin and constipation; gas and bloating; irregular periods; pain and spasms. Vata types should avoid dry, dehydrated and frozen foods, and limit cold foods and beverages.

Please Note: The most important thing to know about vata is that it leads the other doshas. Vata generally goes out of balance first, which causes the early stages of illness and disease. More than half of all illnesses are vata disorders. Balancing vata is important for everyone, because when vata is in balance, pitta and kapha are usually in balance as well.

Pitta

Pitta dominant individuals tend to be of medium build and well proportioned. They have a moderate to good amount of physical energy, endurance and stamina. They also tend to be intelligent, well organized and disciplined, with a sharp wit and a good ability to focus and concentrate. They are very ambitious and driven by nature, but can also become irritable and demanding when not balanced.

Fire is a characteristic of pitta, and it can show up either as red hair or a fiery temper. Since pitta types tend to be warm, they can go out of balance with overexposure to heat or the sun. Also, their eyes have a tendency to be sensitive to light. Pitta types tend to have a strong digestive system but should be careful not to abuse it. Their heat makes them particularly thirsty, and they should make certain not to dilute their digestive juices (a.k.a. digestive fire) by drinking too much liquid during mealtimes. Pitta individuals should avoid acid forming foods, and keep salty, sour, and spicy foods to a minimum.

The pitta dosha leads us to crave moderation, purity and peace. We rely on pitta to regulate our intake of food, water and air. Any toxic substances, such as alcohol and tobacco, show up as a pitta imbalance. Toxic emotions such as anger, jealousy, impatience and intolerance should also be kept in check in order to keep pitta in balance for optimum health.

Kapha

Kapha dominant individuals tend to have strong and sturdy structures with wide, heavy frames. This provides them with a good reserve of physical strength, endurance and stamina. Kaphas innate strength supports their natural resistance to disease and positive outlook on life. Kapha types are affectionate, calm and loyal, but when out of balance, can become self-righteous, stubborn and lazy.

The Kapha dosha is slow. Kapha types learn slowly, with a methodical approach, causing them to retain information rather well with a good understanding of it. They also have a tendency to speak slowly. In addition, kapha types tend to be slow eaters with rather slow digestion. Kapha individuals should avoid overeating, and limit heavy, oily and fatty foods.

Kapha dosha controls the moist tissues of the body. Therefore, a kapha imbalance may show up as a cold, allergies or asthma. This tends to be worse during kapha season, which is March through June. Cold and wet weather aggravate kapha. Kapha types should get lots of exercise and avoid lounging or napping after meals.

The kapha dosha teaches us steadiness, groundedness and a sense of well-being. Kapha types tend to need provoking in order to stimulate their adventurous side. In order to keep kapha types in balance, they need to work on not dwelling in the past or resisting change.

Please Note: There are a number of great books and sites that are dedicated to, or at the very least make reference to, dosha constitutional types; but because of the raw, vegetarian lifestyle I lead, my interest was sparked the most after reading *Conscious Eating*, second edition by Dr. Gabriel Cousens. This book became my blueprint for change. It may seem biased, I know, but when it comes to learning about your own personal constitution and what the very best foods and practices are (or not) for your constitutional type, then I cannot say enough about this book. Dr. Gabriel Cousens is a genius. Even if your intention is not to become a raw vegan or raw vegetarian, this book can be‐ 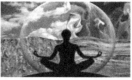 come your manual for living a long, healthy and vibrant life. It is full of original research, sci‐entific data, and nutritional and lifestyle guidelines that anyone can learn from and follow in order to start rejuvenating and balancing their life.

Determining Your Dosha(s)

To help determine your Ayurvedic constitution, feel free to take the questionnaire I devel‐oped below. For comparison purposes, there are many other versions of dosha quizzes and questionnaires to be found in books and on the internet.

For each statement, circle your score from 0 – 3 (please see below). Once completed, add up each column (dosha) to reveal your constitutional type or combination.

You may wish to go through this quiz twice if you have experienced drastic characteris‐tic/trait changes. You can first go through and answer the questions according to what phys‐ical and psychological traits describe what you were like for the majority of your lifetime. This will give you a better understanding of your underlying constitution from birth. Then you can go through a second time and answer according to what your physical and psycho‐logical characteristics are presently. When you view both sets of scores side by side, this will hopefully give you an idea of where your imbalances lie and what areas you can work on. Please do yourself a favor by answering honestly and truthfully. Do not answer according to what you wish to be.

Please Note: This simple questionnaire is intended to help individuals determine the rela‐tive strength of their vata, pitta, and kapha doshas. It is to be used for informational purpos‐es only and is in no way intended to substitute an assessment of your constitution by a quali‐fied healthcare practitioner well versed in the area of Ayurveda.

0 = does not apply to me at all

1 = applies to me on a minimal level

2 = applies to me on a moderate level

3 = applies to me most of the time

Characteristics	Vata Elements of Space and Air	Pitta Elements of Fire and Water	Kapha Elements of Earth and Water
Physical Frame	I am thin, slender and lanky; not much muscular definition; taller or shorter than average 0 1 2 3	I am of medium build; symmetrical; good muscular development 0 1 2 3	I have a broad build and frame; good muscular development; short and stocky or tall and sturdy 0 1 2 3

| **Body Weight** | It is difficult for me to gain weight; tend to be underweight; bony

0 1 2 3 | I can gain and lose weight fairly easily; moderate; good muscle definition

0 1 2 3 | It is difficult for me to lose weight; tend to be overweight, heavy; gain weight easy

0 1 2 3 |
|---|---|---|---|
| **Body Temperature** | My hands and feet are usually cold; prefer warm, moist weather over cold and dry

0 1 2 3 | I am usually warm, regardless of the season; prefer cool to moderate environments

0 1 2 3 | I am adaptable to most environments but do not like cold, damp weather

0 1 2 3 |
| **Skin** | My skin is thin, dry, cool to touch; tends to be rough and cracks

0 1 2 3 | My skin is soft, moist; fair to rosy complexion; warm to touch; tends to be oily in t-zone; prone to freckles and moles; sensitive

0 1 2 3 | My skin is thick, moist smooth; cool to touch; tends to be oily to normal; prone to acne

0 1 2 3 |
| **Hair** | My hair is dry, thin, brittle; tends to be frizzy, kinky or course; may be light or dark in color, but usually very dark

0 1 2 3 | My hair is red, light brown or blonde in color; tends to be soft, wavy or fine; neither dry nor oily; prone to premature graying or thinning

0 1 2 3 | My hair is thick, full and lustrous; tends to be wavy; slightly oily; usually darker in color, but can be medium blonde

0 1 2 3 |
| **Eyes** | My eyes are small; tend to feel dry; dull; usually dark in color

0 1 2 3 | My eyes are medium; sharp, focused with penetrating gaze; usually light in color (light gray, blue or green)

0 1 2 3 | My eyes are large and round; usually blue or brown; tend to have thick, full eyelashes

0 1 2 3 |
| **Face Shape** | My face is oval

0 1 2 3 | My face is triangular; pointed features (nose, chin and jaw line)

0 1 2 3 | My face is round

0 1 2 3 |

Forehead Size	Small 0 1 2 3	Medium 0 1 2 3	Large 0 1 2 3
Mouth/Lips	My mouth is small; thin lips; tend to be dry and cracked 0 1 2 3	My mouth and lips are average in size; soft 0 1 2 3	My mouth is large; full lips; smooth 0 1 2 3
Teeth/Gums	Crooked, uneven teeth; protruding; sensitive to heat and cold; receded gums 0 1 2 3	Even teeth of medium size; often off white to yellow in color; gums are soft, bleed easy and prone to canker sores 0 1 2 3	Even, large teeth; gleaming, white in color; gums are strong and healthy 0 1 2 3
Hands	My hands are usually dry, rough; slender fingers 0 1 2 3	My hands are usually soft, pink, moist; medium fingers; soft nails 0 1 2 3	My hands are generally wide, firm; thick fingers 0 1 2 3
Fingernails	Dry, thin and cracking 0 1 2 3	Medium, soft and pink 0 1 2 3	Wide, thick, strong and white 0 1 2 3
Joints	My joints are small; prominent; tend to crack 0 1 2 3	My joints are medium; flexible 0 1 2 3	My joints are large; sturdy; well-padded and lubricated 0 1 2 3
Energy Level	My energy fluctuates and usually comes in bursts 0 1 2 3	My energy level is moderate to high 0 1 2 3	My energy level is steady 0 1 2 3

Activity Level: Stamina, Strength & Endurance	I am very active, but lose physical stamina rather quickly; low to poor strength and endurance; rarely sweat 0 1 2 3	I enjoy physical activity; have medium stamina, strength and endurance; sweat easily, profusely 0 1 2 3	Tend to avoid physical activity, but can work long hours and maintain a high level of stamina and endurance; strong; sweat minimally 0 1 2 3
Actions	I walk fast and talk fast; always on the go; I become distracted easily; don't always finish what I start; flighty 0 1 2 3	My actions are very thought-out, goal oriented and precise; list maker; like to see things through to the end; motivated 0 1 2 3	I am a "go with the flow" type; like a relaxed, slower pace; take my time accomplishing things; do not like to rush 0 1 2 3
Sleep	I do not require a lot of sleep; light sleeper; toss and turn; tend to wake up easily; prone to insomnia 0 1 2 3	I require a moderate amount of sleep; can sleep rather soundly; I usually fall back to sleep easily if something wakes me up 0 1 2 3	I like to sleep a lot; heavy sleeper; sleep long and deep; slow to wake up; prone to oversleeping 0 1 2 3
Appetite	My appetite is irregular; sometimes I forget to eat; tend to eat quickly 0 1 2 3	My appetite is very strong; need to eat regularly, otherwise tend to get irritable 0 1 2 3	My appetite is steady to low; eat slowly; I enjoy food, but can easily skip meals 0 1 2 3
Bowel Movements	I tend to be bloated, gassy, constipated; have small, hard stools 0 1 2 3	I have regular bowel movements; soft stools (too loose at times); rapid digestion 0 1 2 3	My bowel movements are highly regular; moderate and solid in size; slow digestion 0 1 2 3
Voice/Speech	My voice tends to be high-pitched, weak and often hoarse; fast speech 0 1 2 3	I have a strong voice; can get loud at times; speech is moderate, clear and precise 0 1 2 3	My voice tends to be low-pitched, deep-toned and pleasant; slow speech 0 1 2 3

Thoughts	My thoughts are often scattered; find it difficult to bring my ideas to fruition; wishful thinker; often find myself escaping into a fantasy world 0 1 2 3	My thoughts are articulate logical and rational; goal oriented; passion driven; realistic; always thinking and focused on the future 0 1 2 3	My thoughts are usually well organized; methodical; thoroughly thought-out; often find myself thinking in the past 0 1 2 3
Decision Making Style	I change my mind frequently; indecisive 0 1 2 3	I am decisive, determined; ready to persevere; natural born innovator, self-starter, leader 0 1 2 3	I often let others make decisions and take the lead; premeditated and purposeful 0 1 2 3
Admirable Traits	I am excitable, creative and imaginative; enjoy artistic forms of expression 0 1 2 3	I am a perfectionist; well organized; productive; proficient; passionate; good sense of humor 0 1 2 3	I am big-hearted, caring and compassionate; nurturing, generous and devoted 0 1 2 3
Emotions & Response to Stress	I tend to be fearful, anxious and nervous; worry a lot and panic when under stress 0 1 2 3	I tend to be become irritable, impatient, and angry when things do not go my way; critical of myself and others; argumentative and demanding when under stress 0 1 2 3	I become sentimental quite easily; tend to let negative emotions build up rather than addressing them; slow to forgive and forget; detach and withdraw when under stress 0 1 2 3
Mood	My mood often fluctuates for no reason; random mood swings; inconsistent 0 1 2 3	My mood is often organized, focused and driven; self-controlled 0 1 2 3	My mood is often relaxed, easy going; consistent 0 1 2 3

Mind	My mind is active and often restless; races a lot; compulsive 0 1 2 3	I have a strong intellect; enjoy learning new things; intense, yet controlled 0 1 2 3	I tend to be easy going, calm and level minded; not easily angered; patient 0 1 2 3
Memory	I learn quickly and easily, but tend to forget just as quickly and easily; good short-term memory; poor long-term 0 1 2 3	My memory is sharp and clear; have no problem learning quickly and easily; good short-term memory; moderate long-term 0 1 2 3	I don't learn as quickly as others, but once learned I rarely forget; excellent long-term memory 0 1 2 3
Dreams	My dreams often involve flying or running; anxious and restless in nature; prone to nightmares 0 1 2 3	My dreams are often vivid and in color; involve action, conflict, passion and/or violence 0 1 2 3	My dreams are often short; involve romance 0 1 2 3
Lifestyle	I tend to lead an erratic lifestyle; unpredictable 0 1 2 3	I tend to lead a very active lifestyles; workhorse 0 1 2 3	I tend to have a relaxed and slow-paced lifestyle; home oriented 0 1 2 3
Personality: Positive & Negative Traits	I tend to be open-minded, spontaneous and free-spirited; can be chaotic and changeable 0 1 2 3	I tend to be self-assured, bold and confident; can be over-zealous and too intense at times 0 1 2 3	I tend to be well grounded, sensible and serous; can be reluctant to change or release possessions 0 1 2 3
Financial Style	I spend money as quickly as I earn it; impulsive; I tend not to save; poor 0 1 2 3	I efficiently manage my money; I save and enjoy buying luxuries, but only when appropriate 0 1 2 3	I spend money on what I really need; I'm frugal; economical by nature; tend to be an avid saver 0 1 2 3

Hobbies	I enjoy travel and adventure; I like the arts (dance, music, theater, drawing and/or painting) 0 1 2 3	I enjoy exercise, vigorous activity, competitive sports and/or politics; I like a good challenge 0 1 2 3	I like leisure time and activities; I enjoy nature, gardening, reading and/or knitting 0 1 2 3
TOTALS	1st Vata: _____	1st Pitta: _____	1st Kapha: _____

Add the 1st total from each column above and combine it with the 2nd total below for a final total in the very last box.

Health disorders & Illness tendencies (Check ALL that apply in all three categories and then add each column up for your total.)	I am prone to: o Pain and stiffness of the low back and joints (arthritis) o Hypertension o Tachycardia (fast or irregular heart rate) o A dry cough and sore throat o Constipation o Anxiety and/or depression o Fatigue o Memory and neurological disorders	I am prone to: o Inflammatory skin disorders and/or infections o Inflammatory arthritis o Blood shot or burning eyes o Anemia o Digestive disorders (diarrhea, ulcers, gastritis, heartburn hemorrhoids) o Excessive body heat o Fevers o Insomnia	I am prone to: o Allergies and/or colds o Sinus Congestion and/or headaches o Respiratory problems o Lethargy o Digestive disorders (slow and sluggish) o Obesity o Water retention o Atherosclerosis (hardening of the arteries)
TOTALS	2nd Vata: _____	2nd Pitta: _____	2nd Kapha: _____

Combine your totals for 1st and 2nd.

TOTAL (Add the two totals above for a final total. The highest total number is your dominant dosha type.) (**Please Note:** the second highest total number is your secondary dosha type.)	Final Total for Vata: _____	Final Total for Pitta: _____	Final Total for Kapha: _____

Balancing the Doshas Through Taste

Dosha	Most Balancing	Most Aggravating
Vata (Space & Air)	Sweet, Sour and Salty	Bitter, Pungent and Astringent
Pitta (Fire & Water)	Sweet, Bitter and Astringent	Sour, Salty and Pungent
Kapha (Earth & Water)	Pungent, Bitter and Astringent	Sweet, Sour and Salty

The Six Tastes: Sweet, Sour, Salty, Bitter, Pungent & Astringent

According to Ayurveda, all the important nutrients that we need to sustain life are contained in a meal that consists of all six tastes. Use the following table to help educate yourself on which tastes and their food sources best balance your constitution.

Taste	Primary Qualities & Actions	Food Sources
Sweet **(Earth & Water)** **Decreases Vata** **Decreases Pitta** **Increases Kapha**	Qualities: Cooling; moistening; creates heaviness and oiliness Actions: Builds tissues; calms nerves; increases saliva; soothes mucous membranes and burning sensations; relieves thirst; and has beneficial effects on skin, hair and the voice	Sweet fruits and natural sugars (such as raw honey); many grains and legumes; milk products; certain vegetables (including beets, carrots, sweet potatoes and yams); herbs and spices (such as basil, fennel, licorice root, peppermint and slippery elm)
Sour **(Fire & Water)** **Decreases Vata** **Increases Pitta** **Increases Kapha**	Qualities: Heating; moistening; creates heaviness and oiliness Actions: Stimulates digestion; helps circulation and elimination; increases absorption of minerals; cleanses and nourishes vital tissues; energizes the body; strengthens the heart; relieves thirst; maintains acidity; and sharpens the senses	Sour fruits (like citrus); yogurt and fermented foods (including miso, sauerkraut and vinegar); herbs and spices (such as caraway, cloves and coriander)
Salty **(Fire & Water)** **Decreases Vata** **Increases Pitta** **Increases Kapha**	Qualities: Heating; moistening; creates heaviness Actions: Improves the flavor of food; stimulates digestion; lubricates tissues; liquefies mucous; maintains mineral balance; aids in the elimination of waste material; and calms nerves	Natural salts (such as sea salt and Himalayan rock salt) and celery

Taste	Primary Qualities & Actions	Food Sources
Bitter (Air & Space) **Increases Vata** **Decreases Pitta** **Decreases Kapha**	Qualities: Cooling; drying; creates lightness Actions: Stimulates the appetite; is a powerful detoxifying agent; has antibiotic, anti-parasitic, and antiseptic qualities; helps reduce weight, water retention, skin rashes, fever, burning sensations and nausea	Green leafy vegetables (including cabbage, dandelion, kale and spinach); other vegetables (such as eggplant, rhubarb and zucchini); certain fruits (including bitter melon, grapefruits and olives); herbs and spices (such as fenugreek and turmeric); coffee and tea
Pungent (Air & Fire) **Increases Vata** **Increases Pitta** **Decreases Kapha**	Qualities: Heating; drying; creates lightness Actions: Stimulates digestion, dispels gas and improves metabolism; aids circulation; promotes sweating and detoxification; clears sinuses; cleanses the blood; and relieves muscle pain	Chili peppers; garlic; onions; radishes; herbs and spices (such as asafoetida, cayenne, ginger and mustard)
Astringent (Air & Earth) **Increases Vata** **Decreases Pitta** **Decreases Kapha**	Qualities: Cooling; drying; firming; creates lightness Actions: Absorbs water, tightens tissues, dries fats	Legumes (such as beans and lentils); fruits (including unripe bananas, cranberries, pears, pomegranates and dried fruit); vegetables (such as artichokes, asparagus, broccoli, cauliflower and turnip); grain-like seeds (including buckwheat and quinoa); spices and herbs (such as basil, marjoram and turmeric); coffee and tea

Please Note: It is recommended to include the six tastes in each meal for optimum health and balance. This can be made easy by simply adding a squeeze of lemon or lime to a dish (which satisfies the sour taste); and by adding a side salad to a meal (which satisfies the bitter and astringent tastes).

APPENDIX G

Yin-Yang Balance

Chinese philosophy defines yin and yang as two opposite, but complementary forces, which must always be in balance.

Everything in the universe has yin and yang aspects – light and dark, hot and cold, female and male, interior and exterior, front and back, etc. – all of which are necessary for life to exist.

According to traditional Chinese medicine (TCM), health is a state of harmony and balance in which our lifestyle and food choices are vitally important. Wow! What a contrastive viewpoint when compared to Western medicine and its ideas about nutrition and wellness. The science and wisdom behind TCM is based on knowing the chemical composition of foods and the biochemical pathways of the body, whereas our Western nutrition philosophy believes in grouping all foods into just three categories (protein, carbohydrates and fat) and then taking the "one-size-fits-all" approach when it comes to proper nutrition and serving size recommendations.

When we become more conscious of our mental and physical state of health, and learn to appreciate and understanding the energetic of food, we too can make better food and activity choices to restore vigor and speed the healing process. In accordance with the ancient healing art of Chinese medicine, an imbalance can come from an excess, or deficiency, of yin (cold) or yang (heat).

Please Note: The following is just a brief overview of yin and yang patterns of imbalance, along with some food choices that may help in restoring harmony within. It is for educational purposes only, and is in no way intended to substitute an assessment of your constitution by a qualified healthcare practitioner well versed in the area of Chinese medicine.

Use the following table as a guide to help figure out if you tend to be more yin (meaning your body constitution is more cold) or whether you tend to be more yang (meaning your body constitution is more warm/hot). In addition, you may also present with signs of dampness or dryness. If so, you may need to further refine your food choices. If you feel that none clearly define you, then your constitution may be neutral at the present time.

Please keep in mind our body constitution is forever changing; therefore, adjusting food choices with the change in seasons, lifestyle changes and different life situations may be necessary.

Yin Patterns of Imbalance Signs of Excess Cold	Yang Patterns of Imbalance Signs of Excess Heat
I often feel chilled	I often feel warm
I tend to get quiet and withdrawn	I tend to be talkative
I dress warm and like the heat	I get uncomfortable in hot weather
I have soft muscles	I tend to wear short sleeves
My complexion is pale	My complexion is ruddy
I have a slow metabolism	I'm prone to headaches, nose bleeds and bleeding gums
My health tends to be worse in cold weather	I'm prone to fever blisters and canker sores
I prefer warm food and drinks	My blood pressure tends to be high
I become anxious and/or depressed easily	I become angry, impatient and/or resentful easily
I'm often tired and sleep (nap) a lot	My sleep is often restless and I tend to have disturbing dreams
I rarely get thirsty	I get thirsty often and crave cold drinks
My urine is usually clear	I tend to have dark urine
I often have loose stools	I often have hard stools

Signs of Excess Dampness	Signs of Excess Dryness
I strongly dislike humidity	I tend to have dry skin and/or dandruff
My health worsens in damp environments	I get flushed cheeks, especially after exercise
I retain fluids easily	I often have a dry throat and/or eyes
I'm overweight	I have a thin, lanky body type
My eyes and face are often puffy and swollen	I'm pone to night sweats
I experience a heaviness, especially in my lower body	I'm experiencing menopause
I'm prone to abdominal bloating	I can easily become both hot or cold
I experience brain fog	I prefer warm liquids in small sips
I often have a stuffy nose or postnasal drip	I tend to crave sweets

I become short of breath easily	I crave salt often
I'm not usually thirsty or hungry	I become easily stressed, irritated and/or flustered
My urine often appears cloudy	I'm often constipated

Please Note: Dampness can be associated with cold or heat and is usually exacerbated when living in a damp climate and/or damp living conditions.

How to Balance Yin (cold)

A cold pattern often occurs in vegetarians or those who eat primarily raw foods (which is especially true if they live in cold climates). Cold can also set in with age and may be combined with dampness. Regular aerobic exercise is imperative, as it warms your core and increases blood flow. Beneficial vegetables include winter squashes, many root vegetables, radishes, onions, garlic and chili peppers. Even certain leafy green herbs are considered warming, such as cilantro, mustard greens and parsley. Nuts and seeds are warming, as are certain herbs and spices such as cayenne, cinnamon, ginger, mustard seed and turmeric. Also, it is advisable to keep your drinking water (which is naturally yin) at room temperature and drink more warming teas and herbal tisanes throughout the day.

How to Balance Dampness

Dampness can be brought on by eating on the go, eating out a lot (especially at fast food establishments), and/or from a diet rich in heavy foods, fried foods, processed and refined foods, and foods loaded with sugar and salt. Aerobic exercise is often necessary for drying a damp constitution. As far as beneficial foods go, bitter foods are at the top of the list. Bitter foods include: cruciferous vegetables such as broccoli, Brussels sprouts, cabbage, cauliflower, collard greens and kale, as well as endive and escarole.

How to Balance Yang (heat)

A heat pattern often shows up in hot weather or with an increase in stress. Ideal activities for balancing the agitated nature of a heat imbalance involve meditation, swimming, walks in nature and yoga. Excellent foods include leafy green vegetables, cucumbers, celery, sea vegetables and tomatoes. Vegetables of all kinds are helpful, whereas meats should be limited. Other cooling foods include: apples, citrus, melons, pears, sprouts and lots of water. Peppermint is a nice and soothing, beneficial cooling herb.

How to Balance Dryness

Dryness is a sign of yin deficiency. Having sufficient yin signifies having a sufficient amount of hormones, skin oils, saliva, digestive juices and lubricating secretions. Dryness tends to set in when women hit menopause and when men hit andropause. Skin and hair become drier; nails feel more brittle and crack; hormonal secretions decrease; etc. Beneficial activities include gardening, meditation, yoga, and simply walking about out in nature. Healthful food choices include beneficial fats, such as avocado, nuts, seeds, coconut oil and olive oil. Other moistening foods include: many sweet fruits, green beans, peas, sweet potatoes, yams and sea vegetables.

Please Note: Menopausal symptoms can get complicated, but essentially they are a deficiency in yin. Although having hot flashes may feel like excess heat (yang), it is actually a sign of diminishing yin. In other words, deficient yin may be masquerading as excess yang when in actuality yang may be either normal or also deficient as well. Stress also depletes yin, causing dryness.

In traditional Chinese medicine (TCM), the balance of yin and yang in the body is often determined by the food we eat more than any other single factor. Yin foods tend to be cooling and/or moistening for the body, whereas yang foods tend to be heating and/or drying. Please beware; there are many exceptions to this general rule. I suggest using this chart for educational purposes, and to help with making better food choices and balancing combinations when balancing yin and yang is your goal. Please keep in mind, this chart is in no way a substitute for consulting with a TCM practitioner, who can tailor a food and herb plan according to your individual needs and health concerns.

Food Balance Chart TCM

	COLD	COOL	NEUTRAL	WARM	HOT
FRUITS	Bananas Cranberries Grapefruits Melons Persimmons Star Fruits	Apples Lemons/Limes Mangos Mulberries Oranges Pears Strawberries Tangerines	Apricots Avocados Figs Grapes Papayas Pineapples Plums Pomegranates	Blackberries Blueberries Cherries Coconuts Dates Guavas Jackfruits Kiwis Kumquats Longans Lychees Peaches Raspberries	Durians
VEGETABLES	Bamboo Shoots Bitter Gourds Bok Choy Dandelion Lettuce Sea Vegetables Tomatoes	Artichokes Asparagus Broccoli Cauliflower Collards Cucumbers Eggplants Escarole Endive Mushrooms Okra Radishes Rutabagas Spinach Sprouts Summer Squash Swiss Chard Turnips	Alfalfa Sprouts Beets Brussels Sprouts Cabbage Celery Carrots Cilantro Corn Kohlrabi Olives Potatoes Pumpkin Shiitake String Beans	Garlic Mustard Greens Onions Parsley Peppers Sweet Potatoes Winter Squash Yams	

	COLD	COOL	NEUTRAL	WARM	HOT
		Watercress			
		Zucchini			
LEGUMES		Lima Beans	Adzuki Beans	Black Beans	
		Mung Beans	Black-Eyed Peas		
		Sprouts	Broad Beans		
			Chickpeas		
			Kidney Beans		
			Lentils		
			Peanuts		
			Pinto Beans		
			Red Beans		
			Soy Beans		
			Split Peas		
GRAINS		Barley	Amaranth	Oats	
		Bran	Blue Corn	Quinoa	
		Pasta	Brown Rice	Spelt	
		Wheat	Buckwheat		
			Couscous		
			Millet		
			Rye		
			Wild Rice		
			White Rice		
NUTS / SEEDS			Pumpkin Seeds	All other nuts/seeds are neutral /warm	
			Sesame Seeds		
			Flax Seeds		
			Sunflower Seeds		
MEAT / POULTRY		Duck	Beef	Chicken	Lamb
			Bison	Ham	Venison
			Goose	Turkey	
			Pork		
			Quail		

	COLD	COOL	NEUTRAL	WARM	HOT
FISH		Clams Codfish Crab Scallops Whitefish	Catfish Herring Mackerel Salmon Sardines Tuna	Anchovies Lobster Mussels Shrimp	Trout
SWEETNERS	White Sugar Artificial Sweeteners	Cane Sugar Maple syrup	Honey Molasses	Brown Sugar	
HERBS / SPICES		Marjoram Peppermint		Basil Caraway Cardamom Cloves Coriander Cumin Dill Fennel Ginger (fresh) Nutmeg Oregano Rosemary Sea Salt Sage Spearmint Star Anise Thyme Turmeric	Cinnamon Horseradish Garlic Ginger (dry) Mustard Seed Pepper (black, cayenne, chilies, etc.)
DAIRY	Ice Cream Yogurt	Ice Cream Yogurt Cow's Milk Products	Cow's Milk Products Human's Milk Most Soft Cheeses	Goat's Milk Products	Most Hard Cheeses

	COLD	COOL	NEUTRAL	WARM	HOT
EGGS		Egg Whites		Egg Yolks	
OILS	Vegetable oils	Sesame Oil	Olive Oil	Butter Coconut Oil Ghee	
FOOD PREP	Fermenting	Blanching Raw	Boiling Poaching Sautéing (with water) Steaming	Baking Deep Frying Frying Grilling Pressure Cooking Roasting Sautéing (with oil)	Baking Deep Frying Frying Grilling Pressure Cooking Roasting Sautéing (with oil)
OTHER	Caffeinated Soda Drugs (stimulants) Hard Alcohol (most)	Beer Green Tea Oolong Tea Water		Black Tea Chocolate Coffee Miso Tobacco Vinegar Wine (some)	Drugs (sedatives)

5 Tastes of TCM	
Bitter	Cold/Cool & Dry
Pungent	Warm/Hot & Dry
Salty	Warm/Hot & Moist
Sour	Warm/Hot & Moist
Sweet	Cold/Cool & Moist

Please Note: Many properties of a food can affect its yin or yang qualities. These include: its freshness, nutrient content, acidity versus alkalinity, how it is prepared, how and where it grows, toxins it contains, level of life force energy, etc.

Quick Tips:

- In general, vegetables tend to be energetically yin and meats tend to be energetically yang, but the way in which these foods are prepared can often change the amount of yin or yang energy it has dramatically. Take vegetables for example, frying and sautéing them will increase yang energy, making them much less yin. A better option would be to lightly steam them. The same goes for clams or scallops, which tend to be yin. If you deep fry them, yang is going to increase dramatically. So what happens with grilled or roasted beef and chicken? Their energy is going to become very yang. I mention this, because depending on what your intention is when choosing certain foods and herbs, you can unintentionally (or intentionally for that matter) alter its energy.
- Anyone experiencing increased dampness (regardless of being too yin or too yang) needs to go easy on the foods and herbs with sweet, sour and/or salty tastes, as these tend to be more moistening.
- Bitter foods and herbs tend to be drying and more cold, which is great for treating damp and heat conditions, but contraindicated for individuals who are too cold and/or too dry.
- Salty and sour foods and herbs tend to be warming and moistening, making them great for treating cold and dry conditions, but they should be limited when there are hot and damp conditions present. Also, the sour taste tends to be a bit more warming and moistening than salty, which may be important to some.
- In Ayurveda, pungent is a recognized taste, but in TCM there is only sour. Please note their different properties: astringent is cooling and drying, whereas sour is warming and moistening.
- There are many versions of yin-yang food lists and charts to be found, and don't be surprised to find some contradictions and discrepancies. For instance, I've seen alcoholic beverages (such as wine) listed as yin, and in other places listed as yang. It may depend on its acidity, dryness or color – but I cannot be certain. I've also seen breads, sugary baked goods, and other processed and refined flour products listed as either yin or yang. For discrepancies like these, I just go with common sense. These foods are way too acidic and not health giving at all; therefore, you won't find them on my shopping list.
- In addition, there are always exceptions to the rule (for instance salty sea vegetables are considered yin by many, whereas certain mushrooms are considered yang). My best advice is to be more aware of the extremes and do your best to combine foods well so that you don't continuously off-balance the scales.
- Being a raw vegetarian, when I need warmth, I add warm and hot herbs and spices to my dishes. I also enjoy making teas and elixir drinks with warming herbs and medicinal mushrooms.

ABOUT THE AUTHOR

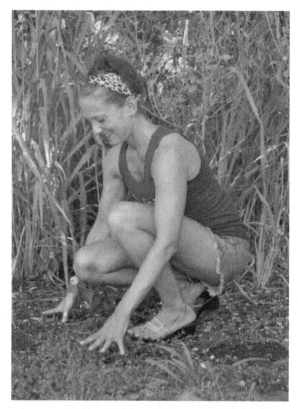

Karen A. Di Gloria (born and raised north of Boston, MA) is considered by friends, family and peers to be the "eternal nurse." Although she has left the field of conventional medicine behind her, Karen's passion for helping others live a quality life has never shined brighter. Her years of experience as an oncology nurse and desire to achieve abundant health were the catalyst for a radical career change.

Karen co-owned and operated Rawk Star Café, Inc. – a raw food café and superfood marketplace in the Tampa Bay area for over seven years. She now follows her true passion as a Quantum Reflex Analysis (QRA) Practitioner and Certified Biofeedback Specialist. She has earned her Raw Nutrition Certification through BodyMind Institute and her Whole Life Coach Certification through the International Training Institute of Health. Karen's fusion of knowledge, achievements and experience make her well qualified to offer nutritional and holistic wellness coaching to those truly ready for a lifestyle change.

"Nobody can go back and start a new beginning, but anyone can start today and make a new ending." – Maria Robinson

REBEL WITH A CAUSE!

My goals as a raw food and wellness coach are to help clients create nutrition and lifestyle habits that have the ability to turn <u>on</u> health-promoting genes, and turn <u>off</u> genes which can make you susceptible to illness and disease. How can someone make a positive shift and gain control of their health naturally? The solution is proper daily exercise, yoga and meditation; a diet based primarily on fresh, organic fruits and vegetables; the highest quality plant-based proteins and fats; medicinal quality superfoods, superfruits and superherbs; and 100% excipient free nutritional supplements. Your genes are just a blueprint, and only you influence what you build from that blueprint.

> *"We are not victims of our genes, but masters of our fate."*
> – Dr. Bruce Lipton

Defy your **<u>D</u>etoxify** and cleanse your body

<u>N</u>ourish and balance your immune system

<u>A</u>dapt to all life's stressors – physical, emotional and environmental

The following is a sampling of the tried, tested and trusted companies I choose to work with when assisting clients on their journey back to true health and vitality. I thank each and every one for their ongoing dedication and commitment to the core values of integrity, honesty, fairness, openness, respect and responsibility.

- ★ Arrowhead Health Works
- ★ Dragon Herbs
- ★ Fungi Perfecti (Host Defense)
- ★ Manitoba Harvest
- ★ Modifilan
- ★ New Horizon Health / Longevity Warehouse / David Wolfe Foods
- ★ Phi Sciences
- ★ Premier Research Labs
- ★ Purium
- ★ Remedylink
- ★ Sunwarrior
- ★ SurThrival
- ★ Ultimate Superfoods/Ojio

For more information about me and the modalities I use, including articles, recipes, pictures, videos, and to stay cutting edge on revolutionary advancements in whole food nutrition and energy medicine, please visit the following links:

- ★ www.frequencyfreedom.com
- ★ www.woke-wellness.com
- ★ www.facebook.com/supernaturawlnewtrition
- ★ www.youtube.com/user/skoolofrawk